TRANSCULTURAL HEALTH CARE

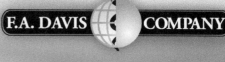
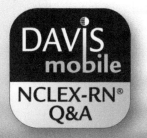
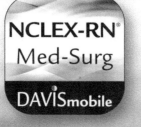
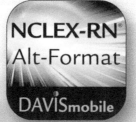
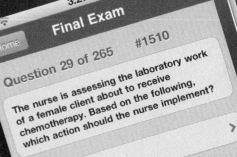

4th Edition

TRANSCULTURAL HEALTH CARE

A Culturally Competent Approach

Larry D. Purnell
Phd, RN, FAAN

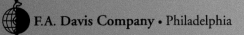
F.A. Davis Company • Philadelphia

F. A. Davis Company
1915 Arch Street
Philadelphia, PA 19103
www.fadavis.com

Revised Index

Printed in the United States of America

Last digit indicates print number: 10 9 8 7 6 5 4 3

Publisher, Nursing: Robert G. Martone
Director of Content Development: Darlene D. Pedersen
Project Editor: Victoria White
Electronic Project Manager: Tyler Baber
Design and Illustrations Manager: Carolyn O'Brien

As new scientific information becomes available through basic and clinical research, recommended treatments and drug therapies undergo changes. The author(s) and publisher have done everything possible to make this book accurate, up to date, and in accord with accepted standards at the time of publication. The author(s), editors, and publisher are not responsible for errors or omissions or for consequences from application of the book, and make no warranty, expressed or implied, in regard to the contents of the book. Any practice described in this book should be applied by the reader in accordance with professional standards of care used in regard to the unique circumstances that may apply in each situation. The reader is advised always to check product information (package inserts) for changes and new information regarding dose and contraindications before administering any drug. Caution is especially urged when using new or infrequently ordered drugs.

Library of Congress Cataloging-in-Publication Data

Transcultural health care : a culturally competent approach / [edited by] Larry D. Purnell. — 4th ed.
    p. ; cm.
Includes bibliographical references and index.
ISBN 978-0-8036-3705-4
I. Purnell, Larry D.
[DNLM: 1. Cultural Competency—United States. 2. Delivery of Health Care—United States. 3. Cultural Diversity—United States. 4. Ethnic Groups—United States. W 84 AA1]

362.1089—dc23

2012016099

Foreword

Knowing is not enough, we must apply.
Willing is not enough, we must do.
Goethe

Goethe's quote is considered a call to action by organizations as prestigious as the Institute of Medicine, and it remains one of my favorite quotes today. It has such incredible implications for health care, particularly as we struggle with the extended time it takes to translate research into practice. In fact, oftentimes, despite strong evidence, we are slow in enacting the changes we need to improve the health care and nursing we deliver. In some cases we are waiting for the "indisputable" evidence, and in other cases we are simply being resistant to change. But occasionally the need for change is thrust upon us, momentum builds, and the realization emerges that there isn't a need to prove the obvious before acting but a need to act as the obvious is all around us. This has become the case with cultural competence in health care.

My *knowing* about the importance of cultural competence developed as I grew up in my bilingual, bicultural Puerto Rican family, where perspectives about health and health care were incredibly varied, and at times at odds with Western medicine. My *knowing* grew, as I trained to be a health-care professional in underserved and diverse settings such as Newark, New Jersey, and New York City, where we saw patients from all cultures, classes, and racial/ethnic backgrounds. What became crystal clear to me was that while we were learning the best medications to treat hypertension or the most advanced algorithms for diagnosing and treating disease, if we couldn't communicate effectively with our patients or get them to buy into, agree with, and cooperate with what we were trying to accomplish, then all that medical knowledge was worth nothing. Whether a doctor, a nurse, or other health professional, caring for patients required an understanding of the sociocultural factors that might impact their health beliefs and behaviors, ranging from how they presented their symptoms, to how they viewed disease and illness, to what informed their health care, diagnostic, and treatment choices. Cases where we couldn't bring our knowledge to bear to ease suffering or cure disease because of "cultural differences" with patients were the ones that kept us up at night and were the most frustrating and disappointing

of all. Along the way I also learned to appreciate that we *all* have culture and that the tools and skills I needed to learn to communicate clearly with patients wouldn't just be helpful in the care of those who were culturally different from me, but to any patient with whom I interacted. For at the end of the day, there were always three cultures in the room—my culture; the patient's culture; and the cultures of medicine, nursing, and other health professions—making every encounter cross-cultural in one way or another.

Despite these almost daily epiphanies during my training, there were few resources available that might provide me with guidance on how to become an effective communicator and caregiver in this new world I was entering. Fortunately, this has changed. New models have been developed, leaders have emerged, and health-care professionals no longer need to go blindly into cross-cultural encounters without guidance, as there are real and practical approaches that facilitate improved understanding, communication, and care. *Knowing is not enough, we must apply.*

Transcultural Health Care: A Culturally Competent Approach builds on a framework for cultural competence—which is essential in the care of the individual—by bringing together health-care providers of various backgrounds and disciplines to share their knowledge, expertise, and experiences in the field with particulars about different populations. This information is presented to provide details about the social and cultural fabric of different cultural groups, with the important caveat that it is not to be used to stereotype patients within these groups, as each patient is an individual and diversity can be as extensive within groups as it is among groups. It is from this principle—that learning background information about cultural groups can help health-care providers both develop a "radar" for potential pitfalls when caring for them *and* serve as a springboard for inquiry with the individual patient—that *Transcultural Health Care* emerges.

Why is this book, and this edition, so timely? In the past, arguments about the importance of cultural competence were based primarily on making the case that our nation was becoming increasingly diverse and that as health-care professionals we need to be prepared to care for patients of different sociocultural backgrounds. This is an important argument, no doubt. Shortly thereafter, research began to emerge demonstrating that being inattentive to cultural issues in the clinical setting leads to lower quality of care for specific populations, such as racial and ethnic minorities—a term that became known as *disparities* in health care. Yet what has evolved more recently is a burgeoning literature documenting the impact of cultural factors on health-care quality, cost, and safety. New research demonstrates that when we are not skilled or prepared to care for patients from diverse backgrounds, they may, when compared to their Caucasian counterparts, suffer more medical errors with greater clinical consequences; have longer hospital stays for the same common clinical conditions; and may have more unnecessary tests ordered—all due to language or cultural barriers between health-care providers and patients. With health-care reform and payment reform on the horizon, we *literally* can no longer afford to be ill prepared to meet the needs of an increasingly diverse nation.

As we look toward the future, we see signs of a breakthrough occurring. More and more is being written about the topic of cultural competence. Students who years ago had to be convinced of the importance of this issue are now arriving more sensitized about cultural competence than ever before and are demanding to build their skills in the field. More research is being conducted on cultural competence and its impact on quality, safety, and cost. Additional areas are being cross-linked to cultural competence, such as patient-centeredness and health literacy. New quality measures and accreditation standards are being developed, and in some states cultural competence training has become a condition of health professional licensure. There is little doubt that the field of cultural competence is moving from the margin to the mainstream and from a luxury to a necessity. As individual providers, we must all do our part to ensure that we are delivering high-quality care to any patient we see, regardless of her or his race, ethnicity, culture, socioeconomic class, or language proficiency. *Transcultural Health Care: A Culturally Competent Approach* helps us build the radar to identify and understand key cross-cultural issues among diverse populations and, when applied with the tools and skills that are essential for exploring the sociocultural perspectives of the individual patient, positions us for success. Now it is time for us to learn the lessons and skills so gracefully shared with us in this book to make a difference in patients' lives. *Willing is not enough, we must do.*

Joseph R. Betancourt, MD, MPH
Director, The Disparities Solutions Center and
Director of Multicultural Education,
Massachusetts General Hospital
Associate Professor of Medicine,
Harvard Medical School
Cofounder, Manhattan Cross-Cultural Group

Preface

The Purnell Model for Cultural Competence and its accompanying organizing framework continue to be used in education, clinical practice, administration, and research. The Model and selected chapters have been translated into Arabic, Flemish, French, Korean, Portuguese, Spanish, Turkish, and Korean, attesting to its value on a worldwide basis. In addition, many health-care organizations have adapted the organizing framework as a cultural assessment tool, and numerous students in the United States and overseas have used the Model to guide research for theses and dissertations. The Model is increasingly being used as a guide to help ensure organizational cultural competence.

This fourth edition of *Transcultural Health Care: A Culturally Competent Approach* has been revised based upon responses from students, faculty, and practicing health-care professionals such as nurses, physicians, emergency medical technicians, nutritionists, and people in noetic sciences. In addition, this edition is divided into two units. Unit 1, Foundations for Cultural Competence: Individual and Organizational, has the following features:

- An expanded chapter on the overview of transcultural diversity and health care
- A separate chapter on the Purnell Model for Cultural Competence, with specific questions in the organizing framework instead of objectives
- A separate chapter on individual competence and evidence-based practice
- A separate chapter on organizational cultural competence
- A separate chapter on global health

Unit 2 is entitled Aggregate Data for Cultural-Specific Groups. As in previous editions, we have made a concerted effort to use nonstereotypical language when describing cultural attributes of specific cultures, recognizing that there are exceptions to every description provided and that the differences within a cultural group are determined by variant cultural characteristics. One important change on the Model is that the primary and secondary characteristics of culture are now called "variant cultural characteristics" at the suggestion of gay, lesbian, and transgendered communities.

The first time a cultural term is used in a chapter, it is in boldface type and is defined in the glossary. Because faculty and clinical practitioners have found the Appendix—Cultural, Ethnic, and Racial Diseases and Illnesses—valuable, it remains in the book. Abstracts are included in the main textbook for each culturally specific full chapter located on Davis Plus.

Space and cost concerns limit the number of chapters that are included in the book; therefore, additional cultural groups are on Davis Plus. Also on Davis Plus are student resources such as review questions, Web sites of interest, case studies, and reflective exercises. Additional faculty resources on Davis Plus include PowerPoint slides with clicker check questions for each chapter and a question bank.

Specific criteria were used for identifying the groups represented in the book and those included in electronic format. Groups included in the book were selected based on any of the following six criteria:

- The group has a large population in North America, such as people of Appalachian, Mexican, German, and African American heritage.
- The group is relatively new in its migration status, such as people of Haitian, Somali, and Arab heritage.
- The group is widely dispersed throughout North America, such as people of Iranian, Korean, Hindu, and Filipino heritage.
- The group is of particular interest to readers, such as people from Amish heritage.
- The group is of particular interest to students and staff from other countries, such as European Americans.

A particular strength of each chapter is that it has been written by individuals who are intimately familiar with the specific culture. Again, we have strived to portray each culture comprehensively, positively, and without stereotyping. We hope you enjoy the book.

Larry D. Purnell

Contributors

Richard Adair, MD
Adjunct Professor of Medicine
University of Minnesota
Minneapolis, Minnesota

Karen Aroian, PhD, RN, FAAN
Director of Research and Chatlos Endowed Professor
University of Florida College of Nursing
Orlando, Florida

Linda Ciofu Baumann, PhD, RN, FAAN
University of Wisconsin-Madison
Madison, Wisconsin

Joseph R. Betancourt, MD, MPH
Director of Disparities Solutions Center
Massachusetts General Hospital
Boston, Massachusetts

Josepha Campinha-Bacote, PhD, MAR,
    PMHCNS-BC, CTN-A, FAAN
Transcultural Healthcare Consultant
Transcultural C.A.R.E. Associates
Blue Ash, Ohio

Marga Simon Coler, EdD, Dr. Causa Honoris,
    FAAN, APRN-BC
Professor Emeritus
University of Connecticut
South Hadley, Massachusetts

Jessie M. Colin, PhD, RN, FAAN
Professor and Director of Nursing PhD, Nursing
    Administration and Nursing Education Programs
Barry University
Miami Shores, Florida

Tina A. Ellis, RN, MSN, CTN
Nursing Instructor
Florida Gulf Coast University
Fort Myers, Florida

Myriam Gauthier, MSN
Graduate Student in Nursing
Faculté des sciences infirmières, Université Laval
Pavillon Ferdinand-Vandry, Québec

Rauda Gelazis, RN, PhD
Retired, Associate Professor
Ursuline College
Pepper Pike, Ohio

Homeyra Hafizi, MSN, RN, COHN/S, LHRM
Coordinator, Employee Health and Workers'
    Compensation
Wuesthoff Health System/HMA
Rockledge, Florida

Laurie B. Hartjes, PhD, RN, PNP-BC
Educational Design Consultant
Lodestone Safety International
Beverly, Massachusetts

Keiko Hattori, RN, PhD
Assistant Professor
Kawasaki University of Medical Welfare
Kurashiki, Okayama, Japan

Sandra M. Hillman, PhD, MS, BS, RN
Associate Professor
College of Mount Saint Vincent
Bronx, New York

David Hodgins, MSN, RN, CEN
Indian Health Service
Shiprock, New Mexico

Olivia Hodgins, RN, PhD, MSA, BSN
Map Instructor and Nurse Executive
Indian Health Service
San Fidel, New Mexico

Kathleen Huttlinger, PhD, RN
Associate Director for Graduate Programs
New Mexico State University
Las Cruces, New Mexico

Eun-Ok Im, PhD, MPH, RN, CNS, FAAN
Professor and Marjorie O. Rendell Endowed
    Professor
University of Pennsylvania
Philadelphia, Pennsylvania

Misae Ito, RN, MW, MSN, PhD
Professor
Kawasaki University of Medical Welfare
Kurashiki, Okayama, Japan

Jayalakshmi Jambunathan, PhD, MSN, BSN, MA BSc
Professor, CON UW Oshkosh
Director, Research and Evaluation and Assistant Dean
UW Oshkosh
Oshkosh, Wisconsin

Galina Khatutsky, MS
Research Analyst
RTI International
Waltham, Massachusetts

Sema Kuguoglu, PhD, BSN, RN
Professor Emeritus, University of Mamara
Funded Professor, University of Gazikent
Istanbul and Gaziantep, Turkey

Anahid Kulwicki, PhD, RN, FAAN
Professor and Associate Dean for Research
Director of the PhD in Nursing Program
Florida International University
Miami, Florida

Ginette Lazure, PhD
Professeure titulaire
Université Laval
Pavillon Ferdinand-Vandry
Médecine, Québec

Stephen R. Marrone, EdD, RN-BC, CTN-A
Deputy Nursing Director
State University of New York
SUNY Downstate Medical Center
Brooklyn, New York

Susan Mattson, RNC-OB, CTN-OB, PhD, FAAN
Professor Emerita
Arizona State University College of Nursing and Health Innovation
Scottsdale, Arizona

Afaf Ibrahim Meleis, PhD, DrPS (hon), FAAN
Margaret Bond Simon Dean of Nursing
University of Pennsylvania School of Nursing
Philadelphia, Pennsylvania

Mahmoud Hanafi Meleis, PhD, PE
Retired Nuclear Engineer
Philadelphia, Pennsylvania

Cora Munoz, PhD, RN
Professor Emerital Adjunct Professor
Capital University
Columbus, Ohio

Irena Papadopoulos, PhD, MA (Ed), BA, RN, RM, NDN, FHEA
Professor
Middlesex University
Highgate Hill, London, UK

Ghislaine Paperwalla, BSN, RN
Research Nurse in Immunology
Veterans Administration Medical Center
Miami, Florida

Jeffrey R. Ross, MAT, MA, BFA
ESL Teacher and Tutor
Springfield School System and the University of Akron
Akron, Ohio

Ratchneewan Ross, PhD, MSc (Public Health), RN
Associate Professor and Director of International Activities
Kent State University
Kent, Ohio

Susan W. Salmond, EdD, RN, CNE, CTN
Dean and Professor
University of Medicine and Dentistry of New Jersey
Newark, New Jersey

Stephanie Myers Schim, PhD, RN, PHCNS-BC
Associate Professor
Wayne State University College of Nursing
Detroit, Michigan

Janice Selekman, DNSc, RN
Professor Nursing
University of Delaware
Newark, DE

Jessica A. Steckler, MS, RN-BC
CEO
The Firm of Jessica A. Steckler
Erie, Pennsylvania

Marshelle Thobaben, RN, PHN, MS, FNP, PMHNP
Department Chair, Professor
Humboldt State University
Arcata, California

Hsiu-Min Tsai, RN, PhD
Dean of Academic Affairs and Associate Professor
Chang Gung University of Science and Technology
Tao-Yuan, Taiwan

Anna Frances Z. Wenger, PhD, RN, FAAN
Professor and Director Emeritus of Nursing
Goshen College
Goshen, Indiana

Marion R. Wenger, PhD
Professor of Linguistics and Foreign Languages
Goshen College
Goshen, Indiana

Cecilia A. Zamarripa, RN, CWON
University of Pittsburgh Medical Center
Pittsburgh, Pennsylvania

Rick Zoucha, APRN, BC, DNSc, CTN
Associate Professor
Duquesne University School of Nursing
Pittsburgh, Pennsylvania

Reviewers

Kristie Berkstresser, MSN, RN, CNE, BC
Assistant Professor of Nursing
HAAC—Central Pennsylvania's Community College
Lancaster, Pennsylvania

Judy Shockey Carter, MSN Ed, RN
Assistant Professor
Anderson University
Anderson, Indiana

Sabrina L. Dickey, RN, BSN, MSN
Assistant Faculty in Nursing
Florida State University
Tallahassee, Florida

David N. Ekstrom, PhD, RN
Associate Professor
Pace University, College of Health Professions
Lienhard School of Nursing
New York, New York

Mary L. Padden, RNC, APN-C, FN-CSA
Assistant Professor, Nursing
Cumberland County College
Vineland, New Jersey

Priscilla L. Sagar, EdD, RN, ACNS-BC, CTN
Professor of Nursing
Mount Saint Mary College
Newburgh, New York

Lisabeth M. Searing, PhD, MSN, RN
Assistant Professor
Illinois Wesleyan University, School of Nursing
Bloomington, Illinois

Gale Sewell, RN, MSN, CNE
Assistant Professor
Indiana Wesleyan University
Marion, Indiana

Jeanine Tweedie, MSN, RN, CNE
Nursing Faculty
Hawaii Pacific University
Kaneohe, Hawaii

Mai-Neng Lee Xiong, BSN
Director of Nursing
People Incorporated Mental Health Services
St. Paul, Minnesota

Table of Contents

Contents – Davis*Plus*

Introduction

The Purnell Model for Cultural Competence and its organizing framework continue to be used in education, clinical practice, administration, and research by nurses, physicians, and other health-care providers. The Model has been translated into Arabic, Flemish, French, German, Korean, Portuguese, Spanish, and Turkish. Health-care organizations have adapted the organizing framework as a cultural assessment tool and to guide research for theses and dissertations in the United States and overseas. The Model's usefulness has been established in the global arena, recognizing and including the client's culture in assessments, health-care planning, interventions, and evaluations. The Model has proven useful with organizational cultural competence as well.

Transcultural Health Care: A Culturally Competent Approach continues to be revised based upon feedback from students and clinical health-care providers, as well as educators from associate degree, baccalaureate, master's, and doctoral programs. Their reviews and suggestions are appreciated.

This edition has been divided into two units. Unit 1 contains five chapters. Chapter 1, Transcultural Diversity and Health Care, gives an overview of transcultural health and nursing care along with essential terminology related to culture. Chapter 2 is an extensive description the Purnell Model for Cultural Competence, along with recommended questions to ask and observations to make when doing a cultural assessment or formulating questions for qualitative research. Chapter 3, Individual Competence and Evidence-Based Practice, includes international standards on culturally competent care and an extensive section on searching literature for evidence-based cultural research. Chapter 4, Organizational Cultural Competence, provides a crosswalk with the Purnell Model and CLAS Standards. Chapter 5, Perspectives on Nursing in a Global Context, addresses health-care organizations that have a global context, the forces that shape global health and nursing, and international migration.

Unit 2 consists of aggregate data on culturally specific groups, 18 of which are covered in the book and an additional 14 on DavisPlus. We continue to make a concerted effort to use nonstereotypical language when describing cultural attributes of specific cultures, recognizing that there are exceptions to every description provided. Aggregate data are true for the group but not necessarily for the individual. Therefore, readers are encouraged to look at the variant cultural characteristics when viewing aggregate data on any population. An attempt has been made to include both the sociological and anthropological perspectives of culture.

Given the world diversity and the diversity within cultural groups, it is impossible to cover each group more extensively. Space and cost concerns limit the number of chapters that are included in the book; therefore, additional cultural groups, PowerPoint slides, interactive exercises, test banks, useful Web sites, and additional case studies are included on Davis*Plus*.

Specific criteria were used for identifying the groups represented in the book and those included in electronic format. Groups included in the book were selected based on any of the following six criteria:

- The group has a large population in North America, such as people of African American, Appalachian, Chinese, German, Irish, and Mexican heritage.
- The group is relatively new in its migration status, such as people of Arab, Haitian, and Cuban heritage.
- The group is widely dispersed throughout North America, such as people of Filipino, Hindu, Iranian, and Korean heritage.
- The group has little written about it in the health-care literature, such as people of Guatemalan, Russian, Somali, and Thai heritage.
- The group holds significant disenfranchised status, such as American Indians.
- The group was of particular interest to readers in previous editions, such as people from Amish heritage.

We have strived to portray each culture positively and without stereotyping. Individual chapter authors made every attempt to incorporate the latest research at the time of writing.

Larry D. Purnell

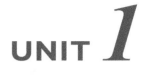

UNIT *1*

FOUNDATIONS FOR CULTURAL COMPETENCE

Individual and Organizational

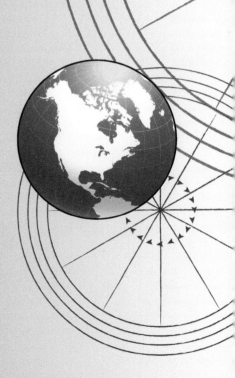

Chapter 1

Transcultural Diversity and Health Care

Larry D. Purnell

The Need for Culturally Competent Health Care

Cultural competence has become one of the most important initiatives in health care in the United States and throughout most of the world. Diversity has increased in many countries due to wars, discrimination, political strife, worldwide socioeconomic conditions, and the creation of the European Union. Some of the diversity is driven by actual numbers of immigrants, but other dimensions come from the visibility of the "new ethnics" and the waning of the social ideology of the "melting pot" (O'Neil, 2008). Instead of the term *melting pot*, meaning everyone is expected to blend, many believe the term *salad bowl* is more appropriate because people can stand out and be seen as individuals. Health ideology and health-care providers have learned that it is just as important to understand the patient's culture as it is to understand the physiological responses in illness, disease, and injury. The health-care provider may be very knowledgeable about laboratory values and standard treatments and interventions for diabetes mellitus, heart disease, and asthma, but if the recommendations are not compatible with the patient's own health beliefs, dietary practices, and views toward wellness, the treatment plan is less likely to be followed (Giger et al., 2007). To this end, a number of worldwide initiatives have addressed cultural competence as a means for improving health and health care, decreasing disparities, and increasing patient satisfaction. These initiatives come from the U.S. Office of Minority Health, the Institute of Medicine, *Healthy People 2020*, the National Quality Forum, the Joint Commission, The American Medical Association, the American Association of Colleges of Nursing, and other professional organizations. Educational institutions—from elementary schools to colleges and universities—are also addressing cultural

diversity and cultural competency as they relate to disparities; health promotion and wellness; illness, disease, and injury prevention; and health maintenance and restoration.

Many countries are now recognizing the need for addressing the diversity of their societies. Societies that used to be rather homogeneous, such as Portugal, Norway, Sweden, Korea, and selected areas in the United States and the United Kingdom, are now facing significant internal and external migration, resulting in ethnic and cultural diversities that did not previously exist, at least not to the degree they do now. Several European countries, such as Denmark, Italy, Poland, the Czech Republic, Latvia, the United Kingdom, Sweden, Norway, Finland, Italy, Spain, Portugal, Hungary, Belgium, Greece, Germany, the Netherlands, and France, either have in place or are developing national programs to address the value of cultural competence in reducing health disparities (Judge, Platt, Costongs, & Jurczak, 2005).

Whether people are internal migrants, immigrants, or vacationers, they have the right to expect the health-care system to respect their personal beliefs, values, and health-care practices. Culturally competent health care from providers and the system, regardless of the setting in which care is delivered, is becoming a concern and expectation among consumers. Diversity also includes having a diverse workforce that more closely represents the population the organization serves. Health-care personnel provide care to people of diverse cultures in long-term-care facilities, acute-care facilities, clinics, communities, and patients' homes. All health-care providers—physicians, nurses, nutritionists, therapists, technicians, home health aides, and other caregivers—need similar culturally specific information. For example, all health-care providers communicate, both verbally and nonverbally; therefore, all health-care providers and ancillary staff need to have similar information and skill development to communicate effectively with diverse populations. The manner in which the information is used may differ significantly based on the discipline, individual experiences, and specific circumstances of the patient, provider, and organization. If providers and the system are competent, most patients will access the health-care system when problems are first recognized, thereby reducing the length of stay, decreasing complications, and reducing overall costs.

A lack of knowledge of patients' language abilities and cultural beliefs and values can result in serious threats to life and quality of care for all individuals (Joint Commission, 2010). Organizations and individuals who understand their patients' cultural values, beliefs, and practices are in a better position to be co-participants with their patients in providing culturally acceptable care. Having ethnocultural-specific knowledge, understanding, and assessment skills to work with culturally diverse patients ensures that the health-care provider can conduct a more targeted assessment. Providers who know culturally specific aggregate data are less likely to demonstrate negative attitudes, behaviors, ethnocentrism, stereotyping, and racism. The onus for cultural competence is on the health-care provider and the delivery system in which care is provided. To this end, health-care providers need both general and specific cultural knowledge when conducting assessments, planning care, and teaching patients about their treatments and prescriptions.

World Diversity and Migration

As of January 2011, the world's population estimate reached 6.8 billion people, with a median age of 27.7 years. The population is expected to approach 7.6 billion by 2020 and 9.3 billion by 2050. The estimated population growth rate remains relatively stable at 1.13 percent, with 19.86 births per 1000 population; 8.7 deaths per 1000 population; and an infant mortality rate of 44.13 per 1000 population, down from 48.87 in 2005. Worldwide life expectancy at birth is currently 66.12 years, up from 64.77 years in 2005 (*CIA World Factbook,* 2011). The ten largest urban populations where significant migration occurs are Tokyo, Japan with 36.7 million; Delhi, India with 22.2 million; São Paulo, Brazil with 20.3 million; Mexico City, Mexico with 19 million; New York–Newark, United States with 19.4 million; Shanghai, China with 16.6 million; Kolata, India with 15.6 million; Dhaka, Bangladesh with 14.7 million; and Karachi, Pakistan with 13.1 million (*CIA World Factbook,* 2011).

As a first language, Mandarin Chinese is the most popular, spoken by 12.65 percent of the world's population, followed by Spanish at 4.93 percent, English at 4.91 percent, Arabic at 3.1 percent, Hindi at 2.73 percent, Portuguese at 2.67 percent, Bengali at 2.71 percent, Russian at 2.16 percent, Japanese at 1.83 percent, and Standard German at 1.35 percent. Only 82 percent of the world population is literate. When technology is examined, more people have a cell phone than a landline—with a ratio of 3:1. Over 1.6 billion people are Internet users, up by 62 percent from 2005 (*CIA World Factbook,* 2011). Language literacy has serious implications for immigration. Over two-thirds of the world's 785 million illiterate adults are found in only eight countries: Bangladesh, China, Egypt, Ethiopia, India, Indonesia, Nigeria, and Pakistan. Of all the illiterate adults in the world, two-thirds are women; extremely low literacy rates are concentrated in three regions: the Arab states, South and West Asia, and Sub-Saharan Africa, where around one-third of the men and half of all women are illiterate (2005 est.) (*CIA World Factbook,* 2011).

The United Nations High Commissioner for Refugees estimated in December 2006, the latest year for which figures are available, a global population of 8.8 million registered refugees, the lowest number in 30 years, and as many as 24.5 million internally displaced persons in more than 50 countries. The actual global population of refugees is probably closer to 10 million given the estimated 1.5 million Iraqi refugees displaced throughout the Middle East. Migrants represent approximately 190 million people or 2.9 percent of the world population, up from 175 million in the year 2000. Moreover, international migration is decreasing, while internal migration is increasing, especially in Asian countries (U.N. Refugee Agency, 2009).

In 1997, the International Organization for Migration studied the costs and benefits of international migration. A comprehensive update has not been undertaken since that time. According to the report, ample evidence exists that migration brings both costs and benefits for sending and receiving countries, although these are not shared equally. Trends suggest a greater movement toward circular migration with substantial benefits to both home and host countries. The perception that migrants are more of a burden on than a benefit to the host country is not substantiated by research. For example, in the Home Office Study (2002) in the United Kingdom, migrants contributed US$4 billion more in taxes than they received in benefits. In the United States, the National Research Council (1998) estimated that national income had expanded by US$8 billion because of immigration. Thus, because migrants pay taxes, they are not likely to put a greater burden on health and welfare services than the host population. However, undocumented migrants run the highest health risks because they are less likely to seek health care. This not only poses risks for migrants but also fuels sentiments of xenophobia and discrimination against all migrants.

> ▶ *What evidence do you see in your community that migrants have added to the economic base of the community? Who would be doing their work if they were not available? If migrants (legal or undocumented) were not picking vegetables (just one example), how much more do you think you would pay for the vegetables?*

U.S. Population and Census Data

As of 2010, the U.S. population was over 308 million, an increase of 16 million since the 2000 census. The 2010 census data include changes designed to more clearly distinguish Hispanic ethnicity as not being a race. In addition, the Hispanic terms have been modified to include *Hispanic* (used more heavily on the East Coast), *Latino* (used more heavily in California and the West Coast), and *Spanish*. The most recent census data estimate that 65.1 percent of the U.S. population are white, 15.8 percent are Hispanic/Latino, 12.9 percent are black, 4.6 percent are Asian, 1.0 percent are American Indian or Alaskan Native, and 0.2 percent are Native Hawaiian or other Pacific Islander. These groupings will be more specifically reported as the census data are analyzed. The categories as used in the 2010 U.S. Census are as follows:

1. *White* refers to people having origins in any of the original peoples of Europe and includes Middle Easterners, Irish, German, Italian, Lebanese, Turkish, Arab, and Polish.
2. *Black,* or *African American,* refers to people having origins in any of the black racial groups of Africa and includes Nigerians and Haitians or any person who self-designates this category regardless of origin.
3. *American Indian* and *Alaskan Native* refer to people having origins in any of the original peoples of North, South, or Central America and who maintain tribal affiliation or community attachment.
4. *Asian* refers to people having origins in any of the original peoples of the Far East, Southeast Asia, or the Indian subcontinent. This category includes the terms *Asian Indian, Chinese, Filipino, Korean, Japanese, Vietnamese, Burmese, Hmong, Pakistani,* and *Thai*.
5. *Native Hawaiian* and *other Pacific Islander* refer to people having origins in any of the original peoples of Hawaii, Guam, Samoa, Tahiti, the Mariana Islands, and Chuuk.
6. *Some other race* was included for people who are unable to identify with the other categories.
7. In addition, the respondent could identify, as a write-in, with two races (U.S. Census Bureau, 2010).

The Hispanic/Latino and Asian populations continue to rise in numbers and in percentage of the overall population; however, although the black/African American, Native Hawaiian and Pacific Islanders, and American Indian and Alaskan Natives groups continue to increase in overall numbers, their percentage of the population has decreased. Of the Hispanic/Latino population, most are Mexicans, followed by Puerto Ricans, Cubans, Central Americans, South Americans, and Dominicans. Salvadorans are the largest group from Central America. Three-quarters of Hispanics live in the West or South, with 50 percent of the Hispanics living in just two states: California and Texas. The median age for the entire U.S. population is 41.8 years, and the median age for Hispanics is 27.2 years (U.S. Census Bureau, 2010). The young age of Hispanics in the United States makes them ideal candidates for recruitment into the health professions, an area with crisis-level shortages of personnel, especially of minority representation.

Before 1940, most immigrants to the United States came from Europe, especially Germany, the United Kingdom, Ireland, the former Union of Soviet Socialist Republics, Latvia, Austria, and Hungary. Since 1940, immigration patterns to the United States have changed: Most are from Mexico, the Philippines, China, India, Brazil, Russia, Pakistan, Japan, Turkey, Egypt, and Thailand. People from each of these countries bring their own culture with them and increase the cultural mosaic of the United States. Many of these groups have strong ethnic identities and maintain their values, beliefs, practices, and languages long after their arrival. Individuals who speak only their indigenous language are more likely to adhere to traditional practices and live in ethnic enclaves and are less likely to assimilate into their new society. The inability of immigrants to speak the language of their new country creates additional challenges for healthcare providers working with these populations. Other countries in the world face similar immigration challenges and opportunities for diversity enrichment. However, space does not permit a comprehensive analysis of migration patterns.

> ▶ *What changes in ethnic and cultural diversity have you seen in your community over the last 5 years? Over the last 10 years? Have you had the opportunity to interact with these newer groups?*

Racial and Ethnic Disparities in Health Care

A number of organizations have developed documents addressing the need for cultural competence as one strategy for eliminating racial and ethnic disparities. In 2005, the Agency for Healthcare Research and Quality (AHRQ) released the "Third National

Healthcare Disparities Report" (AHRQ, 2005), which provided a comprehensive overview of health disparities in ethnic, racial, and socioeconomic groups in the United States. This report was a companion document to the "National Healthcare Quality Report" (2006), which was an overview of quality health care in the United States. *Healthy People 2010*'s (www.healthypeople.gov) goals were to increase the quality and the length of a healthy life and to eliminate health disparities. Healthy People provided science-based, 10-year national objectives for improving the health of all Americans. For 3 decades, Healthy People has established benchmarks and monitored progress over time in order to (1) encourage collaborations across communities and sectors, (2) empower individuals toward making informed health decisions, and (3) measure the impact of prevention activities (http://www.healthypeople.gov/2020/about/default.aspx).

The *Healthy People 2020* (www.healthypeople2020.gov) report had a renewed focus on identifying, measuring, tracking, and reducing health disparities through determinants of health such as the social and economic environment, the physical environment, and the person's individual characteristics and behaviors.

Although the term *disparities* is often interpreted to mean racial or ethnic disparities, many dimensions of disparity exist in the United States, particularly in health. If a health outcome is seen in a greater or lesser extent among different populations, a disparity exists. Race or ethnicity, sex, sexual identity, age, disability, socioeconomic status, and geographic location all contribute to an individual's ability to achieve good health. During the past two decades, one of *Healthy People's* overarching goals focused on disparities. Indeed, in *Healthy People 2000,* the goal was to reduce health disparities among Americans; in *Healthy People 2010,* it was to completely eliminate, not just reduce, health disparities; and in *Healthy People 2020,* the goal was expanded to achieve health equity, eliminate disparities, and improve the health of all groups.

Healthy People 2020 defines a *health disparity* as "a particular type of health difference that is closely linked with social, economic, and/or environmental disadvantage." Health disparities adversely affect groups of people who have systematically experienced greater obstacles to health based on their racial or ethnic group; religion; socioeconomic status; gender; age; mental health; cognitive, sensory, or physical disability; sexual orientation or gender identity; geographic location; or other characteristics historically linked to discrimination or exclusion. In addition, powerful, complex relationships exist among health and biology, genetics, and individual behavior, and among health and

health services, socioeconomic status, the physical environment, discrimination, racism, literacy levels, and legislative policies. These factors, which influence an individual's or population's health, are known as determinants of health (*Healthy People 2020*).

> ▶ *What health disparities have you observed in your community? To what do you attribute these disparities? What can you do as a professional to help decrease these disparities?*

More specific data on ethnic and cultural groups are included in individual chapters. As can be seen by the overwhelming data, much more work needs to be done to improve the health of the nation. Space does not permit an extensive discourse on racial and ethnic disparities in other countries, but documents with frequent updates that include other countries, conditions, and policies are listed as a resource on DavisPlus.

Culture and Essential Terminology
Culture Defined

Anthropologists and sociologists have proposed many definitions of *culture*. For the purposes of this book, which is primarily focused on individual cultural competence instead of the culturally competent organization, **culture** is defined as the totality of socially transmitted behavioral patterns, arts, beliefs, values, customs, lifeways, and all other products of human work and thought characteristics of a population of people that guide their worldview and decision making. Health and health-care beliefs and values are assumed in this definition. These patterns may be explicit or implicit, are primarily learned and transmitted within the family, are shared by most (but not all) members of the culture, and are emergent phenomena that change in response to global phenomena. Culture, a combined anthropological and social construct, can be seen as having three levels: (1) a tertiary level that is visible to outsiders, such as things that can be seen, worn, or otherwise observed; (2) a secondary level, in which only members know the rules of behavior and can articulate them; and (3) a primary level that represents the deepest level in which rules are known by all, observed by all, implicit, and taken for granted (Koffman, 2006). Culture is largely unconscious and has powerful influences on health and illness.

An important concept to understand is that cultural beliefs, values, and practices are learned from birth: first at home, then in the church and other places where people congregate, and then in educational settings. Therefore, a 3-month-old female child from Russian Ashkenazi Jewish heritage who is adopted by a European American family and reared in a dominant European American environment will have a European American worldview. However, if that child's heritage has a tendency toward genetic/hereditary conditions, they would come from her Russian Jewish ancestry, not from European American genetics.

▶ *Who in your family had the most influence in teaching you cultural values and practices? Outside the family, where else did you learn about your cultural values and beliefs? What cultural practices did you learn in your family that you no longer practice?*

When individuals of dissimilar cultural orientations meet in a work or a therapeutic environment, the likelihood for developing a mutually satisfying relationship is improved if both parties attempt to learn about one another's culture. Moreover, race and culture are not synonymous and should not be confused. For example, most people who self-identify as African American have varying degrees of dark skin, but some may have white skin. However, as a cultural term, *African American* means that the person takes pride in having ancestry from both Africa and the United States; thus, a person with white skin could self-identify as African American.

Important Terms Related to Culture

Attitude is a state of mind or feeling about some aspect of a culture. Attitudes are learned; for example, some people think that one culture is better than another. No one culture is "better" than another; they are just different, and many different cultures share the same customs. A belief is something that is accepted as true, especially as a tenet or a body of tenets accepted by people in an ethnocultural group. A belief among some cultures is that if you go outside in the cold weather with wet hair, you will catch a cold. Attitudes and beliefs do not have to be proven; they are unconsciously accepted as truths. **Ideology** consists of the thoughts and beliefs that reflect the social needs and aspirations of an individual or an ethnocultural group. For example, some people believe that health care is the right of all people, whereas others see health care as a privilege.

The literature reports many definitions of the terms *cultural awareness, cultural sensitivity,* and *cultural competence.* Sometimes, these definitions are used interchangeably, but each has a distinct meaning. **Cultural awareness** has to do with an appreciation of the external signs of diversity, such as the arts, music, dress, foods, and physical characteristics. **Cultural sensitivity** has to do with personal attitudes and not saying things that might be offensive to someone from a cultural or ethnic background different from the

health-care provider's. **Cultural competence** in health care is having the knowledge, abilities, and skills to deliver care congruent with the patient's cultural beliefs and practices. Increasing one's consciousness of cultural diversity improves the possibilities for health-care practitioners to provide culturally competent care.

▶ *What activities have you done to increase your cultural awareness and competence? How do you demonstrate that you are culturally sensitive?*

One progresses from unconscious incompetence (not being aware that one is lacking knowledge about another culture), to conscious incompetence (being aware that one is lacking knowledge about another culture), to conscious competence (learning about the patient's culture, verifying generalizations about the patient's culture, and providing cultural-specific interventions), and, finally, to unconscious competence (automatically providing culturally congruent care to patients of diverse cultures). Unconscious competence is difficult to accomplish and potentially dangerous because individual differences exist within cultural groups. To be even minimally effective, culturally competent care must have the assurance of continuation after the original impetus is withdrawn; it must be integrated into, and valued by, the culture that is to benefit from the interventions.

Developing mutually satisfying relationships with diverse cultural groups involves good interpersonal skills and the application of knowledge and techniques learned from the physical, biological, and social sciences as well as the humanities. An understanding of one's own culture and personal values and the ability to detach oneself from "excess baggage" associated with personal views are essential for cultural competence. Even then, traces of ethnocentrism may unconsciously pervade one's attitudes and behavior. **Ethnocentrism**—the universal tendency of human beings to think that their ways of thinking, acting, and believing are the only right, proper, and natural ways (which most people practice to some degree)—can be a major barrier to providing culturally competent care. Ethnocentrism perpetuates an attitude in which beliefs that differ greatly from one's own are strange, bizarre, or unenlightened and, therefore, wrong. Values are principles and standards that are important and have meaning and worth to an individual, family, group, or community. For example, the dominant U.S. culture places high value on youth, technology, and money. The extent to which one's cultural values are internalized influences the tendency toward ethnocentrism. The more one's values are internalized, the more difficult it is to avoid the tendency toward ethnocentrism.

▶ *Given that everyone is ethnocentric to some degree, what do you do to become less ethnocentric? With which groups are you more ethnocentric? If you were to rate yourself on a scale of 1 to 10, with 1 being only a little ethnocentric and 10 being very ethnocentric, what score would you give yourself? What score would your friends give you? What score would you give your closest friends?*

The Human Genome Project (2003) determined that 99.9 percent of all humans share the same genes. One-tenth percent of genetic variations account for the differences among humans, although these differences may be significant when conducting health assessments and prescribing medications and treatments. Ignoring this small difference, however, is ignoring the beliefs, practices, and values of a small ethnic or cultural population to whom one provides care. However, the controversial term *race* must still be addressed when learning about culture. Race is genetic in origin and includes physical characteristics that are similar among members of the group, such as skin color, blood type, and hair and eye color (Giger et al., 2007). People from a given racial group may, but do not necessarily, share a common culture. Race as a social concept is sometimes more important than race as a biological concept. Race has social meaning, assigns status, limits or increases opportunities, and influences interactions between patients and clinicians. Some believe that race terminology was invented to assign low status to some and privilege, power, and wealth to others (American Anthropological Association, 1998). Thus, perhaps the most significant aspect of race is social in origin. Moreover, one must remember that even though one might have a racist attitude, it is not always recognized because it is ingrained during socialization and leads to ethnocentrism.

▶ *How do you define race? What other terms do you use besides race to describe people? In what category did you classify yourself on the last census? What categories would you add to the current census classifications?*

Worldview is the way individuals or groups of people look at the universe to form basic assumptions and values about their lives and the world around them. Worldview includes cosmology, relationships with nature, moral and ethical reasoning, social relationships, magicoreligious beliefs, and aesthetics.

Any **generalization**—reducing numerous characteristics of an individual or group of people to a general form that renders them indistinguishable—made about the behaviors of any individual or large group of people is almost certain to be an oversimplification. When a generalization relates less to the actual observed behavior than to the motives thought to underlie the behavior (i.e., the *why* of the behavior), it is likely to be oversimplified. However, generalizations can lead to **stereotyping**, an oversimplified conception, opinion, or belief about some aspect of an individual or group. Although generalization and stereotyping are similar, functionally, they are very different. Generalization is a starting point, whereas stereotyping is an endpoint. The health-care provider must specifically ask questions to determine these values and avoid stereotypical views of patients. See the section on Variant Characteristics of Culture in this chapter.

▶ *Everyone engages in stereotypical behavior to some degree. We could not function otherwise. If someone asks you to think of a nurse, what image do you have? Is the nurse male or female? How old is the nurse? How is the nurse dressed? Is the nurse wearing a hat? How do you distinguish a stereotype from a generalization?*

Within all cultures are subcultures and ethnic groups whose values/experiences differ from those of the dominant culture with which they identify. Indeed, subcultures share beliefs according to the *variant characteristics* of culture, as described later in this chapter. In sociology, anthropology, and cultural studies, a **subculture** is defined as a group of people with a culture that differentiates them from the larger culture of which they are a part. Subcultures may be distinct or hidden (e.g., gay, lesbian, bisexual, and transgendered populations). If the subculture is characterized by a systematic opposition to the dominant culture, then it may be described as a counterculture. Examples of subcultures are Goths, punks, and stoners, although popular lay literature might call these groups cultures instead of subcultures. A counterculture would include cults (Merriam Webster Online Dictionary, 2010).

The terms *transcultural* versus *cross-cultural* have been hotly debated among experts in several countries but especially in the United States. Specific definitions of these terms vary. Some attest that they are the same, whereas others say they are different. Historically, nursing seems to favor the word *transcultural*. Indeed, the term has been credited to a nurse anthropologist, Madeleine Leininger, in the 1950s (Leininger & McFarland, 2006), and it continues to be popular in the United States, the United Kingdom, and many European countries. The term *cross-cultural* can be traced to anthropologist George Murdock in the 1930s and is still a popular term used in the social sciences, although the health sciences have used it as well. The term implies comparative interactivity among cultures.

Cultural humility, another term found in cultural literature, focuses on the process of intercultural exchange, paying explicit attention to clarifying the professional's values and beliefs through self-reflection and incorporating the cultural characteristics of the professional and the patient into a mutually beneficial and balanced relationship (Trevalon & Murray-Garcia, 1998). This term appears to be most popular with physicians and some professionals from the social sciences.

Cultural safety is a popular term in Australia, New Zealand, and Canada, although it is used elsewhere. Cultural safety expresses the diversity that exists within cultural groups and includes the social determinants of health, religion, and gender, in addition to ethnicity (*Guidelines for Cultural Safety*, 2005). **Cultural leverage** is a process whereby the principles of cultural competence are deliberately invoked to develop interventions. It is a focused strategy for improving the health of racial and ethnic communities by using their cultural practices, products, philosophies, or environments to facilitate behavioral changes of the patient and professional (Fisher et al., 2007).

Acculturation occurs when a person gives up the traits of his or her culture of origin as a result of contact with another culture. Acculturation is not an absolute, and it has varying degrees. Traditional people hold onto the majority of cultural traits from their culture of origin, which is frequently seen when people live in ethnic enclaves and can get most of their needs met without mixing with the outside world. Bicultural acculturation occurs when an individual is able to function equally in the dominant culture and in one's own culture. People who are comfortable working in the dominant culture and return to their ethnic enclave without taking on most of the dominant culture's traits are usually bicultural. Marginalized individuals are not comfortable in their new culture or their culture of origin. **Assimilation** is the gradual adoption and incorporation of characteristics of the prevailing culture (Portes, 2007).

Enculturation is a natural conscious and unconscious conditioning process of learning accepted cultural norms, values, and roles in society and achieving competence in one's culture through socialization. Enculturation is facilitated by growing up in a particular culture, and it can be through formal education, apprenticeships, mentorships, and role modeling (Clarke & Hofsess, 1998).

Individualism, Collectivism, and Individuality

All cultures worldwide vary along an individualism and collectivism scale and are subsets of broad worldviews. A continuum of values for individualistic and collectivistic cultures includes orientation to self or group, decision making, knowledge transmission, individual choice and personal responsibility, the concept of progress, competitiveness, shame and guilt, help-seeking, expression of identity, and interaction/communication style (Hofstede, 1991; Hofstede & Hofstede, 2005).

Elements and the degree of individualism and collectivism exist in every culture. People from an individualist culture will more strongly identify with the values at the individualistic end of the scale. Moreover, individualism and collectivism fall along a continuum, and some people from an individualistic culture will, to some degree, align themselves toward the collectivistic end of the scale. Some people from a collectivist culture will, to some degree, hold values along the individualistic end of the scale. Acculturation is a key component of adopting individualistic and collectivistic values. Those who live in ethnic enclaves usually, but not always, adhere more strongly to their dominant cultural values, sometimes to such a degree that they are more traditional than people in their home country. Acculturation and the variant characteristics of culture determine the degree of adherence to traditional individualistic and collectivist cultural values, beliefs, and practices (Hofstede, 1991; Hofstede & Hofstede, 2005).

Communicating, assessing, counseling, and educating a person from an individualistic culture, where the most important person in society is the individual, may require different techniques than for a person in a collectivist culture where the group is seen as more important than the individual (Hofstede & Hofstede, 2005). The professional must not confuse individualism with individuality—the degree that varies by culture and is usually more prevalent in individualistic countries. **Individuality** is the sense that each person has a separate and equal place in the community and where individuals who are considered "eccentrics or local characters" are tolerated (Purnell, 2010).

Some highly individualistic cultures include traditional European American (in the United States), British, Canadian, German, Norwegian, and Swedish, to name a few. Some examples of collectivist cultures include traditional Arabic, Amish, Chinese, Filipino, Korean, Japanese, Latin American, Mexican, American Indians (and most other indigenous Indian groups), Taiwanese, Thai, Turkish, and Vietnamese. Far more world cultures are collectivistic than are individualistic. It may be difficult for a nurse who is from a highly collectivist culture to communicate with patients and staff in highly individualistic cultures, such as the United States and Germany (Hofstede & Hofstede, 2005).

Cultures differ in the extent to which health and information are explicit or implicit. In low-context cultures, great emphasis is placed on the verbal mode, and many words are used to express a thought. Low-context cultures are individualistic. In high-context cultures, much of the information is implicit where fewer words are used to express a thought, resulting in more of the message being in the nonverbal mode. Great emphasis is placed on personal relationships. High-context cultures are collectivistic (Hofstede, 1991; 2001).

Consistent with individualism, individualistic cultures encourage self-expression. Adherents to individualism freely express personal opinions, share many personal issues, and ask personal questions of others to a degree that may be seen as offensive to those who come from a collectivistic culture. Direct, straight forward questioning is usually appreciated with individualism. However, the professional should take cues from the patient before this intrusive approach is initiated. Small talk before getting down to business is not always appreciated. Individualistic cultures usually tend to be more informal and frequently use first names. Ask the patient by what name he or she prefers to be called. Questions that require a "yes" or "no" answer are usually answered truthfully from the patient's perspective. In individualistic cultures that value autonomy and productivity, one is expected to be a productive member of society. Among collectivistic cultures, people with a mental or physical disability are *more likely* to be hidden from society to "save face," and the cultural norms and values of the family unit mean that the family provides care in the home (Purnell, 2001).

Indeed, it is absolutely imperative to include the family, and sometimes the community, in health care for effective counseling; otherwise, the treatment plan may falter. However, among many Middle Eastern and other collectivistic cultures, family members with mental or physical disabilities are hidden from the community for fear that children in the family might not be able to obtain a spouse if the condition is known. For other impairments, such as HIV, the condition may be kept from public view, not because of confidentiality rights but for fear that news of the condition will spread to other family members and the community.

The greater the perceived cultural stigma, the more likely the delay in seeking counseling, resulting in the condition being more severe at the time of treatment. Individualistic cultures socialize their members to view themselves as *independent*, separate, distinct individuals, where the most important person in society is self. A person feels free to change alliances and not feel bound by any particular group (shared identity). Although they are part of a group, they are still free to act independently within the group and less likely to engage in "groupthink." In individualism, competition, whether individual or group, permeates every aspect of life. Separateness, independence, and the capacity to express one's own views and opinions are both explicitly valued and implicitly assumed.

In individualistic cultures, a person's identity is based mainly on one's personal accomplishments, career, and challenges. A high standard of living supports self-efficiency, self-direction, self-advocacy, and independent living. Decisions made by elders and people in hierarchal positions may be questioned or not followed because the ideal is that all people expect to, and are expected to, make their own decisions about their lives. Moreover, people are personally responsible and held accountable for their decisions. Improving self, doing "better" than others (frequently focused on material gains), and making progress on a community or national level are expected. If one fails, the blame and shame are on the individual alone.

In collectivistic cultures, people are socialized to view themselves as members of a larger group, family, school, church, educational setting, workplace, and so on. They are bound through the expectations of loyalty and personal and familial lifetime protective ties. Children are socialized where priority is given to connections and interrelationship with others as the basis of psychological well-being. Older people and those in hierarchical positions are respected, and people are less likely to openly disagree with them. Parents and elders may have the final say in their children's careers and life partners. The focus is not on the individual but on the group.

Collectivism is characterized by not drawing attention to oneself, and people are not encouraged to ask controversial questions about themselves or others. When one fails, shame may be extended to the family, and external explanations, spiritual, superiors, or fate may be given. To avoid offending someone, people are expected to practice smooth interpersonal communication by not openly disagreeing with anyone and being evasive about negative issues. Among most collectivist cultures, disagreeing with or saying "no" to a health-care professional is considered rude. In fact, in some languages, there is no word for "no." If you ask a collectivist patient if she knows what you are asking, if she understands you, and if she knows how to do something, she will always answer "yes." But "yes" could mean (a) I hear you, but I do not understand you; (b) I understand you, but I do not agree with what you are saying; and (c) I know how to do that, but I might not do it. Repeating what has been prescribed does not ensure understanding; instead, ask for a demonstration or some other response that is more likely to determine understanding.

Variant Characteristics of Culture

Great diversity exists within a cultural group. Major influences that shape people's worldviews and the degree to which they identify with their cultural group of origin are called the "variant characteristics of culture." Some variant characteristics cannot be changed, while others can. They include but are not limited to the following:

- *Nationality:* One cannot change his or her nationality, but over time many people have changed their names to better fit into society or to decrease discrimination. For example, many Jews changed the spelling of their last names during and after World War II to avoid discrimination.
- *Race:* Race cannot be changed, but people can and do make changes in their appearance, such as with of cosmetic surgery.
- *Color:* Skin color cannot usually be changed on a permanent basis.
- *Age:* Age cannot be changed, but many people go to extensive lengths to make themselves look younger. One's worldview changes with age. In some cultures, older people are looked upon with reverence and increased respect. Age difference with the accompanying worldview is frequently called the *generation gap*.
- *Religious affiliation:* People can and do change their religious affiliations or self-identify as atheists. However, if someone changes his or her religious affiliation—for example, from Judaism to Pentecostal or Baptist to Islam—a significant stigma may occur within their family or community.
- *Educational status:* As education increases, people's worldview changes and increases their knowledge base for decision making.
- *Socioeconomic status:* Socioeconomic status can change either up or down and can be a major determinant for access to and use of health care.
- *Occupation:* One's occupation can change. Of course, an occupation can be a health risk if employment is in a coal mine, on a farm, or in a high-stress position. In addition, someone who is educated in the health professions would not have as much difficulty with health literacy.
- *Military experience:* People who have military experience may be more accustomed to hierarchical decision making and rules of authority.
- *Political beliefs:* Political affiliation can change according to one's ideology. One of the major reasons for migration is ideological and political beliefs.

- *Urban versus rural residence:* People can change their residence with concomitant changes in ideology with different health risks and access to health care.
- *Enclave identity:* For people who primarily live and work in an ethnic enclave where they can get their needs met without mixing with the world outside, they may be more traditional than people in their home country.
- *Marital status:* Married people and people with partners frequently have a different worldview than those without partners.
- *Parental status:* Often, when people become parents—having children, adopting, or taking responsibility for raising a child—their worldview changes, and they usually become more futuristic.
- *Sexual orientation:* Sexual orientation is usually stable over time, but some people are bisexual. In addition, people who are incarcerated may engage in same-sex activity but return to a heterosexual lifestyle when released from prison. Gender reassignment is now a possibility for some, although a significant stigma may occur.
- *Gender issues:* Men and women may have different concerns in regards to type of work and work hours, pay scales, and health inequalities.
- *Physical characteristics:* One's physical characteristics may have an effect on how people see themselves and how others see them and can include such characteristics as height, weight, hair color and style, and skin color.
- *Immigration status (sojourner, immigrant, or undocumented status):* Immigration status and length of time away from the country of origin also affect one's worldview. People who voluntarily immigrate generally acculturate and assimilate more easily. Sojourners who immigrate with the intention of remaining in their new homeland for only a short time on work assignments or refugees who think they may return to their home country may not have the need or desire to acculturate or assimilate. Additionally, undocumented individuals (illegal immigrants) may have a different worldview from those who have arrived legally. Many in this group remained hidden in society so they will not be discovered and returned to their home country.
- *Length of time away from the country of origin:* Usually, the longer people are away from their culture of origin, the less traditional they become as they acculturate and assimilate into their new culture.

Some examples of how variant cultural characteristics change one's worldview follow.

Consider two people with the following variant characteristics. One is a 75-year-old devout Islamic female from Saudi Arabia, and the other is a 19-year-old African American fundamentalist Baptist male from Louisiana. Obviously, the two do not look alike, and they probably have very different worldviews and beliefs, many of which come from their religious tenets and country of origin.

The variant cultural characteristics of being a single transsexual urban business executive will most likely have a different worldview from that of a married heterosexual rural secretary who has two teenagers. In another case, a migrant farm worker from the highlands of Guatemala with an undocumented status has a different perspective than an immigrant from Mexico who has lived in New York City for 10 years.

Ethics Across Cultures

As globalization grows and population diversity with nations increases, health-care providers are increasingly confronted with ethical issues related to cultural diversity. At the extremes stand those who favor multiculturalism and postmodernism versus those who favor humanism. Internationally, multiculturalism asserts that no common moral principles are shared by all cultures. Postmodernism asserts a similar claim against all universal standards, both moral and immoral. The concern is that universal standards provide a disguise, whereas dominant cultures destroy or eradicate traditional cultures.

Humanism asserts that all human beings are equal in worth, that they have common resources and problems, and that they are alike in fundamental ways (Macklin, 1999). Humanism does not put aside the many circumstances that make individuals' lives different around the world. Many similarities exist as to what people need to live well. Humanism says that certain human rights should not be violated. Macklin (1998) asserts that universal applicability of moral principles is required, not universal acceptability. Beaucamp (1998) concurs that fundamental principles of morality and human rights allow for cross-cultural judgments of immoral conduct. Of course, there is a middle ground.

Throughout the world, practices are claimed to be cultural, traditional, and beneficial, even when they are exploitative and harmful. For example, female circumcision, a traditional cultural practice, is seen by some as exploiting women. In many cases, the practice is harmful and can even lead to death. Although empirical, anthropological research has shown that different cultures and historical eras contain different moral beliefs and practices, it is far from certain that what is right or wrong can be determined only by the beliefs and practices within a particular culture or subculture. Slavery and apartheid are examples of civil rights violations.

Accordingly, codes of ethics are open to interpretation and are not value-free. Furthermore, ethics belong to the society, not to professional groups. Ethics and ethical decision making are culturally bound. The Western ethical principles of patient autonomy, self-determination, justice, do no harm, truth telling, and promise-keeping are highly valued, but not all cultures—non-Western societies—place such high regard on these values. For example, in Russia, the truth is optional, people are expected to break their promises, and most students cheat on examinations. Cheating on a business deal is not necessarily considered dishonorable (Birch, 2006).

In health organizations in the United States, advance directives give patients the opportunity to decide about their care, and staff members are required to ask patients about this upon admission to a health-care facility. Western ethics, with its stress on individualism, asks this question directly of the patient. However, in collectivist societies, such as among some ethnic Chinese and Japanese, the preferred person to ask may be a family member. In addition, translating health forms into other languages can be troublesome because a direct translation can be confusing. For example, "informed consent" may be translated to mean that the person relinquishes his or her right to decision making.

Some cultural situations occur that raise legal issues. For instance, in Western societies, a competent person (or an alternative such as the spouse, if the person is married) is supposed to sign her or his own consent for medical procedures. However, in some cultures, the eldest son is expected to sign consent forms, not the spouse. In this case, both the organization and the family can be satisfied if both the spouse and the son sign the informed consent.

Instead of Western ethics prevailing, some authorities advocate for universal ethics. Each culture has its own definition of what is right or wrong and what is good or bad. Accordingly, some health-care providers encourage international codes of ethics, such as those developed by the International Council of Nurses (2010). These codes are intended to reflect the patient's culture and whether the value is placed on individualism or collectivism. Most Western codes of ethics have interpretative statements based on the Western value of individualism. International codes of ethics do not contain interpretative statements but, rather, let each society interpret them according to its culture. As our multicultural society increases its diversity, health-care providers need to rely upon ethics committees that include members from the cultures they serve.

As the globalization of health-care services increases, providers must also address very crucial issues, such as cultural imperialism, cultural relativism, and cultural imposition. **Cultural imperialism** is the practice of extending the policies and practices of one group (usually the dominant one) to disenfranchised and minority groups. An example is the U.S. government's forced migration of Native American tribes to reservations with individual allotments of lands (instead of group ownership), as well as forced attendance of their children at boarding schools attended by white people. Proponents of cultural imperialism appeal to universal human rights values and standards (Purnell, 2001).

Cultural relativism is the belief that the behaviors and practices of people should be judged only from the context of their cultural system. Proponents of cultural relativism argue that issues such as abortion, euthanasia, female circumcision, and physical punishment in child rearing should be accepted as cultural values without judgment from the outside world. Opponents argue that cultural relativism may undermine condemnation of human rights violations, and family violence cannot be justified or excused on a cultural basis (Purnell, 2001).

Cultural imposition is the intrusive application of the majority group's cultural view upon individuals and families (Universal Declaration of Human Rights, 2001). Prescription of special diets without regard to patients' cultures and limiting visitors to immediate family, a practice of many acute-care facilities, border on cultural imposition (Purnell, 2001).

▶ *What practices have you seen that might be considered a cultural imposition?*
What practices have you seen that might be considered cultural imperialism?
What practices have you seen that might be considered cultural relativism?
What have you done to address them when you have seen them occurring?

Health-care providers must be cautious about forcefully imposing their values regarding genetic testing and counseling. No group is spared from genetic disease. Advances in technology and genetics have found that many diseases, such as Huntington's chorea, have a genetic basis. Some forms of breast and colon cancers, adult-onset diabetes, Alzheimer's disease, and hypertension are some of the newest additions. Currently, only the well-to-do can afford broad testing. Advances in technology will provide the means for access to screening that will challenge genetic testing and counseling. The relationship of genetics to disability, individuals with a disability, and those with a potential disability will create moral dilemmas of new complexity and magnitude.

Many questions surround genetic testing. Should health-care providers encourage genetic testing? What is, or should be, done with the results? How do we approach testing for genes that lead to disease or disability? How do we maximize health and well-being without creating a eugenic devaluation of those who have a disability? Should employers and third-party payers be allowed to discriminate based on genetic potential for illness? What is the purpose of prenatal screening and genetic testing? What are the assumptions for state-mandated testing programs? Should parents and individuals be allowed to "opt out" of testing? What if the individual does not want to know the results? What if the results could have a deleterious outcome to the infant or the mother? What if the results got into the hands of insurance companies that then denied payment or refused to provide coverage? Should public policy support genetic testing, which may improve health and health care for the masses of society? Should multiple births from fertility drugs be restricted because of the burden of cost, education, and health of the family? Should public policy encourage limiting family size in the contexts of the mother's health, religious and personal preferences, and the availability of sufficient natural resources (such as water and food) for future survival? What effect do these issues have on a nation with an aging population, a decrease in family size, and decreases in the numbers and percentages of younger people? What effect will these issues have on the ability of countries to provide health care for their citizens? Health-care providers must understand these three concepts and the ethical issues involved because they will increasingly encounter situations in which they must balance the patient's cultural practices and behaviors with health promotion and wellness, as well as illness, disease, and injury prevention activities for the good of the patient, the family, and society. Other international issues that may be less controversial include sustainable environments, pacification, and poverty (Purnell, 2001).

REFERENCES

Agency for Healthcare Research and Quality (AHRQ). (2005). *Third national healthcare disparities report.* U.S. Department of Health and Human Services. AHRQ Publication No. 060. Retrieved from http://health-equity.pitt.edu/371/

Agency for Healthcare Research and Quality (AHRQ). (2006). *National healthcare quality report.* Retrieved from http://www.ahrq.gov/

American Anthropological Association. (1998). *Statement on race: Position paper.* Retrieved from http://www.aaanet.org/stmts/racepp.htm

Beaucamp, T. (1998). The mettle of moral fundamentalism: A reply to Robert Baker. *Kennedy Institute of Ethics Journal, 8*(4), 389–401.

Birch, D. (2006, October 27). In Russia, the truth is optional. *Baltimore Sun,* pp. 2F, 6F.

Centers for Disease Control. (1985). *Perspectives on disease prevention and health promotion.* Retrieved from www.cdc.gov/mmwr/preview/mmwrthml/00000688.htm

CIA World Factbook. (2011). *World.* Retrieved from https://www.cia.gov/library/publications/the-world-factbook/geos/xx.html

Clarke, L., & Hofsess, L. (1998). Acculturation. In S. Loue (Ed.), *Handbook of immigrant health* (pp. 37–59). New York: Plenum Press.

Council of New Zealand. (2005). *Guidelines for cultural safety: The treaty of Waitangi and Maori health.* Retrieved from http://www.nursingcouncil.org.nz

Fisher, T.L., Burnet, D.L., Huang, E.S., Chin, T.L., & Cagney, K.A. (2007). Cultural leverage: Interventions using culture to narrow racial disparities in health care. *Medical Care Research Review, 64* (5 suppl. 243S–282S).

Giger, J., Davidhizar, R., Purnell, L., Taylor Harden, J., Phillips, J., & Strickland, O. (2007). American Academy of Nursing Expert Panel Report: Developing cultural competence to eliminate health disparities in ethnic minorities and other vulnerable populations. *Journal of Transcultural Nursing, 18*(2), 95-102.

Healthy People 2010. (2005). Retrieved from http://www.healthy-people.gov

Healthy People 2010. (2001). *Companion document for lesbian, gay, bisexual, and transgender health.* Retrieved from http://www.lgbthealth.net

Healthy People 2020. Retrieved from www.healthypeople2020.gov

Hofstede, G. (1991). *Cultures and organizations: Software of the mind.* New York: McGraw-Hill.

Hofstede, G. (2001). *Culture's consequences: Comparing values, behaviors, institutions, and organizations across nations* (2nd ed.). Thousand Oaks, CA: Sage.

Hofstede, G., & Hofstede, J. (2005). *Cultures and organizations: Software of the mind* (2nd ed.). New York: McGraw-Hill.

Home Office Study. (2002). Retrieved from http://news.google.com/news?q=Home+Office+Study++United+Kingdom&hl=en&lr=&sa=Xoi=news&ct=title

Human Genome Project. (2003). Retrieved from http://www.ornl.gov/sci/techresources/Human_Genome/home.shtml

International Council of Nurses. (2010). *Ethics.* Retrieved from http://www.icn.ch/publications/ethics/

Joint Commission. (2010). Effective Communication, Cultural Competence and Family Centered Care: A Roadmap for Hospitals.

Judge, K., Platt, S., Costongs, C., & Jurczak, K. (2005). Health inequalities: A challenge for Europe. Retrieved from http://eurohealthnet.eu/sites/eurohealthnet.eu/files/publications/pu_2.pdf

Koffman, J. (2006). Transcultural and ethical issues at the end of life. In J. Cooper (Ed.), *Stepping into palliative care* (pp. 171–186). Abington, UK: Radcliffe Publishing Ltd.

Leininger, M., & McFarland, M. (2006). *Culture care diversity and universality: A worldwide theory.* Burlington, MA: Jones and Bartlett.

Macklin, R. (1998). A defense of fundamental principles and human rights: A reply to Robert Baker. *Kennedy Institute of Ethics Journal, 8*(4), 389–401.

Macklin, R. (1999). *Against relativism: Cultural diversity and the search for ethical universals in medicine.* New York: Oxford University Press.

Merriam Webster Online Dictionary: Subculture versus counter-culture. (2010). Retrieved from http://www.merriam-webster.com/dictionary/counterculture

National Research Council. (1998). Retrieved from www.nation-alacademies.org/news.nsf/isbn/0309063566?OpenDocument

National Standards of Cultural and Linguistic Services. (2007). Retrieved from http://minorityhealth.hhs.gov/templates/browse.aspx?lvl=2&lvlID=15

O'Neil, E. (2008). Preface. In L. Purnell & B. Paulanka, *Transcultural health care: A culturally competent approach* (3rd ed.). Philadelphia: F.A. Davis Co.

Portes, A. (2007). Migration, development and segmented assimilation: A conceptual review of evidence. *Annals of American Academy of Political and Social Science, 610,* 73–97.

Purnell, L. (2001). Cultural competence in a changing health-care environment. In N. L. Chaska (Ed.), *The nursing profession: Tomorrow and beyond* (pp. 451–461). Thousand Oaks, CA: Sage Publications.

Purnell, L. (2010). Cultural rituals in health and nursing care. In P. Esterhuizen & A. Kuckert (Eds.), *Diversiteit in de verpleeg-kunde* [*Diversity in nursing*] (pp. 130–196). Amsterdam: Bohn Stafleu van Loghum.

Trevalon, M., & Murray-Garcia, J. (1998). Cultural humility versus cultural competence. *Journal of Health Care for the Poor and Underserved, 9*(2), 117–125.

U.N. Refugee Agency. (2009). Retrieved from http://www.unhcr.org

Universal Declaration of Human Rights. (2001). Retrieved from www.amnesty.org

U.S. Census Bureau. (2010). *Demographic profiles.* Retrieved from 2010.census.gov/news/press-kits/demographic-profiles.html

DavisPlus *For case studies, review questions, and additional information, go to*
http://davisplus.fadavis.com

Chapter 2

The Purnell Model for Cultural Competence

Larry D. Purnell

This chapter presents the Purnell Model for Cultural Competence, its organizing framework, and the assumptions upon which the model is based. The model provides a comprehensive, systematic, and concise framework for learning and understanding culture. The empirical framework of the model provides a basis for health-care providers, educators, researchers, managers, and administrators in all health disciplines to provide holistic, culturally competent, therapeutic interventions; health promotion and wellness; illness, disease, and injury prevention; health maintenance and restoration; and health teaching across educational and practice settings.

The purposes of this model are the following:

- Provide a framework for all health-care providers to learn concepts and characteristics of culture. Define circumstances that affect a person's cultural worldview in the context of historical perspectives.
- Provide a model that links the most central relationships of culture.
- Interrelate characteristics of culture to promote congruence and to facilitate the delivery of consciously sensitive and competent health care.
- Provide a framework that reflects such human characteristics as motivation, intentionality, and meaning.
- Provide a structure for analyzing cultural data.
- View the individual, family, or group within their unique ethnocultural environment.

Assumptions Upon Which the Model Is Based

The major explicit assumptions upon which the model is based are as follows:

- All health-care professions need similar information about cultural diversity.

- All health-care professions share the meta-paradigm concepts of global society, family, person, and health.
- One culture is not better than another culture; they are just different.
- Core similarities are shared by all cultures.
- Differences exist within, between, and among cultures.
- Cultures change slowly over time.
- The variant cultural characteristics (see Chapter 1) determine the degree to which one varies from the dominant culture.
- If patients are coparticipants in their care and have a choice in health-related goals, plans, and interventions, their compliance and health outcomes will be improved.
- Culture has a powerful influence on one's interpretation of and responses to health care.
- Individuals and families belong to several subcultures.
- Each individual has the right to be respected for his or her uniqueness and cultural heritage.
- Caregivers need both culture-general and culture-specific information in order to provide culturally sensitive and culturally competent care.
- Caregivers who can assess, plan, intervene, and evaluate in a culturally competent manner will improve the care of patients for whom they care.
- Learning culture is an ongoing process that increases by working with diverse encounters.
- Prejudices and biases can be minimized with cultural understanding.
- To be effective, health care must reflect the unique understanding of the values, beliefs, attitudes, lifeways, and worldviews of diverse populations and individual acculturation patterns.
- Differences in race and culture often require adaptations to standard interventions.

- Cultural awareness improves the caregiver's self-awareness.
- Professions, organizations, and associations have their own culture, which can be analyzed using a grand theory of culture.
- Every patient contact is a cultural encounter.

Overview of the Theory, the Model, and the Organizing Framework

The Purnell Model has been classified as holographic and complexity theory because it includes a model and organizing framework that can be used by all health-care providers in various disciplines and settings. The model is a circle: the outer rim represents global society, the second rim represents community, the third rim represents family, and the inner rim represents the person (Fig. 2-1). The interior of the circle is divided into 12 pie-shaped wedges depicting cultural domains and their concepts. The dark center of the circle represents unknown phenomena. Along the bottom of the model, a jagged line represents the nonlinear concept of cultural consciousness. The 12 cultural domains (constructs) provide the organizing framework of the model. Following the discussion of each domain, a table provides statements that can be adapted as a guide for assessing patients in various settings. Accordingly, health-care providers can use these same questions to better understand their own cultural beliefs, attitudes, values, practices, and behaviors.

Macro Aspects of the Model

The macro aspects of this interactional model include the metaparadigm concepts of a global society, community, family, person, and conscious competence. The theory and model are conceptualized from biology, anthropology, sociology, economics, geography, history, ecology, physiology, psychology, political science, pharmacology, and nutrition, as well as theories from communication, family development, and social support. The model can be used in clinical practice, education, research, and the administration and management of health-care services or to analyze organizational culture.

Phenomena related to a global society include world communication and politics; conflicts and warfare; natural disasters and famines; international exchanges in education, business, commerce, and information technology; advances in health science; space exploration; and the expanded opportunities for people to travel around the world and interact with diverse societies. Global events that are widely disseminated by television, radio, satellite transmission, newsprint, and information technology affect all societies, either directly or indirectly. Such events create chaos while consciously and unconsciously forcing people to alter their lifeways and worldviews.

Think of a recent event that has affected global society, such as a conflict or war, health advances in technology, possible environmental exposure to health problems, or volcanic eruptions. How did you become aware of this event? How has this event altered your views and other people's views of worldwide cultures?

In the broadest definition, community is a group of people who have a common interest or identity that goes beyond the physical environment. Community includes the physical, social, and symbolic characteristics that cause people to connect. Bodies of water, mountains, rural versus urban living, and even railroad tracks help people define their physical concept of community. Today, however, technology and the Internet allow people to expand their community beyond physical boundaries through social and professional networking sites. Economics, religion, politics, age, generation, and marital status delineate the social concepts of community. Symbolic characteristics of a community include sharing a specific language or dialect, lifestyle, history, dress, art, or musical interest. People actively and passively interact with the community, necessitating adaptation and assimilation for equilibrium and homeostasis in their worldview. Individuals may willingly change their physical, social, and symbolic community when it no longer meets their needs.

How do you define your community in terms of objective and subjective cultural characteristics? How has your community changed over the last 5 to 10 years? The last 15 years? The last 20 years? If you have changed communities, think of the community in which you were raised.

A **family** is two or more people who are emotionally connected. They may, but do not necessarily, live in close proximity to one another. Family may include physically and emotionally close and distant consanguineous relatives, as well as physically and emotionally connected and distant non–blood-related significant others. Family structure and roles change according to age, generation, marital status, relocation or immigration, and socioeconomic status, requiring each person to rethink individual beliefs and lifeways.

Whom do you consider family? Are they all blood related? How have they influenced your culture and worldview? Who else has helped instill your cultural values?

A person is a biopsychosociocultural being who is constantly adapting to her or his community. Human beings adapt biologically and physiologically with the aging process; psychologically in the context of social relationships, stress, and relaxation; socially as they interact with the changing

The Purnell Model for Cultural Competence

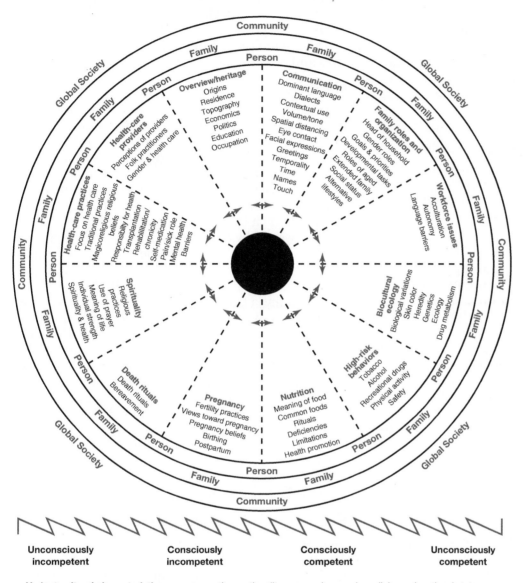

Unconsciously incompetent   **Consciously incompetent**   **Consciously competent**   **Unconsciously competent**

Variant cultural characteristics: age, generation, nationality, race, color, gender, religion, educational status, socioeconomic status, occupation, military status, political beliefs, urban versus rural residence, enclave identity, marital status, parental status, physical characteristics, sexual orientation, gender issues, and reason for migration (sojourner, immigrant, undocumented status).

Unconsciously incompetent: not being aware that one is lacking knowledge about another culture
Consciously incompetent: being aware that one is lacking knowledge about another culture
Consciously competent: learning about the client's culture, verifying generalizations about the client's culture, and providing culturally specific interventions
Unconsciously competent: automatically providing culturally congruent care to clients of diverse cultures

Figure 2-1 The Purnell Model for Cultural Competence. *(Adapted with permission from Larry Purnell, Newark, DE.)*

community; and culturally within the broader global society. In highly individualistic cultures (see Chapter 1), a person is a separate physical and unique psychological being and a singular member of society. The self is separate from others. However, in highly collectivistic cultures, the individual is defined in relation to the family or other group rather than a basic unit of nature.

> ▶ *In what ways have you adapted (1) biologically and physiologically to the aging process, (2) psychologically in the context of social relationships, (3) socially in your community, and (4) culturally within the broader society?*

Health, as used in this book, is a state of wellness as defined by the individual within his or her cultural group. Health generally includes physical, mental, and spiritual states because group members interact with the family, community, and global society. The concept of health, which permeates all metaparadigm concepts of culture, is defined globally, nationally, regionally, locally, and individually. Thus, people can speak about their personal health status or the health status of the nation or community. Health can also be subjective or objective in nature.

> *How do you define health? Is health the absence of illness, disease, injury, and/or disability? How does your profession define health? How does your nation or community define health? How do these definitions compare with your original cultural heritage?*

Micro Aspects of the Model

On a micro level, the model's organizing framework consists of 12 domains and their concepts, which are common to all cultures. These 12 domains are interconnected and have implications for health. The utility of this organizing framework comes from its concise structure, which can be used in any setting and applied to a broad range of empirical experiences and can foster inductive and deductive reasoning in the assessment of cultural domains. Once cultural data are analyzed, the practitioner can fully adopt, modify, or reject health-care interventions and treatment regimens in a manner that respects the patient's cultural differences. Such adaptations improve the quality of the patient's health-care experiences and personal existence.

The Twelve Domains of Culture

These are the 12 domains that are essential for assessing the ethnocultural attributes of an individual, family, or group:

1. Overview, inhabited localities, and topography
2. Communication
3. Family roles and organization
4. Workforce issues
5. Biocultural ecology
6. High-risk behaviors
7. Nutrition
8. Pregnancy and childbearing practices
9. Death rituals
10. Spirituality
11. Health-care practices
12. Health-care providers

Overview, Inhabited Localities, and Topography

This domain includes concepts related to the country of origin, the current residence, and the effects of the topography of both the country of origin and the current residence on health, economics, politics, reasons for migration, educational status, and occupations. Learning about a culture includes becoming familiar with the heritage of its people and understanding how discrimination, prejudice, and oppression influence value systems and beliefs used in everyday life.

Heritage and Residence

Heritage and residence includes ancestry as the country of origin; where they were born, if different from the country of origin; and other places they have lived. For example, one's ancestry might be German as the country of origin but born in the United States and lived or worked in Asia or Central American, where that person might have been exposed to tropical diseases unknown in the United States. Likewise, the topography and physical environment of one's residence may increase one's chances of being inflicted with an can we leave in disease? There is a difference between a disease and an illness and we have both here. illness such as malaria from swampy areas, asthma from polluted inner-city environments, or cancer if exposed to radioactive fallout. Regardless of one's environment and lifestyle, one heritage may be an increased risk for genetic and hereditary diseases that are common among French Canadians, the Amish, and Ashkenazi Jews (see specific chapters on these cultural groups).

One's occupation can also have deleterious effects on health if exposed to asbestos, working in farming with pesticides, or in textile factories with increased risk for respiratory, eye, and ear infections. A complete health history may be required because people might have worked in several occupations over a lifetime.

Reasons for Migration and Associated Economic Factors

The social, economic, religious, and political forces of the country of origin play an important role in the development of the ideologies and the worldview of individuals, families, and groups and are often a major motivating force for emigration. People emigrate for better economic opportunities; because of religious and political oppression and ethnic cleansing; as a result of environmental disasters, such as earthquakes and hurricanes in their home countries; and by forced relocation, such as with slaves and indentured servants. Others have emigrated for educational opportunities and personal ideologies or a combination of factors. Most people emigrate in the hope of a better life, but the individual or group personally defines this ideology.

A common practice for many immigrants is to relocate to an area that has an established population with similar ideologies that can provide initial support, serve as cultural brokers, and orient them to their new culture and health-care system. When immigrants settle and work exclusively in predominantly ethnic communities, primary social support is enhanced, but acculturation and assimilation into the wider society may be hindered. Although ethnic enclaves assist them with acculturation (to an extent), they may need extra help in adjusting to their new homeland's language as well as securing access to health-care services, living accommodations, and employment opportunities. Further, people who move voluntarily are likely to experience less difficulty with acculturation than people who are forced to emigrate. Some individuals immigrate with the intention of remaining in this country only a short time, making money, continuing their education, and returning home, whereas others immigrate with the intention of relocating permanently.

▶ *What is your cultural heritage? How might you find out more about it? How does your cultural heritage influence your current beliefs and values about health and wellness? What brought you/your ancestors to your current country of residence? Why did you/your ancestors emigrate?*

Educational Status and Occupations

The value placed on formal education differs among cultural and ethnic groups and is often related to their socioeconomic status in their homeland and their abilities and reasons for emigrating. Some people place a high value on formal education; however, some do not stress formal education because it is not needed for employment in their homeland. Consequently, they may become engulfed in poverty, isolation, and enclave identity, which may further limit their potential for formal educational opportunities and planning for the future.

In regard to learning styles, the Western system places a high value on the student's ability to categorize information using linear, sequential thought processes. However, not everyone adheres to this pattern of thinking. Others have spiral and circular thought patterns that move from concept to concept without being linear or sequential; therefore, they may have difficulty placing information in a stepwise methodology, which is common in individualistic cultures. When someone is unaware of the value given to such behaviors, the person may seem disorganized, scattered, and faulty in their cognitive patterns, resulting in increased difficulty with written and verbal communications.

Some educational systems stress application of content over theory. Most European educational programs emphasize theory over practical application, and Arab education emphasizes theory with little attention given to practical application. As a result, Arab students are more proficient at tests requiring rote learning than at those requiring conceptualization and analysis. Being familiar with the individual's personal educational

values and learning modes allows health-care providers, educators, and employers to adjust teaching strategies for patients, students, and employees. Educational materials and explanations must be presented at a level consistent with the patient's educational capabilities and within their cultural framework and beliefs (see Chapter 3).

▶ *How strongly do you believe in the value of education? Who in your life is responsible for instilling this value? Do you consider yourself to be a more linear/sequential learner or a random-patterned learner?*

Immigrants bring job skills from their homelands and traditionally seek employment in the same or similar trades. Sometimes, these job skills are inadequate for the available jobs in the new society; thus, immigrants are forced to take low-paying jobs and join the ranks of the working poor and economically disadvantaged. Immigrants to America are employed in a broad variety of occupations and professions; however, limited experiential, educational, and language abilities of more recent immigrants often restrict employment possibilities. More importantly, experiential backgrounds sometimes encourage employment choices that are identified as high risk for chronic diseases, such as exposure to pesticides and chemicals. Others may work in factories that manufacture hepatotoxic chemicals, in industries with pollutants that increase the risk for pulmonary diseases, and in crowded conditions with poor ventilation that increase the risk for tuberculosis or other respiratory diseases.

Understanding patients' current and previous work background is essential for health screening. For example, newer immigrants who worked in malaria-infested areas in their native country, such as Egypt, Italy, Turkey, and Vietnam, may need health screening for malaria. Those who worked in mining, such as in Ireland and Poland, may need screening for respiratory diseases. Those who lived in overcrowded and unsanitary conditions, such as with refugees and migrant workers, may need to be screened for such infectious diseases as tuberculosis, parasitosis, and respiratory diseases. *Table 2-1* identifies guidelines for assessing the cultural domain *overview, inhabited localities, and topography.*

Communication

Perhaps no other domain has the complexities as that of communication. Communication is interrelated with all other domains and depends on verbal language skills that include the dominant language, dialects, and contextual use of the language, as well as paralanguage variations such as voice volume, tone, intonations, reflections, and willingness to share thoughts and feelings. Other important communication characteristics include nonverbal communications, such as eye

II▶ Table 2-1 | **Overview and Heritage**

Suggested Question	Sample Rationale/Example
1. Where do you currently live?	Someone living in a wooded area with deer is at an increased risk for Lyme disease.
2. What is your ancestry?	Ashkenazi Jewish population has a high incidence of genetic and hereditary health conditions.
3. Where were you born?	Immigrants from Eastern Europe near Chernobyl have an increased risk for genetic mutations and hereditary defects related to radioactive contamination.
4. How many years have you lived in the United States (or other country, as appropriate)?	Length of time away from the home country may determine the degree of assimilation and acculturation.
5. Were your parents born in the United States (or other country, as appropriate)?	Generation may determine the degree of assimilation and acculturation.
6. What brought you (your parents/ancestors) to the United States (or other country, as appropriate)?	Refugees may have post-traumatic stress disorders related to their stay in refugee camps and suffered from rape, torture, and a host of infectious and communicable diseases such as tuberculosis.
7. Describe the land or countryside where you live. Is it mountainous, swampy, etc.?	People living in swampy areas are at increased incidence for malaria.
8. Have you lived in other places in the United States/world?	People immigrating from or who have recently visited parts of Central American may be at increased for and need to be assessed for arthropod-borne diseases.
9. What is your income level?	Income level has implications for affording medications, dressings, and prescriptive devices.
10. Does your income allow you to afford the essentials of life?	Determines the ability to afford healthy diets.
11. Do you have health insurance?	Refer to social services for financial support.
12. Are you able to afford health insurance on your salary?	The working poor cannot afford health insurance.
13. What is your educational level (formal/informal/self-taught)?	Educational level may determine ability to understand health prescriptions.
14. What is your current occupation? If retired, ask about previous occupations.	A person may currently be retired or may now work as a salesperson but previously worked as a coal miner, increasing the risk of black lung disease.
15. Are there (were there) any particular health hazards associated with your job(s)?	People working in home remodeling may be at risk for asbestosis.
16. Have you been in the military?	People who served in the military may suffer from post-traumatic stress syndrome or diseases contracted in their military experiences.
17. Are you married?	Part of a standard assessment.
18. How many children do you have?	Part of a standard assessment.

contact, facial expressions, use of touch, body language, spatial distancing practices, and acceptable greetings; temporality in terms of past, present, or future orientation of worldview; clock versus social time; and the name format and the degree of formality in the use of names. Communication styles may vary among insiders (family and close friends) and outsiders (strangers and unknown health-care providers). Hierarchical relationships, gender, and some religious beliefs affect communication.

Dominant Language and Dialects

The health-care provider must be aware of the dominant language and the difficulties that dialects may cause when communicating in the patient's native language. For example, English is a monochromic, low-contextual language in which most of the message is in the verbal mode, and verbal communication is frequently seen as being more important than nonverbal communication. Thus, people for whom English is the dominant language are more likely to miss the more subtle nuances of communication. Accordingly, if a misunderstanding occurs, both the sender and the receiver of the message take responsibility for the miscommunication.

English differs somewhat in its pronunciation, spelling, and choice of words from English spoken in Great Britain, Australia, and other English-speaking countries. Within each country, several dialects can exist, but generally the differences do not cause a major concern with communications. However, accents and dialects within a country, region, or local area can cause misunderstanding; for example, the "Elizabethan English" that is spoken in parts of the United States and the English spoken in Glasgow, Scotland, are both completely different from the English spoken in Central London. The Spanish spoken in Spain differs from the versions spoken in Puerto Rico, Panama, or Mexico, which has as many as 50 different dialects. In such cases, dialects that vary widely may pose substantial problems for health-care providers and interpreters in obtaining accurate health data, in turn increasing the difficulty of making accurate diagnoses.

> *What is your dominant language? Do you have difficulty understanding other dialects of your dominant language? Have you traveled abroad where you had difficulty understanding the dialect or accent? What other languages beside your dominant language do you speak?*

When speaking in a nonnative language, health-care providers must select words that have relatively pure meanings, be certain of the voice intonation, and avoid the use of regional slang and jargon to avoid being misunderstood. Minor variations in pronunciation may change the entire meaning of a word or a phrase and result in inappropriate interventions.

Given the difficulty of obtaining the precise meaning of words in a language, it is best for health-care providers to obtain someone who can interpret the meaning and message, not just translate the individual words. Remember, translation refers to the written word, and interpretation refers to the spoken word. Children should never be used as interpreters for their family members. Not only does it have a negative bearing on family dynamics, but sensitive information may not be transmitted. (See Chapter 3 for guidelines for using interpreters.)

Those with limited language ability may have inadequate vocabulary skills to communicate in situations in which strong or abstract levels of verbal skills are required, such as in the psychiatric setting. Helpful communication techniques with diverse patients include displaying tact, consideration, and respect; gaining trust by listening attentively; addressing the patient by preferred name; and showing genuine warmth and openness to facilitate full information sharing. When giving directions, be explicit. Give directions in sequential procedural steps (e.g., first, second, third). Do not use complex sentences with conjunctions or contractions.

> *Give some examples of problems communicating with patients who did not speak or understand English. What did you do to promote effective communication?*

Before trying to engage in more sensitive areas of the health interview, the health-care provider may need to start with social exchanges to establish trust if time permits, use an open-ended format rather than yes or no closed-response questions, elicit opinions and beliefs about health and symptom management, and focus on facts rather than feelings. An awareness of nonverbal behaviors is essential to establishing a mutually satisfying relationship.

The context within which a language is spoken is an important aspect of communication. Some languages are low in context, and most of the message is explicit, requiring many words to express a thought. Other languages are highly contextual, with most of the information either in the physical context or internalized, resulting in the use of fewer words with more emphasis on unspoken understandings.

Voice volume and tone are important paralanguage aspects of communication. A loud voice volume may be interpreted as reflecting anger, when in fact a loud voice is merely being used to express their thoughts in a dynamic manner. Thus, health-care providers must be cautious about voice volume and tones when interacting with diverse cultural groups so that their intentions are not misunderstood.

> *On a scale of 1 to 10, with 1 being low and 10 being high, where do you place yourself in the scale of high-contextual versus low-contextual communication? Do you tend to use a lot of words to express a thought? Do you know family members/friends/acquaintances who are your opposite in terms of low-contextual versus high-contextual communication? Does this sometimes cause concerns in communication? Do you think biomedical language is high or low context?*

Cultural Communication Patterns

Communication includes the willingness of individuals to share their thoughts and feelings. Some cultures encourage people to disclose very personal information about themselves, such as information about sex, drugs, and family problems. In some cultures, having well-developed verbal skills is seen as important, whereas in other cultures, the person who has very highly developed verbal skills is seen as having suspicious intentions. Some cultures willingly share their thoughts and feelings among family members and close friends, but they may not easily share thoughts, feelings, and health information with "outsiders" (i.e., health-care providers) until they get to know them. By engaging in small talk and inquiring about family members before addressing the patient's health concerns, health-care providers can help establish trust and, in turn, encourage more open communication and sharing of important health information.

▶ *How willing are you to share personal information about yourself? How does it differ with family, friends, or strangers? Do you tend to speak faster, slower, or about the same rate as the people around you? What happens when you meet someone who speaks much more rapidly or much more slowly than you do? Do you normally speak in a loud or low voice volume? How do you respond when someone speaks louder or softer than you do?*

Touch, a method of nonverbal communication, has substantial variations in meaning among cultures. For the most part, individualistic cultures are low-touch cultures, which have recently been reinforced by sexual harassment guidelines and policies. For many, even casual touching may be seen as a sexual overture and should be avoided whenever possible. People of the same sex (especially men) or opposite sex do not generally touch each other unless they are close friends. It is recognized that the low-touch individualistic culture has variations within the United States according to age and location. However, among most collectivist cultures, two people of the same gender can touch each other without it having a sexual connotation, although modesty remains important. Always explain the necessity and ask permission before touching a patient for a health examination. Being aware of individual practices regarding touch is essential for effective health assessments.

Personal space needs to be respected when working with multicultural patients and staff. Among more individualistic cultures, conversants tend to place at least 18 inches of space between themselves and the person with whom they are talking. Most collectivist cultures require less personal space when talking with each other (Hall, 1990). They are quite comfortable standing closer to each other than are people from individualistic cultures; in fact, they interpret physical proximity as a valued sign of emotional closeness. Patients who stand very close and stare during a conversation may offend some health-care practitioners. These patients may interpret health-care providers as being cold because they stand so far away, perhaps appearing as being standoffish. Thus, an understanding of personal space and distancing characteristics can enhance the quality of communication among individuals.

▶ *How comfortable are you with being touched on the arm or shoulder by friends? By people who know you well? Do you consider yourself to be a "person who touches frequently" or do you rarely touch friends? Can you think of groups in the clinical setting for whom therapeutic touch is not appropriate?*

Regardless of the class or social standing of the conversants, people from individualistic cultures are expected to maintain direct eye contact without staring. A person who does not maintain eye contact may be perceived as not listening, not being trustworthy, not caring, or being less than truthful. Among some traditional collectivist cultures, sustained eye contact can be seen as offensive; further, a person of lower social class or status is expected to avoid eye contact with superiors or those with a higher educational status. Thus, eye contact must be interpreted within its cultural context to optimize relationships and health assessments.

The use of gestures and facial expressions varies among cultures. Most Americans gesture moderately when conversing and smile easily as a sign of pleasantness or happiness, although one can smile as a sign of sarcasm. A lack of gesturing can mean that the person is too stiff, too formal, or too polite.

▶ *What are your spatial distancing practices? How close do you stand to family? Friends? Strangers? Does this distancing remain the same with the opposite gender? Do you maintain eye contact when speaking with people? Is it intense? Does it vary with the age or gender of the person with whom you are conversing? What does it mean when someone does not maintain eye contact with you? How do you feel in this situation?*

Preferred greetings and acceptable body language also vary among cultural groups. An expected practice for many cultures in business is to extend the right hand when greeting someone for the first time. More elaborate greeting rituals occur in Asian, Arab, and Latin American countries and are covered in individual chapters.

Although many people consider it impolite or offensive to point with one's finger, many do so and do not see it as impolite. In other cultures, beckoning is done by waving the fingers with the palm down, whereas extending the thumb, like thumbs-up, is considered a vulgar sign. Among some cultures, signaling for someone to come by using an upturned finger is a provocation, usually done to a dog. Among the Navajo, it is considered rude to point; rather, the Navajo shift their lips toward the desired direction.

▶ *Do you tend to use your hands a lot when speaking? Can people tell your emotional state by your facial expressions?*

Temporal Relationships

Temporal relationships—people's worldview in terms of past, present, and future orientation—vary among individuals and among cultural groups. Some cultures, usually highly individualistic ones, are future-oriented, and people are encouraged to sacrifice for today and work to save and invest in the future. The future is important in that people can influence it. Fatalism, the belief that powers greater than humans are in control, may be seen as negative; however, to many others, it is seen as a fact of life not to be judged. Other cultures are regarded as a past-oriented society, in which laying a proper foundation by providing historical background information can enhance communication. However, for people in many societies, temporality is balanced among past, present, and future in the sense of respecting the past, valuing and enjoying the present, and saving for the future.

Differences in temporal orientation can cause concern or misunderstanding among health-care providers. For example, in a future-oriented culture, a person is expected to delay purchase of nonessential items to afford prescription medications. However, in less future-oriented cultures, the person buys the nonessential item because it is readily available and defers purchasing the prescription medication. The attitude is, why not purchase it now; the prescription medication can be purchased later.

Most people from individualistic cultures see time as a highly valued resource and do not like to be delayed because it "wastes time." When visiting friends or meeting for strictly social engagements, punctuality is less important, but one is still expected to appear within a "reasonable" time frame. In the health-care setting, if an appointment is made for 9 a.m., the person is expected to be there at 8:45 a.m. so she or he is ready for the appointment and does not delay the health-care provider. For immigrants from rural settings, time may be even less important. These individuals may not even own a timepiece or be able to tell time. Expectations for punctuality can cause conflicts between health-care providers and patients, even if one is cognizant of these differences. These details must be carefully explained to individuals when such situations occur. Being late for appointments should not be misconstrued as a sign of irresponsibility or not valuing one's health.

▶ *How timely are you with professional appointments? With social engagements? What does it mean to you when people are chronically late? Can you give examples indicating that you are past oriented? Present oriented? Future oriented? Do you consider yourself more one than the other?*

Format for Names

Names are important to people, and name formats differ among cultures. The most common Western system is to have a first or given name, a middle name, and then the family surname. The person would usually write the name in that order. In formal situations, the person would be addressed with a title of Mr., Mrs., Ms., or Miss and the last name. Friends and acquaintances would call the person by the first name or perhaps a nickname. Married women may take their husband's last name, keep their maiden name, or use both their maiden and married names. However, in some cultures, the family or surname name comes first, followed by the given name and then the middle name. The person would usually write and introduce himself or herself in that order. Married women usually keep their maiden name. Other name formats are even more complex and may include a given name, a middle name, the father's family name, and the mother's maiden name. When a woman marries, she may keep all these names plus add the surname of her husband. She may choose any name she wants for legal purposes. When in doubt, the health-care provider needs to ask which name is used for legal purposes. Such extensive naming formats can create a challenge for health-care workers keeping a medical record when they are unaware of differences in ethnic recording of names. See individual chapters for name formats. Table 2-2 identifies guidelines for assessing the cultural domain communication.

▶ *How do you prefer to be addressed or greeted? Does this change with the situation? How do you normally address and greet people? Do your responses change with the situation?*

Family Roles and Organization

The cultural domain of family roles and organization affects all other domains and defines relationships among insiders and outsiders. This domain includes concepts related to the head of the household, gender roles, family goals and priorities, developmental tasks of children and adolescents, roles of the aged and extended family members, individual and family social status in the community, and acceptance of alternative lifestyles, such as single parenting, nontraditional sexual orientations, childless marriages, and divorce. Family structure in the context of the larger society determines acceptable roles, priorities, and the behavioral norms for its members.

Head of Household and Gender Roles

An awareness of family decision-making patterns (i.e., patriarchal, matriarchal, or egalitarian) is important for determining with whom to speak when health-care decisions have to be made. Among many cultures, it is acceptable for women to have a career and for men to assist with child care, household domestic chores, and cooking responsibilities. Both parents work in many families, necessitating placing children in child-care facilities. In some families, fathers are responsible for deciding when to seek health care for family members, but mothers may have significant influence on final decisions.

II▶ Table 2-2 | **Communication**

Suggested Question	Sample Rationale/Example
1. What is your full name?	Part of a standard assessment. Hispanics/Latinos have an extended name format that includes a first name, middle name, father's last name, and mother's last name, with an additional last name of the husband if a woman is married.
2. What is your legal name?	Complex naming can make it difficult for medical record keeping. Explain that the legal name is needed for accurate medical records.
3. By what name do you wish to be called?	Helps establish trust and increases comfort level of the patient.
4. What is your primary language?	Determining the preferred language for consent forms and discharge instructions.
5. Do you speak a specific dialect?	A dialect-specific interpreter is preferred.
6. What other languages do you speak?	Sometimes a second or third language may be helpful for interpretation if the preferred language interpreter is not available.
7. Do you find it difficult to share your thoughts, feelings, and ideas with family? Friends? Health-care providers?	Additional time may be needed to establish trust and get full disclosure, especially with sensitive topics.
8. Do you mind being touched by friends? Strangers? Health-care workers?	Asking permission and explaining the rationale before touching reinforces the trust relationship.
9. How do wish to be greeted? Handshake? Nod of the head, etc.?	Demonstrates respect and helps establish trust.
10. Are you usually on time for appointments?	Explain rationale for the expectation of timeliness: will not be seen and have to reschedule and may still be charged for the appointment.
11. Are you usually on time for social engagements?	Ask only if question is pertinent.
12. Observe the patient's speech pattern. Is the speech pattern high- or low-context?	Patients from high-context cultures place greater value on silence and implicit communication and may take more time to give a response.
13. Observe the patient when physical contact is made. Does he/she withdraw from the touch or become tense?	Being aware of the patient's level of comfort helps establish trust. Reinforce the necessity and ask permission before touching.
14. How close does the patient stand when talking with family members? With health-care providers?	Spatial distancing is culture bound. Do not take offense if a patient stands closer or farther away than what you are accustomed to.
15. Does the patient maintain eye contact when talking with the health-care provider?	Some avoid eye contact with people in hierarchal positions as a sign of respect. The health-care provider is in a hierarchal position.

Among many, the decisions may be egalitarian, but the male's role in the family is to be the spokesperson for the family. The health-care provider, when speaking with parents, should maintain eye contact and direct questions about a child's illness to both parents.

▶ *How would you classify the decision-making process in your family—patriarchal, matriarchal, or egalitarian? Does it vary by what decision has to be made? Are gender roles prescribed in your family? Who makes the decisions about health and health care?*

Prescriptive, Restrictive, and Taboo Behaviors for Children and Adolescents

Every society has prescriptive, restrictive, and taboo practices for children and adolescents. Prescriptive beliefs are things that children or teenagers *should do* to have harmony with the family and a good outcome in society. Restrictive practices are things that children and teenagers *should not do* to have a positive outcome. Taboo practices are those things that, if done, are likely to cause significant concern or negative outcomes for the child, teenager, family, or community at large.

For some Western cultures, a child's individual achievement is valued over the family's financial status. This is different from some non-Western cultures in which attachment to family may be *more important* than the need for children to excel individually. At younger ages, rather than having group toys, each child has his or her own toys and is taught to share them with others. Individualistic cultures encourage autonomy in children, and after completing homework assignments (with which parents are expected to help), children are expected to contribute to the family by doing chores, such as taking out the garbage, washing dishes, cleaning their own room, feeding and caring for pets, and helping with cooking. They are not expected to help with heavy labor at home, except in rural farm communities.

In Western cultures, children are allowed and encouraged to make their own choices, including managing their own allowance money and deciding who their friends might be—although parents may gently suggest one friend as a better choice than another. Children and teenagers are permitted and encouraged to have friends of both the same and opposite genders. They are expected to be well behaved, especially in public. They are taught to stand in line—first come, first served—and to wait their turn. As they reach the teenage years, they are expected to refrain from premarital sex, smoking, using recreational drugs, and drinking alcohol until they leave the home. However, this does not always occur, and teenage pregnancy and the use of recreational alcohol and drugs remain high. When children become teenagers, most are expected to get a job, such as babysitting, delivering newspapers, or doing yard work to make their own spending money, which they manage as a way of learning independence. The teenage years are also seen as a time of natural rebellion

In Western cultures, when young adults become 18 or complete their education, they usually move out of their parents' home (unless they are in college) and live independently or share living arrangements with nonfamily members. If the young adult chooses to remain in the parents' home, then she or he might be expected to pay rent. However, young adults are generally allowed to return home, as needed, for financial or other purposes. Individuals over the age of 18 are expected to be self-reliant and independent, which are virtues in the Western cultures.

This differs from most collectivist cultures in which children are expected to live at home with their parents until they marry because dependence, not independence, is the virtue.

Adolescents have their own subculture, with its own values, beliefs, and practices that may not be in harmony with those of their dominant culture. Being in harmony with peers and conforming to the prevalent choice of music, clothing, hairstyles, and adornment may be especially important to adolescents. Thus, role conflicts can become considerable sources of family strain in many more traditional families who may not agree with the values of individuality, independence, self-assertion, and egalitarian relationships. Many teens may experience a cultural dilemma with exposure outside the home and family

▶ *Were you taught to be independent and autonomous or dependent in your family? Was there more emphasis on the individual or on the group?*

Family Goals and Priorities

In most cultures, family goals and priorities are centered on raising and educating children. During this stage, young adults make a personal commitment to a spouse or significant other and seek satisfaction through productivity in career, family, and civic interests. In most societies, young adulthood is the time when individuals work on Erikson's developmental tasks of *intimacy versus isolation* and *generativity versus stagnation.*

Western cultures place a high value on children, and many laws have been enacted to protect children who are seen as the "future of the society." In most collectivist cultures, children are desirable and highly valued as a source of family strength, and family members are expected to care for one another more so than in Western cultures.

Collectivistic cultures have great reverence for the wisdom of older people, and families eagerly make space for them to live with extended families. Children are expected to care for elders when they are unable to care for themselves. A great embarrassment may occur to family members when they cannot take care of their older family members.

The concept of extended family membership varies among societies. The extended family is extremely important, especially in collectivist cultures, and health-care decisions are often postponed until the entire family is consulted. The extended family may include biological relatives and nonbiological members who are considered brothers, sisters, aunts, or uncles. In some cultures, the influence of grandparents in decision making is considered more important than that of the parents.

Individualistic cultures also place a high value on egalitarianism, nonhierarchical relationships, and equal treatment regardless of their race, color, religion, ethnicity, educational or economic status, sexual orientation, or country of origin. However, these beliefs are theoretical and not always seen in practice. For example, throughout the world, women usually have a lower status than men, especially when it comes to prestigious positions and salaries. Most top-level politicians and corporate executive officers are white men. Subtle classism does exist, as evidenced by comments referring to "working-class men and women." Many Western cultures are known for their informality and for treating everyone the same. They call people by their first names very soon after meeting them, whether in the workplace, in social situations, in classrooms, in restaurants, or in places of business. Some readily talk with waitstaff and store clerks and call them by their first names, considering this respectful behavior. Formality can be communicated by using the person's last (family) name and title such as Mr., Mrs., Miss, Ms., or Dr. To this end, achieved status is more important than ascribed status. What one has accumulated in material possessions, where one went to school, and one's job position and title are more important than one's family background and lineage. However, in some families ascribed status has equal importance to achieved status. Without a caste or class system, theoretically one can move readily from one socioeconomic position to another. To some, if formality is maintained, it may be seen as pompous or arrogant, and some even deride the person who is very formal. However, formality is a sign of respect in many other cultures.

> *What were prescriptive behaviors for you as a child? As a teenager? As a young adult? What were restrictive behaviors for you as a child? As a teenager? As a young adult? What were taboo behaviors for you as a child? As a teenager? As a young adult? How are elders regarded in your culture? In your family?*

Alternative Lifestyles

The traditional family is nuclear, with a married man and woman living together with one or more unmarried children. This concept of family is becoming a more varied community, including unmarried people, both women and men, living alone; single people of the same or different genders living together with or without children; single parents with children; and blended families consisting of two parents who have remarried, with children from their previous marriages and additional children from their current marriage.

However, in some cultures, the traditional family is extended, with parents, unmarried children, married children with their children, and grandparents all sharing the same living space or at least living in very close proximity.

The newest category of family, domestic partnerships, is sanctioned by many states in the United States and grants some of the rights of traditional married couples to unmarried heterosexual, homosexual, older people, and disabled couples who share the traditional bond of the family. Some states in the United States, as well as some countries, allow gay and lesbian couples to marry and adopt children.

Social attitudes toward homosexual activity vary widely, and homosexual behavior occurs in societies that deny its presence. Homosexual behavior carries a severe stigma in some societies. Discovering that one's son or daughter is homosexual is akin to a catastrophic event for some, whether it is a collectivistic or individualistic culture.

> *Do you consider your family nuclear or extended? How close are you to your extended family? How is status measured in your family? By money or by some other attribute? What are your personal views of two people of the same gender living together in a physical relationship? What about heterosexual couples? Does divorce cause a stigma in your culture? In your family?*

When the health-care provider needs to provide assistance and make a referral for a person who is gay, lesbian, bisexual, or transsexual, a number of options are available. Some referral agencies are local, whereas others are national, with local or regional chapters. Many are ethnically or religiously specific. See DavisPlus for the links to the local and regional offices of some national organizations. Table 2-3 identifies guidelines for assessing the cultural domain *family roles and organization.*

Workforce Issues
Culture in the Workplace

A fourth domain of culture is workforce issues. Differences and conflicts that exist in a homogeneous culture may be intensified in a multicultural workforce. Factors that affect these issues include language barriers, degree of assimilation and acculturation, and issues related to autonomy. Moreover, such concepts as gender roles, cultural communication styles, health-care practices of the country of origin, and selected concepts from all other domains affect workforce issues in a multicultural work environment.

Timeliness and punctuality are two culturally based attitudes that can create serious problems in the multicultural workforce. In most Western cultures, people are expected to be punctual on their job, with formal meetings, and with appointments. With social engagements, punctuality is not as important. However, in many cultures, punctuality is not stressed unless one is meeting with officials or it is required for transportation schedules, such as for trains or air travel. Timeliness for social engagements may not be taken seriously and may simply begin when most of the people arrive. The lack of adherence to meeting time demands in other countries is often in direct opposition to the Western concept and the ethic for punctuality.

> *How timely are you in reporting to work? Do you see people in the workforce who do not report to work on time? What problems does it cause if they are not on time? What would you do as a supervisor to encourage people to report to work on time?*

Clinical professionals trained in their home countries now occupy a significant share of technical and laboratory positions in health-care facilities in many counties throughout the world. Service

> *How important are technical skills and verbal skills in your work environment? Does your organization encourage more formal or more informal communication? Why? Do you believe that everything needs to be proven scientifically? Do you value a more direct or indirect style of communication?*

Ⅰ▷ Table 2-3 Family Roles and Organization

Suggested Question	Sample Rationale/Example
1. Who makes most of the decisions in your family?	If the decision maker is not accessed, no decision will be made and time will be wasted.
2. What types of decisions do(es) the female(s) in your family make?	In many traditional families, the female usually makes decision about the household and child care.
3. What types of decisions do(es) the male(s) in your family make?	In many traditional families, the male usually makes decisions about affairs outside the household, but not always.
4. What are the duties of the women in the family?	Determining the division of labor can become important when illness occurs.
5. What are the duties of the men in the family?	Determining the division of labor can become important when illness occurs.
6. What should children do to make a good impression for themselves and for the family?	A child's behavior in the Appalachian and Greek cultures can bring shame upon the family.
7. What should children **not** do to make a good impression for themselves and for the family?	Among traditional Koreans, children are expected to do well in school, or shame may come to the family.
8. What are children forbidden to do?	Among traditional Germans, taboo behaviors include talking back to elders and touching another person's possessions.
9. What should young adults do to make a good impression for themselves and for the family?	Among Somalis, young adults are expected to marry and assist older family members.
10. What should young adults **not** do to make a good impression for themselves and for the family?	Among traditional Mexican families, young adults should not dress in a provocative manner; otherwise, shame can come to them or their family.
11. What are adolescents forbidden to do?	A taboo behavior for young female adults in Haiti is engaging in sexual activity before marriage.
12. What are the priorities for your family?	For lower socioeconomic families, the priority may be having adequate food and shelter, with stress on the present.
13. What are the roles of older adults in your family? Are they sought for their advice?	Among traditional Turks, no decision is made until after seeking the advice of older adults.
14. Are there extended family members in your household? Who else lives in your household?	Most traditional Asian cultures live in extended family arrangements in their home country.
15. What are the roles of extended family members in this household?	Extended family members provide significant financial and social support and are important sources for child care.
16. What gives you and your family status?	Status for some is having material necessities.
17. Is it acceptable to you for people to have children out of wedlock?	Among traditional Arab families, shame may occur if a pregnancy occurs outside of marriage.
18. Is it acceptable to you for people to live together and not be married?	Among many Asian cultures, a man and woman living together without being married may cause them to be rejected by their family.
19. Are you accepting of gay, lesbian, or transgendered people?	Not all cultures and individuals are accepting of gay, lesbian, or gender reassignment populations.
20. What is your sexual preference/orientation?	Lesbians have more risk factors for breast cancer than heterosexual women.

employees, such as food preparation workers, nurse aides, orderlies, housekeepers, and janitors, represent the most culturally diverse component of hospital workforces. These unskilled and semiskilled positions are among the most attainable for new immigrants.

▶ *Does your workforce (class) reflect the ethnic and racial diversity of the community? Why? Why not? What might you do to increase this diversity?*

Issues Related to Autonomy

Cultural differences related to assertiveness influence how health-care providers view one another. In most Western individualistic cultures, professionals are expected to be assertive with other professionals for the benefit of the patient. However, in some collectivist and patriarchal societies, women, for example, may be unprepared for the level of sophistication and autonomy expected in individualistic cultures. Educational training for health-care providers varies significantly throughout the world.

Language ability in a new country may not meet the standards expected in the workforce, especially in the health-care environment and in positions where highly developed verbal skills are required. Thus, the newer immigrant—for whom the language of the host country is new—may need extra time in translating messages and formulating replies.

When individuals speak in their native language at work, it may become a source of contention for both patients and health-care providers. Most employees do not want to exclude or offend others, but it is easier to speak in their native language to articulate ideas, feelings, and humor among themselves. Negative interpretations of behaviors can be detrimental to working relationships in the health-care environment. Some foreign graduates, with limited aural language abilities, may need to have care instructions written or procedures demonstrated.

▶ *Does your profession encourage autonomy in the workforce? Does your current work (class) encourage autonomy and independence? Do you see any cultural or gender differences in autonomy? Do people speak different languages at work? What difficulty does this cause?*

Generational Differences in the Workforce

Not only is the workforce becoming more multicultural in most countries, but over the last decade, increased interest has been found in the professional literature regarding generational differences in the workforce. Most of the literature on generational differences describes the dominant culture of the United States, with little mention as to how these differences might coincide with the multiethnic workforce. However, these descriptions do not always "fit" the generalizations as well as they do for the dominant, nonethnic, nonimmigrant populations. Table 2-4 identifies guidelines for assessing the cultural domain *workforce issues.*

▶ *How many generations are in your work group (class)? Are their beliefs and practices similar to or different from what is reported in the literature? Do the generational differences cause conflict? Which generation takes the lead in resolving conflicts when they arise?*

Biocultural Ecology

The domain *biocultural ecology* identifies specific physical, biological, and physiological variations in ethnic and racial origins. These variations include skin color and physical differences in body habitus; genetic, hereditary, endemic, and topographic diseases; psychological makeup of individuals; and differences in

the way drugs are metabolized by the body. No attempt is made here to explain or justify any of the numerous, conflicting, and highly controversial views and research about racial variations in drug metabolism and genetics.

Skin Color and Other Biological Variations

Skin coloration is an important consideration for health-care providers because anemia, jaundice, and rashes require different assessment skills in dark-skinned people than in light-skinned people. To assess for oxygenation and cyanosis in dark-skinned people, the practitioner must examine the sclera, buccal mucosa, tongue, lips, nail beds, palms of the hands, and soles of the feet rather than relying on skin tone alone. Jaundice is more easily determined in Asians by assessing the sclera rather than relying on the overall change in skin color. Health-care providers must establish a baseline skin color (by asking a family member or someone known to the individual), use direct sunlight (if possible), observe areas with the least amount of pigmentation, palpate for rashes, and compare skin in corresponding areas. With people who are generally fair-skinned, prolonged exposure to the sun places them at an increased risk for skin cancer.

▶ *Do you have difficulty assessing rashes, bruises, and sunburn in people with a skin color different from yours? Do you have difficulty assessing jaundice and oxygenation in people with a skin color different from yours? How does your assessment of skin differ between patients with light versus dark skin? Do you take precautions and protect yourself against the sun? Why? Why not?*

Variations in body habits occur among ethnic and racially diverse individuals in terms of bone density, length of long bones, and shoulder and hip width, but do not usually cause a concern for health-care providers. However, bone density is greater in whites than in Asian and Pacific Islanders; osteoporosis is lowest in black males and highest in white females. Given diverse gene pools, this type of information is often difficult to obtain, and much of the research is inconclusive.

Diseases and Health Conditions

Some diseases are more prevalent and endemic in certain racial or ethnic groups, especially with migration. Specific health problems are covered in individual chapters in this book and in the Appendix. In general, many adverse health conditions are a result of genetics, lifestyle, and the environment. Genetic conditions occur among families in all races, but some conditions, such as Tay-Sachs disease, hemophilia, and cystic fibrosis, are more common among particular ethnic and racial groups.

ⅠⅠ▷ Table 2-4 Workforce Issues

Suggested Question	Sample Rationale/Example
1. Do you usually report to work on time?	Not all cultures espouse timeliness in reporting to work. If timeliness is important, this must be explicitly explained along with consequences.
2. Do you usually report to meetings on time?	If timeliness is important for attendance at meetings, this must be explicitly explained.
3. What concerns do you have about working with someone of the opposite gender?	Strict orthodox separation of the sexes may cause disharmony if men and women are expected to work in close proximity.
4. Do you consider yourself a "loyal" employee?	Among the Japanese, an employer may expect absolute loyalty, and employees remain with the same company their entire lives.
5. What do you do when you do not know how to do something related to your job?	Among many traditional Koreans, when an employee does not know how to do something, rather than admitting it, they may go to a co-worker of the same nationality (if available).
6. Do you consider yourself to be assertive in your job?	Traditional Asians are sometimes not seen as assertive as some American employers would like. Most professionals are assertive, but in a different way from assertiveness in individualistic cultures.
7. What difficulty does English (or another language) give you in the workforce?	Low verbal and written literacy may have implications for accuracy in fulfilling job requirements.

▷ *What are the most common illnesses and diseases in your family? In your community? What might you do to decrease the incidence of illness and diseases in your family? In your community?*

Lifestyle causes include cultural practices and behaviors that can generally be controlled—for example, smoking, diet, and stress. Environmental causes refer to factors (e.g., air and water pollution) and situations over which the individual has little or no control (e.g., presence of malarial or dengue mosquitoes, exposure to chemical and pesticides, access to care, and associated diseases).

▷ *Are you aware of any outbreaks of new illnesses or diseases in your community? In other parts of the world? How might these outbreaks have been prevented?*

Variations in Drug Metabolism

Information regarding drug metabolism among racial and ethnic groups has important implications for health-care providers when prescribing medications. Besides the effects of (1) smoking, which accelerates drug metabolism; (2) malnutrition, which affects drug response; (3) a high-fat diet, which increases absorption of antifungal medication, whereas a low-fat diet renders the drug less effective; (4) cultural attitudes and beliefs about taking medication; and (5) stress, which affects catecholamine and cortisol levels on drug metabolism, studies have identified some specific alterations in drug metabolism among diverse racial and ethnic groups. Information for specific groups is included in each chapter. Health-care providers need

to investigate the literature for ethnic-specific studies regarding variations in drug metabolism, communicate these findings to other colleagues, and educate their patients regarding these side effects. Medication administration is one area in which health-care providers see the importance of culture, ethnicity, and race. Table 2-5 identifies guidelines for assessing the cultural domain *biocultural ecology*.

▷ *Why is it important for health-care providers to be aware of variations in drug metabolism in the body? What conditions besides genetics have an influence on drug metabolism?*

High-Risk Behaviors

High-risk behaviors include use of tobacco, alcohol, or recreational drugs; lack of physical activity; increased calorie consumption; unsafe driving practices; failure to use seat belts and helmets; failure to take precautions against human immunodeficiency virus (HIV) and sexually transmitted infections (STIs); and high-risk recreational activities. High-risk behaviors occur in all ethnocultural groups, with the degree and types of high-risk behaviors varying.

Alcohol consumption crosses all cultural and socioeconomic groups. Enormous differences exist among ethnic and cultural groups around the use of and response to alcohol. Even in cultures in which alcohol consumption is taboo, it is not ignored. However, alcohol problems are not simply a result of how much people drink. When drinking is culturally approved, it is typically done more by men than women and is more often a social, rather than a solitary, act. The group in which drinking is most frequently practiced is usually composed of same-age social peers

II▶ Table 2-5   Biocultural Ecology

Suggested Question	Sample Rationale/Example
1. Are you allergic to any medications?	Part of a standard assessment.
2. What problems did you have when you took over-the-counter medications?	Part of a standard assessment. Ask about medicines purchased in or outside the United States because a variety that require a prescription in the United States can be purchased over the counter in other countries.
3. What are the major illnesses and diseases in your family?	Part of a standard assessment.
4. Are you aware of any genetic diseases in your family?	Middle Eastern as well as other populations have many hereditary and genetic illnesses.
5. What are the major health problems in the country from which you come (if appropriate)?	Certain diseases and illnesses have a higher incidence among some groups compared with other groups; for example, thalassemia are more common among people with Mediterranean ancestry.
6. With what race do you identify?	National agenda are addressing racial and ethnic disparities.
7. Observe skin coloration and physical characteristics.	To assess for rashes on people with dark skin, the health-care provider may need to palpate rather than rely on visual cues.
8. Observe for and ask about physical handicaps and disabilities.	Many people do not disclose handicaps or disabilities upon initial encounter unless specifically asked, especially learning disabilities.

(Peele & Brodsky, 2001). Studies on increasing controls on the availability of alcohol to decrease alcohol consumption, with the premise that alcohol-related problems occur in proportion to per capita consumption, have not been supported. Furthermore, countries with temperance movements have greater alcohol-related behavior problems than do countries without temperance movements (Purnell & Foster, 2003a; 2003b).

Countries in which drinking alcoholic beverages is integrated into rites and social customs, and in which one is expected to have self-control and sociability, have lower rates of alcohol-related problems than those of countries and cultures in which ambivalent attitudes toward drinking prevail (Purnell & Foster, 2003a; 2003b). Hilton's (1987) study demonstrated a clear and distinct difference in the alcohol abuse rate by socioeconomic status. The conclusion of many studies suggests that alcohol-related violence is a learned behavior, not an inevitable result of alcohol consumption (Purnell & Foster, 2003a; 2003b).

Health-Care Practices

Obesity and being overweight are a result of an imbalance between food consumed and physical activity. National data have shown an increase in the calorie consumption of adults and no change in physical activity patterns. However, obesity is a complex issue related to lifestyle, environment, and genes. Many underlying factors have been linked to the increase in obesity, such as increased portion sizes; eating out more often; increased consumption of sugar-sweetened drinks; increased television, computer, electronic gaming time; changing labor markets; and fear of crime, which prevents outdoor exercise.

The practice of self-care by using folk and magico-religious practices before seeking professional care may also have a negative impact on the health status of some individuals. Overreliance on these practices may mean that the health problem is in a more advanced stage when a consultation is sought. Such delays make treatment more difficult and prolonged. Selected complementary and alternative health-care practices are addressed in this chapter under the domain *healthcare practices* and in each culture-specific chapter.

The cultural domain of *high-risk behaviors* is one area in which health-care providers can make a significant impact on patients' health status. High-risk health behaviors can be controlled through ethnic-specific interventions aimed at health promotion and health-risk prevention. This can be accomplished through educational programs in schools, business organizations, churches, and recreational and community centers, as well as through one-on-one and family counseling techniques. Taking advantage of public communication technology can enhance participation in these programs if they are geared to the unique needs of the individual, family, or community. Table 2-6 identifies guidelines for assessing the cultural domain *high-risk behaviors*.

▶ *In which high-risk health behaviors do you engage? What do you do to control or reduce your risk? Which high-risk health behaviors do you see most frequently in your family? In your community? What might you do to help decrease these high-risk behaviors?*

Nutrition

The cultural domain of *nutrition* includes much more than merely having adequate food for satisfying hunger. This domain also comprises the meaning of

ⅡⅠ Table 2-6 **High-Risk Health Behaviors**

Suggested Question	Sample Rationale/Example
1. How many cigarettes a day do you smoke?	A smoking history is standard for any assessment. Because smoking carries a stigma among some, ask this question without a judgmental attitude.
2. Do you smoke a pipe (or cigars)?	Part of a smoking assessment.
3. Do you chew tobacco?	Chewing tobacco is a common practice in rural areas and increases the risk for oropharyngeal cancer.
4. How much alcohol do you drink each day? Ask about wine, beer, spirits, coffee, energy drinks.	Part of a standard assessment.
5. What recreational drugs do you use?	Recreational drug use is part of a standard assessment. In order for the patient to disclose this sensitive information, ask in a nonjudgmental manner.
6. Do you exercise each day? What type? How long?	Physical activity or lack thereof is part of a standard assessment for health promotion and wellness.
7. Do you use seat belts/helmets?	Part of a standard assessment.
8. What precautions do you take to prevent getting a sexually transmitted infection/HIV?	Part of a standard assessment and an opportunity to evaluate high-risk patients.

food to the culture; common foods and rituals; nutritional deficiencies and food limitations; and the use of food for health promotion and wellness, illness and disease prevention, and health maintenance and restoration. Understanding a patient's food choices and preparation practices is essential for providing culturally competent dietary counseling. Health-care providers may be considered professionally negligent when prescribing, for example, an American diet to a Hispanic or an Asian patient whose food choices and mealtimes may be different from American food patterns.

Meaning of Food

Food and the absence of food—hunger—have diverse meanings among cultures and individuals. Cultural beliefs, values, and the types of foods available influence what people eat, avoid, or alter to make food congruent with cultural lifeways, and food offers cultural security and acceptance. Food plays a significant role in socialization and can denote caring or lack of caring or closeness.

▶ *What are your personal beliefs about weight and health? Do you agree with the dominant American belief that thinness correlates with desirability and beauty? What does food mean in your culture besides satisfying hunger?*

Common Foods and Food Rituals

Traditional food habits are basic to satisfactory nutrition to most people. Perhaps a traditional diet does not really exist for some people; rather, they have favorite foods and preparation practices that health-care providers need to assess for effective dietary

recommendations for health illness and disease prevention and health promotion and wellness. Most immigrants bring their favorite foods with them when they relocate, including preferred mealtimes. Food choices may vary according to the region of the country, urban versus rural residence, and weekdays versus weekends. In addition, food choices vary by marital status, economic status, climate changes, religion, ancestry, availability, and personal preferences.

Specific food pyramids have been developed by several organizations and are available for Vietnamese, African American, Chinese, Cuban, Puerto Rican, Navajo, Jewish, and Asian Indians, to name a few. They are included in culture-specific chapters and can also be found on the Internet by going to a search engine and typing in "multicultural food pyramid." Several ethnic food pyramids are also on Davis*Plus*.

Many older people and people living alone, regardless of cultural background, do not eat balanced meals. They state that they do not take the time to prepare a meal, even though most American homes have labor-saving devices, such as stoves, microwave ovens, refrigerators, and dishwashers. For those who are unable to prepare their own meals because of disability or illness, most communities have a Meals on Wheels program through which community and church organizations deliver, usually once a day, a hot meal along with a cold meal for later and food for the following morning's breakfast. Socioeconomic status may dictate food selections—for example, hamburger instead of steak, canned or frozen vegetables and fruit rather than fresh produce, and fish instead of shrimp or lobster. Special occasions and holidays are frequently associated with ethnic-specific foods. Many religious groups are required to fast during specific holiday seasons. However, health-care providers may need to remind patients that fasting is not required during times of illness or pregnancy.

Given the intraethnic variations of diet, it is important for health professionals to inquire about the specific diets of their patients. Expecting the patient to eat according to an American mealtime schedule and to select American foods from an exchange list may be unrealistic for patients of different cultural backgrounds. Counseling about food-group requirements, intake restrictions, and exercise must respect cultural behaviors and individual lifeways. Culturally congruent dietary counseling, such as changing amounts and preparation practices while including preferred ethnic food choices, can reduce the risk for obesity, cardiovascular disease, and cancer. Whenever possible, determining a patient's dietary practices should be started during the intake interview.

▶ *In what food rituals does your family engage? Do you have specific foods and rituals for holidays? What would happen if you changed these rituals? Do food patterns change for you by the season? During the week versus the weekend?*

Dietary Practices for Health Promotion

The nutritional balance of a diet is recognized by most cultures throughout the world. Most cultures have their own distinct theories of nutritional practices for health promotion and wellness, illness and disease prevention, and health maintenance and restoration. Common folk practices and selected diets are recommended during periods of illness and for prevention of illness or disease. For example, cultures subscribe to the hot-and-cold (opposites) theory of food selection to prevent illness and maintain health. Although each of these cultural groups has its own specific name for the hot-and-cold theory of foods, the overall belief is that the body needs a balance of opposing foods. These practices are covered in culture-specific chapters.

▶ *What do you eat to maintain your health? What does a healthy diet mean to you? Do you agree with the U.S. Department of Agriculture Food Pyramid? Why? Why not? What do you eat when you are ill?*

Nutritional Deficiencies and Food Limitations

Because of limited socioeconomic resources or limited availability of their native foods, immigrants may eat foods that were not available in their home country. These dietary changes may result in health problems when they arrive in a new environment. This is more likely to occur when individuals immigrate to a country where they do not have native foods readily available and do not know which new foods contain the necessary and comparable nutritional ingredients.

Consequently, they do not know which foods to select for balancing their diet.

Enzyme deficiencies exist among some ethnic and racial groups. For example, many people are lactose-intolerant and are unable to drink milk or eat dairy products to maintain their calcium needs. Thus, the health-care provider may need to assist patients and their families in identifying foods high in calcium when they are unable to purchase their native foods. In general, the wide availability of foods in the United States reduces the risks of these disorders as long as people have the means to obtain culturally nutritious foods. Recent emphasis on cultural foods has resulted in larger grocery stores having sections designated for ethnic goods and in small businesses selling ethnic foods and spices to the general public. The health-care provider's task is to determine how to assist the patient and identify alternative foods to supplement the diet when these stores are not financially or geographically accessible. Table 2-7 identifies guidelines for assessing the cultural domain *nutrition*.

▶ *What enzyme deficiencies run in your family? Do you have any difficulty getting your preferred foods? What other food limitations do you have?*

Pregnancy and Childbearing Practices

The cultural domain *pregnancy and childbearing practices* includes culturally sanctioned and unsanctioned fertility practices; views toward pregnancy; and prescriptive, restrictive, and taboo practices related to pregnancy, birthing, and the postpartum period.

Many traditional, folk, and magico-religious beliefs surround fertility control, pregnancy, childbearing, and postpartum practices. The reason may be the mystique that surrounds the processes of conception, pregnancy, and birthing. Ideas about conception, pregnancy, and childbearing practices are handed down from generation to generation and are accepted without validation or being completely understood. For some, the success of modern technology in inducing pregnancy in postmenopausal women and others who desire children through in vitro fertilization and the ability to select a child's gender raises serious ethical questions about parenting.

Fertility Practices and Views Toward Pregnancy

Commonly used methods of fertility control include natural ovulation methods, birth control pills, foams, Norplant, the morning-after pill, intrauterine devices, tubal ligation or sterilization, vasectomy, prophylactics, and abortion. Although not all of these methods are acceptable to all people, many women use a combination of fertility control methods. The most extreme examples of fertility control are sterilization and

Table 2-7 Nutrition

Suggested Question	Sample Rationale/Example
1. Are you satisfied with your weight?	Not all cultures adhere to or believe in the U.S. weight recommendations.
2. Which foods do you eat to maintain your health?	Food choices are seen as a means for promoting health.
3. Which foods do you avoid to maintain your health?	Each culture has certain foods people avoid for maintaining their health.
4. Do you avoid specific foods? Why do you avoid these foods?	Kosher Jews do not eat pork.
5. Which foods do you eat when you are ill?	Common foods eaten when ill among many cultures include toast and tea or ginger ale when ill.
6. Which foods do you avoid when you are ill?	If the health-care provider recommends a food that the person culturally or personally avoids, it may not be followed.
7. Why do you avoid these foods (if appropriate)?	This is usually a culturally learned practice.
8. For what illnesses do you eat certain foods?	People drink a "hot toddy" for a cold or minor illness. The ingredients vary, but generally include tea, lemon or lime, sugar or honey, and some type of alcohol, such as whiskey or rum.
9. Which foods do you eat to balance your diet?	Many cultures adhere to specific foods for balancing a diet; frequently related to opposite qualities of food such as the hot-and-cold theories.
10. Which foods do you eat every day?	Incorporating these foods into dietary prescriptions will increase compliance with dietary instructions.
11. Which foods do you eat every week?	Incorporating these foods into dietary prescriptions will increase compliance with dietary instructions.
12. Which foods do you eat that are part of your cultural heritage?	Including culturally preferred foods into nutritional recommendations increases compliance.
13. Which foods are high-status foods in your family/culture?	High-status foods vary according to cost and availability.
14. Which foods are eaten only by men? Women? Children? Teenagers? Older people?	Among some Guatemalan highland indigenous populations, men primarily eat eggs for the added protein value. The belief is that because men do heavy labor, they need more protein. However, they are supposed to share the protein foods on their plates with children.
15. How many meals do you eat each day?	Many Turks eat 4 to 6 times a day, but in smaller amounts than most European Americans do.
16. What time do you eat each meal?	May have implications for medication administration.
17. Do you snack between meals?	Snacks can be a significant source of added calories.
18. What foods do you eat when you snack?	Many snacks are not considered healthy food choices.
19. What holidays do you celebrate?	Holidays are a time for special meals and a time when many people overconsume calories.
20. Who usually buys the food in your household?	Many times it is just as important to talk with the person who purchases the food as it is with the person who prepares the meals. In migrant worker camps, the person who prepares the meals is not the person who purchases food for the group. If one member of the group needs a special diet, such as with a diabetic, the purchaser of the food needs to be included in nutritional education.
21. Who does the cooking in your household?	The person who does the cooking should be included in dietary counseling and education for special diets.
22. Do you have a refrigerator?	For the homeless and those in severe poverty, proper food storage must be taken into consideration.
23. How do you cook your food?	Preparation practices with butter, lard, etc., can add significant calories to meals.
24. How do you prepare meat?	Preparation practices can add significant calories.
25. How do you prepare vegetables?	Preparation practices add significant calories to meals, such as adding butter or bacon fat to vegetables.
26. What do you drink with your meals?	Beverages can add significant calories to meals. Be sure to ask if sugar is added to beverages, including natural juices.
27. Do you drink special teas?	Teas are used by many people for health promotion and wellness and in times of illness.
28. Do you have any food allergies/intolerances?	Many American Indians and Asians have lactose intolerance.
29. Are there certain foods that cause you problems when you eat them?	Looking for allergies or side effects of specific foods to avoid in dietary counseling.
30. How does your diet change with each season?	For those who live in colder climates, fresh fruits and vegetables may be too expensive in the colder months.

abortion. Sterilization in the United States is now strictly voluntary; however, some countries still perform involuntary sterilization to control birth rates and to control conception in people with mental retardation or deformities. Abortion remains a controversial issue in many countries and religions. For example, in some countries, women are encouraged to have as many children as possible, and abortion is illegal. However, in other countries, abortion is commonly used as a means of limiting family size for a variety of reasons. The "morning-after pill" also continues to be controversial to some.

Fertility practices and sexual activity, sensitive topics for many, is one area in which "outside" health-care providers may be more effective than health-care providers known to the patient because of the concern about providing intimate information to someone they know. Some of the ways health-care providers can promote a better understanding of practices related to family planning include using videos in the native language and videos and pictures of native ethnic people, using material written at the individual's level of education, and providing written instructions in both English and the native language. Health-care providers should avoid family planning discussions on the first encounter; such information may be better received on subsequent visits when some trust has developed. Approaching the subject of family planning obliquely may make it possible to discuss these topics more successfully.

> ▶ *Does pregnancy have a special meaning in your culture? Is fertility control acceptable in your culture? Do most people adhere to fertility control practices in your culture? What types of fertility control are acceptable? Unacceptable?*

Prescriptive, Restrictive, and Taboo Practices in the Childbearing Family

Most societies have prescriptive, restrictive, and taboo beliefs for maternal behaviors and the delivery of a healthy baby. Such beliefs affect sexual and lifestyle behaviors during pregnancy, birthing, and the immediate postpartum period. Prescriptive practices are things that the mother should do to have a good outcome (healthy baby and pregnancy). Restrictive practices are those things that the mother should not do to have a positive outcome (healthy baby and delivery). Taboo practices are those things that, if done, are likely to harm the baby or mother.

One prescriptive belief is that women are expected to seek preventive care, eat a well-balanced diet, and get adequate rest to have a healthy pregnancy and baby. A restrictive belief is that pregnant women should refrain from being around loud noises for prolonged periods of time. Taboo behaviors during pregnancy include smoking, drinking alcohol, drinking large amounts of caffeine, and taking recreational drugs—practices that are sure to cause harm to the mother or baby.

A taboo belief common among many cultures is that a pregnant woman should not reach over her head because the baby may be born with the umbilical cord around its neck. A restrictive belief among others is that permitting the father to be present in the delivery room and seeing the mother or baby before they have been cleaned can cause harm to the baby or mother. If the father is absent from the delivery room or does not want to see the mother or baby immediately after birth, it does not mean that he does not care about them. However, in many cultures, the father is often encouraged to take prenatal classes with the expectant mother and provide a supportive role in the delivery process; fathers with opposing beliefs may feel guilty if they do not comply. The woman's female relatives provide assistance to the new mother until she is able to care for herself and the baby. Additional cultural beliefs carried over from cultural migration and American diversity include the following:

- If you wear an opal ring during pregnancy, it will harm the baby.
- Birthmarks are caused by eating strawberries or seeing a snake and being frightened.
- Congenital anomalies can occur if the mother sees or experiences a tragedy during her pregnancy.
- Nursing mothers should eat a bland diet to avoid upsetting the baby.
- The infant should wear a band around the abdomen to prevent the umbilicus from protruding and becoming herniated.
- A coin, key, or other metal object should be put on the umbilicus to flatten it.
- Cutting a baby's hair before baptism can cause blindness.
- Raising your hands over your head while pregnant may cause the cord to wrap around the baby's neck.
- Moving heavy items can cause your "insides" to fall out.
- If the baby is physically or mentally abnormal, God is punishing the parents.

In some other cultures, the postpartum woman is prescribed a prolonged period of recuperation in the hospital or at home, something that may not be feasible in the United States because of the shortened length of confinement in the hospital after delivery.

The health-care provider must respect cultural beliefs associated with pregnancy and the birthing process when making decisions related to the health care of pregnant women, especially those practices that do not cause harm to the mother or baby. Most cultural practices can be integrated into preventive teaching in a manner that promotes compliance.

Table 2-8 identifies guidelines for assessing the cultural domain *pregnancy and childbearing practices*.

> ▶ *What are some prescriptive practices for pregnant women in your culture? What are some restrictive practices for pregnant women in your culture? What are some taboo practices for pregnant women in your culture? What special foods should a woman eat to have a healthy baby in your culture? What foods should be avoided? What foods should a nursing mother eat postpartum? What foods should she avoid?*

Death Rituals

The cultural domain *death rituals* includes how the individual and the society view death and euthanasia, rituals to prepare for death, burial practices, and bereavement. Death rituals of ethnic and cultural groups are the least likely to change over time and may cause concerns among health-care personnel. Some staff may not understand the value of customs with which they are not familiar, such as the ritual washing of the body. Death practices, beliefs, and rituals vary significantly among cultural and religious groups. To avoid

▶ Table 2-8 Pregnancy and Childbearing Practices

Suggested Question	Sample Rationale/Example
1. How many children do you have?	Part of a standard assessment.
2. Have you ever had an abortion? Stillbirth? Miscarriage?	Part of a standard OB/GYN assessment.
3. What do you use for birth control?	Each cultural and religious group has acceptable and unacceptable methods of birth control.
4. What does it mean to you and your family when you are pregnant?	In some cultures, a woman is not a true woman and has not reached her potential until she becomes pregnant.
5. What special foods do you eat when you are pregnant?	Although there are no specifically prescribed foods for a pregnant Polish woman, she is expected to eat for two.
6. What foods do you avoid when you are pregnant?	Chinese women are reluctant to take iron because they believe it will make delivery more difficult.
7. What activities do you avoid when you are pregnant?	A belief among many traditional Panamanians is that a pregnant woman should not walk in the moonlight for fear the baby will be born with a cleft lip or palate.
8. Do you do anything special when you are pregnant?	Korean women are expected to work hard during pregnancy to help ensure having a smaller baby.
9. Do you eat nonfood substances when you are pregnant?	Eating nonfood substances, pica, is common among many cultural groups. One example is clay, which can interfere with iron absorption.
10. Who do you want with you when you deliver your baby?	Some women prefer their mothers or another female family member rather than their husbands.
11. In what position do you want to be when you deliver your baby?	Traditional Indian women in Guatemala prefer to deliver in a squatting position rather than in the supine position. Negotiating for the position during delivery may be necessary in some organizations.
12. What special foods do you eat after delivery?	Hindu women are restricted to liquids, rice, gruel, and bread.
13. What foods do you avoid after delivery?	Guatemalan women avoid eating spicy foods because the milk will cause irritability in the baby.
14. What activities do you avoid after you deliver?	Russian women should do no strenuous activity after delivery to prevent any complications.
15. Do you do anything special after delivery?	Traditional Japanese women should not wash their hair for several days postpartum
16. Who will help you with the baby after delivery?	Looking for home support for the mother.
17. What bathing restrictions do you have after you deliver?	Many Egyptian women may be reluctant to bathe postpartum because air may get into the mother and cause illness. However, a sponge bath is acceptable.
18. Do you want to keep the placenta?	Some American Indians bury the placenta outside their home to keep away evil spirits.
19. What do you do to care for the baby's umbilical cord?	A common practice among Mayans is to place a coin or metal object, held on with an abdominal binder, to prevent the umbilicus from protruding when the baby cries.

cultural taboos, health-care providers must become knowledgeable about unique practices related to death, dying, and bereavement.

Death Rituals and Expectations

For many health-care providers educated in a culture of mastery over the environment, death is seen as one more disease to conquer, and when this does not happen, death becomes a personal failure. Thus, for many, death does not take a natural course because it is "managed" or "prolonged," making it difficult for some to die with dignity. Moreover, death and responses to death are not easy topics for many to verbalize. Instead, many euphemisms are used rather than verbalizing that the person died—for example, "passed away," "no longer with us," and "was visited by the Grim Reaper." The individualistic cultural belief in self-determination and autonomy extends to people making their own decisions about end-of-life care. Mentally competent adults have the right to refuse or decide what medical treatment and interventions they wish to extend life, such as artificial life support and artificial feeding and hydration.

> ▶ *What terms do you use when referring to death? Why do you use these terms? What specific burial practices do you have in your family/culture?*

Among most Westerners, the belief is that a dying person should not be left alone, and accommodations are usually made for a family member to be with the dying person at all times. Health-care personnel are expected to care for the family as much as for the patient during this time. Most people are buried or cremated within 3 days of the death, but extenuating circumstances may lengthen this period to accommodate family and friends who must travel a long distance to attend a funeral or memorial service. The family can decide whether to have an open casket—so family and friends can view the deceased—or a closed casket. Significant variations in burial practices occur with other ethnocultural groups throughout the world.

Responses to Death and Grief

Numerous countries have been launching major initiatives to help patients die as comfortably as possible without pain. As a result, more people are choosing to remain at home or to enter a hospice for end-of-life care where their comfort needs are better met. When death does occur, some people conservatively control their grief, although women are usually more expressive than men. For many, especially men, they are expected to be stoic in their reactions to death, at least in public. Generally, tears are shed, but loud wailing and uncontrollable sobbing rarely occur. The belief is that the person has moved on to a better existence and

does not have to undergo the pressures of life on earth. Regardless of the gender or culture, bereavement is a very private issue, and there are no norms; people grieve in their own way.

Variations in the grieving process may cause confusion for health-care providers, who may perceive some patients as overreacting and others as not caring. The behaviors associated with the grieving process must be placed in the context of the specific ethnocultural belief system in order to provide culturally competent care. Caregivers should accept and encourage ethnically specific bereavement practices when providing support to family and friends. Bereavement support strategies include being physically present, encouraging a reality orientation, openly acknowledging the family's right to grieve, accepting varied behavioral responses to grief, acknowledging the patient's pain, assisting them to express their feelings, encouraging interpersonal relationships, promoting interest in a new life, and making referrals to other resources, such as a priest, minister, rabbi, or pastoral care. Table 2-9 identifies guidelines for assessing the cultural domain *death rituals*.

> ▶ *How do men grieve in your culture? How do women grieve in your culture? Do you have a living will or advance directive? Why? Why not? Are you an organ donor? Why? Why not? Is there a specific time frame for bereavement?*

Spirituality

The domain *spirituality* involves more than formal religious beliefs related to faith and affiliation and the use of prayer. For some people, religion has a strong influence over and shapes nutrition practices, health-care practices, and other cultural domains. Spirituality includes all behaviors that give meaning to life and provide strength to the individual. Furthermore, it is difficult to distinguish religious beliefs from cultural beliefs because for some, especially the very devout, religion guides the dominant beliefs, values, and practices even more than their culture does.

Spirituality, a component of health related to the essence of life, is a vital human experience that is shared by all humans. Spirituality helps provide balance among the mind, body, and spirit. Trained and traditional religious leaders provide comfort to both the patient and the family. Spirituality does not have to be scientifically proven and is patterned unconsciously from a person's worldview. Accordingly, people may deviate somewhat from the majority view or position of their formally recognized religion.

Dominant Religion and Use of Prayer

Of the major religions in the world, 33 percent of people are Christians (17 percent are Roman

IID Table 2-9   Death Rituals

Suggested Question	Sample Rationale/Example
1. What special activities need to be performed to prepare for death?	When death is impending, Muslims want the bed to face toward Mecca.
2. Would you want to know about your impending death?	A belief among traditional Somalis is that a person might give up hope if impending death is made known.
3. What is your preferred burial practice? Interment, cremation?	Patient's wishes should be granted.
4. How soon after death does burial occur?	For traditional Jews, burial is before sundown the next day.
5. How do men grieve in your culture?	In some cultures, men are expected to be stoical and maintain control of their emotions. Expressions of grief have a wide variation.
6. How do women grieve in your culture?	In some cultures, women are expected to be histrionic with their grief to demonstrate their care for the deceased loved one. Expressions of grief have a wide variation.
7. What does death mean to you?	Among Hindus, death means rebirth.
8. Do you believe in an afterlife?	Many Christians believe that there is a better life after death.
9. Are children included in death rituals?	The Amish include children in all aspects of dying and burial.

Catholic); 16 percent are Muslim; 13 percent are Hindu; 6 percent are Buddhists; 12 percent are non-religious; and over 2 percent are atheist (*CIA World Factbook*, 2011).

Many people migrate for religious freedom. Furthermore, specific religious groups are concentrated regionally within a country. Unlike in many countries that support a specific church or religion and in which people discuss their religion frequently and openly, religion is not an everyday topic of conversation for most Americans. The health-care provider who is aware of the patient's religious practices and spiritual needs is in a better position to promote culturally competent health care. The health-care provider must demonstrate an appreciation of and respect for the dignity and spiritual beliefs of patients by avoiding negative comments about religious beliefs and practices. Patients may find considerable comfort in speaking with religious leaders in times of crisis and serious illness.

Prayer takes different forms and different meanings. Some people pray daily and may have altars in their homes. Others may consider themselves devoutly religious and say prayers only on special occasions or in times of crisis or illness. Health-care providers may need to make special arrangements for individuals to say prayers in accordance with their belief systems.

▶ *With what religion do you identify? Do you consider yourself devout? Do you need anything special to pray? When do you pray? Do you pray for good health? How do religiosity and spirituality differ for you? What gives meaning to your life? How are spirituality, religiosity, and health connected for you?*

Meaning of Life and Individual Sources of Strength

What gives meaning to life varies among and within cultural groups and among individuals. To some people, their formal religion may be the most important facet of fulfilling their spirituality needs, whereas for others, religion may be replaced as a driving force by other life forces and worldviews. Among other people, family is the most important social entity and is extremely important in helping meet their spiritual needs. For others, what gives meaning to life is good health and well-being. For a few, spirituality may include work or money.

A person's inner strength comes from different sources. For some, inner self is dependent on being in harmony with one's surroundings, whereas for others, a belief in a supreme being may give personal strength. For most people, spirituality includes a combination of these factors. Knowing these beliefs allows health-care providers to assist individuals and families in their quest for strength and self-fulfillment.

Spiritual Beliefs and Health-Care Practices

Spiritual wellness brings fulfillment from a lifestyle of purposeful and pleasurable living that embraces free choices, meaning in life, satisfaction in life, and self-esteem. For some, ritual dancing and herbal treatments (combined with prayers and songs) are performed for total body healing and the return of spirits to the body. Practices that interfere with a person's spiritual life can hinder physical recovery and promote physical illness.

Health-care providers should inquire whether the person wants to see a member of the clergy even if she or he has not been active in church. Religious emblems should not be removed because they provide solace to the person, and removing them may increase or cause anxiety. A thorough assessment of spiritual life is essential for the identification of solutions and resources that can support other treatments. Table 2-10 identifies guidelines for assessing the cultural domain *spirituality*.

Health-Care Practices

Another domain of culture is *health-care practices*. The focus of health care includes traditional, magico-religious, and biomedical beliefs; individual responsibility for health; self-medicating practices; and views toward mental illness, chronicity, rehabilitation, and organ donation and transplantation. In addition, responses to pain and the sick role are shaped by specific ethnocultural beliefs. Significant barriers to health care may be shared among cultural and ethnic groups.

Health-Seeking Beliefs and Behaviors

For centuries, people's health has been maintained by a wide variety of healing and medical practices. Currently, most of the world is undergoing a paradigm shift from one that places high value on curative and restorative medical practices with sophisticated technological care to one of health promotion and wellness; illness, disease, and injury prevention; health maintenance and restoration; and increased personal responsibility. Most believe that the individual, the family, and the community have the ability to influence their health. However, among other populations, good health may be seen as a divine gift from a superior being, with individuals having little control over health and illness.

Table 2-10	**Spirituality**
Suggested Question	Sample Rationale/Example
1. What is your religion?	Part of a standard assessment.
2. Do you consider yourself deeply religious?	Religion may have more influence than the culture.
3. How many times a day do you pray?	Islam requires prayer five times a day.
4. What do you need to say your prayers?	If possible, Muslims need a prayer rug.
5. Do you meditate?	Meditation can be used for relaxation and for pain control.
6. What gives strength and meaning to your life?	For some, the most important thing in their life is family.
7. In what spiritual practices do you engage for your physical and emotional health?	Prayer, meditation, yoga, and quiet time are some examples.

The primacy of patient autonomy is generally accepted as an enlightened perspective in individualistic cultures. To this end, advance directives, such as "durable power of attorney" or a "living will" are an important part of medical care. Accordingly, patients can specify their wishes concerning life and death decisions before entering an inpatient facility. The durable power of attorney for health care allows the patient to name a family member or significant other to speak for the patient and make decisions when or if the patient is unable to do so. The patient can also have a living will that outlines the person's wishes in terms of life-sustaining procedures in the event of a terminal illness. Most inpatient facilities have forms that patients may sign, or they can elect to bring their own forms, many of which are available on the Internet. Most countries and cultural groups engage in preventive immunization for children. Guidelines for immunizations were developed largely as a result of the influence of the World Health Organization (WHO). Specific immunization schedules and the ages at which they are prescribed vary widely among countries and can be obtained from the WHO website (see DavisPlus). However, some religious groups, such as Christian Scientists, do not believe in immunizations. Beliefs like this, which restrict optimal child health, have resulted in court battles with various outcomes.

Responsibility for Health Care

The world is moving to a paradigm in which people take increased responsibility for their health. In a society in which individualism is valued, people are expected to be self-reliant. In fact, people are expected to exercise some control over disease, including controlling the amount of stress in their lives. If someone does not maintain a healthy lifestyle and then gets sick, some believe it is the person's own fault. Unless someone is very ill, she or he should not neglect social and work obligations.

The health-care delivery system of the country of origin and degree of individualism and collectivism may shape patients' beliefs regarding personal responsibility for health care. Most countries in the world have some kind of basic universal coverage for their citizens, although access and quality may vary significantly from rural and urban settings and for vulnerable populations.

▶ *What do you do to take responsibility for your health? Do you take vaccines yearly to prevent the flu or other illnesses? Do you have adequate health insurance? Do you have regular checkups with your health-care provider?*

A potential high-risk behavior in the self-care context includes self-medicating practices. Self-medicating behavior in itself may not be harmful, but when combined with or used to the exclusion of prescription medications, it may be detrimental to the person's health. A common practice with prescription medications is for people to take medicine until the symptoms disappear and then discontinue the medicine prematurely. This practice commonly occurs with antihypertensive medications and antibiotics. No culture is immune to self-medicating practices; almost everyone engages in it to some extent.

Each country has some type of control over the purchase and use of medications. The United States is more restrictive than many countries and provides warning labels and directions for the use of over-the-counter medications. In many countries, pharmacists may be consulted before physicians for fever-reducing and pain-reducing medicines. In parts of Central America, a person can purchase antibiotics, intravenous fluids, and a variety of medications over the counter; most stores sell medications, and vendors sell drugs in street-corner shops and on public transportation systems. People who are accustomed to purchasing medications over the counter in their native country frequently see no problem in sharing their medications with family and friends. To help prevent contradictory or exacerbated effects of prescription medications and treatment regimens, health-care providers should ask about patients' self-medicating practices. One cannot ignore the ample supply of over-the-counter medications in pharmacies worldwide, the numerous television advertisements for self-medication, and media campaigns for new medications, encouraging viewers to ask their doctor or health-care provider about a particular medication.

▶ *In what self-medicating practices do you engage? What makes you decide when to see your health-care provider when you have an illness?*

Folk and Traditional Practices

Some societies and individuals favor traditional, folk, or magico-religious health-care practices over biomedical practices and use some or all of them simultaneously. For many, what are considered alternative or complementary health-care practices in one country may be mainstream medicine in another society or culture. In the United States, interest has increased in alternative and complementary health practices. The U.S. government has a National Center for Complementary and Alternative Medicine at the National Institutes of Health that has awarded millions of dollars in grants to bridge the gap between traditional and nontraditional therapies.

▶ *In the context of Western medicine, in what complementary and alternative practices have you practiced? For what conditions have you used them? Were they helpful? How willingly do you accept other people's traditional practices?*

As an adjunct to biomedical treatments, many people use acupuncture, acupressure, acumassage, herbal therapies, and other traditional treatments. Some cultural groups and individuals commonly visit traditional healers because modern medicine is viewed as inadequate. Examples of folk medicines include covering a boil with axle grease, wearing copper bracelets for arthritis pain, swallowing wild turnip root and honey for a sore throat, and drinking herbal teas. The Chinese subscribe to the yin-and-yang theory of treating illnesses, and Hispanic groups believe in the hot-and-cold theory of foods for treating illnesses and disease. Traditional schools of pharmacy in many countries sell folk remedies. Most people practice folk medicine in some form; they may use family remedies passed down from previous generations.

An awareness of combined practices when treating or providing health education to individuals and families helps ensure that therapies do not contradict one another, intensify the treatment regimen, or cause an overdose. At other times, they may be harmful, conflict with, or potentiate the effects of prescription medications. Many times, these traditional, folk, and magico-religious practices are and should be incorporated into the plans of care for patients. Inquiring about the full range of therapies being used, such as food items, teas, herbal remedies, nonfood substances, over-the-counter medications, and medications prescribed or loaned by others, is essential so that conflicting treatment modalities are not used. If patients perceive that the health-care provider does not accept their beliefs, they may be less compliant with prescriptive treatment and less likely to reveal their use of these practices.

Barriers to Health Care

For people to receive adequate health care, a number of considerations must be addressed. Several studies in the United States have identified that a lack of fluency in language is the primary barrier to receiving adequate health care in the United States (Institute of Medicine, 2001; Joint Commission, 2010a; 2010b; The Disparities Solutions Center, 2010). One can only deduce that this is true for other countries as well. Other barriers include the following:

- *Availability:* Is the service available and at a time when needed? For example, no services exist after 6 p.m. for someone who needs suturing of a minor laceration. Clinic hours coincide with patients' work hours, making it difficult to schedule appointments for fear of work reprisals.
- *Accessibility:* Transportation services may not be available, or rivers and mountains may make it difficult for people to obtain needed health-care services when no health-care provider is available in

their immediate region. It can be difficult for a single parent with four children to make three bus transfers to get one child immunized.

- *Affordability:* The service is available, but the patient does not have financial resources.
- *Appropriateness:* Maternal and child services are available, but what might be needed are geriatric and psychiatric services.
- *Accountability:* Are health-care providers accountable for their own education and do they learn about the cultures of the people they serve? Are they culturally aware, sensitive, and competent?
- *Adaptability:* A mother brings her child to the clinic for an immunization. Can she get a mammogram at the same time or must she make another appointment?
- *Acceptability:* Are services and patient education offered in a language preferred by the patient?
- *Awareness:* Is the patient aware that needed services exist in the community? The service may be available, but if patients are not aware of it, the service will not be used.
- *Attitudes:* Adverse subjective beliefs and attitudes from caregivers mean that the patient will not return for needed services until the condition is more compromised. Do health-care providers have negative attitudes about patients' home-based traditional practices?
- *Approachability:* Do patients feel welcomed? Do health-care providers and receptionists greet patients in the manner in which they prefer? This includes greeting patients with their preferred names.
- *Alternative practices and practitioners:* Do biomedical providers incorporate patients' alternative or complementary practices into treatment plans?
- *Additional services:* Are child- and adult-care services available if a parent must bring children or an aging parent to the appointment with them?
- *Literacy:* Language has been identified as the biggest barrier to health care, and not just for those for whom English is a second language. See Chapter 3 to identify patients with health literacy needs.

Health-care providers can help reduce some of these barriers by calling an area ethnic agency or church for assistance, establishing an advocacy role, involving professionals and laypeople from the same ethnic group as the patient, using cultural brokers, and organizationally providing culturally congruent and linguistically appropriate services. If all of these elements are in place and used appropriately, they have the potential of generating culturally responsive care.

▶ *Looking at the list of barriers to health care, which apply to you? How can you decrease these barriers? What are the barriers to health care in your community?*

Cultural Responses to Health and Illness

Significant research has been conducted on patients' responses to pain, which has been called the "fifth vital sign." Most health-care professionals believe that patients should be made comfortable and not have to tolerate high levels of pain. Accrediting bodies, such as the Joint Commission, survey organizations to ensure that patients' pain levels are assessed and that appropriate interventions are instituted.

A number of studies related to pain and the ethnicity/culture of the patient have been completed. Most of the studies have come from end-of-life care. Some of the salient research findings follow:

- Sixty-five percent of "minority" patients have inadequate pain control versus 30 percent of "nonminority" patients (Anderson et al., 2002; Cleeland et al., 1994; 1997; Foley, 2000).
- A patient's ethnicity has a greater influence on the amount of opioid prescribed by the clinician than on the amount of opioid self-administered by the patient (Ng, Dimsdale, Rollnik, & Shapiro, 1996).
- Communication between patient and health-care provider influences pain diagnosis and treatment (American Academy of Pain Medicine, 2004; Purnell & Paulanka, 2005).
- The brain's pain-processing and pain-killing systems vary by race and ethnicity (American Academy of Pain Medicine, 2004).
- Few minority patients are told in advance about possible side effects of pain medicine and how to manage them (Anderson et al., 2002).
- African American and Hispanic patients with severe pain are less likely than white patients to be able to obtain needed pain medicine because pharmacies do not carry the medicines (Morrison, Wallenstein, Natale, Senzel, & Huang, 2001).
- African Americans are less likely to have their pain recorded (Bernabei et al., 1998).
- Inadequate education of pain and analgesia expectations may contribute to poor pain relief in the Asian populations (Kuhn et al., 1990).
- Disparities in pain management and quality care at end of life exist among African American women in general and, specifically, those with breast cancer (Payne, Medina, & Hampton, 2003).
- Hispanic patients are more likely to describe pain as "suffering," the emotional component. African Americans are more likely to describe pain as "hurts," the sensory component (Anderson et al., 2002).
- Socioeconomic factors negatively influence prescribing pain medicine.
- Pain does not have the same debilitating effect for patients from Eastern cultures as it does for patients from Western cultures (Kodiath & Kodiath, 1992).

- Stoicism, fatalism, family, and spirituality have a positive impact on Hispanics and pain control (Purnell & Paulanka, 2005).
- Chinese, Korean, and Vietnamese patients do not favor taking pain medicine over a long period of time.
- Vietnamese Canadians prefer herbal therapies over prescription pain medicine (Voyer, Rail, Laberge, & Purnell, 2005).
- Haitians, Haitian Americans, and Haitian Canadians combine herbal therapies with prescription medicine without telling the health-care provider (Voyer et al., 2005).
- Black, Hispanic, and Asian women receive less epidural analgesia than do white women (Rust et al., 2004).
- Cultural background, worldview, and variant characteristics of culture influence the pain experience.
- The greater the language differences, the poorer the pain control.
- For Asians, tolerating pain may be a way of atoning for past sins.

Pain scales are in different languages and with faces appropriate to the language and ethnicity of the patient (Pain Source Book, 2005). Additional resources for pain are the American Pain Foundation, The American Pain Society, the Boston Cancer Pain Education Center (in 11 languages), and the OUCHER Pain scale for children (OUCHER!, n.d.), all of which are available on the Internet. Health-care practitioners must investigate the meaning of pain to each person within a cultural explanatory framework to interpret diverse behavioral responses and provide culturally competent care. The health-care provider may need to offer and encourage pain medication and explain that it will help the healing progress.

▶ *What is your first line of intervention when you are having pain? When do you decide to see a health-care practitioner when you are in pain? What differences do you see between yourself and others when they are in pain? Where did you learn your response to pain? Do you see any difference in the clinical setting in response to pain among ethnic and cultural groups? Between men and women?*

The manner in which mental illness is perceived and expressed by a cultural group has a direct effect on how individuals present themselves and, consequently, on how health-care providers interact with them. In some societies, mental illness may be seen by many as not being as important as physical illness. Mental illness is culture-bound; what may be perceived as a mental illness in one society may not be considered a mental illness in another. For some, mental illness and severe physical handicaps are considered a disgrace and taboo. As a result, the family is likely to keep the

mentally ill or handicapped person at home as long as they can. This practice may be reinforced by the belief that all individuals are expected to contribute to the household for the common good of the family, and when a person is unable to contribute, further disgrace occurs. In some cultures, children with a mental disability are stigmatized, and the lack of supportive services may cause families to abandon their loved ones because of the cost of long-term care and the family's desire and desperate need for support. Such children may be kept from the public eye in hope of saving the family from stigmatization.

▶ *What are your perceptions about mental illness? Does mental illness have the same value as physical illness and disease? When you are having emotional difficulties, what is your first line of defense? Have you observed different attitudes/responses from providers regarding physical and mental illnesses?*

Rehabilitation and occupational health services focus on returning individuals with handicaps to productive lifestyles in society as soon as possible. The goal of the health-care system is to rehabilitate everyone: convicted criminals, people with alcohol and drug problems, as well as those with physical conditions. To establish rapport, health-care practitioners working with patients suffering from chronic disease must avoid assumptions regarding health beliefs and provide rehabilitative health interventions within the scope of cultural customs and beliefs. Failure to respect and accept patients' values and beliefs can lead to misdiagnosis, lack of cooperation, and alienation of patients from the health-care system.

▶ *Do you see physically challenged individuals as important as nonphysically challenged individuals in terms of their worth to society? What are your beliefs about rehabilitation? Should everyone have the opportunity for rehabilitation?*

Sick role behaviors are culturally prescribed and vary among ethnic societies. Traditional individualistic cultural practice calls for fully disclosing the health condition to the patient. However, traditional collectivistic families may prefer to be informed of the bad news first, and then slowly break the news to the sick family member. Given the ethnocultural acceptance of the sick role, health-care providers must assess each patient and family individually and incorporate culturally congruent therapeutic interventions to return the patient to an optimal level of functioning.

▶ *What do you normally do when you have a minor illness? Do you go to work (class) anyway? What would make you decide not to go to work or class? Does the sick role have a specific meaning in your culture?*

Blood Transfusions and Organ Donation

Most religions favor organ donation and transplantation and transfusion of blood or blood products. Jehovah's Witnesses do not believe in blood transfusions. Some individuals and cultures choose not to participate in organ donation or autopsy because of their belief that they will suffer in the afterlife or that the body will not be whole on resurrection. Information about kidney transplants and ethnicity can be found at the National Kidney Foundation's website and in individual chapters in this book. Health-care providers may need to assist patients in obtaining a religious leader to support them in making decisions regarding organ donation or transplantation.

Some people do not sign donor cards because the concept of organ donation and transplantation is not customary in their homelands. Health-care providers should supply information regarding organ donation on an individual basis, be sensitive to individual and family concerns, explain procedures involved with organ donation and procurement, answer questions factually, and explain involved risks. A key to successful marketing approaches for organ donation is cultural awareness. Table 2-11 identifies guidelines for assessing the cultural domain *health-care practices*.

▶ *Are you averse to receiving blood or blood products? Why? Why not? Are you an organ donor? Why? Why not?*

Health-Care Providers

The domain *health-care providers* includes the status, use, and perceptions of traditional, magico-religious,

▮▶ Table 2-11 Health-Care Practices

Suggested Question	Sample Rationale/**Example**
1. In what prevention activities do you engage to maintain your health?	A strong value in the dominant European American culture is to have regularly scheduled health checkups, including self breast examinations, mammograms, and colonoscopies.
1. Who in your family takes responsibility for the family's health?	Among Arabs, family, not the individual, has the primary responsibility for a person's health-seeking care.
2. What over-the-counter medicines do you use?	All cultural groups and individuals use over-the-counter medication; some use them to the exclusion of prescription medicines.
3. What herbal teas and folk medicines do you use?	Panamanians, like many Hispanic/Latino populations, use a wide variety of herbal teas for many health conditions.
4. For what conditions do you use herbal medicines?	Iranians use a variety of berries, leaves, seeds, and dried flowers steeped in hot or cold water and drunk for digestive problems.
5. What do you usually do when you are in pain?	African Americans may see pain and suffering as inevitable and something that is to be endured.
6. How do you express your pain?	Among Mexicans, being able to endure pain is seen as a sign of strength.
7. How are people in your culture viewed or treated when they have a mental illness?	Having a mental illness in many Arab cultures is seen as a stigma; therefore, the person with a mental illness may be well cared for but kept hidden from society.
8. How are people with physical disabilities treated in your culture?	The Amish approach disability as a community responsibility, and those with a disability are incorporated into all family and social activities.
9. What do you do when you are sick? Stay in bed; continue your normal activities, etc.?	For many from the European American culture, a belief is "if you are not dead," take something for relief and continue with your daily routines.
10. What are your beliefs about rehabilitation?	Studies demonstrate that for Germans, if rehabilitation is needed to function at maximum capacity, then all rehab exercises are done.
11. How are people with chronic illnesses viewed or treated in your culture?	For most Arabs, if a chronic illness is debilitating, family members readily assume that person's responsibilities.
12. Are you averse to blood transfusions?	Besides a religious prohibition for a Jehovah's Witness to receive blood, many people do not want a blood transfusion for fear of contracting HIV/AIDS.
13. Is organ donation acceptable to you?	Jewish law views organ transplants for four perspectives: the recipient, the living donor, the cadaver donor, and the dying donor. Because life is sacred, if the recipient's life can be prolonged without considerable risk, then the transplant is favorably viewed.
14. Are you an organ donor?	Part of a standard assessment.
15. Would you consider having an organ transplant if needed?	Organ donation and transplantation among Muslims are individual decisions.

ID Table 2-11 **Health-Care Practices** *Continued from page 42*

Suggested Question	Sample Rationale/**Example**
16. Are health-care services readily available to you?	The health-care provider needs to be aware of access problems for health care and make attempts to improve access.
17. Do you have transportation problems accessing needed health-care services?	Many organizations have vouchers for public transportation.
18. What traditional health-care practices do you use? Acupuncture, acupressure, cai gao, moxibustion, aromatherapy, coining, etc.?	If the health-care provider is familiar with traditional practices within the culture, more specific information can be obtained.

and biomedical health-care providers. This domain is interconnected with communications, family roles and organization, and spirituality. In addition, the gender of the health-care provider may be significant for some people.

Traditional Versus Biomedical Providers

Most people combine the use of biomedical health-care providers with traditional practices, folk healers, and/or magico-religious healers. The health-care system abounds with individual and family folk practices for curing or treating specific illnesses. A significant percentage of all care is delivered outside the perimeter of the formal health-care arena. Many times herbalist-prescribed therapies are handed down from family members and may have their roots in religious beliefs. Traditional and folk practices often contain elements of historically rooted beliefs.

▶ *What alternative health-care providers do you see for your health-care needs besides traditional allopathic-care providers? For what conditions do you use nonallopathic providers? Do you think traditional health-care providers are as valuable as allopathic health-care providers?*

The traditional practice in the United States is to assign staff to patients regardless of gender differences, although often an attempt is made to provide a same-gender health-care provider when intimate care is involved, especially when the patient and caregiver are of the same age. However, health-care providers should recognize and respect differences in gender relationships when providing culturally competent care because not all ethnocultural groups accept care from someone of the opposite gender. Health-care providers need to respect patients' modesty by providing adequate privacy and assigning a same-gender caregiver whenever possible.

▶ *Do you prefer a same-gender health-care provider for your general health care? Do you mind having an opposite-gender provider for intimate care? Why? Why not? Do you prefer Western-trained health-care providers or does it not make any difference?*

Status of Health-Care Providers

Health-care providers are perceived differently among ethnic and cultural groups. Individual perceptions of selected health-care providers may be closely associated with previous contact and experiences with health-care providers. In many Western societies, health-care providers, especially physicians, are viewed with great respect, although recent studies show that this is declining among some groups. Although many nurses in the United States do not believe they are respected, public opinion polls usually place patients' respect of nurses higher than that of physicians. The advanced practice role of registered nurses is gaining respect as more of them have successful careers and the public sees them as equal or preferable to physicians and physician assistants in many cases.

▶ *Does one type of health-care provider have increased status over another type? Should all health-care providers receive equal respect, regardless of educational requirements? Does the ethnicity or race of a provider make any difference to you? Why? Why not?*

Depending on the country of origin and experience of working with professional nurses, some physicians may misunderstand the assertive behavior of Western-educated nurses because in their home country, nurses were not expected to be assertive. Some patients perceive older male physicians as being of higher rank and more trustworthy than younger health professionals, especially for patients who come from a collectivist culture where they are taught from a very early age to respect elders and to show deference to nurses and physicians, regardless of gender or age.

Evidence suggests that respect for professionals is correlated with their educational level. In some cultures, the nurse is expected to defer to physicians. In many countries, the nurse is viewed more as a domestic than as a professional person, and only the physician commands respect. Health beliefs are not border bound. People bring their beliefs with them upon migration.

In some cultures, folk and magico-religious health-care providers may be deemed superior to biomedically

ID Table 2-12 **Health-Care Providers**

Suggested Question	Sample Rationale/Example
1. What health-care providers do you see when you are ill? Physicians, nurses?	Not all patients see Western allopathic practitioners for illnesses, at least not as first access. Some use Western providers and traditional providers simultaneously.
2. Do you prefer a same-sex health-care provider for routine health problems? For intimate care?	Among Orthodox Jewish Islamic patients, a same-sex provider should be assigned unless it is an emergency.
3. What healers do you use besides physicians and nurses?	If the health-care provider is familiar with the specific culture, better/more pointed questions can be asked. Among many Hispanics/Latinos, folk practitioners are consulted for the evil eye and other conditions.
4. For what conditions do you use healers?	Many American Indians use a variety of traditional healers. Being able to integrate traditional healers with allopathic professionals will increase compliance with recommendations.

Adapted from Purnell, L. (2009). *Guide to culturally competent health care.* Philadelphia: F.A. Davis Co.; and Purnell, L. (2011). Models and theories focused on culture. In J.B. Butts and K.L. Rich (Eds.), *Philosophies and theories for advanced practice nursing.* Sudbury, MA: Jones & Bartlett Learning.

educated physicians and nurses. It may be that folk, traditional, and magico-religious health-care providers are well known to the family and provide more individualized care. In such cultures, health-care providers take time to get to know patients as individuals and engage in small talk totally unrelated to the health-care problem to accomplish their objectives. Establishing satisfactory interpersonal relationships is essential for improving health care and education in these ethnic groups. Table 2-12 identifies the guidelines for assessing the cultural domain *health-care practitioners*.

REFERENCES

American Academy of Pain Medicine. (2004). Retrieved from www.painmed.org

Anderson, K., Richman, S., Hurley, J., Palos, G., Valero, V., Mendoza, T., et al. (2002). Cancer pain management among underserved minority outpatients: Perceived needs and barriers to optimal control. *Cancer, 94*(8), 2295–2304.

Bernabei, R., Gambassi, G., Lapane, K., Landi, F., Gasonis, C., Dunlop, R., et al. (1998). Management of pain in elderly patients with cancer. *Journal of the American Medical Association, 279*(23), 1877–1882.

CIA World Factbook. (2011). *The World.* Retrieved from https://www.cia.gov/library/publications/the-worldfactbook/geos/xx.html

Cleeland, C., Gonin, R., Baez, L., Loehrer, P., & Pandya, K. (1997). Pain and treatment of pain in minority patients with cancer: The Eastern Cooperative Oncology Group Minority Outpatient Pain Study. *Annals of Internal Medicine, 127*(9), 813–816.

Cleeland, C., Gonin, R., Hatfield, A., Edmonson, J., Blum, R., Steward, J., et al. (1994). Pain and its treatment in outpatients with metastatic cancer. *New England Journal of Medicine, 330,* 592–596.

Foley, K. (2000). Controlling cancer pain. *Hospital Practice, 35*(4), 111–112.

Hall, E. (1990). *The silent language.* New York: Anchor Books.

Hilton, M. (1987). Demographic characteristics and the frequency of heavy drinking as predictors of drinking problems. *British Journal of Addiction, 82,* 913–925.

Institute of Medicine. (2001). *Crossing the quality chasm.* Retrieved from http://www.iom.edu/Reports/2001/Crossing-the-Quality-Chasm-A-New-Health-System-for-the-21st-Century.aspx

Joint Commission. (2005). *Pain source book.* Retrieved from www.painsourcebook.ca

Joint Commission. (2010a). *Advancing effective communication, cultural competence, and family centered care: A roadmap for hospitals.* Joint Commission.

Joint Commission. (2010b). *Patient-centered communication standards and EPs.* Joint Commission.

Kodiath, M., & Kodiath, A. (1992). A comparative study of patients with chronic pain in India and the United States. *Clinical Nursing Research, 3,* 278–291.

Kuhn, S., Cooke, K., Collins, M., Jones, J., & Mucklow, J. (1990). Perceptions of pain relief after surgery. *British Medical Journal, 300,* 1687–1690.

Morrison, R.S., Wallenstein, S., Natale, D.K., Senzel, R.S., & Huang, L.L. (2001). "We don't carry that"—Failure of pharmacies in predominantly nonwhite neighborhoods to stock opioid analgesics. *New England Journal of Medicine, 342*(14), 1023–1026.

Ng, B., Dimsdale, J., Rollnik, J., & Shapiro, H. (1996). The effect of ethnicity on prescriptions for patient-controlled analgesia for post-operative pain. *Pain, 66*(1), 9–12.

Payne, R., Medina, E., & Hampton, J. (2003). Quality of life concerns in patients with breast cancer: Evidence for disparity of outcomes and experiences in pain management and palliative care among African-American Women. *Cancer, 97*(1 Suppl), 311–317.

Peele, S., & Brodsky, A. (2001). *Alcohol and society.* Retrieved from http://www.peele.net OUCHER! (N.D.). Retrieved from http://www.oucher.org/

Purnell, L., & Foster, J. (2003a). Cultural aspects of alcohol use: Part I. *The Drug and Alcohol Professional, 3*(3), 17–23.

Purnell, L., & Foster, J. (2003b). Cultural aspects of alcohol use: Part II. *The Drug and Alcohol Professional, 2*(3), 3–8.

Purnell, L. & Paulanka, B. (2005). *Guide to culturally competent health care.* Philadelphia: F. A. Davis Company.

Rust, G., Nembhard, W., Nichols, M., Omole, R., Minor, P., et al. (2004). Racial and ethnic disparities in the provision of epidural analgesia to Georgia Medicaid beneficiaries during labor and delivery. *American Journal of Obstetrics and Gynecology, 191,* 456–462.

The Disparities Solutions Center at Massachusetts General Hospital. (2010). *Improving quality and achieving equity: A guide for hospital leaders.* Boston, MA: The Disparities Solutions Center at Massachusetts General Hospital.

Voyer, P., Rail, G., Laberge, S., & Purnell, L. (2005). Cultural minority older women's attitudes toward medication and implications for adherence to a drug regimen. *Journal of Diversity in Health and Social Care, 2*(1), 47–61.

DavisPlus For case studies, review questions, and additional information, go to
http://davisplus.fadavis.com

Chapter 3

Individual Cultural Competence and Evidence-Based Practice

Larry D. Purnell and Susan Salmond

Individual Cultural Competence

Self-Awareness and Health Professions

Culture has a powerful unconscious impact on patients and health professionals. Culture in health-care settings is extremely complex for the following reasons:

- Each patient has a culture.
- Each health-care provider has a culture that may be different from that of the patient.
- Each profession, nursing, medicine, physical therapy, occupational therapy, and social work, to name a few, has a culture.
- Each specialty such as medicine, surgery, gerontology, psychiatry, hospice/palliative care, pediatrics, rehabilitation, to name a few, has a subculture of the dominant professional culture.
- Each organization has a culture with subcultures within each organization.

When all these competing cultures and subcultures are combined, a significant mismatch may occur, creating an increased complexity of providing culturally competent care.

The way health-care providers perceive themselves as competent providers is often reflected in the way they communicate with patients. Thus, it is essential for health-care providers to think about their cultures, their behaviors, and their communication styles in relation to their perceptions of cultural differences. They should also examine the impact their beliefs have on others, including patients and coworkers, who are culturally diverse. Before addressing the multicultural backgrounds and unique individual perspectives of each patient, health-care providers must first address their own personal and professional knowledge, values, beliefs, ethics, and life experiences in a manner that optimizes interactions and assessment of culturally diverse individuals.

Self-knowledge and understanding promote strong professional perceptions that free health-care professionals from prejudice and allow them to interact with others in a manner that preserves personal integrity and respects uniqueness and differences among individual patients. The process of professional development and diversity competence begins with *self-exploration* or critical reflection. Although the literature provides numerous definitions of *self-awareness*, discussion of research integrating the concept of self-awareness with multicultural competence is minimal. Many theorists and diversity trainers imply that self-examination or awareness of personal prejudices and biases is an important step in the cognitive process of developing cultural competence (Boyle & Andrews, 2011; Calvillo et al., 2009; Giger et al., 2007). However, discussions of emotional feelings elicited by this cognitive awareness are somewhat limited, given the potential impact of emotions and conscious feelings on behavioral outcomes.

> ▶ *In your opinion, why is there conflict about working with culturally diverse patients? What attitudes are necessary to deliver quality care to patients whose culture is different from yours?*

Self-awareness in cultural competence is a deliberate and conscious cognitive and emotional process of getting to know yourself: your personality, your values, your beliefs, your professional knowledge standards, your ethics, and the impact of these factors on the various roles you play when interacting with individuals different from yourself. Critically analyzing our own values and beliefs in terms of how we see differences enables us to be less fearful of others whose values and beliefs are different from our own (Calvillo et al., 2009). The ability to understand oneself sets the stage for integrating new knowledge related to cultural differences into the health-care provider's knowledge base, perceptions of health, interventions, and the impact these factors have on the various roles of professionals when interacting with multicultural patients.

> ▶ *What have you done in the last 5 to 10 years to increase your self-awareness? Has increasing your self-awareness resulted in an increased appreciation for cultural diversity? How might you increase your knowledge about the diversity in your community? In your school?*

Measuring Individual Cultural Competence

Much has been debated, especially since the early 1990s, about objectively measuring individual competence. Most tools for measuring cultural competence are self-reported and subjective in nature. A number of tools have been developed to assess individual and organizational cultural competence. Some have been validated and are specific to a discipline or area of practice, whereas others are more general in nature. To select one that more specifically meets your needs, go to an Internet search engine such as www.scholar.google.com and enter "cultural competence measurement" or "cultural competence assessment tools" in the search field. The Office of Minority Health also has a document on Cultural Competence Standards (www.omhrc.gov). In general, cultural competence is a journey involving the willingness and ability of an individual to deliver culturally congruent and acceptable health and nursing care to the patients to whom one provides care. To this author, individual cultural competence can be arbitrarily divided among cultural general approaches, the clinical encounter, and language.

The American Academy of Nursing with representatives from the Transcultural Nursing Society has developed Standards of Practice for Culturally Competent Nursing Care based on social justice (Douglas et al., 2011). Box 3-1 lists the 12 standards,.

Cultural General Approaches

A number of general approaches exist to help health-care providers achieve cultural competence, including the following:

1. Developing an awareness of one's own existence, sensations, thoughts, and environment without letting it have an undue influence on those from other backgrounds.
2. Continuing to learn cultures of patients to whom one provides care.
3. Demonstrating knowledge and understanding of the patient's culture, health-related needs, and meanings of health and illness.
4. Accepting and respecting cultural differences in a manner that facilitates the patient's and the family's ability to make decisions to meet their needs and beliefs.

5. Recognizing that the health-care provider's beliefs and values may not be the same as the patient's.
6. Resisting judgmental attitudes such as "different is not as good."
7. Being open to new cultural encounters.
8. Recognizing that variant cultural characteristics determine the degree to which patients adhere to the beliefs, values, and practices of their dominant culture.
9. Having contact and experience with the communities from which patients come.
10. Being willing to work with patients of diverse cultures and subcultures.
11. Accepting responsibility for one's own education in cultural competence by attending conferences, reading literature, and observing cultural practices.
12. Promoting respect for individuals by discouraging racial and ethnic slurs among coworkers.
13. Intervening with staff behavior that is insensitive, lacks cultural understanding, or reflects prejudice.
14. Having a cultural general framework for assessment as well as having cultural-specific knowledge about the patients to whom care is provided.

The Clinical Encounter

The clinical encounter is a rich area for learning about and becoming more culturally competent. As clinical practice begins seeing increasing numbers of diverse patients and families, health-care providers increase their knowledge base and skills. Some specific approaches that are helpful in becoming more culturally competent are:

- Adapting care to be congruent with the patient's culture.
- Responding respectively to all patients and their families (includes addressing patients and family members as they prefer, formally or informally).
- Collecting cultural data on assessments.
- Forming generalizations as a method for formulating questions rather than stereotyping.
- Recognizing culturally based health-care beliefs and practices.
- Knowing the most common diseases and illnesses affecting the unique population to whom care is provided.
- Individualizing care plans to be consistent with the patient's cultural beliefs.
- Having knowledge of the communication styles of patients to whom you provide care.
- Accepting varied gender roles and childrearing practices from patients to whom you provide care.
- Having a working knowledge of the religious and spirituality practices of patients to whom you provide care.

▶ Box 3-1 | **Standards of Practice for Culturally Competent Nursing Care**

- **Standard 1: Social Justice**
  Professional nurses shall promote social justice for all. The applied principles of social justice guide decisions of nurses related to the patient, family, community, and other health-care professionals. Nurses will develop leadership skills to advocate for socially just policies.
- **Standard 2: Critical Reflection**
  Nurses shall engage in critical reflection of their own values, beliefs, and cultural heritage in order to have an awareness of how these qualities and issues can impact culturally congruent nursing care.
- **Standard 3: Knowledge of Cultures**
  Nurses shall gain an understanding of the perspectives, traditions, values, practices, and family systems of culturally diverse individuals, families, communities, and populations for whom they care, as well as knowledge of the complex variables that affect the achievement of health and well-being.
- **Standard 4: Culturally Competent Practice**
  Nurses shall use cross-cultural knowledge and culturally sensitive skills in implementing culturally congruent nursing care.
- **Standard 5: Cultural Competence in Healthcare Systems and Organizations**
  Healthcare organizations should provide the structure and resources necessary to evaluate and meet the cultural and language needs of their diverse patients.
- **Standard 6: Patient Advocacy and Empowerment**
  Nurses shall recognize the effect of healthcare policies, delivery systems, and resources on their patient populations, and shall empower and advocate for their patients as indicated. Nurses shall advocate for the inclusion of their patients' cultural beliefs and practices in all dimensions of their health care when possible.
- **Standard 7: Multicultural Workforce**
  Nurses shall actively engage in the effort to ensure a multicultural workforce in health-care settings. One measure to achieve a multicultural workforce is through strengthening of recruitment and retention effort in the hospital and academic setting.
- **Standard 8: Education and Training in Culturally Competent Care**
  Nurses shall be educationally prepared to promote and provide culturally congruent health care. Knowledge and skills necessary for ensuring that nursing care is culturally congruent shall be included in global health-care agendas that mandate formal education and clinical training, as well as required ongoing, continuing education for all practicing nurses.
- **Standard 9: Cross-Cultural Communication**
  Nurses shall use culturally competent verbal and nonverbal communication skills to identify patient's values, beliefs, practices, perceptions, and unique health-care needs.
- **Standard 10: Cross-Cultural Leadership**
  Nurses shall have the ability to influence individuals, groups, and systems to achieve positive outcomes of culturally competent care for diverse populations.
- **Standard 11: Policy Development**
  Nurses shall have the knowledge and skills to work with public and private organizations, professional associations, and communities to establish policies and standards for comprehensive implementation and evaluation of culturally competent care.
- **Standard 12: Evidence-Based Practice and Research**
  Nurses shall base their practice on interventions that have been systematically tested and shown to be the most effective for the culturally diverse populations that they serve. In areas where there is a lack of evidence of efficacy, nurse researchers shall investigate and test interventions that may be the most effective in reducing the disparities in health outcomes.

- Having an understanding of the family dynamics of patients to whom you provide care.
- Using faces and language pain scales in the ethnicity and preferred languages of the patients.
- Recognizing and accepting traditional, complementary, and alternative practices of patients to whom you provide care.
- Incorporating patient's cultural food choices and dietary practices into care plans and
- Incorporating patient's health literacy into care plans and health education initiatives.

Language Interpretation, Health Literacy, and Translation

Language

Language ability, as mentioned previously, is the biggest barrier to effective health-care access, diagnosis, assessment, and comprehension of medication and health prescription instructions. Strategies for improving language ability for effective communication with patients and family follow:

- Developing skills and using interpreters (includes sign language) with patients and families who have limited English proficiency.
- Providing patients with educational documents that are translated into their preferred language.
- Providing discharge instructions at a level the patient and the family understand and in the language the patient and the family prefer.
- Providing medication and treatment instructions in the language the patient prefers.
- Using pain scales in the preferred language of the patient.

▶ *Look at the list of activities that promote individual cultural competence. Which of these activities have you used to increase your cultural competence? Which ones can you easily add to increase your cultural competence? Which ones are the most difficult for you to incorporate?*

Provider cross-cultural skills and interpreter services, and written patient materials in different languages and at a low level of health literacy, ensure that patients understand their options, choices, costs, and benefits. The health-care provider and the organization should become familiar with the Code of Ethics for Medical Interpreters (1987) and make this National Standards on Interpreting in Health Care (2007).

One of the biggest barriers to effective health care, in addition to access, is health literacy, and this is not just for people for whom English is a second language. Over 40 percent of adults have significant literacy challenges, and 88 percent of adults have less than "proficient" health literacy skills. Communication difficulties may lead to misdiagnosis and inappropriate treatment, and may limit the process of truly informed consent. Communication problems are the most frequent cause of serious adverse events, as recorded by the Joint Commission. Furthermore, patients with limited English proficiency have longer hospital stays than English speakers for some common medical and surgical conditions (Joint Commission, 2010). In addition, patients may not understand discharge instructions, and some may be afraid to seek care due to language barriers and embarrassment or cultural differences. Recognizing that a patient needs help reading or completing admission forms can be a sensitive issue, and staff should obtain the necessary information without embarrassing the patient. Some recommendations for interpretation are shown in Box 3-2.

Health Literacy

The health-care provider has a responsibility to determine if a patient has low health literacy. Patients with low health literacy may have great difficulty understanding their health information, participating in treatment decisions, and following through with treatment plans. Some comments by patients that might indicate low literacy include forgetting their glasses, wanting another family member to complete forms, and wanting to take forms home to complete them. Health-care providers should ask the patient if he or she needs assistance in completing forms and offer to assist the patient. Alternative media, such as a video with pictures and diagrams can help to reinforce key points. It is a good idea to have the patient or the responsible family member demonstrate the procedure to show that the patient understands (Joint Commission, 2010).

▶▶ Box 3-2   Recommendations for Working with an Interpreter

- Use interpreters who can decode the words and provide the meaning behind the message.
- Use dialect-specific interpreters whenever possible.
- Use interpreters trained in the health-care field.
- Give the interpreter time alone with the patient.
- Provide time for translation and interpretation.
- Use same-gender interpreters whenever possible.
- Maintain eye contact with both the patient and the interpreter to elicit feedback; read nonverbal cues.
- Speak slowly without exaggerated mouthing, allow time for translation, use the active rather than the passive tense, wait for feedback, and restate the message. Do not rush; do not speak loudly.
- Use as many words as possible in the patient's language and nonverbal communication when unable to understand the language.
- Use phrase charts and picture cards if available.
- During the assessment, direct your questions to the patient, not to the interpreter.
- Ask one question at a time, and allow interpretation and a response before asking another question.
  Be aware that interpreters may affect the reporting of symptoms, insert their own ideas, or omit information.
    Remember that patients can usually understand more than they can express; thus, they need time to think in their own language. They are alert to the health-care provider's body language, and they may forget some or all of their English in times of stress.
- Avoid the use of relatives, who may distort information or not be objective.
- Avoid using children as interpreters, especially with sensitive topics.
- Avoid idiomatic expressions and medical jargon.
- If a certified interpreter is unavailable, the use of an uncertified interpreter may be acceptable; however, the difficulty might be omission of parts of the message or distortion of the message, including transmission of information not given by the speaker and messages not being fully understood.
- If available, use an interpreter who is older than the patient.
- Review responses with the patient and interpreter at the end of a session.
- Be aware that social class differences between the interpreter and the patient may result in the interpreter's not reporting information that he or she perceives as superstitious or unimportant.

Translation

Whereas interpretation is verbal, translation is written. Sometimes a patient may have adequate verbal skills for understanding health-related information but not have adequate reading skills. To help ensure health literacy of written materials, present materials at a fifth-grade or lower reading level, use bulleted points for crucial information, and translate materials into the patient's referred language (Office of Disease Prevention and Health Promotion, 2011). In addition, use information from the National Network of Libraries of Medicine (2011) that includes health information for professionals and the public.

25

Use national- and state-level data on sexual orientation from Web sites such as http://www.census.org and http://www.gaydata.org to develop initiatives that address the health concerns of gay and lesbian patients (Joint Commission, 2010).

Evidence-Based Practice and Culturally Congruent Best Practices

The mandate for evidence-based practice (EBP) to reduce the "know-do" gap (Antes, Sauerland, & Seiter, 2006) between known science and implementation in practice has been driven by the demand for improved safety and quality outcomes for clients (Box 3-3). This has necessitated a culture shift from an opinion-based culture grounded in intuition, clinical experience/expertise, and pathophysiological rationale (Swanson, Schmitz, & Chung, 2010) to a culture of EBP in which there is conscientious, explicit, and judicious use of current best evidence in making decisions about the care of individuals or groups of patients. Evidence alone does not constitute EBP, but rather evidence is one component needed to inform decision making. Evidence-based practice is put in action when evidence, clinical expertise, clinical context, and patient preferences and values inform one another in a positive way (Kitson, 2002). No one component is the most important; rather, the weight given to each component varies according to the clinical situation (Melnyk, Fineout-Overholt, Stilwell, & Williamson, 2009). Figure 3-1 portrays the dynamic nature of the process as it combines the four core components contributing to clinical decision making. Table 3-1 summarizes the components of EBP and the actions and resources needed to facilitate its implementation.

Understanding the Four Components of Evidence-Based Practice

The four components of EBP, all of which contribute to the best patient outcomes, are best research

---

ID Box 3-3 Quality and Safety Education for Nurses

The Institute of Medicine (IOM) *Health Profession Education Report* on safety and quality in the United States' health-care system has fueled a number of organizations and commissions to address quality and safety in education for health professionals. A few of these are listed as follows and further described on DavisPlus Web Resources:

• Quality and Safety Education for Nurses (QSEN)
• National Quality Forum (NQF)
• Agency for Health Research and Quality (AHRQ)
• Institute for Healthcare Improvement (IHI)
• National Association of Healthcare Quality (NAHQ)

   Although some of the initiatives are discipline-specific with well-developed documents for including content and teaching strategies for quality and safety, the overarching principles are the same for all professions. The IOM's initial five core areas are as follows:

• Delivering patient-centered care
• Working as part of interdisciplinary teams
• Practicing evidence-based medicine
• Focusing on quality improvement
• Using information technology

   The Robert Wood Johnson Foundation funded the American Association of Colleges of Nursing (AACN) to develop teaching strategies that address the IOM's competencies, which included safety as a separate core area. The task force convened by the AACN enhanced the essentials of baccalaureate education that included the knowledge, skills, and attitudes required to meet the education needs of QSEN (www.aacn.nche.edu).

Patient-Centered Care

Patient-centered care accounts for and recognizes that the patient and family are co-participants to ensure culturally competent care and that their cultural preferences, values, and needs are addressed (see cultural general approaches and the clinical encounter in this chapter). In order for preferences to be adequately addressed, culturally acceptable communication is a core requirement for developing trust with full disclosure (Institute for Patient and Family Centered Care: www.ipfcc.org) (see the section on communication in Chapter 2). Health-care providers must respect patients' expertise and recognize that beliefs and values of the health-care providers may not be the same as those of the patients.

Teamwork and Cultural Care

Teamwork and collaboration are extremely important processes in culture. Given the complexity of the culture of the patient, the cultures of individual team members, the cultures of the professions and specialties, and the culture of the organization (see Chapter 4), to function effectively, mutual respect and shared decision making are essential (Cronenwett et al., 2007).

Evidence-Based Practice

Evidence-based practice (EBP) has proven to be difficult to integrate into cultural care because the available literature on EBP is still in its infancy with few large studies. Best practices in clinical care integrate clinical expertise and patient/family preferences for optimal delivery (see the section on EBP in this chapter).

Continues on page 50

IID Box 3-3 **Quality and Safety Education for Nurses** *Continued from page 49*

Quality Improvement

Quality improvement in cultural care is a combination of individual and organizational cultural competence (see Chapter 4). Quality cultural care cannot occur without the support of the organization in which care is delivered and should include expertise from the community it serves.

Health Literacy and Safety

Safety and minimizing risk are concerns on multiple levels, but specific to cultural aspects are health literacy and interpretation and translation services (see language interpretation, translation, and health literacy in this chapter). Health-care providers in all professions must discuss safety issues with their patients in both home and environmental contexts with patients' occupations—for example, the use of pesticides with people who work in agricultural environments.

Informatics

Informatics and information technology include the ability of health-care providers to access cultural information, specifically knowing where to obtain cultural general and specific information. Information must be obtained from recognized peer-reviewed literature, professional organizations and associations, and other credible sources whose content has been validated.

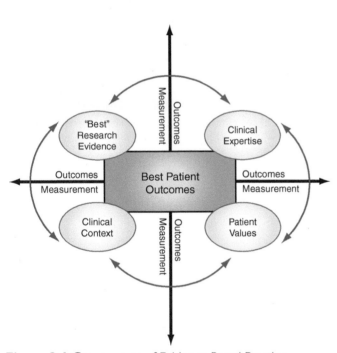

Figure 3-1 Components of Evidence-Based Practice

evidence, clinical expertise, patient preferences and values, and clinical context (see Figure 3-1).

Best Evidence

Locating Best Evidence from the Literature When one considers that there are more than 1500 new articles and 55 new clinical trials per day, the impossibility of staying current in all of the conditions and situations that patients present with becomes apparent. Practicing from an evidence-based (EB) perspective requires the clinician to recognize these knowledge limitations and to reflect on their ongoing practice to determine what evidence they are relying on and when they need evidence. Ask "why" things are being done as they are, "whether" there is evidence supporting the approach, or "what" the evidence suggests may be best in this clinical situation and "whether" there are likely to be cultural considerations that necessitate examining evidence specific to your cultural group (Salmond, 2007). **Asking Clinical Questions to Retrieve Evidence** Practicing from an EB perspective requires asking clinical questions and searching for the evidence to guide practice. There is a technique to asking clinical questions so that the evidence can be retrieved quickly and

IID Table 3-1 **The Evidence-Based Practice Process**

	Components	Resources/Change Needed
Identify best evidence	*Clinical inquiry:* What knowledge is needed? *Informed skepticism:* Why are we doing it this way? Is there a better way to do it? What is the evidence for what we do? Would doing this be as effective as doing that? (Salmond, 2007)	• Shift from "know how" and doing to "know why" • Reflect on what information is needed to provide "best" care • Generate questions about practice and care • Role model clinical inquiry at report, rounds, conferences • Use interdisciplinary case reviews to evaluate actual care • Include clinical librarians as members of teams participating in clinical rounds and conferences

II▷ Table 3-1 The Evidence-Based Practice Process *Continued from page 50*

	Components	Resources/Change Needed
	Convert information needs from practice into focused, searchable questions (patient intervention-comparison-outcome [PICO] framework).	• Consider recurring clinical issues, need for information, negative incidents/events as sources for questions or information needs • Identify clinical issues sensitive to nursing interventions • Narrow broad clinical issues/questions into searchable, focused questions • Use the mnemonic PICO to frame questions • Specify population of interest by using the specific cultural group identifier or broader terms such as multiethnic, multicultural
	Search databases for highest level of evidence in a timely manner	• Use evidence-searching skills to target relevant focused evidence • Begin search with filtered resources • Understand the match between question and design • Search strategies: key terms, multiple databases, point-of-care data • Use assistance of clinical librarian • Clinical Practice Guidelines available at www.clearinghouse.gov
	Use critical appraisal process to determine strength and validity of evidence and relevance to one's practice	• Demonstrate knowledge of research design • Demonstrate knowledge of statistics • Use critical appraisal tools to guide process of research critique • Utilize journal clubs • Summarize findings from evaluation, resolving conflicting evidence
Clinical experience and expertise	Use clinical expertise to determine how to use evidence in care of patient and how to manage patient in absence of evidence or presence of conflicting evidence	• Consider evidence in relation to own patient population • Consider cost-benefit ratio • Consider multidimensionality of patient and clinical situation in relation to evidence that is often reductionistic • Ensure holistic assessment and planning inclusive of the social and cultural context
Patient values and preferences	Demonstrate ability to perform a culture assessment and identify patient preferences and values that inform the clinical decision.	• Understand culture-general and culture-specific knowledge to guide interactions with patient • Use interview skills to avoid culture imposition and seek client's true preferences • Communicate evidence and treatment options considering patient values and preferences using decision aids when available • Involve patient and family in both information giving and decision making
Translation evidence from total process into clinical decisions and strategies for best patient outcomes	Use all four components in clinical decision-making process and implementation of clinical decision	• Provide plan of care based on evidence, clinical judgment, patient preferences, and organizational context • Use implementation frameworks for translating evidence into practice throughout an organization or care site including the community
Monitor patient outcomes	Use outcome tools to track patient outcomes	• Develop audit systems to track patient outcomes • Make clinical outcomes accessible electronically for analysis • Analyze outcomes and effectiveness of "evidence-based" clinical intervention

efficiently. The key is to ask focused questions. Who is the *population* of *interest*? What is the *intervention* or *phenomenon of interest*? What is the *outcome of interest*? If the broad interest is duration of breastfeeding, it should be narrowed further. Determine if evidence for a particular cultural or social group is needed, and specify this population by using key words as outlined in Table 3-2. Narrow down what the intervention of interest is—for example, barriers to breastfeeding, interventions to support breastfeeding, or educational and support programs to encourage breastfeeding. Finally, for quantitative studies, select an outcome that defines how success of the program will be meas-

ured—for example, initiation of breastfeeding, exclusive breastfeeding, or duration of breastfeeding. Putting it all together, the question might be "Does a structured *doula* program (support program) affect the initiation of breastfeeding among urban minority women?" or "What is the experience of breastfeeding for teenage mothers?" Table 3-2 provides a quick reference to asking clinical questions.

The question has been asked, and the goal is to search for the "best" evidence. Best evidence is usually found in clinically relevant research that has been conducted using sound methodology (Sackett, 2000). For the busy clinician, the key is to know how to find

II▶ Table 3-2   Locating Evidence Sources

Asking Clinical Questions and Search Terms to Locate Practices with Cultural Variation	1. Include your specific phenomena of interest or intervention of interest: (breastfeeding, literacy, patient education, type of drug, exercise regimen)
	2. Include your population and/or group interest: Consider who you are interested in, age, gender, diagnosis (middle-aged obese women, adolescents, elders residing in the community), cultural group that could include:
	  • culture (or specific culture group, i.e., Hispanic, Muslim), cross-cultural, transcultural
	  • ethnocultural, multicultural, multiethnic groups
	  • minority, ethnic minority groups
	  • immigrants, newcomers
	  • country of interest (i.e., Canada, Vietnam, Tanzania)
	3. Include outcome of interest (breastfeeding duration, breastfeeding satisfaction, weight loss, quality of life, HbA1c levels, adherence to low-sodium diet)
	4. Include type of information desired
	  • Systematic review
	  • Clinical practice guidelines
	  • Research Method (i.e., randomized controlled trial, qualitative)

Systematic Reviews	Cochrane Collaboration Library: **http://www2.cochrane.org/reviews/** Campbell Collaboration Library: **http://www.campbellcollaboration.org/library.php** Joanna Briggs Institute Library: **http://www.joannabriggs.edu.au** Agency for Healthcare Research & Quality: **http://www.ahrq.gov/clinic/epcindex.htm** *International Journal of Evidence Based Healthcare* Bibliographic Databases (select systematic reviews, meta-analysis, or add as search terms)
Evidence-Based Guidelines	National Guideline Clearinghouse: **http://www.guideline.gov/** Guidelines International Network (G-I-N): **http://www.openclinical.org/prj_gin.html**
Bibliographic Databases	Academic Search Premiere PsychARTICLES CINAHL PsychINFO Embase PubMed Medline REHABDATA Proquest Social Science Journals
Grey Literature	New York Academy of Medicine Grey Literature: **http://www.nyam.org/library/online-resources/grey-literature-report/current-grey-literature.html** WorldWideScience.org: **http://worldwidescience.org/** World Health Organization: **http://www.who.int/topics/** Pan American Health Organization: **http://new.paho.org/** Family Health International: **http://www.fhi.org/en/AboutFHI/index.htm** United Nations Educational, Scientific and Cultural Organization: **http://portal.unesco.org/culture** Kaiser Permanente Institute for Health Research: **http://www.kpco-ihr.org/index.htm** Kaiser Family Foundation: **http://www.kff.org/** Scirus for Scientific Information: **http://www.scirus.com/**

II▶ Table 3-2   Locating Evidence Sources *Continued from page 52*

	Health Sciences Online: **http://hso.info/hso/cgi-bin/query-meta?v%3aframe=form&frontpage= 1&v%3aproject=HSO&**
	Culture Link Network: **http://www.culturelink.org/dbase/index.html**
Internet Searching	**www.google.com**
	www.altheweb.com
Journals Specific to Evidence-Based Care	*Clinical Evidence*
	Evidence-Based Nursing, Evidence-Based Mental Health, Evidence-Based Healthcare
	Electronic Journals on Evidence-Based Practice: **http://www.wcpt.org/node/29660**
Patient Decision Aids	Ottowa Hospital Research Institute: **http://decisionaid.ohri.ca/index.html**
	Dartmouth Hitchcock Center for Shared Decision Making: **http://patients.dartmouth-hitchcock.org/shared_decision_making/decision_aid_library.html**
	Foundation for Informed Medical Decision Making: **http://www.fimdm.org/about.php**
	Mayo Clinic Shared Decision Making National Resource Center: http://shareddecisions.mayoclinic.org/

this evidence. Haynes (2006) suggests beginning with sources where the clinician can access filtered evidence that has already been critically appraised and determined to be of sufficient rigor to be considered for application into practice. These include systematic reviews, critically appraised topics (guidelines), and critically appraised individual articles.

Because one study is generally not enough to change practice, the best evidence often comes from systematic reviews that have pooled the primary research data for assessment and summarization. By using a systematic review, the clinician can generally rely on the fact that a comprehensive search for all available information has taken place, that the information has been screened for relevance to the clinical question, and that the information has been appraised for the rigor of the research. The studies actually included in the final summarization or synthesis are appraised to be of high quality and pooled together, providing more precise, powerful, and convincing conclusions. Sources for systematic reviews (see Table 3-2) include the AHRQ, Cochrane Collaboration, Campbell Collaboration, and Joanna Briggs libraries. Bibliographic databases should also be searched. The *International Journal of Evidence Based Healthcare* is a publication dedicated to systematic reviews.

Practice Guidelines Practice guidelines (preferably based on systematic reviews) translate research findings into systematically developed statements to assist health-care providers and patients in making decisions about appropriate health care for specific clinical circumstances. Guidelines are just what the name implies: a guide to inform health-care providers in applying best practice, not a cookbook where a recipe must be followed. Sources for guidelines include AHRQ and the guideline.gov Web site and the Guidelines International Network (see Table 3-2). Guidelines

can be specific to a disease condition such as asthma management (Management of Asthma Working Group, 2009) or HIV prevention (Kaplan, Benson, Holmes, Brooks, Pau, & Masur, 2009), or they can address broader program and intervention issues such as programming for HIV prevention for adolescents (Family Health International, 2010) or population-specific recommendations (Foggs, 2008).

In the absence of systematic reviews or practice guidelines, search for single studies using bibliographic databases (see Table 3-2). Many EB journals, such as *Evidence-Based Nursing, Evidence-Based Medicine,* and *Evidence-Based Mental Health,* provide filtered literature synopses of primary research providing the reader with a summary, an appraisal, and recommendations for translation into practice. To review filtered literature, a single-paper search should be done in these journals by adding the journal in the key word search.

If the question is still unanswered after searching the filtered literature, search for primary studies (nonfiltered) by searching the bibliographic databases. If there are journals that commonly carry articles related to the topic, include the journal title in the electronic search or hand-search the journal. The *Journal of Transcultural Nursing* may be a helpful source for information on culture.

Articles retrieved from nonfiltered sources need to be critically appraised to determine scientific rigor prior to use in practice. This requires determining whether the best or strongest design was used for the particular questions and whether the study design was rigorous. For questions of intervention (e.g., "In African Americans with newly diagnosed hypertension, what is the best diuretic treatment in lowering blood pressure?"), randomized controlled trials are the best type of design, followed by cohort studies, case-controlled studies, case series, and descriptive studies. For questions about meaning or understanding an experience (e.g., "What is the experience of marginalization in new African immigrants?"), qualitative studies are the best design. Rigor is assessed by reviewing the article for its adherence to design principles. There are many tools to assist in this process. One good source is the CASP International (www.caspinternational.org), which has a tool for the different study design types.

Grey Literature. Another source of evidence that can provide valuable information, especially in the area of culture, is *grey literature*, which consists of material that is not formally published by commercial publishers or peer-reviewed journals. It includes technical reports, fact sheets, state-of-the-art reports, conference proceedings, and other documents from institutions, organizations, government agencies, Internet-based materials and sites, and other forms of media (newspapers, films, published photographs) and the like. The "grey" non-peer-reviewed literature is an important source of information on culture because there are few peer-reviewed publications on specific diseases and cultural implications or diseases and management among the culturally and linguistically diverse. It is important that grey literature be authenticated as reliable and accurate as far as this can be assessed.

At the New York Academy of Medicine there has been a push by public health and health policy researchers for the Academy Library to obtain grey literature and to add it to the catalog (Gray, 1998). This has developed into the New York Academy of Medicine's *Grey Literature Report*, a bimonthly online report targeting researchers, health-care providers, practitioners, students, and the lay public who are interested in public health, health and science policy, health of minorities, vulnerable and special populations (children, women, uninsured, elderly), and those areas of general medicine and disease in which the Academy has research interests. Other key grey literature sites are listed in Table 3-2. Examples of valuable grey literature reports relevant to understanding the impact of culture on health decision making or reporting on cultural health issues include *Cross-Cultural Considerations in Promoting Advance Care Planning in Canada* (Con, 2008); *Culture and Mental Health in Haiti: A Literature Review* (WHO/PAHO, 2010); and *2010 National Healthcare Disparities Report* (Agency for Healthcare Research and Quality, 2010).

Best Clinical Expertise

Although locating and drawing from best evidence is important, by itself it cannot direct practice. One reason for this is the lack of quality evidence on topics of interest. This is especially true for evidence on social and cultural influences on health and health outcomes. Very few studies have been devoted to ethnic minority groups. Although legislation was passed in the early 1990s requiring NIH-funded researchers to include ethnic minorities as subjects in numbers adequate to allow for valid subgroup analyses of differences in effect by ethnic group, it is still difficult to get ethnic minority groups to participate in research (Hulme, 2010). A second reason is that there is poor fit between our patients in actual practice and those studied in research studies. Most studies control for one or two variables, whereas in practice our patients' problems can be very complex and their value systems very different. Mosley (2009) articulates that "we are living in a spectrum from good evidence at one end to no evidence at the other. We spend most of our lives in the gray area in the middle with somewhat adequate evidence, and we are often not really sure what is good evidence and what is not for the findings to be put into practice." Navigating this gray area requires clinicians to use their practical knowledge, professional-craft knowledge, or practical know-how (Rycroft-Malone, Seers, Titchen, Harvey, Kitson, & McCormack, 2004).

Evidence informs clinicians. Clinicians rely on their clinical judgment and expertise to thoroughly assess the patient and differentiate nuances that influence treatment perspectives. Unfortunately, in health care significant emphasis is placed on assessment of the biophysical domain, with much less attention paid to psychological, cultural, and social factors that clearly affect health behaviors and outcomes. Clinical expertise must be holistic and recognize the social and cultural determinants of health (McMurray, 2004) and evidence this in an inclusive skill set for cultural assessment and culturally competent interaction. The clinician must be able to evaluate and adapt research evidence and clinical guidelines in light of not only the clinical presentation but in response to social and cultural values of the client. They must use their clinical acumen to question why the client is or is not responding to treatment and use a holistic framework to determine whether there are intervening biophysical, psychological, social, or cultural considerations that have not been accounted for that could be influencing outcomes and then make necessary adjustments (Shah & Chung, 2009).

Patient Values and Preferences

It is insufficient to simply blend expertise and evidence because at the heart of the issue is the patient. Although critics of EBP have indicated that there is too great an emphasis on empirical evidence and clinical expertise, the reality is that EBP that integrates all four components is complementary with patient-centered care. Practicing from an EB perspective requires the clinician to recognize the uniqueness of the patient and family and to value the patient as a co–decision maker in selection of interventions or approaches toward his or her improved health.

The individual's or group's beliefs about health and illness must be understood if one is to design interventions that are likely to have an impact on health behavior. Their definitions of health and their perceptions of the importance of health states such as mobility, freedom from pain, prolonged life expectancy, and preservation of faculties are important to define because they are valued differently, and these values influence both clinician recommendations and patient decisions. Failure to consider these patient preferences and practicing from a medical model value system leads to unintentional bias toward a professional's view of the world (Kitson, 2002). If EBP is to be value-added, it is critical to ensure that the users of the knowledge—the health-care providers—become active shapers of knowledge and action (Clough, 2005). Health-care providers must be prepared to make "real-time" adjustments to their approach to care based on patient feedback.

Culture embodies a way of living, a worldview targeting our beliefs about human nature, interpersonal relationships, relationships of people to nature, time or the temporal focus of life, and ways of living one's life (activity). Health-care providers armed with this culture-general knowledge are more open to multiple ways of being, and it serves as a framework for building culture-specific knowledge. It is important to understand the factors that an individual from one cultural group believes cause different types of illnesses and the culture-specific remedies to treat those illnesses. Although not easy to assess, Hulme (2010) provides questions to determine an individual's explanatory model for health conditions. Questions address the patients' perception of what they think caused the problem, why they think it started, and when it started; what they think their sickness does to them; how they perceive the severity and duration of the illness; what they expect from the treatment; the main problems the illness has caused them; and their fears about the illness.

When designing counseling and prevention programs for communities and populations, it is important to be guided by the notion that best practices in counseling and prevention programs do not automatically translate intact across cultural lines (Giihert, Harvey, & Belgrave, 2009). Adaptations of best practices to integrate culture-specific approaches can become an active ingredient in enhancing outcomes. Giihert and colleagues (2009) identified that Africentric interventions and culturally congruent practices targeting African American populations have demonstrated significantly greater positive outcomes across several important behavioral health areas, including increases in positive child, adolescent, and family development; improved outcomes for incarcerated individuals; and decreases in substance abuse and HIV risk behavior. Cultural translation is the process of adapting EB guidelines or best practice to be congruent with select populations of interest and should be

undertaken when there is "variability across groups, when cultural or contextual processes influence risk or protection from target problems, or when the external validity of evidence-based interventions is jeopardized by differences in engagement (e.g., participation rates, attrition, and compliance)" (DePue et al., 2010).

Understanding and integrating patient values require attention to salient ethnocultural factors, such as beliefs, language, and traditions. Developing a relationship with the patient; listening to the patient's expectations, concerns, and beliefs; and informing the patient of the evidence is the beginning to making the patient central to the decision-making process. With this base it is possible for a professional's perspective as health-care provider and the patient's preferences and characteristics to be weighed equally in the decision-making process, a process known as shared decision making. In shared decision making, the clinician contributes technical expertise, while the patient is the expert on his or her own needs, situations, and preferences. Bringing the two together advances the goal of the decision-making process to match care with patient preferences and to shift the locus of decision making from solely the clinician to the patient (Johnson, Kim, & Church, 2010).

Shared decision making is called for when there is no clearly indicated "best" therapeutic option or in preference-sensitive situations or situations where the best choice depends on the patients' values or their preferences for the benefits, harms, and scientific uncertainties of each option (Godolphin, 2009). It is the process of interacting with patients who wish to be involved in arriving at an informed, values-based choice among two or more medically reasonable alternatives. Examples of preference-sensitive situations include the following:

1. Should I have knee replacement surgery for my arthritis?
2. Should I take warfarin to prevent a stroke?
3. Should I take allergy shots?
4. Should I have an MRI for low back pain?
5. Should I stop taking my antidepressants and take herbal treatments?
6. Facilitating shared decision making involves communicating individualized information on treatment options, treatment outcomes, and probabilities of the benefits and risks and having patients reflect and discuss their personal values or the importance they place on benefits versus harms so that a decision on the best strategy can be reached.
7. Hulme (2010) emphasizes that not involving patients in shared decision making because of perceptions of inability to pay or different cultural models is paternalistic at best and an example of institutional racism at worst.
8. Clinicians need to partake in shared decision making with all patients and be willing to discuss options congruent with culture.

To assist clinicians with shared decision making, EB patient decision aids (PtDAs) have been developed. PtDAs are tools that help people become involved in decision making by providing information about the options and outcomes and by clarifying personal values (Godolphin, 2009). They aid people in making specific and deliberative choices among options by providing information about the options and outcomes that are relevant to a person's health status. In randomized trials, PtDAs have improved patient knowledge, improved the proportion of patients with realistic perceptions of the chances of benefits and risks, reduced decisional conflict/uncertainty, and prevented overuse of options that informed patients do not value (O'Connor, Llewellyn-Thomas, & Flood, 2004). They are different from traditional patient education material because they present balanced, personalized information about options in enough detail for patients to make informed judgments about the personal value of the options (O'Connor et al., 2007). They are designed to complement, rather than replace, counseling from a health-care provider.

O'Connor and colleagues (2004) found that decision aids had the following core elements: tailored information provision, exercises that support values clarification, and guidance in how to arrive at decisions. For a patient, a decision-making aid can help to clarify what he or she wants in a treatment, to weigh the pros and cons of different options, and to understand how the options would affect her or him personally (Edwards & Elwyn, 2009). With the use of a decision-making aid, patients can feel confident that they have the information necessary to make a decision. For clinicians, decision aids can promote more effective counseling by providing the clinician with more accurate, structured, and complete information; reducing the need to memorize information; and helping ensure compliance with standards (Elwyn, Frosch, Volandes, Edwards, & Montori, 2010).

The Ottowa Hospital Research Institute has as one of its primary missions practice-changing research with an emphasis on knowledge translation, clinical decision rules, and patient decision aids. It is a leader in shared decision-making research and has a tool for a general decision guide that can be used for any health or social decision, as well as nearly 300 decision aids on specific treatment topics. Other developers of PtDAs include the Foundation for Informed Medical Decision Making and its commercial partner Health Dialog, Healthwise, the Mayo Clinic, and the Dartmouth Hitchcock Center for Shared Decision Making. The National Cancer Institute and the Centers for Disease Control and Prevention are compiling and managing clearinghouses of decision aids. Searches for decision aids can be done by keying in the terms *decision aid, patient decision aid, decision guide,* or *patient decision guide* and the condition of interest.

To ensure quality in PtDA development, the CREDIBLE quality standards acronym can be used to evaluate the tool as shown in Table 3-3. The criteria were developed as part of the Cochrane Systematic Review of Patient Decision Aids.

Clinical Context

The clinical context encompasses the setting in which okay health care is provided or the environment in which the proposed change is to be implemented (McCormack, Kitson, Harvey, Rycroft-Malone, Titchen, & Seers, 2002). Drennan (1992) argues that culture, or "the way things are done around here," at

▶ Table 3-3   CREDIBLE Criteria for Evaluating Patient Aids

C	Competently Developed	• Are the essential components that promote quality decision making included? • Are the credentials of developers included in the decision aid or supporting materials? • Is the development process adequate? A complete development process includes a needs assessment and review by a panel of experts and a panel of potential users.
R	Recently Updated	• Does the developer have an update policy or evidence review process that is continuous or at least every two years?
E	Evidence-Based	• Is there a link to an evidence review group, or is the process that was used to identify and appraise evidence described? • Are references to scientific studies or systematic overviews used to support statements describing benefits/harms?
DI	Disclosures of Conflicts of Interest	• Is there disclosure of sponsorship and conflict of interest?
BL	Balanced Presentation of Options, Benefits, and Harms	• Is there a balanced presentation of potential harms and benefits? • Do the majority of users find it balanced?
E	Decision Aid Is Efficacious at Improving Decision Making	• Do evaluations show that the decision aid improves knowledge? • Do evaluations show that the decision aid is acceptable to users? • Do evaluations show other benefits? • Do evaluations show that it was free from adverse effects? • Do evaluations include a randomized controlled trial?

the individual, team, and organizational levels creates the context for practice and change. Organizational culture is a paradigm—a way of thinking about the organization, comprising a linkage of basic assumptions, values, and artifacts (Schein, 1992) and having its own belief system, paradigms, customs, and language. In addition to organizational culture, the medical culture also has a powerful influence on treatment approaches and modalities. The medical culture values objectivity, cause and effect, biophysical care, and, in many cases, the power of their own expertise and status. These cultures may be resistant to new paradigms calling for EBP. Additionally, these values may be in opposition to patient values, creating clashes between providers and patients.

A largely unexplored disparity currently exists between the beliefs and expectations of health-care providers and patients, particularly when there is also a disparity between the cultures/ethnicity of the two (Asthma and Allergy Foundation of America, 2005; Enarson & Ait-Khaled, 1999; Walker, Weeks, McAvoy, & Demetriou, 2005). Viewing biomedicine as a culture in itself, such that interactions between patients and health-care providers become a communication between cultures or transactions between worldviews, appears to be a necessary process in establishing a trusting and effective partnership and thus improving the health outcomes of patients.

The clinical context also includes the environment in which health behaviors are enacted. As such it goes beyond the traditional health-care organizational setting and includes the home, residential care, the neighborhood, and the broader community. The importance of context is becoming more apparent, with a greater emphasis on implementation science or the study of methods to promote the transfer of research findings into routine health-care policy and practice. However, evidence on which interventions work in specific contexts is not readily available.

Clearly, more research is needed that focuses on the contextual realities of implementation. It is believed that better attention to context will result in testable approaches to facilitate knowledge into action in real-world settings. Innovative approaches have been developed and can serve as models for clinicians. Three examples include the Centers for Disease Control and Prevention's (CDC) 's DEBI (Diffusion of Effective Behavioral Interventions , 2001) project (www.effectiveinterventions.org), the RE-AIM framework, and the Health Care Innovations Exchange.

The DEBI project was designed to bring science-based, community, group, and individual-level HIV prevention interventions to community-based service providers and state and local health departments and has documented many innovations for implementation science approaches. It provides strategies for community, group, and structural interventions to facilitate

adoption of health behaviors that will reduce the spread of HIV.

The RE-AIM (2011) framework (www.re-aim.org) was first used as a model to encourage consistent reporting of research results, then as a way to organize reviews of the existing literature on health promotion and disease management in different settings, and, subsequently, as a model to translate research into practice and to help plan programs and improve their chances of working in real-world settings. It is a valuable framework for understanding the relative strengths and weaknesses of different approaches to health promotion and chronic disease self-management, such as in-person counseling, group education classes, telephone counseling, and Internet resources in a variety of contexts. These are the five steps to translate research into action:

1. Identify strategies to effectively **Reach** your target population.
2. Test the **Effectiveness** or efficacy in the target population.
3. Develop strategies to facilitate **Adoption** of strategies by target settings or institutions.
4. Ensuring that the intervention is **Implemented** consistently.
5. **Maintenance** of intervention effects in individuals and settings over time.

Reach and efficacy are individual levels of impact. In order to reach beyond the individual level to gain wider translation, it is necessary to consider organizational strategies: adoption and implementation. Maintenance can be at both individual and organizational levels of impact.

Finally, AHRQ, Health Care Innovations Exchange is a web-based repository of evidence aimed at increasing the rate of implementation of new and better ways of delivering health care toward its mission to improve the quality of health care and reduce disparities. It offers busy health professionals and researchers a variety of opportunities to share, learn about, and ultimately adopt EB innovations and tools suitable for a range of health-care settings and populations (http://www.innovations.ahrq.gov/about.aspx).

The abundance of new evidence that has *not* been successfully translated into practice is a critical reminder of the importance of context and the strength of the existing culture. Difficult questions remain to be addressed. What should be done with health-care providers who cannot or will not adapt to EBP? How will lack of interdisciplinary collaboration be approached? How will it be handled if long-standing treatment approaches show no evidence of fostering improvement? What is the individual's responsibility compared with the organization's and community's responsibilities in ensuring readiness for EBP? What are the best approaches for facilitating knowledge translation in different contexts? Knowing the answer to some of these questions will influence outcomes of getting knowledge into practice.

Evidence-based practice is not research-directing practice but evidence-informing practice. The clinician evaluates best evidence in light of his or her clinical expertise, patient preferences, and clinical context to make decisions about patient or program management. Health-care providers practicing from an EB perspective need the skills to acquire and evaluate evidence, make decisions about adaptation of evidence, or plan to be congruent with the patient values and clinical context.

REFERENCES

Agency for Healthcare Research and Quality. (2010). *2010 National healthcare disparities report.* U.S. Department of Health and Human Services. Rockville, MD. Retrieved from http://www.ahrq.gov/qual/nhdr10/nhdr10.pdf

Antes, G., Sauerland, S., & Seiler, C. M. (2006). Evidence-based medicine—From best research evidence to a better surgical practice and health care. *Archives of Surgery, 391,* 61–67.

Asthma and Allergy Foundation and the National Pharmaceutical Council. (2005). *Asthma and Allergy Foundation of America. Ethnic disparities in the burden and treatment of asthma.* National Pharmaceutical Council.

Boyle, J., & Andrews, M. (2011). *Transcultural concepts in nursing* (5th ed.). Philadelphia: Lippincott.

Calvillo, E., Clark, L. Ballantyne, J., Pacquiao, D., Purnell, L., & Villarruel, A. (2009). Cultural competency in baccalaureate education. *Journal of Transcultural Nursing, 20*(2), 137–145.

CASP International. (2011). Retrieved April 8, 2011 from http://www.caspinternational.org/?o=1012

Clough, E. (2005). Foreword. In J. Burr and P. Nicholson (Eds.), *Researching health care consumers, critical approaches* (pp. ix–xi). Basingstoke, UK: Palgrave (MacMillan).

International Medical Interpreters Association. (1987). *Code of ethics for medical interpreters.* Retrieved from http://www.imiaweb.org/uploads/pages/376.pdf

Con, A. (2008). *Cross-cultural considerations in promoting advance care planning in Canada.* Retrieved from http://www.bccancer.bc.ca/NR/rdonlyres/E17D408A-C0DB-40FA-9682-9DD914BB771F/28582/COLOUR030408_Con.pdf

Cronewett, L., Sherwood, G., Pohl, J., Barnsteiner, J., Moore, S., Sullivan, D.T., Ward, D., & Warren, J. (2009). Quality and safety education for advanced nursing practice. *Nursing Outlook, 57*(6), 338–348.

DePue, J.D., Rosen, R.K., Batts-Turner, M., Bereolos, N., House, M. Held, R.F., Nu'usolia, O., Tuitele, J., Goldstein, M.G., & McGarvey, S.T. (2010). Cultural translation of interventions: Diabetes care in American Samoa. *American Journal of Public Health, 100*(11), 2085–2093.

Douglas, M., Pierce, J., Rosenkoetter, M., Clark Callister, L., Hattar-Pollara, M., Lauderdale, J., Milstead, J., Nardi, D., Pacquiao, D., & Purnell, L. (2011). Standards of practice for culturally competent nursing care. *Journal of Transcultural Nursing, 22*(4), 317–334.

Drennan, D. (1992). *Transforming company culture.* London: McGraw-Hill.

Edwards, A., & Elwyn, G., eds. (2009). *Shared decision-making. Achieving evidence-based patient choice.* Oxford: Oxford University Press.

Elwyn, G., Frosch, D., Volandes, A.E., Edwards, A., & Montori, V.M. (2010). Investing in deliberation: A definition and classification of decision support interventions for people facing difficult health decisions. *Medical Decision Making, 30,* 701–711.

Enarson, D.A., & Ait-Khaled, N. (1999) Cultural barriers to asthma management [commentary] *Pediatric Pulmonology, 28,* 297–300.

Family Health International. (2010). *Evidence-based guidelines for youth peer education.* Retrieved from http://www.fhi.org/NR/rdonlyres/einc2hb5no52blspygp6gksckcgdvpa6b76gfevo7k537fzyc53zrangjrhxisliwsagwqjeju7kfn/peeredguidelines.pdf

Foggs, M.B. (2008). Guidelines management of asthma in a busy urban practice. *Current Opinions in Pulmonary Medicine, 14*(1), 46–56.

Giger, J., Davidhizar, R., Purnell, L., Taylor Harden, J., Phillips, J., & Strickland, O. (2007). American Academy of Nursing Expert Panel Report: Developing cultural competence to eliminate health disparities in ethnic minorities and other vulnerable populations. *Journal of Transcultural Nursing, 18*(2), 95–102.

Giihert, D.J., Harvey, Á.R., & Belgrave, F.Z. (2009). Advancing the Africentric paradigm shift discourse: Building toward evidence-based Africentric interventions in social work practice with African Americans. *Social Work, 54*(1), 243–252.

Godolphin, W. (2009). Shared decision making. *Healthcare Quality, 12,* 186–190.

Gray, B. (1998). Sources used in health policy research and implications for information retrieval systems. *Journal of Urban Health, 75*(4), 842–852.

Haynes, R.B. (2006). Of studies, syntheses, synopses, summaries and systems: The "5S" evolution of information services for evidence-based health care decisions. *American·Collge of Physicians (ACP) Journal Club, 145*(3), A8–A9.

Hulme, P.A. (2010). Cultural considerations in evidence-based practice. *Journal of Transcultural Nursing, 21*(3), 271–280.

Johnson, S.L., Kim, Y.W., Church, K. (2010). Towards client-centered counseling: Development and testing of the WHO Decision-Making Tool, *Patient Education and Counseling, 81,* 355–361.

Joint Commission. *Advancing effective communication, cultural competence and family centered care: A roadmap for hospitals.* (2010). Joint Commission.

Kaplan, J.E., Benson, C., Holmes, K.H., Brooks, J.T., Pau, A., & Masur, H. (2009). Centers for Disease Control and Prevention (CDC), National Institutes of Health, HIV Medicine Association of the Infectious Diseases Society of America. Guidelines for prevention and treatment of opportunistic infections in HIV-infected adults and adolescents: Recommendations from CDC, the National Institutes of Health, and the HIV Medicine Association of the Infectious Diseases Society of America. *MMWR Recommendation Report, 10,* 58(RR-4), 1–207.

Kitson, A. (2002). Recognizing relationships: Reflections on evidence-based practice. *Nursing Inquiry, 9*(3), 179–186.

Management of Asthma Working Group. (2009). *VA/DoD clinical practice guideline for management of asthma in children and adults.* Washington, DC: Department of Veteran Affairs, Department of Defense.

McMurray, A. (2004). Culturally sensitive evidence-based practice. *Collegian, 11,* 14–18.

McCormack, B., Kitson, A., Harvey, G., Rycroft-Malone, J., Titchen, A., & Seers, K. (2002). Getting evidence into practice: The meaning of "context." *Journal of Advanced Nursing, 38*(1), 94–104.

Melnyk, B.M., Fineout-Overholt, E., Stillwell, S.B., & Williamson, K.M. (2009). Igniting a spirit of inquiry: An essential foundation for evidence-based practice. *American Journal of Nursing, 109*(11), 49–52.

Mosley, C. (2009). Evidence-based medicine: The dark side. *Journal of Pediatric Orthopedics, 29*(8), 839–843.

National Assessment of Adult Literacy. (2003). Retrieved from http://nces.ed.gov/naal/

National Council on Interpreting in Health Care. (2007). Retrieved from www.ncihc.org/

National Network of Libraries of Medicine. (2011). Retrieved from http://nnlm.gov/

New York Academy of Medicine. (2011). *Grey literature report.* Retrieved from http://www.nyam.org/library/online-resources/grey-literature-report/

O'Connor, A.M., Stacey, D., Entwistle, V., Llewellyn-Thomas, H., Rovner, D., Holmes-Rovner, M., Tait, V., Tetroe, J., Fiset, V., Barry, M., & Jones J. (2004). *Decision aids for people facing health treatment or screening decisions. Cochrane Review, Issue 1.* Chichester, UK: John Wiley & Sons, Ltd.

O'Connor, A.M., Llewellyn-Thomas, H.A., & Flood, A.B. (2004). Modifying unwarranted variations in health care: Shared decision making using patient decision aids. *Health Affairs, no. (2004).* Retrieved from http://content.healthaffairs.org/content/early/2004/10/07/hlthaff.var.63.citation

O'Connor, A.M., Wennberg, J.E., Legare, F., Llewellyn-Thomas, H.A., Mouton, B.W., Sepucha, K.R., Sodano, A.G., & King, J.S. (2007). Toward the "Tipping Point": Decision aids and informed patient choice. *Health Affairs, 26*(3), 716–725.

Ottowa Hospital Research Institute. (2011). Retrieved from http://decisionaid.ohri.ca/AZinvent.php

RE-AIM: Reach, Effectiveness, Adaptation, Implementation, and Effectiveness. (2011). Retrieved April 8, 2011 from http://www.re-aim.org/about-re-aim.aspx

Rycroft-Malone, J., Seers K., Titchen, A., Harvey, G., Kitson, A., & McCormack, B. (2004). *Journal of Advanced Nursing, 47*(1), 81–90.

Sackett, D. (2000). *Evidence-based medicine: How to practice and teach EB* (2nd ed.). Amsterdam, The Netherlands: Churchill Livingtone.

Salmond, S. (2007). Advancing evidence-based practice: A primer. *Orthopaedic Nursing, 26*(2), 114–123.

Schein, E. H. (1992). *Organizational culture and leadership* (2nd ed). San Francisco, CA: Jossey-Bass.

Shah, H.M., & Chung, K.C. (2009). Archie Cochrane and his vision for evidence-based medicine. *Plastic and Reconstructive Surgery, 124*(3), 982–988.

Swanson, J.A., Schmitz, D., & Chung, K.C. (2010). How to practice evidence-based medicine. *Plastic & Reconstructive Surgery, 126*(1), 286–294.

Walker, C., Weeks, A., McAvoy, B., & Demetriou, E. (2005). Exploring the role of self-management programs in caring for people from culturally and linguistically diverse backgrounds in Melbourne, Australia. *Health Expect, 8,* 315–323.

World Health Organization/Pan American Health Organization (HO/PAHO). (2010). *Culture and mental health in Haiti: A literature review.* Geneva: WHO. Retrieved from http://www.who.int/mental_health/emergencies/culture_mental_health_haiti_eng.pdf

DavisPlus *For case studies, review questions, and additional information, go to* **http://davisplus.fadavis.com**

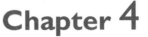

Chapter 4

Organizational Cultural Competence

Stephen R. Marrone

Throughout the world, an emerging consensus is that cultural competence is an essential component of accessible, socially responsive, and fiscally efficient quality health care. According to the Institute of Medicine (2002), the key component that affects health disparities is the cultural competency of the health-care provider. However, providing culturally competent care has been hindered to some extent by a dearth of systematic approaches and organizational support.

Cultural competence does not relate solely to the care of patients, families, and the community; it is also applicable to educational, health-care, and professional organizations. As described in the Purnell Model (see Chapter 2), the workforce issues domain can be used to assess organizational culture and cultural issues among staff.

The purpose of this chapter, therefore, is to provide an overview of the requisite organizational infrastructure designed to create and sustain cultural competency. The National Standards for the Delivery of Culturally and Linguistically Appropriate Health Care Services (Office of Minority Health, 2001), the Cultural Competence Assessment Profile (HRSA, 2002), and the Purnell Model for Cultural Competence, provide the organizing framework for this chapter.

Health Disparities

Racial and ethnic diversity among health-care providers correlates with the delivery of quality care to diverse patient populations (Betancourt, Green, Carrillo, & Ila, 2003). Evidence demonstrates that racial concordance between minority patients and minority physicians is associated with greater patient satisfaction and higher self-rated quality of care (Saha, Komaromy, Koepsell, & Bindman, 1999). Evidence also supports that minority patients prefer minority physicians regardless of practice

location or other geographic issues (Saha, Taggart, Kamaromy, & Bindman, 2000). Spanish-speaking patients, for example, report greater satisfaction when care is provided by Spanish-speaking providers than by non–Spanish-speaking providers (Morales, Cunningham, Brown, Liu, & Hays, 1999). Likewise, African-American patients report more satisfaction with care when their physician utilizes an inclusive, participatory decision-making approach to health care (Cooper-Patrick et al., 1999). However, other surveys report that not all patients prefer a health-care provider of the same background (Robert Wood Johnson Foundation, 2011).

Health disparities data suggest that members of minority groups experience a disproportionately higher rate of illness, more severe complications, and increased mortality and morbidity related to cardiovascular disease, diabetes, asthma, and cancer (OMH, 2002). Multiple factors external to the health-care system influence health disparities—namely, lower socioeconomic status of minorities, hazardous jobs with increased incidence of injury, lower educational and literacy levels, lack of or inadequate health insurance, fear of the health-care system, overuse of over-the-counter medications and home remedies, and the use of the emergency department for care. A systemic review of the literature entitled *Unequal Treatment: Confronting Racial/Ethnic Disparities in Health Care*, conducted by the Institute of Medicine, reported the findings of more than 175 studies that illustrated racial and ethnic disparities in the diagnosis and treatment of multiple medical conditions, even when analyses were controlled for socioeconomic status, insurance status, site of care, stage of disease, comorbidities, and age (IOM, 2003).

The root causes of health disparities relate to a disconnect between patients' health beliefs, values, preferences, and behaviors and those of the dominant health-care system (Coleman-Miller, 2000). This lack of fit includes variations in patient recognition of symptoms; thresholds for seeking care; the ability to communicate symptoms to a provider who understands their meaning; the ability to understand the prescribed treatment plan, including use of medications; expectations of care; access to and utilization of diagnostic and therapeutic procedures; and adherence to preventive measures (Einbinder & Schulman, 2000). These core factors are considered to be the primary influencers for decision making among patients and health-care providers, physicians in particular, and the degree to which patients access and interact with the health-care delivery system (Public Health Reports, 2003). Emphasis on cultural competency in health care and culturally competent health-care organizations has emerged as a result of these findings.

Culturally Competent Health-Care Organizations

Cultural competence in health care has been defined as "a set of congruent behaviors, attitudes, and policies that come together in a system, agency, or among professionals and enable that system, agency, or those professionals to work effectively in cross-cultural situations" (HRSA, 2002, p. 3). The tenets of cultural competency are not specific to one health-care discipline and must be inclusive of all professional disciplines, as well as clerical, technical, and unlicensed assistive personnel. Hence, the provision of culturally safe care relies on all members of the health-care team receiving consistent and comparable information about the needs of the diverse patients, families, and communities they serve (Public Health Reports, 2003). It is important to understand that cultural competency is a process and not a result (Purnell, Davidhizar, Giger, Fishman, Strickland, & Allison, 2011). To be effective, health care must reflect the unique understanding of the values, beliefs, attitudes, lifeways, and worldviews of diverse populations and individual acculturation patterns (Purnell, 2008).

A culturally competent health-care organization incorporates culture at all levels to meet culturally unique needs (Purnell et al., 2011). Culturally competent health-care organizations outperform their competitors by achieving and sustaining greater performance and outcomes measures and increased market share as evidenced by improved consumer access to care. Enhanced quality of care reduces health disparities and improves health outcomes for vulnerable and underserved populations. Thus, greater patient and staff satisfaction leads to an increased consumer market share to and secures financial sustainability of the organization (Marrone, 2010).

> ▶ *Examining where you work/go to school, what evidence can you find that the mission and philosophy of the organization include statements on diversity and inclusion? Is the board of trustees reflective of the diversity of the community and patient population?*

Culturally competent health-care delivery organizations provide consumers with effective, understandable, and respectful care provided in ways that fit with their cultural values and beliefs and in the consumer's preferred language. To achieve this goal, organizations develop, implement, and promote a written strategic plan that outlines clear goals, policies, operational plans, and management accountability/oversight mechanisms to provide culturally and linguistically appropriate services. Consequently, to ensure the design of an evidence-based strategic plan, the organization conducts initial and ongoing organizational self-assessments of diversity-related activities. It integrates cultural and linguistic competence-related measures into internal audits, performance improvement programs, patient satisfaction assessments, and outcomes-based evaluations. Finally, it collects and updates information related to consumers' race, ethnicity, and spoken and written language(s) and integrates this information into the organization's data management system. These data help maintain a current demographic, cultural, and epidemiological profile of the community to plan for and implement services that respond to its cultural and linguistic characteristics (OMH, 2001).

> ▶ *Does the organization where you work/go to school have a strategic plan that reflects the needs of the community? What would you recommend to improve organizational competence?*

To determine the need for diversity-related services, it is essential that organizations create a community demographic needs assessment tool to assess the cultural beliefs and language needs of the people who live there. To provide effective patient education, it is necessary to review the language literacy level and the use of culturally respectful images in written and visual (i.e., television or video) patient education materials. Organizations should develop systems that indicate whether language assistance is needed prior to or at the point of entry into the organization (Purnell et al., 2011)

A key ingredient to creating and sustaining organizational cultural competency is to designate *diversity champions* who have acquired the requisite knowledge and skills to provide culturally congruent care at all levels within the organization. Champions can mentor other health-care providers within their discipline and/or department to expand their influence on consumer care and services. Furthermore, culturally competent human resources departments promote patient-centered care by including patient satisfaction measures in employee performance appraisals (Purnell et al., 2011), by establishing diversity-related sentinel events, and by completing a root cause analysis. Culturally competent organizations create their own or revise standardized consumer satisfaction tools to include items related to the provision of culturally and linguistically appropriate care and monitor data at all levels of committee and council meetings throughout the organization. Developing a data bank with best practices and lessons learned need not be complex. The following items have been used successfully:

1. "Did you receive care that was respectful to your cultural and religious beliefs?"
2. "Did you receive care in your preferred language?"
3. "Did you receive care in a language that helped you to make informed decisions?"

To be effective, written satisfaction surveys should be translated into the languages that represent the catchment area for the organization (Purnell et al., 2011).

Andrews (1998) provided the following six-step framework for ensuring organizational cultural competency:

1. Collect demographic and descriptive data of the prevalent cultural, ethnic, linguistic, and spiritual groups represented among patients, families, visitors, the community, and the staff in the service area.
2. Describe the effectiveness of current systems and processes in meeting diverse needs.
3. Assess the organization's strengths and limitations by examining the institution's ethos toward cultural diversity and the presence or absence of a corporate culture that promotes accord among its constituents.
4. Determine organizational need and readiness for change through dialogue with key stakeholders aimed at discovering foci of anticipated support and recognizing areas of potential resistance.
5. Implement strategic plans, policies, and procedures that include measurable benchmarks of success and an ongoing process to ensure that change is maintained.
6. Evaluate actual outcomes against established benchmarks utilizing performance improvement, quality, and customer satisfaction data.

Culturally competent health-care organizations implement strategies to recruit, retain, and promote at all levels of the organization a diverse staff and leadership team that are representative of the demographics of the service area. The goal of recruiting and retaining a diverse workforce that matches the demographics of the service area is to reduce health disparities among vulnerable and underserved populations that often results from discordant consumer–provider

relationships. Culture and language discordance can lead to decreased access to care, decreased quality of care, increased cost of care, decreased patient satisfaction, recidivism, discrimination, and poor health outcomes (American Association of Critical Care Nurses, 2008; Europa, 2010).

▶ *In the organization where you work/go to school, are pictures, posters, and calendars representing the diversity of the patient and staff posted throughout the organization? What additional pictures or posters would you include?*

To reduce discordance between consumers and providers, an organization needs to integrate diversity into the organization's mission statement, strategic plans, and goals (Purnell et al., 2011). A diverse workforce program should include mentoring programs, community-based internships, and collaborations with academic partners such as universities, local schools, training programs, and faith-based organizations. To expand the recruitment base, organizations should recruit at minority health and recruitment fairs, advertise in multiple languages, and list job opportunities in minority publications such as local newspapers and community newsletters (Purnell et al., 2011).

CLAS Standards

The National Standards on Culturally and Linguistically Appropriate Services in Health Care (CLAS Standards) were developed via national consensus by the U.S. Department of Health and Human Services—Office of Minority Health (OMH). The CLAS Standards were intended to guide health-care organizations in the provision of safe care and services that were culturally, ethnically, linguistically, and spiritually appropriate and effective. The guiding principles and associated actions and interventions of culturally and linguistically appropriate health-care services are intended to be integrated throughout the organization and designed, implemented, and evaluated in partnership with the communities being served (OMH, 2001).

The 14 CLAS Standards are organized according to the following themes (OMH, 2001):

1. Standards 1–3 reflect culturally competent care.
2. Standards 4–7 refer to language access services, such as interpreter and translation services.
3. Standards 8–14 outline organizational support for cultural competence in health care. These standards are currently under revision and therefore will not be repeated here in their entirety.

Cultural Competence Assessment Profile

The Cultural Competence Assessment Profile, funded by the U.S. Department of Health and Human Services—Health Resources and Services Administration (HRSA), was developed to answer the question "How do we know cultural competence when we see it?" (HRSA, 2002). The Profile is based on evidence from foundational work in organizational cultural competency such as the CLAS Standards and provides the infrastructure to conceptualize how to assess cultural competence at the organizational level. Essentially, the profile is intended to gather information based on the specific performance and outcomes characteristics that should be evident across the health-care continuum in a culturally competent organization. The Profile can assist organizations by providing a framework to organize activities related to the cultural competence and quality monitoring for compliance with cultural competence standards (HRSA, 2002).

The Assessment Profile was built on the following assumptions:

- Organizational cultural competence is an integral component of patient-centered care and can contribute to improving access to care, quality of care, and health outcomes.
- Health-care organizations drive the development and maintenance of individual provider cultural competence and the environment of care.
- Cultural competence is a business imperative that supports organizational branding and increases the organization's market share among diverse cultural groups, thereby leading to continuous service and process improvements (HRSA, 2002).

The performance areas of the Cultural Competence Assessment Profile include organizational values, governance, planning and monitoring/evaluation, communication, staff development, organizational infrastructure, and services/interventions (HRSA, 2002). Organizational values refer to the organization's viewpoint regarding cultural competence and its commitment to provide culturally congruent care. Governance relates to goal-setting, policy-making, and oversight methods used to help ensure the delivery of culturally congruent care. *Planning, monitoring, and evaluation* include the use of internal and external stakeholders in short- and long-term planning for the delivery of culturally congruent health-care services. *Communication* focuses on the schema through which information is exchanged, vertically and horizontally, with internal and external consumers, executives, and members of the health-care team in order to promote cultural competence. *Staff development* underscores the need for organizations to ensure that staff at all levels of the organization acquire the attitudes, knowledge, and skills for delivering culturally congruent care. *Organizational infrastructure* refers to organizational resources required to hardwire the delivery of culturally congruent care and services throughout the continuum of care. *Services and interventions* relate to an organization's delivery of clinical and community health services that reflect the needs of the diverse consumer groups within the organization's service area (HRSA, 2002).

The Purnell Model

Theories and conceptual models are essential in scientific disciplines because they enable health-care providers to describe, explain, and predict concepts and phenomena. Nursing and health-care theories guide practice, influence decisions and interventions, and provide a framework for evaluating outcomes. Theory serves as the foundation for the provision of culturally congruent care by culturally competent health-care providers.

The Purnell Model is based on theories and evidence derived from organizational, administrative, communication, and family development theories, in addition to anthropology, sociology, psychology, anatomy and physiology, biology, ecology, nutrition, pharmacology, religion, history, economics, political science, and linguistics. Hence, the major assumptions of the Purnell Model that affect organizational cultural competency were developed from a broad perspective, allowing their use across practice disciplines and organizational/environmental contexts. See Chapter 2 for a complete description of the Purnell Model.

The Purnell Model is germane to all health-care disciplines in a variety of environmental contexts. The 12 domains of the Purnell Model can provide an organizing framework for organizational cultural competency as it highlights the importance of interprofessional collaboration with emphasis on patient-centered care, managed care, and case management across the health-care continuum. The model can guide the development of assessment instruments, planning strategies, and individualized patient, family, or community interventions

As outlined in Table 4-1, triangulation among the Purnell Model, current CLAS Standards (OMH, 2002), and the Cultural Assessment Profile (HRSA, 2002) can be used to frame the design of an organizational cultural competency program. The Purnell domain *overview and heritage* supports that culturally competent organizations articulate mission and vision statements, values, a strategic plan, and standard operating procedures (policies and procedures) that reflect the value of diversity. The mission, vision, and values drive the shared governance model that provides for a dedicated chief diversity officer to oversee the activities of a transdisciplinary diversity council. A cultural health assessment should be included in patient history and assessment data at all points of entry into the system. Traditional or folk healing practices that are integrated into the plan of care should be identified.

The Purnell domain *communication* supports organizational efforts to ensure that signage is placed in all

(continued on page 68)

▐▌ Table 4-1 Crosswalk: Purnell Model, CLAS Standards, and Cultural Assessment

Purnell Model Domains[1]	CLAS Standards[2]	Cultural Assessment Profile[3]	Indicators
Overview/Heritage Advocates for the formation of a transdisciplinary diversity council, ethics committee, and patient education committee that include community members and give attention to the health literacy of the service area. A strong community partnerships with key individuals and agencies reflective of the demographics in the service area, and the health-care team should include community members of governing board (Purnell, 2011).	*Standard 1:* Effective, respectful care in preferred language. *Standard 2:* Cultural, demographic, and epidemiological community profile.	*Domains:* Organizational values Governance Staff development Organizational infrastructure	• Mission, vision, values, strategic plan, and standard operating procedures (policies and procedures) that reflect value of diversity • Shared governance model • Dedicated chief diversity officer • Diversity competence program for all levels of staff • History and assessment databases that include traditional and folk healing practices • Cultural health assessment performed by clinical staff • Code of professionalism that outlines diverse behavioral expectations • Breaches trigger a "culture code" for immediate intervention • Transdisciplinary diversity council, ethics committee, and patient education committee that include community members • Community partnerships with key individuals and agencies reflective of the demographics in the service area and the health-care team • Community members of the governing board and decision-making groups • Dynamic demographic data collection and management systems
Communication supports organizational efforts to ensure that signage is placed in all areas in multiple languages related to directions within the organization. Requires that the availability of language assistance services and includes sign language, the translation of critical documents such as consents and patient education materials, pain scales, and communication boards/aids for patients who are not able to speak or understand the dominant language.	Language assistance services *Standard 5:* Notice of language assistance services *Standard 6:* Competence of language assistance services provided by interpreters *Standard 7:* Translated signage and patient materials	*Domain:* Governance	• Signage in multiple languages • Translation of critical documents such as consent forms, patient education materials, pain scales, communication boards • Patient education programs that address diversity of the service area, such as meal planning for diabetes management of Caribbean Americans • Customer service initiatives that address diversity • Maintain an organizational language

II▶ Table 4-1 **Crosswalk: Purnell Model, CLAS Standards, and Cultural Assessment** *Continued from page 64*

Purnell Model Domains[1]	CLAS Standards[2]	Cultural Assessment Profile[3]	Indicators
Family roles and organization Can guide the development of organizational visitation policies, including open visiting hours that address cultural norms and visitor role responsibilities; policies related to diverse decision-making practices, such as informed consent; and the purchase and utilization of racially, ethnically, and age-appropriate toys for infants and children and high-fidelity manikins used in simulation education.	*Standard 1:* Effective, respectful care in preferred language	*Domains:* Organizational values Planning Monitoring, and evaluation Staff development Organizational infrastructure Services and interventions	• Visitation policies, including open visiting hours that address cultural norms and visitor role responsibilities • Protocols for diverse decision-making practices, such as informed consent • Racially, ethnically, and age-appropriate toys and manikins used in simulation education
Workforce issues Supports the development of diversity-related education content and competencies integrated into orientation, in-service education, staff development, and continuing education programs for all levels of staff and the integration and utilization of a standardized communication method such as SBAR (Situation, Background, Assessment, and Recommendation) among the interprofessional healthcare team	*Standard 2:* Recruit, retain, and promote diversity *Standard 3:* Ongoing staff education *Standard 8:* Written strategic plan *Standard 9:* Conduct organizational self-assessment *Standard 10:* Collect demographics and integrate into data management system *Standard 11:* Implement services based on demographic profile *Standard 12:* Collaborative community partnerships *Standard 13:* Culturally relevant conflict management processes *Standard 14:* Inform public of diversity-related initiatives	*Domains:* Organizational values Governance Communication Staff development Organizational infrastructure	• Diversity content and competencies integrated into orientation, in-service education, staff development, and continuing education programs for all levels of staff • Standardized communication methods among caregivers, such as using SBAR or other shared mental and communication models
Biocultural ecology Gives direction to the development of educational programs and clinical practices that recognize physical and genetic variations that have an impact on assessment and treatment plans including preventive services and early screening, and to the design of patient education, counseling, and screening related to known genetic predispositions to diseases and biological variations regarding the pharamcokinetics of medications and other substances.	*Standard 1:* Effective, respectful care in preferred language	*Domains:* Organizational values Planning Monitoring and evaluation Staff development Organizational infrastructure Services and interventions	• Educational programs and clinical practices that recognize physical and genetic variations that affect assessment and treatment plans including preventive services and early screening. • Patient education, counseling, and screening related to known genetic predispositions to diseases and biological variations regarding drug metabolism.

Continues on page 66

⫸ Table 4-1   Crosswalk: Purnell Model, CLAS Standards, and Cultural Assessment *Continued from page 65*

Purnell Model Domains[1]	CLAS Standards[2]	Cultural Assessment Profile[3]	Indicators
High-risk behavior Identifies the need for assessing known high-risk behaviors in the service area and including these behaviors on the risk assessment portions of patient admission histories and health screenings for inclusion in patients' plans of care.	*Standard 1:* Effective, respectful care in preferred language	*Domains:* Organizational values Planning Monitoring and evaluation Staff development Organizational infrastructure Services and interventions	• Assessment for known high risk behaviors in the service area included on admission histories and health screenings to be included in the patients plan of care. • Patient and community education programs that address high-risk behaviors in the catchment area, i.e., smoking cessation, alcohol and drug abuse, teen pregnancy. • Community outreach programs and community partnerships that address high risk behaviors related to morbid and mortality in the service area.
Nutrition Lends importance to creating menu plans that reflect the demographics of the services area, such as offering kosher or halal meals or other ethnic meal choices; formulating policies and procedures that address bringing ethnic foods from home; using hot versus cold foods and drinks during illness and recovery; and establishing flexible meal times to accommodate culturally driven meal time preferences, for example, offering dinner at sundown for fasting during Ramadan for Muslim patients.	*Standard 1:* Effective, respectful care in preferred language.	*Domains:* Organizational values Planning Monitoring ,and evaluation Staff development Organizational infrastructure Services and interventions	• Menu plans that reflect the demographics of the services area, i.e., Kosher, Halal, or other ethnic meal choices. • Policies and procedures that address bring food from home. • Use of hot versus cold foods during illness and recovery. • Flexible meal times to accommodate culturally driven meal time preferences i.e., day time fasting for Muslim patients during Ramadan.
Pregnancy and childbearing practices Supports the development of perinatal practices, policies, and procedures that address diverse birthing practices, including gender roles and responsibilities before, during, and after birth; hot versus cold; and views of birth as a sickness/illness or natural experience.	*Standard 1:* Effective, respectful care in preferred language.	*Domains:* Organizational values Planning Monitoring and evaluation Staff development Organizational infrastructure Services and interventions	Labor and delivery and postpartum policies and procedures that address diverse birthing practices, including gender roles and responsibilities, hot versus cold, and views of birth as a sickness/illness or natural experience
Death rituals Requires that organizations develop plans for the provision of culturally relevant palliative care services, policies, procedures, and staff competencies that address diverse dying and bereavement practices across the lifespan, and culturally relevant counseling services related to death and dying, organ donation, and care of the body at the time of death.	*Standard 1:* Effective, respectful care in preferred language.	*Domains:* Organizational values Planning Monitoring and evaluation Staff development Organizational infrastructure Services and interventions	• Culturally relevant palliative care services. • Policies, procedures, and competencies that address diverse dying and bereavement practices across the lifespan. • Culturally relevant counseling services related to death and dying, organ donation, and care of the body.

IID Table 4-1 | **Crosswalk: Purnell Model, CLAS Standards, and Cultural Assessment** *Continued from page 66*

Purnell Model Domains[1]	CLAS Standards[2]	Cultural Assessment Profile[3]	Indicators
Spirituality Requires organizations to make certain that chaplain services are available for each religion that is represented within the service area. Partnerships with key community religious leaders, including traditional and folk healers should be established in response to the cultural and spiritual needs of consumers and staff.	*Standard 1:* Effective, respectful care in preferred language.	*Domains:* Organizational values Planning Monitoring and evaluation Staff development Organizational infrastructure Services and interventions	• Chaplain services for all dominant religions. • Partnerships with community leaders. • Policies and procedures that address work schedule, meal and medication times, and hours of operation (i.e., clinic visits) in response to cultural and spiritual needs of consumers and staff.
Health-care practice Underscores the need for cultural competent education for all levels of clinical and administrative staff that addresses cultural perspectives of the sick role; medical management, including folk and traditional healing practices. Cultural emphasis on preventive versus acute care can guide the provision of community health and wellness programs to increase access to care, enhance quality of care, improve health outcomes at the individual and community levels, and reduce health disparities.	*Standard 1:* Effective, respectful care in preferred language	*Domains:* Organizational values Staff development	Cultural competency education that addresses cultural perspectives of the sick role, medical management including folk and traditional healing practices, genetic implications for care across the continuum, and cultural emphasis on preventive versus acute.
Health-care provider Highlights the need for a dedicated chief diversity officer to oversee diversity-related initiatives such as the diversity council, affirmative action program, discrimination events, culture codes, and culturally related conflict management and grievance procedures. Additionally, this domain supports the creation of job descriptions that outline role-related cultural competencies, job requirements that specify role specific language proficiency and cultural competencies, and initial and ongoing performance appraisals that include cultural competency requirements.	*Standard 1:* Effective, respectful care in preferred language	*Domains:* Organizational values, Communication, Organizational infrastructure	• Chief Diversity Officer position to oversee diversity-related initiatives. affirmative action, discrimination, culture codes, conflict management, and grievance procedures. • Job descriptions that outline cultural competency. • Job requirements that specify language proficiency and cultural competency. • Initial and ongoing performance appraisals that include cultural competency requirements.

Sources: [1]Purnell et al., 2011.
[2]OMH, 2001.
[3]HRSA, 2002.

areas in multiple languages related to directions within the organization. It also requires that the availability of language assistance services include sign language, the translation of critical documents such as consents and patient education materials, pain scales, and communication boards/aids for patients who are not able to speak or understand the dominant language.

Knowledge and Skill Acquisition

Health-care organizations should ensure that staff at all levels and across all disciplines receive ongoing education related to culturally and linguistically appropriate service delivery (OMH, 2001). To ensure the successful acquisition and maintenance of culturally and linguistically appropriate knowledge and skills, organizations must plan to allocate fiscal resources to educate staff at all levels in order to develop the requisite role-specific competencies for the provision of culturally congruent care. In addition, if bilingual staff express an interest in, and are able to provide, the service, internal and/or external funding sources should be made available to support the training of staff as medical interpreters.

Educational programming and learning outcomes related to cultural competence need to include, principally, the cognitive and affective domains of learning, with, to a lesser degree, the psychomotor domain. The curriculum should follow the educational design principle of *simple-to-complex* and *general-to-specific*. The learning objectives and educational content should be evidence-based and address definitions of cultural competence; discrimination, prejudice, and stereotyping; role-specific performance criteria for the provision of culturally congruent care; and the completion of a cultural health assessment, in general, and specific culture care needs of the most commonly encountered demographics of the service area in particular. Moreover, the education should also include self-reflection, critical thinking, and cross-cultural communication, including the appropriate use of medical interpreters. Generational diversity and the diversity that exists among the health-care team should also be addressed.

Diversity-related education must start in orientation and continue through unit/department-based, population-specific orientation programs. Additionally, diversity education should be woven into annual educational initiatives and performance appraisals using evidence-based assessment instruments to ensure the initial and ongoing maintenance of competency, including the proficiency of trained medical interpreters. To accommodate the variety of learning styles that exist within the health-care team, a variety of educational venues, such as face-to-face classroom interaction, online, Web-based programs, and online and/or hard-copy resources at the point of care should be available. Informal venues such as *lunch-and-learn*,

and including diversity-related topics on staff meeting agenda has been helpful to keep cultural competency visible in daily operations.

▶ *In the organization where you work/go to school, are culturally diversity classes required as part of orientation and on a yearly basis for administrators, professionals, and other health-care providers?*

Transdisciplinary, interprofessional team learning approaches have demonstrated improved communication within the health-care team. Onsite consultation and conferences and workshops conducted by experts in the fields of transcultural nursing, cultural competency, and organizational culture have been reported to help sustain diversity initiatives in fast-paced health-care delivery systems (IOM, 2002; Marrone, 2008). Other successful strategic initiatives within culturally competent organizations that support staff knowledge and skill acquisition include providing staff with incentives such as reward and recognition ceremonies, pins, acknowledgment in organizational newsletters or Web sites, preference to attend external conferences and workshops for staff that have completed initial and ongoing cultural competency education and competency requirements, and incentives for staff to volunteer in the community to learn about community members and the cultures represented within the service area.

Language Assistance Services

Culturally competent health-care organizations must provide language assistance services, including interpreter services, at no cost to the customer with limited English (or dominant language) proficiency at all points of contact and in a timely manner during all hours of operation. In addition, organizations must provide consumers in their preferred language both verbal and written notices informing them of their rights to receive language assistance services. Likewise, organizations must ensure the competence of language assistance provided to limited English proficient (or dominant language) consumers by interpreters and must make available easily understood patient-related materials and post signage in the languages of the commonly encountered groups and/or groups represented in the service area.

▶ *In your work setting, are major patient documents translated into the languages of the clients served? Which languages are included? What other languages would you recommend?*

According to multiple sources, language discordance can lead to decreased access to care, decreased quality of care, increased cost of care, decreased patient satisfaction, recidivism, discrimination, and poor health outcomes (AACN, 2003; 2008; Europa, 2010).

Patients who speak little or no English (or nondominant language) are at greater risk of medical errors or misdiagnosis if they are not provided with an interpreter, are less likely to use preventive care services, and are more likely to use emergency rooms than English (or dominant language) speakers (Cornelio, 2004).

Culturally competent health-care organizations must provide language assistance at all points of entry and care and during all hours of operation. Incorrect interpretation and/or translation can result in patient confusion, threaten patient safety, and cause emotional distress, resulting in increased costs to the organization. Resources for interpretation and translation services include interpretation agencies, community language banks, telephonic services at the point of care, and interactive video- or computer-based services for the deaf or hearing impaired (Tang, 2010). Frequently used techniques to identify the languages spoken within the community and service area—as well as the need for sign language—include information from the local community; community organizations; directly from consumers; national, regional, and community census data; and community needs assessment (Tang, 2010). Critical documents such as informed consent forms, patient education materials, and pain assessment tools, as well as signage and directions within the organization, should be translated into the major languages spoken by the consumers in the service area (Purnell et al., 2011).

▶ *What does your organization do to provide interpreters to patients who do not have a good command of English? What in-house resources are available to staff? Are language interpretation lines used? In what languages is interpretation readily available? What languages are needed but not available?*

There is an emerging body of knowledge related to health literacy and its relationship to patient health, compliance with medical treatment plans, and access to care. Health literacy is the degree to which an individual is able to read, understand, and use information to make health-care decisions (see Chapter 3). Low health literacy can have a negative impact on health outcomes and potentially increase the risk of medical errors. Negative sequelae can be minimized by the use of correctly interpreted and simple printed information with pictures and diagrams (see Chapter 3). Written policies and procedures for the development and purchase of written and/or video/audio patient education materials in the dominant and nondominant languages should be evaluated by a transdisciplinary patient education team, the members of which should include community partners and organizational constituents who are knowledgeable in health literacy and cultural competency (Marrone, 2010; Tang, 2010).

Community Resources and Partnerships

Socially responsible educational, health-care, and professional organizations, must be forged that use a variety of formal and informal mechanisms to facilitate community and consumer involvement in designing, implementing, and evaluating diversity-related initiatives (OMH, 2001). Active, bidirectional, and mutually beneficial partnerships with formal and informal community leaders and key informant interviews and focus group meetings with cultural and spiritual leaders, political and regulatory leaders and accrediting agencies, natural and lay healers, and community elders are all mechanisms to ensure that organizations provide culturally relevant services. Health-care organizations, in particular, need to negotiate with managed care organizations for culturally relevant health services across the continuum of care and advocate on behalf of the vulnerable and underserved populations within the organization's service sector.

Advocacy

Advocacy on behalf of consumer and health-care team diversity is a critical element within the schema of organizational cultural competency. Culturally competent health-care organizations ensure that conflict and grievance resolution processes are culturally and linguistically sensitive and capable of identifying, preventing, and resolving cross-cultural conflicts or complaints by patients/consumers (OMH, 2002). Furthermore, culturally competent health-care organizations establish an environment committed to diversity nondiscrimination through clearly articulated behavioral and performance expectations that are communicated to all levels of staff both verbally and in writing. In essence, culturally competent organizations create and sustain a culture of *zero tolerance* for discrimination in all sectors of the work environment.

▶ *Does the organization where you work/go to school have cultural brokering/mentoring programs for new employees? What strategies would you use to initiate such a program?*

Best practice supports the development of the *chief diversity officer* role to lead all diversity-related organizational initiatives, such as the diversity council. The chief diversity office and diversity council would have the following roles:

• Advise the chief executive team in the development of strategies that support diversifying the organization's workforce.
• Review organizational policies, recruitment practices, patient education materials, and care practices that may have an adverse impact on one or more consumer groups within the service area (Thornicroft, Brohan, Kassam, & Lewis-Holmes, 2008).

- Establish written, evidence-based criteria for hiring external and promoting internal candidates and apply policies consistently to all candidates.
- Revise job standards for job performance to reasonably accommodate individuals with disabilities (Tartaglia, McMahon, West, Belongia, & Shier Beach, 2007).
- Develop policies that address discrimination, conflict management, and grievance resolution processes and incorporate them into the patient bill of rights.
- Educate staff as mediators in cross-cultural conflicts.
- Train or hire patient advocates.
- Post signage that notifies patients and families that a grievance process exists.

> *Does the organization where you work/go to school have culturally appropriate toys available on pediatric units, in the Emergency Department, and in reception areas where children are likely to be? Where might you go to obtain such toys?*

Transparency

Health-care organizations are encouraged to regularly make available to the public information about their progress and successful innovations in implementing diversity initiatives and to provide public notice in their communities about the availability of this information (OMH, 2001). Strategies that have proven beneficial include the following (Marrone, 2010; Purnell et al., 2011):

- Create and distribute brochures to patients/families and include in admissions packets that highlight the attention to and respect for diversity within the organization.
- Include diversity services on patient/family education television channels and in the organization's Web site and brochures.
- Publish articles in professional health-care journals and local/neighborhood periodicals to market diversity services and to share success stories.
- Inform community agencies and local advocacy groups regarding the diversity services that are offered by the organization and the benefits thereof.
- Reach out to professional associations to present and publish diversity-related initiatives and outcomes in the association's publications, on their Web sites, and at local, regional, national, and international conferences.
- Partner with case managers and discharge planners regarding patients with needs related to culture, health literacy, and the ability of ambulatory/community services to provide culturally relevant care following hospitalization.

- Use legislative representative as a vehicle for constituents who need health-care providers who are sensitive to cultural issues.

Outcomes Metrics to Assess Cultural Competence

Several methods have been developed to assess organizational cultural competence. However, to date, consensus has not been achieved regarding which data elements to be measured. Few reliable data collection instruments are available to assess organizational cultural competence (HRSA, 2002). In spite of this limitation, a review of the literature reveals that indicators of cultural competence in health-care delivery organizations typically include organizational values and governance structures, quality monitoring and evaluation, communication, education, services, community involvement, access, health outcomes, financial stability/viability, and data management/data-driven decisions (Joint Commission, 2011; Marrone, 2008).

Outcomes metrics for organizational cultural competency include the following:

1. Organizational Values and Governance Structures
   a. Philosophy, mission, vision, values, and strategic plan that reflect responsiveness to internal and external diversity.
   b. Annual Report Cards that demonstrate accomplishments related to diversity-related initiatives for patients, families, and the community.
2. Quality Monitoring and Evaluation
   a. Increased consumer satisfaction with care and services particularly related to:
      i. providers rated as being actively engaged with the consumer/practitioner partnership, and,
      ii. Increased time with providers during primary care visits.
   b. Improvements in health and wellness status in the service area, particularly related to underserved populations.
   c. Improved public safety in the service area.
   d. Increased compliance with treatment plans.
   e. Decreased medical errors related to informed consent and wrong patient, wrong site/side surgeries or procedures.
3. Communication
   a. Documented use of trained medical interpreters and/or use of language telephone interpretation services for patients who do not understand the primary language of care used within the organization.
   b. Documented use of patient education materials that are culturally sensitive and reflect the health literacy level and language proficiency of the patient/family.

c. Documented use of critical documents, such as consent forms and patient education materials that have been translated into the most frequent languages represented by the demographic data of the service area.

d. Documentation systems that include cultural health assessment data and the integration of assessment findings into a transdisciplinary plan of care.

4. Education
   a. Cultural competency performance criteria that are integrated into performance appraisals for all levels of job descriptions.
   b. Learning outcomes that reflect culturally, ethnically, linguistically, and spiritually relevant health-care interventions, plans of care, and clinical evaluation strategies.

5. Services
   a. Increased access to services by diverse, underserved, and vulnerable populations.
   b. Increase in cultural- and language-related services and programs provided in response to community needs assessment date.

▶ *In the organization where you work/go to school, are food pyramids and food selections available and reflective of the patients' and staffs' languages and culture?*

6. Community Involvement
   a. Community leaders represented among key organizational decision making and stakeholder groups, such as Board of Trustees, Governing Board, Diversity Council, Patient Education Committee, and Ethics Committee.

7. Access
   a. Increased use of preventive services with resultant decreased use in Emergency Department visits for nonemergent health needs.

8. Health Outcomes
   a. Decrease in racial and ethnic health disparities in the service area.

9. Financial Stability/Viability
   a. Decreased health-care costs chiefly related to decreased length of stay (LOS), decreased complications, issues of "noncompliance," decreased Emergency Department visits for nonemergent health issues, and decreased readmissions and recidivism.
   b. Increased revenue principally related to increased use of services by underserved populations and increased throughout related to decreased LOS.
   c. Decreased litigation and malpractice.

10. Data Management
    a. Decreased disparities related to the access and use of health-care services or in received and/or recommended treatment.

b. Review and analysis of consumer satisfaction with care and services data and evidence that information has been used to influence the design/redesign of strategic initiatives and services.

Resources to Support Culturally Competent Health-Care Organizations

Many governmental, regulatory, and professional agencies provide useful information that can assist with the design of an organizational infrastructure that supports cultural competency. The World Health Organization provides technical support to assist countries and regions in addressing priority health issues and engages in partnerships to establish health and care norms and standards; policy, program, and human resources development; and the prevention and control of major communicable diseases (WHO, 2010).

The U.S. Office of Minority Health (OMH) develops health policies and programs that are aimed at protecting the health of minority populations through the elimination of health disparities among vulnerable populations (OMH, 2001). The OMH developed the CLAS Standards in Health Care to guide health-care delivery systems toward meeting the culture care needs of consumers within their respective service areas. The Institute of Medicine (IOM) serves as an independent advisor for health and science policy development. The IOM established Core Competencies for Health Care Professionals that encourage patient-centered care, collaborative interprofessional teams, evidence-based practice, quality improvement, and informatics (IOM, 2002).

The Joint Commission is a U.S. agency with an international affiliate that is aimed at continuously improving the safety and quality of care provided to the public through the accreditation of health-care facilities. The Joint Commission developed evaluation strategies in support of culturally competent organizations. Organizational cultural competency evaluation strategies include the following:

1. Allocating resources to initial and ongoing team-building and cultural training and educational programs, such as the development of interdisciplinary cultural diversity committees and outreach programs to minority nursing and medical organizations.

2. Integrating cultural diversity initiatives into and cited cultural competency standards within all levels of the organization, such as vision and mission statements, strategic objectives, learning outcomes, clinical performance criteria, policies and procedures, documentation systems, and research.

3. Assessing the cultural composition of the staff as compared with the demographics of the community.

4. Developing hiring practices, promotion strategies, and outreach programs that underscore diversity as a priority.
5. Assessing and integrating patient satisfaction, staff satisfaction, quality improvement, and health outcomes data related to cultural, spiritual, and linguistic diversity into all levels of the organizational strategic planning.
6. Utilizing only trained medical interpreters and translators.
7. Integrating patients' health and illness values and traditions into written plans of care and progress notes.
8. Assessing patient/family understanding of teaching and discharge instructions (Joint Commission, 2011).

The Transcultural Nursing Society (2012) is a professional nursing organization that is committed to enhancing the quality of culturally congruent care provided by nurses prepared in transcultural nursing that supports improved health and wellness for people worldwide. The Society developed a certification process for nurses and other health-care professionals that ensures competency in providing culturally competent care. The International Council of Nurses (ICN) (2010) promotes healthy lifestyles, healthy workplaces, and healthy communities by working closely with the national nursing associations representing 130 countries. The Council supports programs that mitigate poverty, pollution, and other underlying causes of illness, includes care strategies that address meeting spiritual and emotional needs, and advocates that prevention, care, and cure are the rights of every human being.

The American Organization of Nurse Executives (AONE) (2011) developed the AONE Guiding Principles for Diversity in Health Care Organizations and the AONE Diversity for Health Care Organizations Toolkit to assist health-care organizations to establish a healthy practice and work environment that reflects the diversity through a commitment to inclusivity, tolerance, and governance structures.

The Future of Culturally Competent Health-Care Organizations

Global geographic migrations resulting in wide-reaching demographic variations are anticipated to grow over the next several decades. These demographic changes amplify the importance of addressing cultural, ethnic, racial, linguistic, and spiritual health disparities. Minority populations that are currently experiencing poorer health status are expected to grow more rapidly, particularly in industrialized countries. Governments and health-care organizations are focusing more on reducing health disparities by ensuring the cultural competency of the health-care system and its providers.

Successful culturally competent health-care organizations utilize evidence-based organizing frameworks that articulate well with one another to ensure the integrity and reliability of diversity-related initiatives. The triangulated framework used in this chapter to illustrate the critical elements of organizational cultural competency included the CLAS Standards, the Purnell Model, and the Cultural Assessment Profile. Collectively, the components provide the road map and guideposts for the delivery of culturally and linguistically appropriate health-care services to diverse consumers.

In summary, hallmark characteristics of culturally competent health-care organizations include the following (Marrone, 2010):

- An organizational infrastructure that respects and celebrates diversity as reflected in the vision, mission, values, strategic plan, standard operating procedures (policies and procedures), quality initiatives, education plan, employee competencies, and clinical and operational performance outcomes
- The design, implementation, and evaluation of a well-structured strategic plan that ensures the provision of culturally, spiritually, and linguistically appropriate services consistent with the demographics of the service area
- Retention, recruitment, and promotion strategies that attract and retain health-care professionals prepared in transcultural concepts at all levels of the organization that are representative of the consumer demographics in the service area
- Availability of diversity-related resources at the point of care
- Education programs that ensure that all levels of staff receive initial and ongoing learning and skill acquisition related to the culture care needs of the consumer demographics in the service area
- Evidence-based assessment strategies that reliably measure access to care, quality of care, health outcomes, and patient and staff satisfaction, and stratify data related to the demographics of the service area
- A network of active partnerships with community leaders and consumer groups that reflect the demographics of the service area who assist the organization in the assessment, planning, implementation, and evaluation of diversity-related initiatives

Finally, essential to the provision of safe, quality language services, culturally competent health-care organizations must develop systems and processes that ensure ongoing self-assessments to determine if consumers are receiving care in their preferred language, maintain a current organizational language data bank that reflects the dynamic changes in languages spoken within the service area, employ trained and validated medical interpreters and translators to provide language assistance services at all points of care and across the continuum of care at no cost to the consumers, and have in place retention and recruitment strategies for diverse staff at all levels of the organization represented in the service area.

Culturally competent organizations must provide patients and visitors with written notices of their right to receive language assistance services; maintain signage in the major languages spoken by consumers, including sign language for the deaf/hearing impaired and Braille for the blind/visually impaired; establish and maintain partnerships with key formal and informal community leaders; safeguard that interpretation and translation services are efficient and accessible at the point of care throughout the continuum of care; and utilize subject matter experts and specialists in transcultural care and cultural competency to guide the language services product development

REFERENCES

American Association of Critical Care Nurses. (2003). Safeguarding the patient and the profession: The value of critical care nurse certification. *American Journal of Critical Care, 12*, 154–164.

American Association of Critical Care Nurses. (2008). *AACN standards for establishing and sustaining healthy work environments.* Retrieved from http://www.aacn.org/wd/hwe/content/resources.pcms?menu=practice American Organization of Nurse Executives. (2011). *Guidelines and toolkit for diversity in health care organizations.* Retrieved from http://www.nursezone.com/nursing-news-events/more-news/AONE-Releases-Online-Tool-Kit-To-Support-Diversity_32546.aspx

Andrews, M.M. (1998). A model for cultural change: Nurse leaders must realize the importance of transculturally based administrative practices. *Nursing Management, 29*, 62–66.

Betancourt, J.R., Green, A.R., Carrillo, J.E., & Ila, O.A. (2003). Defining cultural competence: A practical framework for addressing racial/ethnic disparities in health and health care. *Public Health Reports, 118*, 293–302.

Coleman-Miller B. (2000). A physician's perspective on minority health. *Health Care Financing Review, 21*, 45–56.

Cooper-Patrick, L., Gallo, J.J., Powe, N.R., Steinwachs, D.M., Eaton, W.W., & Ford, D.E.. (1999). Mental health service utilization by African Americans and Whites: The Baltimore epidemiological catchment area follow-up. *Medical Care, 37*(10), 1034–1045.

Cornelio, M. (2004). Quality translation in health care: Kaiser Permanente—Meeting the challenge. *Apuntes, 12*(4), 14–15.

Einbinder, L.C., & Schulman, K.A. (2000). The effect of race on the referral process for invasive cardiac procedures. *Medical Care Research and Review, 1*, 162–177.

Europa. (2010). *Commission takes steps to promote patient safety in Europe* [Press release]. Retrieved from http://europa.eu/rapid/press ReleasesAction.do?reference=IP/08/1973&format=HTML&aged=0&language=EN&guiLanguage=en

Health Resources and Services Administration. (2002). Indicators of cultural competence in health care delivery organizations: An organizational cultural competence assessment profile. U.S. Department of Health and Human Resources. Retrieved from http://www.hrsa.gov/CulturalCompetence/healthdlvr.pdf

Institute of Medicine. (2002). *Unequal treatment: Confronting racial and ethnic disparities in health care.* Washington, DC: National Academies Press.

International Council of Nurses. (2010). *Vision statement.* Retrieved from http://www.icn.ch/visionstatement.htm

Joint Commission. (2011). *Patient safety: About hospitals, language, and culture.* Retrieved from www.jointcommission.org/assets/1/6/hlc_paper.pdf

Marrone, S.R. (2008). Factors that influence critical care nurses' intentions to provide culturally congruent care to Arab Muslims. *Journal of Transcultural Nursing, 19*, 8–15.

Marrone, S.R. (2010). Organizational cultural competency. In M. Douglas & D. Pacquiao (Eds.), *Core curriculum in transcultural nursing and health care.* Thousand Oaks, CA: Sage.

Morales, L.S., Cunningham, W.E., Brown, J.A., Liu, H., & Hays, R.D. (1999). Are Latinos less satisfied with communication by healthcare providers? *Journal of General Internal Medicine, 14*, 409–417.

Office of Minority Health. (2001). *National standards for culturally and linguistically appropriate services.* Retrieved from http://minorityhealth.hhs.gov/templates/browse.aspx?lvl=2&lvlID=15

Office of Minority Health. (2002). *Eliminating racial and ethnic disparities in health: Overview.* Retrieved from http://www.raceandhealth.hhs.gov/sidebars/sbinitover.htm

Public Health Reports. (2003). Defining cultural competence: A practical framework—301. *Public Health Reports.* July–August, Volume 118.

Purnell, L., Davidhizar, R., Giger, G., Fishman, D., Strickland, O., & Allison, D. (2011). A guide to developing a culturally competent organization. *Journal of Transcultural Nursing, (22)*1, 5–14.

Purnell, L.D., & Paulanka, B.J. (2008). *Transcultural health care: A culturally competent approach* (3rd ed.). Philadelphia: F.A. Davis.

Robert Wood Johnson Foundation. (2011). *Getting minority patients' points of view about cultural barriers to health care.* Retrieved from http://www.rwjf.org/reports/grr/055258.htm

Saha, S., Komaromy, M., Koepsell, T.D., & Bindman, A.B. (1999). Patient-physician racial concordance and the perceived quality and use of health care. *Archives in Internal Medicine, 159*, 997–1004.

Saha, S., Taggart, S.H., Komaromy, M., & Bindman, A.B. (2000). Do patients choose physicians of their own race? *Health Affairs, 19*, 76–83.

Tang, G. (2010) Organizational cultural competency: Interpretation services. In M. Douglas & D. Pacquiao (Eds.), *Core curriculum in transcultural nursing and health care.* Thousand Oaks, CA: Sage.

Tartaglia, A., McMahon, B.T., West, S.L., Belongia, L., & Shier Beach, L. (2007). Workplace discrimination and healthcare: The national EEOC ADA research project. *Journal of Vocational Rehabilitation, 27*, 163–169.

Thornicroft, G., Brohan, E., Kassam, A., & Lewis-Holmes, E. (2008). Reducing stigma and discrimination: Candidate interventions. *International Journal of Mental Health Systems, 2*, 1–7.

Transcultural Nursing Society. (2012). *Mission, vision, philosophy, and values.* Retrieved from http://www.tcns.org

World Health Organization. (2010). *Role of WHO in public health.* Retrieved from http://www.who.int/en/

DavisPlus *For case studies, review questions, and additional information, go to*

http://davisplus.fadavis.com

Chapter 5

Perspectives on Nursing in a Global Context

Linda C. Baumann and Laurie B. Hartjes

Overview

The global context of health addresses circumstances that affect populations worldwide, such as quantity and nutritional value of food, air, and water quality; exposure to infectious diseases and environmental toxins; access to essential medications; and gender inequalities. Viewing health without geographic boundaries is a shift from an international health perspective that has emphasized exchanges between national governments. This global perspective affects nursing practice. Globalization has led to a growing interdependence of the world's population and involves the integration of economies, cultures, technologies, and governance (Chapman, 2009). In addition, global health affected by climate change is of such importance to the world's future that all governments must understand the issues and become part of the solution (Gostin, 2008; Narayan, Ali, & Koplan, 2010).

Health is a global priority for a number of reasons:

- Most of the public has been sensitized to the potential for infectious diseases to spread rapidly in a world with extensive travel, human migration, global commerce, and transmission routes that include food, insects, animals, and other vectors.
- There are shared concerns about the societal burdens imposed by an increase in chronic diseases requiring long-term management such as diabetes, cardiovascular disease, and cancer.
- The threat of bioterrorism necessitates surveillance for suspicious clusters of symptoms for populations at a global level.
- Unhealthy populations can destabilize economies, and economic insecurity creates the conditions for poor health.
- Ethical and humanitarian considerations support addressing health from a global perspective (Gostin, 2007). Significant trends that will

influence the work of nurses in the decades ahead are the shift in health conditions from an acute care focus to chronic care, and the increasing number of elderly health consumers (Pruitt & Epping-Jordan, 2005).

Definitions of Health, Global Health, One Health, and Global Nursing

The Preamble to the Constitution of the World Health Organization (WHO) defined *health* as a state of complete physical, mental, and social well-being and not merely the absence of disease or infirmity (WHO, 1946). The Institute of Medicine (IOM) defined global health as health problems, issues, and concerns that transcend national boundaries, may be influenced by circumstances or experiences in other countries, and are best addressed by cooperative actions and solutions (IOM, 1997). A revised definition of *global health* has been proposed based on the evolution of philosophy, attitude, and practice over the past decade:

> Global health is an area for study, research, and practice that places a priority on improving health and achieving equity in health for all people worldwide. Global health emphasizes transnational health issues, determinants, and solutions; involves many disciplines within and beyond the health sciences and promotes interdisciplinary collaboration; and is a synthesis of population-based prevention with individual-level clinical care. (Koplan, Bond, Merson, Reddy, Rodriquez, & Sewankambo, 2009, p. 1995)

Global nursing is the adoption of a global health perspective by nursing professionals interested in seeking collaborative and sustainable solutions to health problems irrespective of national boundaries. These solutions and innovations involve both the professional development of individuals and capacity building in nursing systems at national, regional, and international levels (International Council of Nurses, 2009). This work requires respect for differences in language, culture, customs, and health beliefs. Equally important is the need to approach health issues in partnership with communities by mutually identifying expectations, resources, and strategies for capacity building that are best suited to the specific context (SNV & UNDP, 2009).

The One Health Initiative supports the integration of human medicine, veterinary medicine, and environmental science for the purpose of improving the lives of all species—both human and nonhuman. This recognition of the interconnectedness of all life systems offers new avenues for collaboration and for research questions that will extend our understanding of the dynamic nature of biologic relationships.

Global Health Frameworks

The 1978 World Assembly of the United Nations at Alma-Ata adopted a framework of *Health for All by the Year 2000* with an emphasis on poverty reduction, social justice, and the expansion of primary health-care services. The declaration noted that health was a human right and that countries have the obligation to ensure that all people have access to primary health care (i.e., universal access). This framework identified the essential elements of primary health care (Table 5-1) and endorsed the reallocation of resources to communities to reduce health-care inequality worldwide (WHO & UNICEF, 1978).

Although primary health care has been successfully implemented as a national health policy in some countries, the Alma-Ata declaration failed to achieve its goals in others due to lack of political will, lack of basic resources, and lack of measurable objectives with which to monitor goal achievement. In response to the challenges of implementing universal access to primary health care, the *World Development Report*

(World Bank, 1993) identified the need to invest in health as a cost-effective investment in national development. This report also highlighted the role of the private sector in improving the welfare of populations worldwide.

This philanthropic call to action stimulated foundations and global health leaders to work together to fill a resource gap not otherwise being met. Although there are over 50 philanthropic health organizations with over $96 million in annual donations, the Bill and Melinda Gates Foundation, created in 2000, is among the largest of all the transparently operated charitable foundations in the world, with annual donations of over $2 billion (Health Grants Information Center, 2009). The Gates Foundation was inspired to some degree by the philanthropic history of the Rockefeller Foundation dating back to 1891. Rockefeller donations have targeted substantial global health and welfare problems, such as large United Nations projects and the ambitious (although ultimately unsuccessful) worldwide goal of eradicating yellow fever and malaria. In 2006, Warren Buffet pledged more than $30 billion in stocks to the Gates Foundation, while encouraging other wealthy individuals to give more to charitable causes.

A subsequent framework for addressing the root causes of global health disparities was adopted at the World Assembly in 2000, known as the Millennium Declaration (WHO, 2011). Eight Millennium Development Goals (MDGs) were identified in this declaration to be achieved by 2015 (Table 5.2).

These goals include specific target objectives and measurable indicators. Together these goals aim to reduce poverty, hunger, and ill health and to promote equitable educational opportunities and environmentally sustainable practices. Critics of the MDG framework note that these goals fail to address chronic conditions, disabilities, or unintentional injuries (Fuster & Voute, 2005). Although monitoring has shown that some goals have been partially achieved in some countries, most will fall short of the 2015 targets (WHO, 2011). The *2006 World Health Report* identified shortages of

IID Table 5-1   Essential Elements of Primary Health Care

1. Education concerning prevailing health problems and methods of prevention and control
2. Promotion of the food supply and proper nutrition
3. The provision of safe water and basic sanitation
4. Maternal and child health care, including family planning
5. Immunization against the major infectious diseases
6. Prevention and control of locally endemic diseases
7. Appropriate treatment of common diseases and injuries
8. Provision of essential drugs

World Health Organization and UNICEF. (1978). *Primary health care: Report of the International Conference on Primary Health Care*. Alma-Ata USSR. September 6–12, 1978. Geneva: WHO.

IID Table 5-2   Millennium Development Goals

Goal 1	Eradicate extreme hunger and poverty
Goal 2	Achieve universal primary care
Goal 3	Promote gender equality and empower women
Goal 4	Reduce child mortality
Goal 5	Improve maternal health
Goal 6	Combat HIV/AIDS, malaria, and other diseases
Goal 7	Ensure environmental sustainability
Goal 8	Develop a global partnership for development

World Health Organization. (2011) *2015 millennium development goals*. Retrieved from http://www.un.org/millenniumgoals/

human resources as a critical obstacle to the achievement of the MDGs (WHO, 2006). Despite the challenges and shortcomings, the MDG framework supports an integrated database and a road map for monitoring goal achievement using core targets that are measured locally and nationally, and then shared globally.

Finally, a framework entitled *Smart Global Health Policy* has been proposed to guide the U.S. global health agenda (CSIS, 2010). The following five-point agenda was developed to leverage U.S. influence and past successes to create a healthier and safer world:

1. Maintain the commitment to the fight against HIV/AIDS, malaria, and tuberculosis.
2. Prioritize women and children in U.S. global health efforts.
3. Strengthen prevention and capabilities to manage health emergencies.
4. Ensure that the United States has the capacity to match our global health ambitions.
5. Make smart investments in multilateral institutions.

These three frameworks provide guidance for the development of nursing curricula and practice standards that view health needs, resources, and interventions through a global lens in a world that is increasingly interconnected.

Global Health Organizations

An important role for world governments is to provide health services. When governments lack the resources or political will to meet basic health, welfare, and safety needs, there are hundreds of thousands of national and international organizations that have coalesced to reduce the associated suffering. The organizations focusing on global health issues are often classified as bilateral, multilateral, and nongovernmental.

Bilateral organizations use funding from one government to improve health and welfare elsewhere. The U.S. Agency for International Development (USAID) is a major bilateral organization in the United States that was created in 1961 as an independent federal government agency under the direction of the secretary of state. Objectives of USAID are to assist countries with disaster relief, antipoverty programs, and the implementation of democratic reforms. The President's Emergency Plan for AIDS Relief (PEPFAR) and the President's Malaria Initiative are both USAID programs. More recently, these USAID health programs have become part of an overarching program called the "whole-of-government" umbrella under the Global Health Initiative (GHI) (USAID: Health, 2009). The GHI coordinates U.S. government global health efforts, with $63 billion committed over six years (2009–2014) to help partner countries reform their health systems.

Multilateral (or intergovernmental) organizations are those that receive funding from multiple governments as well as nongovernmental sources, with funding distributed to many different countries. The major multilateral organizations were created by the United Nations (UN) and remain under the UN organizational umbrella, such as the World Health Organization (WHO), the World Bank, the United Nation Children's Fund (UNICEF), and the United Nations Development Programme (UNDP). Other highly visible examples of multilateral organizations are the World Trade Organization (WTO), the European Union (EU), and the Organization for Economic Cooperation and Development (OECD).

Nongovernmental organizations (NGOs) make significant contributions nationally and internationally based on their unique missions. By definition, NGOs are independent from government influence, and they are often in a unique position to address issues not addressed by governments. NGOs were given Consultative Status in 1945 as part of Article 71 of Chapter X of the United Nations Charter. Although new NGOs are being created daily, some have become very large and influential. The Bangladesh Rural Advancement Committee (BRAC) has 120,000 employees, the majority of whom are women, as well as microfinance and education programs in Asia and Africa that reach more than 110 million people. World Vision, a Christian humanitarian organization, is an NGO with an annual budget in the billions of dollars, enough to match the gross domestic products of some countries. Other faith-based organizations also play a role in mitigating threats to health through their support of public health measures to ensure access to safe food, water, and sanitation; housing; direct health services; and schools. Table 5-3 provides brief descriptions of major bilateral, multilateral, and NGO organizations.

Sigma Theta Tau International (STTI) is a professional nursing honor society that strives to connect nurses worldwide to collaborate on issues of common interest. STTI has 469 chapters in 86 countries and a mission of using knowledge, scholarship, service, and learning to improve the health of all. STTI partnerships have yielded a series of think tank conferences, as well as reports such as the *Competency Framework for International Health Consultants*, *Practice Innovations* at Magnet health-care facilities, and the *Global Standards for the Initial Education of Professional Nurses and Midwives* written in partnership with the WHO.

The International Council of Nurses (ICN) is another nursing organization with a global focus. ICN is a federation of more than 130 national nurses associations representing more than 13 million nurses. Founded in 1899, ICN is the oldest and largest organization serving health professionals. Its mission is to ensure quality nursing care for all, sound health policies globally, the advancement of nursing knowledge,

IID Table 5-3 Examples of International Health Organizations

Bilateral Organizations

Peace Corps	U.S. government agency that places volunteers in 139 countries to work on issues ranging from AIDS education to information technology and environmental preservation, and to foster cultural understanding. **www.peacecorps.gov**
U.S. Agency for International Development (USAID)	U.S. government agency that provides economic, development and humanitarian assistance to countries for reasons of poverty, conflict and natural disaster, and to support populations engaging in democratic reforms. **www.usaid.gov**

Multilateral Organizations

Food and Agricultural Organization	UN agency that provides international leadership for combating world hunger. FAO helps countries improve agriculture, forestry, and fisheries practices to ensure good nutrition for all. **www.fao.org**
Pan American Health Organization	UN agency focused on improving the health of the countries of the Americas. Also serves as the Regional Office of the Americas for the World Health Organization. **www.paho.org**
United Nations Children's Fund	UN agency that advocates for children in the areas of nutrition, environment, education, gender equity, health, and public policy. **www.unicef.org**
United Nations High Commissioner for Refugees (UNHCR)	UN agency to protect the rights and well-being of refugees. **www.unhcr.org**
United Nations Program on HIV/AIDS (UNAIDS)	UN partnership that strives to ensure universal access to services for HIV prevention, treatment, care and support. **www.unaids.org**
World Bank	UN-affiliated intergovernmental financial institution that provides low-interest loans, interest-free credits, and grants to developing countries to invest in areas such as education, health, infrastructure, and resource management. **www.worldbank.org**
World Health Organization (WHO)	UN-affiliated intergovernmental agency responsible for shaping the health research agenda, setting norms and standards, articulating evidence-based policy options, providing technical support to countries, and monitoring and assessing health trends. **www.who.int/en/**

Nongovernmental Organizations

CARE International	Relief and development organization that identifies underlying causes of global poverty. Operating in more than 70 countries, CARE responds to emergencies by delivering aid and helping people rebuild their lives. **www.care-international.org**
Health Volunteers Overseas	A network of health-care providers who aim to increase health-care access in low-resource countries. They work to improve access through clinical training and education programs. HVO train, mentor, and support health-care providers in more than 25 countries. **www.hvousa.org**
Human Rights Watch	Investigates and exposes human rights violations and holds oppressors accountable for their crimes. Dedicated to upholding freedom and preventing discrimination. **www.hrw.org**
International Medical Corps	Dedicated to relieving suffering through health-care training and relief and development programs. Builds capacity in underserved communities. **www.internationalmedicalcorps.org**
International Red Cross	Based primarily on the Geneva Conventions of 1864 and 1949, ensures humanitarian protection and assistance for victims of war and armed violence and other emergencies. The goal of ICRC's Health Unit activities is to give people affected by conflict access to basic preventive and curative health care that meets universally recognized standards. **www.icrc.org**
Médecins sans Frontières (Doctors without Borders)	Provides life-saving medical and technical assistance to people affected by natural or man-made disasters and armed conflict. Field staff deliver direct care in more than 60 countries, often in very difficult conditions. **www.msf.org**
Oxfam International	Group of 14 international organizations that work with other local organizations in 98 countries to fight poverty and injustice. Oxfam objectives are guided by the belief that respect for human rights is the key to lifting people from poverty. **www.oxfam.org**
Partners in Health	Strives to create solidarity in health by partnering with poor communities to combat disease and poverty by using a comprehensive and community based approach. Projects are ongoing in 12 countries. **www.pih.org**
Project Hope	Since 1958, has delivered direct healthcare services and health education to people in more than 35 countries, with a goal of creating sustainable approaches. **www.projecthope.org**

Continues on page 78

II▶ Table 5-3	**Examples of International Health Organizations** *Continued from page 77*
\multicolumn{2}{c}{Nongovernmental Organizations}	
World Vision	Christian humanitarian organization that serves close to 100 million people in over 100 countries. Support children, families and communities to help all people reach their full potential by fighting poverty and injustice. www.worldvision.org
\multicolumn{2}{c}{Other Organizations}	
The Gates Foundation	Philanthropic foundation created by Bill and Melinda Gates. Provides key resources to promote health and education in the United States and globally through innovative approaches to pressing problems. www.gatesfoundation.org
The Rockefeller Foundation	First U.S. philanthropic foundation with global perspective, established by John Rockefeller in 1913. Funded the first global initiative to eradicate malaria and yellow fever in the 1940-1950s. www.rockefellerfoundation.org
The Global Fund	Unique international financing partnership between governments, private sector businesses and affected communities that aims to finance programs addressing HIV/AIDS, tuberculosis and malaria. www.theglobalfund.org
President's Emergency Plan for AIDS Relief (PEPFAR)	U.S. government initiative to save the lives of those suffering from HIV/AIDS around the world. Provides the largest commitment by any nation to combat a single disease internationally. www.pepfar.gov

and the presence worldwide of a respected nursing profession and a competent and satisfied nursing workforce.

Forces Shaping Global Health and Nursing

Policy and National Economies

Government policies determine how health services and health research are financed and how health-care services are distributed. Governments also control the licensing and regulation of nurses, globally the largest group of health-care providers. A high national burden of disease results in lost productivity and incurs treatment expenses, as demonstrated by the substantial economic impact of HIV/AIDS, malaria, and tuberculosis in countries with high prevalence (Audibert, Motel, & Drabo, 2010). Failure to prevent or to provide early intervention for noncommunicable diseases (NCDs) similarly has a significant negative impact on national health budgets (Lancet NCD Action Group, 2011).

Although high-income countries perform better across many measures of health, there is no direct relationship between the two. The Organization for Economic Cooperation and Development (OECD) tracks and reports annually on more than 1200 health system measures across 34 industrialized countries. U.S. health-care spending was significantly higher than other industrialized countries, both per capita and as a percentage of gross domestic product (Anderson, & Squires, 2010), yet the United States ranks in the bottom quartile in life expectancy among OECD countries. Such gaps between investment and health outcomes suggest that efficiencies and cost controls are needed by health-care systems in countries across all income levels.

Population Trends

Demographic transition refers to a documented global pattern characterized by a population with high birth and death rates shifting over time to one of lower birth and death rates, resulting in a higher percentage of older adults. Another transition is the shift from predominantly communicable disease to NCDs. This increase in NCDs creates a need for health-care systems and a nursing workforce that can provide continuous monitoring and services that address prevention measures such as lifestyle modifications, especially healthy diets and regular physical activity (WHO, 2002).

Chronic diseases account for 60 percent of all deaths worldwide, and 80 percent of these deaths occur in low-middle-income countries, where they disproportionately affect youth to middle-age individuals who are in the prime productivity period of life (Daar et al., 2007). It is projected that by 2030 the four leading causes of burden of disease will be related to HIV/AIDS, unipolar depressive disorders, ischemic heart disease, and road traffic accidents (WHO, 2004). HIV/AIDS is estimated to be the leading cause of burden of disease in middle- and low-income countries by 2015 (Mathers & Loncar, 2006).

The global burden of disease is measured using a composite indicator called "disability adjusted life years," or DALY, to measure premature death and loss due to illness and disability in a population. DALY data are reported for communicable diseases; maternal and perinatal conditions; nutrition; NCD; injuries and self-inflicted injuries; and violence (World Bank, 1993). The 10 leading risk factor causes of DALYs by country income group (i.e., low, middle, and high income) are shown in Table 5-4. Critics of the DALY measure point out that this objective measure pays little attention to local and cultural conditions. Further,

II▶ Table 5-4 **Ranking of Selected Risk Factors: 10 Leading Risk Factor Causes of DALYS by Income Group, 2004**

	Risk Factor	DALYs (millions)	Percentage of total		Risk Factor	DALYs (millions)	Percentage of total
	World				**Low-income countries***		
1	Childhood underweight	91	5.9	1	Childhood underweight	82	9.9
2	Unsafe sex	70	4.6	2	Unsafe water, sanitation, hygiene	53	6.3
3	Alcohol use	69	4.5	3	Unsafe sex	52	6.2
4	Unsafe water, sanitation, hygiene	64	4.2	4	Suboptimal breastfeeding	34	4.1
5	High blood pressure	57	3.7	5	Indoor smoke from solid fuels	33	4.0
6	Tobacco use	57	3.7	6	Vitamin A deficiency	20	2.4
7	Suboptimal breastfeeding	44	2.9	7	High blood pressure	18	2.2
8	High blood glucose	41	2.7	8	Alcohol use	18	2.1
9	Indoor smoke from solid fuels	41	2.7	9	High blood glucose	16	1.9
10	Overweight and obesity	36	2.3	10	Zinc deficiency	14	1.7
	Middle-income countries*				**High-income countries***		
1	Alcohol use	44	7.6	1	Tobacco use	13	10.7
2	High blood pressure	31	5.4	2	Alcohol use	8	6.7
3	Tobacco use	31	5.4	3	Overweight and obesity	8	6.5
4	Overweight and obesity	21	3.6	4	High blood pressure	7	6.1
5	High blood glucose	20	3.4	5	High blood glucose	6	4.9
6	Unsafe sex	17	3.0	6	Physical inactivity	5	4.1
7	Physical inactivity	16	2.7	7	High cholesterol	4	3.4
8	High cholesterol	14	2.5	8	Illicit drugs	3	2.1
9	Occupational risks	14	2.3	9	Occupational risks	2	1.5
10	Unsafe water, sanitation, hygiene	11	2.0	10	Low fruit and vegetable intake	2	1.3

*Countries grouped by 2004 gross national income per capita—low income (US $825 or less) high income (US $10,066 or more)
Source: World Health Organization. (2009). *Global health risks: mortality and burden of disease attributable to selected major risks.* Geneva, Switzerland: WHO.

DALYs do not account for the subjective experience of someone with a disability and how this might change over time; they do not account for how disability may affect a household or family; and they fail to account for the true burden of disability beyond lost productivity (Nichter, 2008).

Environmental Factors

The forces of globalization, urbanization, and industrialization underlie the rising prevalence of chronic conditions. These phenomena have radically affected dietary patterns, physical activity behaviors, and key behavioral determinants of NCDs (Beaglehole & Yach, 2003; Narayan et al., 2010). Across nations, food choices and levels of physical activity are becoming more homogeneous, characterized by widespread access to calorie-rich but nutrient-poor foods, built environments that pose barriers to active modes of transportation, and occupational trends toward sedentary work (Lancet NCD Group, 2011). It is estimated that 70 percent of the world's population will be urban residents by 2050, resulting in both benefits and challenges (United Nations, 2007).

Through practice and research, nurses are responding to the health threats posed by environmental exposures (Clarke & Butterfield, 2011; Sattler, 2011). This includes the development of new systems to document exposures and health status changes postexposure. On a broader scale, nurses and other health providers are pushing for public policies to mitigate the health-impairing effects of climate change and other ecosystem disruptions such as the depletion of natural resources, including clean air and water. Figure 5-1 provides a framework developed by the Intergovernmental Panel on Climate Change that depicts health as part of the dynamic interactions between the earth's ecosystems and human-scale social and economic systems. This IPCC framework is compatible with a One Health approach in which all parts of a system are considered when doing research and comparing policy alternatives. It is the complexity of dynamic systems that lends support for adhering to the precautionary principle to avoid irreversible and potentially catastrophic changes. This principle states that if an action or policy has a suspected risk of causing harm to the public or to

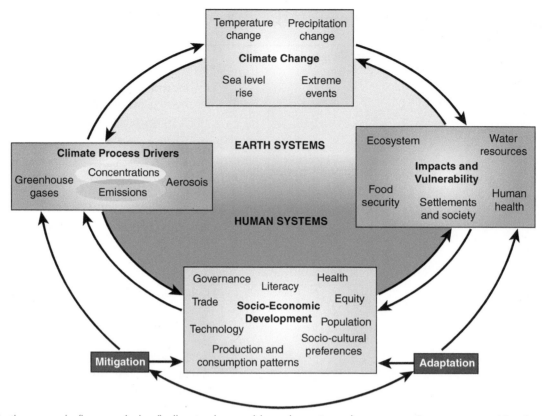

Figure 5-1 Anthropogenic (human-derived) climate change drivers, impacts, and responses. *(Intergovernmental Panel on Climate Change. (2007). Climate change 2007: Synthesis report. Geneva: IPCC. World Health Organization. (2010). Global atlas of the health workforce. Retrieved from http://www.who.int/hrh/workforce_mdgs/en/index.html)*

the environment, in the absence of scientific consensus that the action or policy is harmful, the burden of proof that it is not harmful falls on those taking the action.

Access to Technology

Access to technology is rapidly changing globally. Even in communities where an infrastructure for reliable electricity and phone service does not exist, cell phone penetration is virtually universal. Cell phones and smart phones are being used to deliver health-care services, such as monitoring blood sugar (Cavalcanti, Shirinzadeh, & Kretly, 2008); delivering health education and peer support for healthy behaviors (Piette, 2007, Piette, et al., 2010); and diagnosing diseases that are prevalent in areas with limited access to health-care services, such as malaria. The expansion of Internet access and the development of low-cost health technologies can promote more equitable distribution of health services worldwide. Additionally, electronic health records and integrated systems for sharing health information will increase efficiencies regardless of the site of delivery. The ability to access information anywhere and anytime reduces barriers to the achievement of many global health objectives.

The Global Nursing Workforce

Even though an estimated 35 million nurses and midwives make up the greater part of the global health-care workforce, the demand for nurses currently exceeds supply, and chronic shortages are characteristic of the global nursing workforce (WHO, 2009). It is estimated that there is a global shortage of about 4 million health-care workers (WHO, 2006), and the situation is especially dire in sub-Saharan Africa. Staff shortages in low-resource countries can be attributed to three major forces: (1) an insufficient supply of appropriately trained workers and financially strapped health-care systems that have difficulty with recruitment and retention; (2) substantial numbers of health-care providers who are affected by HIV/AIDS personally and professionally, which has increased the demand for services and has reduced health-care workforce availability, especially in sub-Sahara Africa; and (3) migration patterns that have affected access to health services as more nurses are moving from rural to urban areas, from public health-care systems to private health-care organizations, and from clinical to nonclinical jobs (Laurent, 2011).

The global shortage of nurses is also related to an unprecedented aging of the world population. The older population is growing faster than the total population in virtually all world regions, with a projected doubling of the proportion of older persons by 2050 (United Nations, 2010). In some countries, more than 40 percent of the population will be over 60 years of age in 2050. This change in age demographics will produce profound societal changes that include political representation; family living arrangements; demand for health services; and economic dynamics related to investment, consumption, labor markets, and intergenerational transfers.

The nursing workforce is also aging, with the average age of nurses in the United States at 46 years (American Association of Colleges of Nursing, 2011). The World Health Organization has proposed a model of task shifting to address nurse shortages that are

worsened by this aging of the workforce. Task shifting is the delegation of specific tasks to trained nonprofessional health-care providers (WHO, 2008). Tasks can be shifted from physicians to clinical officers, medical assistants, nurses, or community health workers as appropriate. Task shifting has been successful in providing cost-effective, quality care with high patient satisfaction (Holzemer, 2008).

The uneven ratio of health-care providers to population on a global scale is a significant problem (Figure 5-2). The average nurse-to-population ratio in Europe, the region with the highest ratios, is 10 times that of the lowest regions in Africa and Southeast Asia (Buchan, Kingma, & Lorenzo, 2005). The low availability of nurses in many less developed

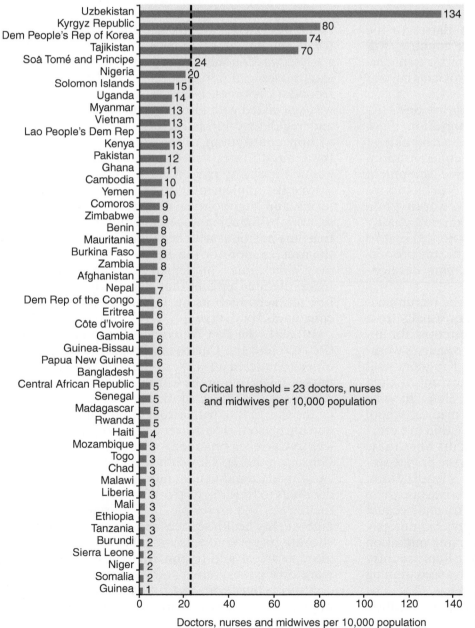

Critical threshold = 23 doctors, nurses and midwives per 10,000 population

Doctors, nurses and midwives per 10,000 population

Figure 5-2 Density of doctors, nurses, and midwives in 49 priority countries. *(World Health Organization. (2010). Global atlas of the health workforce. Retrieved from http://www.who.int/hrh/workforce_mdgs/en/index.html)*

countries is exacerbated by geographic maldistribution with fewer nurses available in rural and remote areas. Without planned and sustained interventions, these wide variances in access to nursing care will undermine attempts to improve health outcomes of world populations.

International Migration

Migration is recognized as a normal activity of a global society. In 1995, almost 100 million (1.8 percent of the world's population) lived outside their countries of birth compared to 175 million (2.9 percent) in 2000 (United Nations, 2004). By 2010, it was estimated that 214 million (3.2 percent) people lived outside their country of origin (United Nations, 2011). International migration has more than doubled from 75 million in 1965 to an estimated 175 million in 2003; (Buchan, Kingma, & Lorenzo, 2005). The United States has the largest professional nurse workforce in the world. It is expected that the migration of nurses to the United States and other high-resource countries will continue, as well as the need for U.S. nurses to understand health-care systems and health problems beyond their borders.

Career mobility and a desire to improve one's living conditions are motivators for migration. *Push* factors that make nursing practice less desirable in one's home country include poor compensation, under-resourced facilities, few career development options, and sociopolitical instability. *Pull* factors include opportunities for increased pay, working in a different culture, and improvement in one's quality of life (Kingma, 2006). Further, remittances sent to families back home represent a significant proportion of the gross national product in many developing nations.

Brain drain is a term used to describe recruitment and migration of health-care providers, usually from low-income countries to developed countries, for improved career options. Foreign-educated nurses working in Australia, Canada, the United Kingdom, and the United States comprise 5 to 10 percent of each country's nursing workforce (Kingma, 2008). In some regions of Africa, over 80 percent of medical school graduates migrate out of the country within five years of graduation. Internal brain drain occurs when those who stay in the home country work in the private sector or for foreign nongovernmental organizations. However, brain drain sometime occurs because there is no work available in the home country and because of bankrupt health-care systems that cannot pay workers. Some positive results of nursing migration are when resources are sent back to the home country or health-care providers return with advanced training and experience (Kirk, 2007).

Challenges associated with international migration include unethical recruitment practices where nurses are misled about working conditions and remuneration and benefits, the need to become familiar with a foreign language and culture, a different health-care system, and drugs and technologies used in other countries. Foreign nurses may be discriminated against based on concern about language proficiency as it relates to patient safety. Gender-based discrimination may be an issue because nursing is often viewed as a female occupation.

Trade and Mutual Recognition Agreements

The nursing workforce in the United States has been affected by the 1994 trilateral trade bloc known as the North American Trade Agreement (NAFTA). NAFTA provides for the movement of goods and services across the borders of Canada, Mexico, and the United States. Health professionals included under the agreement include nurses, clinical laboratory specialists, and physical and occupational therapists.

Squires (2011) explored the effects of NAFTA on the development of Mexican nursing. A thematic analysis was conducted using interviews with 48 Mexican nurses and information from 410 primary and secondary sources. Findings revealed that NAFTA was associated with improvements to the educational and regulatory infrastructures for Mexican nurses without contributing to a mass migration of nurses to the United States and Canada. However, the economic instability caused by the peso crisis of 1995 slowed the implementation of nursing workforce reforms, and later political actions reduced nurses' job security by reducing wages and minimizing access to full-time positions with benefits. This study reaffirms the need to monitor the effects of trade agreements over time, since implementation may contribute to unintended effects that negatively affect frontline workers such as nurses, as well as the health consumers they serve.

In 2001, the Pan American Health Organization (PAHO) and the Caribbean Program Coordination office conducted a review of the scope and impact of nurses' migration in the Caribbean. The strategy that resulted is the Managed Migration Program (MMP) of the Caribbean, with a goal of retaining competent nursing personnel to deliver health programs and services to Caribbean nationals (Salmon, Yan, Hewitt, & Guisinger, 2007). This collaborative effort identified two foundational values: nurses have the right as individuals to freedom of movement within and beyond the region, and all people have the right of access to high-quality health services and programs. The MMP encourages governments and other stakeholders to be more aware of and responsive to six critical nursing workforce issues: terms and conditions of work; recruitment, retention, and training; value of nursing; utilization and deployment; management practices; and policy development.

When considering nursing migration from an even broader perspective, the ICN has developed a credentialing framework that uses Mutual Recognition Agreements (MRAs). These bilateral, international, and regional agreements permit qualifications and credentials to be recognized and accepted across borders. The work to streamline credentialing standards and processes is ongoing to ensure that more MRAs will be available in the future. There is also an effort to reach new global nursing markets in China and Southeast Asia, where the nursing workforce of over 2 million nurses in their twenties can partially alleviate the global shortage of nurses (Nichols, Davis, & Richardson, 2011). In the United States, the nonprofit Commission on Graduates of Foreign Nursing Schools (CGFNS) serves as a clearinghouse for information on international nursing education and licensure. CGFNS is the authorized provider of certification for nurses and other health-care providers seeking employment in the United States.

Nursing Education

The preparation and practice standards for nurses vary significantly by country. Baccalaureate programs are becoming more common, with more than 46 countries requiring the baccalaureate degree as entry level for nursing practice. The baccalaureate degree has not yet been established as the entry-level education for registered nurses universally, despite long-standing advocacy by the ICN and the American Nurses Association to standardize educational pathways. In the United States, there are three educational pathways to achieve a registered nurse level: a two-year associate degree, a three-year diploma, and a baccalaureate degree. The United Kingdom has the two pathways of a nursing diploma or a degree. The Philippines, Denmark, Ireland, New Zealand, and Spain all have one university-based educational pathway to become a registered nurse, even though the required number of credit hours varies among countries.

To promote greater uniformity in the United States, the American Association of Colleges of Nursing (AACN) developed an Essentials series that provides recommendations for baccalaureate, masters, and doctoral curricula. Thus, the achievement of global standards for the education of nurses that has been an ICN vision for more than 100 years has yet to be accomplished.

Because of these multiple paths, if you pick any two countries, you will find problems. Why does nursing preparation in Germany and the United States, or China and the United States, for example, produce a variable skill mix, particularly with the expansion of the role of advanced practice nurses (WHO, 2010)? The goal of global standards for nursing practice is to establish educational criteria to ensure outcomes based on evidence and competency, to promote lifetime learning, and to support nurse competencies that will promote positive population-based health outcomes (WHO, 2009).

Nursing curricula are being shaped by institutional and organizational initiatives that address global health issues. The American Academy of Nursing's (AAN) *Expert Panel on Global Nursing and Health* white paper (Rosenkoetter & Nardi, 2005) examined critical issues such as recruiting international nurses to nursing positions in high-resource countries, faculty and student exchanges, effects of U.S. Citizenship and Immigration Law, and laws governing nursing practice within the public domain. The panel recommended expanding the number of international conferences and exchanges, as well as opportunities and support for collaborative research. This group supports moving curricular references to international nursing into the context of global nursing and health and using technology to increase access to educational materials from any location.

U.S. Nursing Workforce Recommendations

The Future of Nursing: Leading Change, Advancing Health provides a vision of U.S nursing education, regulation, and practice. An appendix to this report entitled *International Models of Nursing* (Nichols et al., 2011) contains six recommendations to address a national and global nursing workforce (Table 5-5).

Nursing education and continued professional development are key elements for addressing global nursing workforce shortages. This has been supported by a push to make academic degrees and quality standards more comparable across countries and to encourage the pursuit of graduate degrees in nursing.

Nurse educators in the United States are increasingly engaged in international partnerships to promote curriculum innovation that is shared across a global faculty network.

II▶ Table 5-5 **Recommendations for the Future U.S. Nursing Workforce**

1. Promote targeted educational investment in foreign educated nurses in the United States
2. Promote baccalaureate education for entry into practice in the United States
3. Harmonize nursing curricula
4. Add global health as subject matter to undergraduate and graduate nursing curricula
5. Establish a national system that monitors and tracks the inflow of foreign nurses, their countries of origin, the settings in which they work, and their education and licensure to ensure a proper skill mix for the U.S. nursing workforce
6. Create an international body to coordinate and recommend national and international workforce policies

Adapted from Institute of Medicine. (2011). The future of nursing: Leading change, advancing health. Washington, DC: The National Academies Press. Appendix J, International Models of Nursing,

These relationships support the development of course content that would include a description of health systems worldwide and information on global patterns of disease, practice conditions, and professional migration.

The formulation of health-care policy can be significantly influenced by a comprehensive database that could assist governmental and private organizations in health planning and policy development by tracking the education, skill mix, and practice and migration patterns of nurses.

In summary, nurses share a common professional history, yet, internationally, education, preparation, regulation, and practice are largely diverse. Market forces have created the demand for a globalized nursing workforce. The WHO developed a set of global standards for competency-based educational criteria and outcomes for the Initial Education of Nurses and Midwives. These evidence-based standards were developed for promoting positive health outcomes, and they acknowledge the progressive nature of education and lifelong learning (WHO, 2009). These standards serve as guidelines for professional nursing regardless of the specific location of the educational program or practice, and they ease the burden placed on nurses who migrate to other countries to practice.

Ethical, Safety, and Health Considerations When Studying or Working Abroad

This final section provides some food for thought for individuals who are planning to study or practice abroad. The increasing numbers of students, faculty, clinicians, and researchers who are pursuing their interests in diverse locations has raised both ethical and practical questions about how to best prepare individuals for work and study in settings that cross national and sociocultural borders. The Working Group on Ethics Guidelines for Global Health Training (WEIGHT) has developed guidelines for institutions, trainees, and sponsors of field-based global health training on ethics and best practices (Crump, Sugarman, & the WEIGHT, 2010). The WEIGHT guidelines encourage institutions to develop structured programs among international partners, including an accounting of the costs and reciprocal benefits associated with these partnerships. Other discussion points are how long-term partnerships can mitigate possible short-term adverse consequences; the characteristics of suitable trainees and supervisors; and how participants should be prepared, including attitudes and risk reduction education. The WEIGHT recommendations include the following actions for global health trainees:

• Recognize that the purpose is learning and possible service. Develop goals and expectations for the experience, and communicate this to the receiving institution or mentor.
• Obtain necessary language skills and become informed about the local social-cultural, political, and historical aspects of the host community.
• Demonstrate cultural competency through personal dress, respect privileged communication, be cognizant of alternate meanings of gestures and body language, and seek a more in-depth understanding of gender and traditional health beliefs in the host setting.
• Meet licensing standards, visa policies, and all other program requirements.
• Follow accepted international guidelines regarding the donation of medication, technology, and other supplies.
• If publications are a possibility, discuss plans for authorship of publications early to determine the degree of collaboration and how it will be credited.
• Be prepared to provide feedback on the training experience and follow-up information on career development.

It's helpful to assess personal attributes so that strengths can be exploited and vulnerabilities acknowledged and compensated for. Good listening skills and an awareness of nonverbal cues are very important in new settings. These will be needed along with good observational skills in general to learn about how various communities perceive the world and approach problems. The ability to weigh options and engage in informed risk-taking is important for making safe decisions while still being able to extend one's experiential base in unfamiliar settings. Finally, the personal characteristics of patience and flexibility will be needed, along with the recognition that feelings of frustration may be cultural in origin. For this reason, an awareness of personal values and cultural assumptions is vital and will need to be reexamined over time.

Venues for learning more about global nursing are the ICN journal *International Nursing Review* and the STTI publication *Journal of Nursing Scholarship*. For students and faculty wishing to study, teach, and conduct research abroad, Fulbright scholarships are an option. The Fulbright Program is the flagship international educational exchange program sponsored by the U.S. government. It is named after the late senator J. William Fulbright (1905–1995), who was the longest serving chair of the Senate Foreign Relations Committee. There have been 300,000 past participants fulfilling its mission to increase mutual understanding between the U.S. citizens and the people of other countries. The Fogarty International Center (FIC) is the U.S. National Institutes of Health (NIH) agency that provides grants and fellowships focused on global health training and research. The FIC mission is to foster partnerships between health research institutions in the United States and abroad while training the next generation of scientists to address global health needs. The FIC was created in 1968 and is named after Representative John E. Fogarty, who was an outspoken advocate for the NIH budget and U.S. global outreach in the health sciences.

When planning to work abroad as a nurse, a travel health consultation is advised to assess risks related to a specific destination and to receive individualized counseling and advice about personal protection practices. This will include a risk assessment to determine the need for immunizations; chemoprophylaxis for malaria; precautions about food and water safety; and personal safety, particularly in countries where roads, vehicles, and infrastructure may be in disrepair (Panosian, 2010). Rabies risk may be substantially higher in some destinations, requiring special precautions and a plan for how to proceed if confronted with a possible exposure. Emergency evacuation insurance is highly recommended, since out-of-pocket costs may vary from a few thousand dollars to over $100,000, depending on the circumstances. Without insurance, this fee must be paid before the evacuation is undertaken.

Nurses globally have more commonalities than differences as they seek to solve problems that range from straightforward to highly complex. The role of a professional nurse, regardless of location, includes advocating for equitable access to health services and essential medication; questioning discriminatory practices based on differences such as age, gender, race, culture, or religion; providing care to the most vulnerable members of society; and providing the education and coaching that empower individuals and families to care for themselves. Although the manner in which nursing advocacy is accomplished will vary depending on local resources, technology, governmental policies, and culture, the goal remains the same: to provide competent and compassionate nursing services based on the best evidence available.

REFLECTIVE EXERCISE 5.1

Rachel Cooper is a nurse practitioner who is departing in two months for an assignment with a Haitian Non-Governmental Organization (NGO) that delivers health-care services within the capital of Port-au-Prince and several neighboring communities. Rachel's preparation began online when she reviewed the CDC recommendations for humanitarian aid workers, as well as specific advice for relief workers going to Haiti. She followed links to the U.S. State Department and the *CIA World Factbook* to read about the Haitian government and health-care system; crime prevention; stress management; heatstroke; and diseases such as hepatitis, typhoid, rabies, tuberculosis,

leptospirosis, HIV, and mosquito-borne malaria and dengue. She plans to avoid travel at night, bring a bike helmet, and register with the U.S. Embassy. She is shopping around for evacuation insurance because the NGO does not provide it. Today Rachel consulted with a travel health specialist for a detailed risk assessment. She was asked about her daytime and nighttime activities; whether the dormitory housing provided air conditioning, window/door screens, or bed nets; and personal health status. Rachel received vaccinations and a prescription for a weekly antimalarial medication. Precautions for food- and water-borne diseases (e.g., cholera) and injury prevention (e.g., traffic accidents, falls, drowning, and violence) were discussed in detail. Rachel is looking forward to this new experience and feels prepared for the health risks she will face in Haiti.

1. What resources are available to U.S. travelers to learn about travel health risks and prevention strategies?
2. For how long after returning to the United States should a traveler be concerned that new symptoms could be related to a travel exposure (i.e., days, weeks, months, years)?
3. What are Rachel's options for emergency evacuation insurance? How much does it cost to be evacuated for health or safety reasons when individuals do not purchase insurance?
4. What cultural issues will Rachel need to be sensitive to while working as a nurse volunteer in Haiti?

REFLECTIVE EXERCISE 5.2

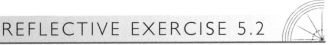

Dr. Lily Lee is a professor of nursing who will spend a semester sabbatical in Kampala, Uganda, to work in diabetes management and to assist with the development of diabetes educational materials. She chose Uganda because over the past five years she has taken nursing and other health science students there for a 3-week immersion experience focused on an overview of health-care, culture, and the environment. While in Uganda, she wants to be part of a recognized organization that can assist her with licensing and credentials requirements, housing, and developing a work plan. She decides to explore a Non-Governmental Organization (NGO) called Health Volunteers Overseas (HVO; www.hvousa.org). She finds the mission statement that describes HVO as a private non-profit organization dedicated to improving the availability and quality of health care in developing countries through the training and education of local health-care providers. Even though there was no posted volunteer opportunity for a nurse in diabetes education, Professor Lee decided to state her specific interest in her application because one of the guiding principles of HVO is not only education about diseases and treatments but to focus on prevention. She was pleased that her application was accepted and now needs to finalize her plans.

Continued

1. What more would Professor Lee want to know about this organization before making a commitment to volunteer for a semester?
2. Once you've visited the Web site, do you think HVO is a good match with Professor Lee's objectives?
3. How will serving as an HVO volunteer be different from her prior visits as a faculty member with students representing her university?
4. What strategies could Professor Lee use to increase the sustainability of her Ugandan project after she is gone?

REFERENCES

American Association of Colleges of Nursing. (2011). *Nursing shortage fact sheet*. Washington, DC: AACN.

Anderson, G.F., & Squires, D.A. (2010). *Measuring the U.S. health care system: A cross-national comparison*. Washington, DC: The Commonwealth Fund.

Audibert, M., Motel, P.C., & Drabo, A. (2010). *Global burden of disease and economic growth*. Clermont-Ferrand, France: Centre d'Etudes et de Recherches sur le Developpement International (CERDI).

Beaglehole, R., & Yach, D. (2003). Globalisation and the prevention and control of non-communicable disease: the neglected chronic diseases of adults. *Lancet, 362*(9387), 903–908.

Buchan, J., Kingma, M., & Lorenzo, F. (2005). *International migration of nurses: Trends and policy implications*. Geneva: ICN.

Cavalcanti, A., Shirinzadeh, B., & Kretly, L.C. (2008). Medical nonrobotics for diabetes control. *Nanomedicine, 4*(2), 127–138.

Chapman, A.R. (2009). Globalization, human rights, and the social determinants of health. *Bioethics, 23*, 97–111.

Clarke, P.N., & Butterfield, P. (2011). Nursing as if the future matters. *Nursing Science Quarterly, 24*(126), 126–129.

Crump, J.A., Sugarman, J., & and the Working Group on Ethics Guidelines for Global Health Training. (2010). Global health training: Ethics and best practice guidelines for training experiences in global health. *American Journal of Tropical Medicine and Hygiene, 83*(6), 1178–1182.

CSIS Commission on Smart Global Health Policy. (2010). *Smart global health policy*. Washington, DC: Center for Strategic and International Studies.

Daar, A.S., Singer, P.A., Persad, D.L., Pramming, S.K., Matthews, D.R., Beaglehole, R., et al. (2007). Grand challenges in chronic non-communicable diseases. *Nature, 450*, 494–496.

Fuster, V., & Voute, J. (2005). MDGs: Chronic diseases are not on the agenda (Comment). *Lancet, 366*, 1512–1514.

Gostin, L.O. (2007). Meeting basic survival needs of the world's least healthy people: Toward a framework convention on global health. *Georgetown Law Journal, 96*(2), 331–392.

Health Grants Information Center. (2009). Retrieved from http://healthgrants.wordpress.com/category/major-philanthropic-foundations/

Holzemer, W.L. (2008). Building a qualified global nursing workforce. *Nursing Care Continuum-Framework and Competencies*. Geneva: International Council of Nurses.

Institute of Medicine (IOM) & Board on International Health. (1997). *America's vital interest in global health: Protecting our people, enhancing our economy, and advancing our international interests*. Washington, DC: National Academy Press.

International Council of Nurses. (2009). *Reducing the gap and improving the interface between education and service: A framework for analysis and solution generation*. Geneva: ICN.

Kingma, M. (2006). *Nurses on the move: Migration and the global health care economy*. Ithaca: ILR Press (Cornell University Press).

Kingma, M. (2008). Nurses on the move: Historical perspective and current issues. *OJIN: The Online Journal of Issues in Nursing, 13*(2), Manuscript 1.

Kirk, H. (2007). Towards a global nursing workforce: The "brain circulation." *Nursing Management, 13*(10), 26–30.

Koplan, J.P., Bond, T.C., Merson, M.H., Reddy, K.S., Rodriguez, M.H., Sewankambo, N.K., et al. (2009). Towards a common definition of global health. *Lancet, 373*, 1993–1995.

Lancet NCD Action Group. (2011). Priority actions for the non-communicable disease crisis. Lancet, published online April 6, 2011. DOI:10.1016/S0140-6736(11)60393-0.

Laurent, C. (2011). Scaling up HIV treatment in resource-limited countries: The challenge of staff shortages. *Journal of Public Health Policy*, 1–8. DOI:10.1057/jphp.2011.8.

Mathers, C.D., & Loncar, D. (2006). Projections of global mortality and burden of disease from 2002 to 2030. *PLOS Medicine, 3*(11), 2011–2030.

Narayan, K.M.V., Ali, M.K., & Koplan, J.P. (2010). Global non-communicable diseases: Where worlds meet. *New England Journal of Medicine, 363*(13), 1196–1198.

Nichols, B.L., Davis, C.R., & Richardson, J.D. (2011). International models of nursing. In Institute of Medicine (Ed.), *The future of nursing: Leading change, advancing health* (Appendix J). Washington, DC: National Academies Press.

Nichter, M. (2008). *Global health*. Tucson, AR: Arizona Press.

Panosian, C. (2010). Courting danger while doing good—protecting global health workers from harm. *New England Journal of Medicine, 363*(26), 2484–2485.

Piette, J. (2007). Interactive behavior change technology to support diabetes self-management: Where do we stand? *Diabetes Care, 30*(10), 2425–2432.

Piette, J.D., Mendoza-Avelares, M.O., Milton, E.C., Lange, I., & Fajardo, R. (2010). Access to mobile communication technology and willingness to participate in automated telemedicine calls among chronically ill patients in Honduras. *Telemedicine Journal and e-Health, 16*(10), 1030–1041.

Pruitt, S.D., & Epping-Jordan, J.E. (2005). Preparing the 21st century global healthcare workforce. *British Medical Journal, 330*(7492), 637–639.

Rosenkoetter, M., & Nardi, D. (2007). American Academy of Nursing expert panel on global nursing and health: White paper on global nursing and health. *Journal of Transcultural Nursing, 18*(4), 305–315.

Salmon, M., Yan, J., Hewitt, H., & Guisinger, V. (2007). Managed migration: The Caribbean approach to addressing nursing services capacity. *Health Services Research, 42*(3), 1354–1372.

Sattler, B. (2011). The greening of a major medical center. *American Journal of Nursing, 111*(4), 60–62.

SNV Netherlands Development Organization & United Nations Development Programme (2009). *Going local to achieve the millennium development goals: Stories from eight countries*. New York: United Nations.

Squires, A. (2011). The North American Free Trade Agreement (NAFTA) and Mexican nursing. *Health policy and planning, 26*(2), 124–132.

United Nations. (2004). *International migration trends*. New York: Population Division, Department of Economic and Social Affairs.

United Nations. (2007). *World urbanization prospects: The 2007 revision (executive summary)*. New York: Department of Economic and Social Affairs.

United Nations. (2010). *World population aging 2009*. New York: Population Division, Department of Economic and Social Affair.

United Nations. (2011). *Migration and human rights. United Nations human rights*. Retrieved from http://www.ohchr.org/EN/Issues/Migration/Pages/MigrationAndHumanRightsIndex.aspx

USAID: Health. (2009). Fact sheet: The U.S. government 's global health initiative. *Retrieved from http://www.usaid.gov/ghi/factsheet.html*

World Bank. (1993). *World development report 1993: Investing in health.*

Washington, DC: World Bank.

World Health Organization. (1946). *Preamble to the Constitution of the World Health Organization as adopted by the International Health Conference*, New York: WHO.

World Health Organization. (2002). *Innovative care for chronic conditions: Building blocks for action*. Geneva: WHO.

World Health Organization. (2004). *The global burden of disease: 2004 update*. Geneva: WHO.

World Health Organization. (2006). *World health report 2006*. Geneva: WHO.

World Health Organization. (2008). *Task shifting: Global recommendations and guidelines*. Geneva: WHO.

World Health Organization. (2009). *Global standards for the initial education of professional nurses and midwives*. Geneva: WHO.

World Health Organization. (2010). *Global atlas of the health workforce*. Retrieved from http://www.who.int/hrh/workforce_mdgs/en/index.html

World Health Organization. (2011). *2015 millennium development goals*. Geneva: WHO.

World Health Organization and UNICEF. (1978). *Primary health care: Report of the International Conference on Primary Health Care*. Alma-Ata USSR. September 6–12, 1978. Geneva: WHO.

DavisPlus *For case studies, review questions, and additional information, go to*
http://davisplus.fadavis.com

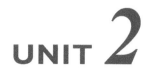

AGGREGATE DATA FOR CULTURAL-SPECIFIC GROUPS

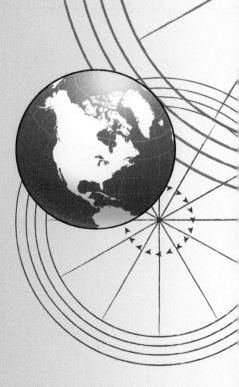

Chapter 6

People of African American Heritage

Josepha Campinha-Bacote

Overview, Inhabited Localities, and Topography

Overview

African Americans are the second largest minority population in the United States, with the Hispanic/ Latino population being the largest (U.S. Department of Health and Human Services, 2009). The population of African Americans, including those of more than one race, was estimated at 40.7 million, comprising 13.5 percent of the total population as of July 1, 2007, according to the Census Bureau (U.S. Department of Commerce, Census Bureau, 2010). This number is projected to rise to 65.7 million (15 percent) of the total population by the year 2050.

African Americans are mainly of African ancestry, but many have non-African ancestors due to the fact that the slave trade resulted in a diaspora from West and Central Africa to many parts of the world, including the West Indies, South America, Central America, and the United States. Over the centuries, in all of parts of the world, the African has mixed with other local ethnic groups. In America this intermixing has largely been with American Indians and European Americans. Although African Americans and African immigrants in the United States share some similarities in respect to phenotype features and experience with racism, discrimination, and prejudices, there are major differences that vary in regard to such factors as sociopolitical history, languages, cultural beliefs, and family life (Chin, 2009, p. 15). Because of the significant diversity that exists among African Americans, health-care providers must be aware of the intracultural variations that exist within this ethnic group.

African Americans have been identified as "Negro," "colored," "black," "black American," "Afro-American," and "people of color." Depending on their cohort group, some African Americans may prefer to identify themselves differently. For example, younger blacks may prefer the term *African American*, whereas elderly African Americans may use the terms *Negro* and *colored*. In contrast, middle-aged African Americans refer to themselves as *black* or *black American*. Although the term *Negro* is not a commonly used today, and many African Americans are offended by its use, the U.S. Census Bureau still included the term *Negro* on the 2010 U.S. Census, along with the terms *black* and *African American*. These different descriptors can cause confusion for those who are attempting to use the politically correct term for this ethnic group. In addition, organizational titles as the National Black Nurses Association, National Center for the Advancement of Blacks in the Health Professions, the National Association for the Advancement of Colored People, and the United College Negro Fund still exist, which clearly depict the differences in how African Americans prefer to be identified. Therefore, it is culturally responsive to ask African Americans what they prefer to be called.

Heritage and Residence

African Americans are largely the descendants of Africans who were brought forcibly to this country as slaves between 1619 and 1860. The literature contains many conflicting reports of the exact number of slaves that arrived in this country. Varying estimates reveal that from 3.5 to 24 million slaves landed in the Americas during the slave trade era. Many slaves who were brought to the American colonies and early United States came from the west coast of Africa, from the Kwa- and Bantu-speaking people. The legacy of African American heritage and history of slavery is often passed on from generation to generation through African American folktales and lived experiences (Taulbert, 1969).

African American slaves were settled mostly in southern states. In 2007, 56 percent of African Americans still live in the South; 19 percent live in the North and Northeast, 9 percent in the West, and 19 percent in the Midwest. In 2008, the 10 states with the largest black populations were New York, Florida, Texas, Georgia, California, North Carolina, Illinois, Maryland, Virginia, and Michigan (U.S. Department of Health and Human Services, 2009). Louisiana is no longer in the top 10 as a result of Hurricane Katrina in 2005. Combined, these 10 states represented 59 percent of the total African American population. Of the 10 largest places in the United States with populations of 100,000 or more, Gary, Indiana, has the largest proportion of blacks—83 percent—followed by Detroit with 82 percent (U.S. Department of Health and Human Services, 2009).

Reasons for Migration and Associated Economic Factors

The Civil War ended slavery in 1865, and particularly in the state of South Carolina, the Reconstruction Act allowed blacks the right to vote and participate in state government. However, most African Americans in the South were denied their civil rights and were segregated. Thus, African Americans lived in poverty and encountered many hardships. After the Civil War, more African Americans migrated from southern rural areas to northern urban areas. Blacks migrated because of a lack of security for life and property. They were unable to get out of debt and support their families despite being successful farmers. Also, World War II was a major catalyst in fostering migration to urban and northern areas, which provided greater economic opportunities and brought African Americans and European Americans into close contact for the first time. Jaynes and Williams (1989) reported that during the 1940s, a net outmigration from the South totaled approximately 1.5 million African Americans (15 percent of the South's black population). Although the migration was viewed as a positive move, many African Americans encountered all the problems of fragmented urban life, racism, poverty, and covert segregation.

Educational Status and Occupations

Before 1954, educational opportunities for African Americans were compromised. School systems were segregated, and blacks were victims of inferior facilities. In fact, in 1910, almost one-third of all blacks were illiterate (Blum et al., 1981). However, in 1954, the Supreme Court decision in *Brown v. Board of Education of Topeka* ruled against the segregation of blacks and whites in the public school systems. Conant (1961) described the plight of African Americans in segregated schools and, to some extent, predicted the long-term social consequences of such a system. His predictions have been borne out as inadequate job opportunities and poor wages, resulting in poverty. Poverty has had a ripple effect on African American

communities, often leading to poorly educated individuals, high dropout rates from school, and drug and alcohol misuse (Ladner & Gourdine, 1992). In many African American communities, this oppressive environment contributes to the existing alcohol and drug problems and the high dropout rate among African Americans, which has been reported as high as 61 percent (Braithwaite, Taylor, & Austin, 2000).

Despite these devastating occurrences, most African American families place a high value on education. In 2008, 81 percent of African Americans age 25 and older had a high school diploma (U.S. Department of Commerce, Bureau of the Census, 2008). The African American family views education as the process most likely to ensure work security and social mobility. Families often make great sacrifices so at least one child can go to college. In African American families, it is not uncommon to see cooperative efforts among siblings to assist one another financially to obtain a college education. For example, as the older child graduates and becomes employed, that child then assists the next sibling, who, in turn, assists the next one. This continues until all of the children who attend college have graduated. Before the civil rights movement, a major emphasis for African Americans in higher education was vocational. The thinking was that if African Americans could learn a trade or vocation, they could become self-sufficient and improve their economic well-being. Preparation for vocational careers is evidenced in the name, mission, and goals of two of the renowned, historically black institutions, Hampton University and Tuskegee University, formerly known as Hampton Institute and Tuskegee Normal and Industrial Institute.

Although African Americans have successfully completed a variety of majors in universities, significant differences exist in the ethnic, racial, and gender makeup of those obtaining higher degrees. In 2008, 18 percent of African Americans had a bachelor's degree or higher, which is 10 percent age points lower than the national average (U.S. Department of Commerce, Bureau of the Census, 2008). Today, African Americans continue to be underrepresented in managerial and professional positions. In addition, the representation of many African Americans and other ethnic groups in the health professions is far below their representation in the general population (Sullivan, 2004). Increasing racial and ethnic diversity among health professionals is critical because evidence indicates that diversity is associated with improved access to care for racial and ethnic minority patients, greater patient choice and satisfaction, and better educational experiences for all students (IOM, 2004).

African Americans represent a large segment of blue-collar workers employed in service occupations (Low-wage labor market, 2006). One reason for this disproportionate representation in professional and managerial positions is believed to be discrimination in employment and job advancement. In 1961, President John F. Kennedy established the Committee on Equal Employment Opportunity to protect minorities from discrimination in employment. However, most African Americans still believe that job discrimination is a major variable contributing to problems they encounter in obtaining better jobs or successful career mobility. With the dismantling of affirmative-action programs, based on misinterpretation of their purpose, this view will, perhaps, continue to gain support.

Most working-class African Americans do not typically advance to the higher socioeconomic levels. Because they are overrepresented in the working class, they are more likely to be employed in hazardous occupations, resulting in occupation-related diseases and illnesses. For example, Michaels (1993) reported that African American males are at a higher risk for developing cancer, which is related to their high representation in the steel and tire industries. According to Clark (1999), genetic factors of greatest importance in the work environment are probably race and gender. Implications are that health-care providers must not only assess African American patients for occupation-related diseases such as cancer and stress-related diseases such as hypertension but must also be familiar with the government's *Healthy People 2010* goals for the health and safety of individuals in the work environment (U.S. Department of Health and Human Services, 1997).

Communication

Dominant Language and Dialects

The dominant language spoken among African Americans is English. Some African Americans use a language that sociolinguists refer to as *African American English* (*AAE*). According to Green (2002) AAE includes the variations of an ethnic and social dialect spoken by African Americans who are members of the working class, street culture, and hip-hop or rap. The two main hypotheses about the origin of AAE are the dialect hypothesis and the Creole hypothesis. The dialect hypothesis supports the position that African slaves, upon arriving in the United States, picked up English very slowly and learned it incorrectly. In turn, these inaccuracies have been passed down through generations. The Creole hypothesis maintains that AAE is the result of a Creole derived from English and various West African Languages.

The major problem that AAE speakers face is prejudice. Most people believe that AAE is inferior to Standard American English (SAE). At times, African Americans who use AAE are misinterpreted as being uneducated. However, it is common for educated African Americans who are extremely articulate in SAE to use AAE when conversing with one another. Thompson, Craig, and Washington (2004) referred to

this ability as *dialect-shifting*. The literature suggests that AAE provides African Americans with a framework for communicating unique cultural ideas and also serves as a way to symbolize racial pride and identity (Allender & Spradley, 2001; Murray & Zentner, 2001).

Over the years, a number of names have been used to describe the different varieties or dialects of AAE. Some of the more common terms are *Black Dialect, Black Folk Speech, Black English, Ebonics, Black Vernacular English* (*BEV*), and *African American Vernacular English* (*AAVE*) (Bland-Stewart, 2005; Green, 2002). Much controversy exists regarding the use of these labels. In December 1996, the Oakland School Board in Oakland, California, passed a resolution to recognize Ebonics as the primary language of African American children and take it into account in their language arts lessons and classrooms (Rickford, 1999). This resolution sparked national debate, and in April 1997, the Oakland School Board dropped the word *Ebonics* from their implementation proposals. Obvious problems occur with defining a language racially because not all African Americans speak these varieties, and some non–African Americans speak them as well.

Cultural Communication Patterns

African American communication has been described as high-context (Cokley, Cooke, & Nobles, 2005). The volume of African Americans' voices is often louder than those in some other cultures; therefore, health-care providers must not misunderstand this attribute and automatically assume this increase in tone is reflecting anger. African American speech is dynamic and expressive, and they communicate more interactively than European Americans. Wood (2009) states that this may explain why some African Americans shout out responses such as "Tell it," "All right," and "Keep talking" during speeches or church sermons. While many European Americans may consider these comments as an interruption, some African Americans regard it as complimentary participation in communication. Body movements are involved when communicating with others. Facial expressions can be very demonstrative. African Americans are reported to be comfortable with a closer personal space than other ethnic groups. Touch is another form of nonverbal communication seen when African Americans are interacting with relatives and extended family members. When interacting with African Americans, the power of touching should not be underestimated for its healing powers (Cokley et al., 2005).

In communicating among themselves, African Americans place a strong value on oral tradition. Oral tradition is the face-to-face transmittal of elements of the African American culture from one generation to another by the spoken word (NMAETC, 2006). One example of this form of communication is story-telling. These stories convey important values and morals on how to live life.

Humor is a form of communication that can serve as a tool to release angry feelings and to reduce stress and ease racial tension. The *dozens*, a social game in which African Americans use humor, is a joking relationship between two African Americans in which each in turn is, by custom, permitted to tease or make fun of the other (Campinha-Bacote, 1993). Frequently, humor is used among the African American population as a preventive mechanism to ward off an anticipated attack. Often, the joking is loud and can be mistaken for aggressive communication if not understood within the context of the African American culture. Being aware of and understanding the function that humor serves in the African American culture can assist health-care providers to formulate culturally responsive health-care interventions. For example, Campinha-Bacote (1993; 1997) documented the effective use of culturally specific humor groups with African American patients with psychiatric disorders.

Many African Americans mistrust health-care providers and express their feelings only to trusted friends or family. What transpires within the family is viewed as private and not appropriate for discussion with strangers. A common phrase that reflects this perspective is "Don't air your dirty laundry in public." Health-care providers must be sensitive to this form of communication in that older and more traditional African Americans may not embrace "talk therapy."

Temporal Relationships

In general, African Americans tend to be more present- than past- or future-oriented. However, the past or future may be valued in specific subgroups of African Americans, such as the elderly, who place greater emphasis on the past than on the present. In contrast, younger and middle-aged African Americans are more present oriented, with evidence of becoming more future oriented, as indicated by the value placed on education.

Some African Americans are more relaxed about time and may not be prompt for their appointments. Within this context, it is more important for them to show up for an appointment than to be on time. What they see as important is the fact that they are there, even though they may arrive 1 or 2 hours late. Therefore, flexibility in timing appointments may be necessary for African Americans, who have a circular sense of time rather than the dominant culture's categorically imperative linear sense of time (Murray & Zentner, 2001).

Format for Names

Most African Americans prefer to be greeted formally as Dr., Reverend, Pastor, Mr., Mrs., Ms., or Miss. They prefer their surname because the family name is highly respected and connotes pride in their family heritage. However, African Americans do not use such formal names when they interact among themselves. An African American youth commonly addresses an unrelated African American who lives in the community as Uncle, Aunt, or Cousin. Adult African Americans may also be called names different from their legal names. Until invited to do otherwise, greet African American patients by using their last name and appropriate title.

Family Roles and Organization
Head of Household and Gender Roles

Although today it is common to find a patriarchal system in African American families, a high percentage of families still have a matriarchal system. The head of the household can be a single mother, grandmother, or aunt. A single head of household is accepted without associated stigma in African American families. When women are unable to provide emotional and physical support for their children, grandmothers, aunts, the church, and extended or augmented families readily provide assistance or take responsibility for the children. One important trend noted today is that a growing number of African American grandparents are functioning in primary parental roles. For example, 44 percent of all children living with grandparents today are African American. Approximately 66 percent of these children have grandparents as the primary caregivers.

Ladner and Gourdine (1992) state, "Single parenting and poverty are viewed as the causal factors in destabilizing the African American family" (p. 208). The poverty rate for African Americans reached 25.8 percent in 2009 (U.S. Department of Commerce, Bureau of the Census, 2008). Forty-one percent of single-mother African American families are living in poverty. Anther contributing factor undermining the African American

REFLECTIVE EXERCISE 6.1

Kesia Crawford, a 6-year-old African American female, is brought into the ER by her grandmother, Mrs. Elvenia Thomas, for vaginal bleeding. The nurse, in an attempt to establish rapport with the grandmother, states, "Shirley, I know you must be very concerned that your granddaughter is experiencing this bleeding." The grandmother immediately becomes defensive in her subsequent responses to the nurse's questions.

1. What are some reasons for Kesia Crawford's vaginal bleeding?
2. How would you conduct a culturally sensitive skin assessment with Kesia Crawford?
3. What may explain why Mrs. Thomas became defensive in her responses to the nurse?

family is the absence of African American males due to high unemployment rates, low life expectancy, and incarceration. Overall, African American men are incarcerated at 6.5 times the rate of white men (U.S. Department of Justice Office of Justice Programs, 2008)

Gender roles and child-rearing practices in the African American family vary widely depending on ethnicity, socioeconomic class, rural versus urban location, and educational achievement. The diverse family structure extends the care of family members beyond the nuclear family to include relatives and nonrelatives. Similar to the pattern in the general society, dual employment of many middle-class African American families requires cooperative teamwork. Many family tasks such as cooking, cleaning, child care, and shopping are shared, requiring flexibility and adaptability of roles.

Because many African American families, especially those with a single head of household, are matrifocal in nature, the health-care provider must recognize women's importance in decision making and disseminating health information. Also, the health-care provider must focus on, and work with, the strengths of African American families, especially single-parent families. Hill (1997) stated that although many African American families headed by single women are economically disadvantaged, they should not be compared or equated with broken or intact families.

Prescriptive, Restrictive, and Taboo Roles for Children and Adolescents

Given African Americans' strong work and achievement orientation, they value self-reliance and education for their children. A dichotomy might exist here, because many parents do not expect to get full benefit from their efforts because of discrimination. Thus, families tend to be more protective of their children and act as a buffer between their children and the outside world.

Respectfulness, obedience, conformity to parent-defined rules, and good behavior are stressed for children. The belief is that a firm parenting style, structure, and discipline are necessary to protect the child from danger outside of the home. In violence-ridden communities, mothers try to keep young children off the streets and encourage them to engage in productive activities. Adolescents are assigned household chores as part of their family responsibility or seek employment for pay when they are old enough, thus learning "survival skills."

Although there has been a decline in the incidence of teen pregnancy, it continues to be a problem in the African American community because of poor pregnancy outcomes such as premature and low-birth-weight infants and obstetric complications. Furthermore, the teenage mother is expected to assume primary responsibility for her child, whereas the extended family becomes a strong support system. Premarital teenage pregnancy

is not condoned in African American families but rather is accepted after the fact. In other instances, the infant may be informally adopted, and someone other than the mother may become the primary caregiver.

Family Roles and Priorities

African American families share a wide range of characteristics, family values, goals, and priorities. An example of a strong family value is the level of respect bestowed upon the elders in the African American community. In this community, the elders, especially grandmothers, are respected for their insight and wisdom. The role of the grandmother is one of the most central roles in the African American family. Grandmothers are frequently the economic support of African American families, and they often play a critical role in child care. It is common to see African American children raised by grandparents; this has contributed to an increase in the number of skipped-generational families seen in the African American community.

Understanding the role of the extended family in the lives of African Americans is essential. Several African American extended-family models exist. Billingsley (1968) divided them into four major types: subfamilies, families with secondary members, augmented families, and nonblood relatives. Subfamily members include nieces, nephews, cousins, aunts, and uncles. Secondary members consist of peers of the primary parents, older relatives of the primary parents, and parents of the primary parents. In an augmented family, the head of the household raises children who are not his or her own relatives. Nonblood relatives are individuals who are unrelated by blood ties but who are closely involved with the family functioning. Nonblood relatives are also referred to as "fictive kin." As a result of long-standing relationships with the family, fictive kin may be serving as the primary caregivers or even as the substitute decision makers and sometimes may be more involved than the related family members (Curriculum Ethnogeriatrics, 2001) Studies have found that African American families exhibit about 70 diverse structural formations versus about 40 among white families (Barbarin, 1983). Barbarin adds that this comparison points to the variability of the African American family structure and to the flexibility of family roles.

Social status is important within the African American community. Certain occupations receive higher esteem than others. For example, African American physicians and dentists tend to have privileged positions. Ministers and clergy also receive respect in the African American community. They have historically held a high status in African American communities and are critical "First Responders" (Cokley et al., 2005).

African Americans who move up the socioeconomic ladder often find themselves caught between two worlds. They have their roots in the African American community, but at times they find themselves interacting more within the European American community. Other African Americans refer to these individuals as "oreos"—a derogatory term that means "black on the outside, but white on the inside." In Frazier's (1957) seminal and controversial publication *Black Bourgeoisie,* he highly criticized middle-class blacks. He argued that African American families who achieve upper-middle-class and middle-class status—the so-called black bourgeoisie—perpetuate a myth of "Negro society." According to Frazier, this term describes behavior, attitudes, and values of a make-believe world created by middle- and upper-class African Americans in order to escape feelings of inferiority in American society.

Alternative Lifestyles

Lesbian and gay relationships undoubtedly occur as frequently among African Americans as in other ethnic groups. A review of the literature reveals that African Americans are less supportive of homosexuality than other racial and ethnic groups, but the reasons have more to do with religion than race. African Americans are markedly more religious on a variety of measures than the U.S. population as a whole, including level of affiliation with a religion, attendance at religious services, frequency of prayer, and religion's importance in life (The Pew Forum on Religion & Public Life, 2009). Negy and Eisenman (2005) reported that while initial results of their study suggested that African Americans had modestly higher homophobia and homonegativity scores than whites, these differences did not hold after controlling for frequency of church attendance, religious commitment, and socioeconomic status. For both ethnic groups, religiosity significantly predicted homophobia and homonegativity.

Acceptance of same-sex relationships varies between and among families. Personal disclosure to friends and family may jeopardize relationships, thereby forcing some to remain closeted. Debate is ongoing about the pros and cons of legitimizing lesbian and gay families, especially when children are involved. Opponents of this family form believe that parental behavior has a profound effect on children's gender identities and establishing family values (Bender, 1998). Single parenting and other alternative lifestyles are discussed in other sections in this chapter.

Workforce Issues
Culture in the Workplace

Although the African American value system reflects a strong emphasis on spirituality, there is also an economic-driven emphasis on materialism. African Americans feel a need to acculturate into mainstream society in order to successfully survive in the workforce. However, this survival is often met with ethnic or racial tension. *Ethnic* or *racial tension* can be defined as a negative workplace atmosphere motivated by prejudicial attitudes about cultural background and/or skin color. Watts (2003) asserts that race is an issue for African Americans, and "the black experience" in America is markedly different from that of other immigrants, specifically in terms of the extended period of the institution of slavery and the issue of skin color as a means for dehumanization of black persons. Watts concludes that matters of race, racism, and racial discrimination persist throughout contemporary American life.

In 2007, the unemployment rate for African Americans was twice that for non-Hispanic whites (8 percent and 4 percent, respectively). This finding was consistent for both men (9 percent compared with 4 percent) and women (8 percent compared with 4 percent) (U.S. Department of Health and Human Services, 2009). Research reveals that African Americans have a long history of workforce disadvantage. While some work organizations are making strides in their efforts to fight against discrimination, African Americans continue to encounter challenges imposed on them through the multifaceted interactions of racially motivated negative attitudes and actions of individual and organizational policies and practices that are not encountered by European Americans. These major problems include such issues as employment process biases, channeling into "minority" positions, lack of access to network and mentors, promotion and advancement difficulties, and emotional and psychological maltreatment (Parks-Yancy, 2010; Queralt, 1996).

African Americans are underrepresented in highly skilled and managerial positions and overrepresented in low-status positions. Middle-class African Americans who hold higher-paying jobs often experience the "glass ceiling" effect, in which access to higher positions is blocked (Bigler & Averhart, 2003). However, Barack Obama, a biracial man born of an African father and European American mother, has instilled hope in African Americans as the first person of color to be elected president of the United States in 2008. Although his presidency appears to demonstrate that the "American Dream" is within reach for African Americans, authors such as Kwate and Meyer (2010) maintain that the problem still persists: "Opportunities *are not* equally distributed and are not allotted solely by meritocratic criteria" (p. 1831). Health-care providers must increase their sensitivity and awareness of cultural nuances and issues that create ethnic or racial tension in the workplace environment, for these factors can have an impact on such stress-related conditions as mental health disorders and hypertension.

Issues Related to Autonomy

Some African American men may experience a difficult time in taking direction from European American supervisors or bosses. This difficulty stems from the era of slavery when African Americans were considered the property of their masters. Many African Americans continue to be frustrated at their lower-level positions and the absence of African American leadership in many workplaces. Lowenstein and Glanville (1995) found that along with historical circumstances, culture and politics affect the employment of African Americans in the health-care industry, often relegating African Americans to nonskilled roles. Today, a large number of African Americans continue to work as nursing assistants, licensed practical nurses (LPNs), or technicians. Thus, if the professional nurse who directs and supervises nonprofessional workers lacks cultural sensitivity toward other ethnic groups, the stage is set for cultural conflict.

Because the dominant language of African Americans is English, they usually have no difficulty communicating verbally with others in the workforce. However, some people may inaccurately view African Americans who exclusively speak AAE as poorly educated or unintelligent. This misinterpretation may affect employment and job promotion where verbal skills are more valued. In addition, the nonverbal communication style (e.g., strong intonation and animated body movements) of some African Americans is often misunderstood and labeled as more aggressive than assertive in comparison with that of other cultural groups.

Biocultural Ecology
Skin Color and Other Biological Variations

African Americans encompass a gene pool of over 100 racial strains. Therefore, skin color among African Americans can vary from light to very dark. As health-care providers, we are trained in the art of using alterations in skin color and deviations from an individual's normal skin tone to aid in our diagnoses. For example, jaundice is a sign of a liver disorder; pink and blue skin changes are associated with pulmonary disease; ashen or gray color signals possible cardiac disease; copper skin tone indicates Addison's disease; and a nonblanchable erythema response signifies the presence of a stage I pressure ulcer (Salcido, 2002). We commonly use these alterations in skin color as potential signals of pathology because we can visualize changes such as the increased blood flow (erythema) that signals such problems as inflammation. However, these acquired assessment skills are based on a Eurocentric rather than a melanocentric approach to skin assessment (Campinha-Bacote, 2007). Sommers (2011) urges health-care providers to cultivate color awareness in regard to assessing the skin of African Americans. Color awareness recognizes that skin color is relevant to health and should not be ignored. Furthermore, by applying color awareness to health assessment, health-care providers can more appropriately manage skin conditions among patients of all skin colors and help reduce disparities in health-care delivery.

Assessing the skin of most African American patients requires clinical skills different from those for assessing people with white skin. For example, pallor in dark-skinned African Americans can be observed by the absence of the underlying red tones that give the brown and black skin its "glow" or "living color." Lighter-skinned African Americans appear more yellowish-brown, whereas darker-skinned African Americans appear ashen. Assessing such conditions as inflammation, cyanosis, jaundice, and petechiae in African Americans may require natural light and the use of different assessment skills. African Americans exhibiting inflammation or petechiae must be assessed by palpation of the skin for warmth, edema, tightness, or induration. If feasible, do not to wear gloves to perform the skin assessment, because they have a tendency to diminish sensitivity to skin temperature changes. To assess for cyanosis in dark-skinned African Americans, the health-care provider needs to observe the oral mucosa or conjunctiva. Jaundice is assessed more accurately in dark-skinned persons by observing the sclera of the eyes, the palms of the hands, and the soles of the feet, which may have a yellow discoloration. In performing a skin assessment it may also be helpful to ask the patient, family, significant other, or caregiver to point out an area of normal skin color, temperature, and texture to serve as a baseline (Sommers, 2011).

Researchers studying forensic sexual assault examinations found data suggesting African American women had a lower incidence of genital injury after rape when compared to European American women (Sommers et al., 2008). However, they maintain that the difference in reported injury prevalence was not related to race or ethnicity but rather due to reduced visibility of injury in dark-skinned women. Their research demonstrated that skin color explained the differences in the numbers of genital injuries than race or ethnicity, concluding that the prevalence of genital injuries in dark-skinned women has likely been underreported because of difficulty seeing the injuries. Sommers (2011) argues that these findings are important given the role of forensic evidence in the criminal justice system; women whose injuries are documented during the forensic examination have better judicial outcomes than women without documented injuries.

The literature also confirms that health-care providers are not doing an adequate job of detecting and reducing pressure ulcer risk in African Americans. According to recent studies, African Americans are at higher risk for developing more severe pressure ulcers and associated mortality and morbidity (Salcido, 2002). The *National Healthcare Disparities Report* (AQHR, 2005) revealed that in both 2002 and 2003, the proportion of high-risk, long-stay, and short-stay residents who had pressure sores was higher among African Americans and Hispanics when compared with non-Hispanic whites. Salcido (2002) asserted that it may be due to our lack of ability to make an early diagnosis of skin in jeopardy of breaking down. Currently, researchers are testing a variety of devices that could be used to detect and diagnose alterations in blood flow, regardless of the color of the patient's skin. These devices include visible and near-infrared spectroscopy, pulse oximetry, laser Doppler, and ultrasound (Matas et al., 2001; Salcido, 2002; Sowa, Matas, Schattka, & Mantsch, 2002).

Several skin disorders are found among the African American population. The major skin disorder is postinflammatory hyperpigmentation, which is the darkening of the skin after resolution of skin trauma, lesions of a dermatosis, or as a result of treatments administered for skin disorders. Hypopigmentary changes have also been noted in these instances. African Americans also have a tendency toward the overgrowth of connective tissue associated with the protection against infection and repair after injury. Keloid formation is one example of this tendency. Diseases such as lymphoma and systemic lupus erythematosus occur in African Americans secondary to this overgrowth of connective tissue.

Certain skin conditions are gender-specific among some African Americans. Pseudofolliculitis barbae ("razor bumps") is more common among African American males. This skin condition results from curved hairs growing back into the skin, causing itchy and painful bumps. African American males should be counseled regarding the best shaving method to keep this disorder to a minimum. Suggestions include the use of electric clippers, a triple-bladed razor, a depilatory, or laser therapy. Melasma ("the mask of pregnancy") is more common among darker-skinned African American females during pregnancy. This condition is characterized by brown spots or patches on the face. Also noted among African American women is alopecia (hair loss) related to the use of chemicals to straighten/relax the hair or from braiding.

African Americans, in general, also experience a disproportionate amount of pigment discoloration, with vertiligo (white patches) being the most common. This autoimmune disease manifests as white patches on the skin and causes skin discoloration and is also associated with diabetes and thyroid disorders. Birthmarks are more prevalent in African Americans, occurring in 20 percent of the African American population compared with 1 to 3 percent in other ethnic groups. One example is mongolian spots, which

are found more often in African American newborns but disappear over time.

African Americans must also be screened for skin cancer. Skin cancer comprises 1 to 2 percent of all cancers in African Americans (Gloster & Neal, 2006). Whereas squamous cell carcinoma is the second most common type of skin cancer in white patients, it is the most common type in patients of African and Asian Indian descent. Basal cell cancer is the second most common skin cancer of African Americans and is associated with chronic sun exposure. This type of skin cancer is more aggressive in African Americans than in whites. While melanoma is uncommon in African Americans, it is often terminal. The overall melanoma survival rate for African Americans is only 77 percent, as compared with 91 percent for whites (Ries et al., 2008). Many African Americans believe that they are not at risk for skin cancer because of their higher concentration of melanin; however, health-care providers must help to dispel this myth and educate African Americans regarding skin cancer protection.

Diseases and Health Conditions

Underwood and colleagues (2005) asserted that African Americans experience an "excessive burden of disease." When examining the relationship of social characteristics such as education, income, and occupation to health indicators, African Americans have worse indicators when compared with those of whites (Navarro, 1997). African Americans are at greater risk for many diseases, especially those associated with low-income, stressful life conditions, lack of access to primary health care, and negating health behaviors such as violence, poor dietary habits, lack of exercise, and lack of importance placed on seeking primary health care early. The Institute of Medicine (IOM)

REFLECTIVE EXERCISE 6.2

Abu Jemison, a 43-year-old African American man, has been admitted to the psychiatric unit with a provisional diagnosis of schizophrenia. His admitting history states that he is having auditory hallucinations (hearing voices from God), exhibiting paranoid behavior, and is aggressive. Mr. Jemison is started on olanzapine (Zyprexa™) 10 mg once a day.

1. What are the cultural factors that may explain his paranoid behavior, auditory hallucinations, and aggressive behavior?
2. What factors must be considered when confirming a diagnosis of schizophrenia?
3. What are the medication issues you must consider since Mr. Jemison has been prescribed the antipsychotic drug Zyprexa™?

report provides health-care providers with overwhelming evidence documenting the severity of health disparities among African Americans (Smedley, Stith, & Nelson, 2002). Whereas previous research attributed the problem of health disparities among African Americans and other minority groups to access-related factors, income, age, comorbid conditions, insurance coverage, socioeconomic status, and expressions of symptoms, the IOM's report cites racial prejudice and differences in the quality of health as possible reasons for increased disparities (Burroughs, Mackey, & Levy, 2002).

In 2007, the leading causes of death in the African American population were heart disease, malignant neoplasms (cancer), cerebral vascular diseases (strokes), unintentional injuries, diabetes mellitus, homicide, nephritis, nephrotic syndrome and nephrosis, chronic lower respiratory diseases, human immunodeficiency virus (HIV) disease, and septicemia (U.S. Department of Health and Human Services, Center for Disease Control and Prevention National Center for Health Statistic, 2010). Although progress has been noted regarding an increase in the life expectancy among African Americans, they continue to fall behind statistics of European Americans. African American men's life expectancy is 70 years compared with 75.9 years for white men, while African American women's life expectancy is 76.8 years compared with 80.8 years for white women (U.S. Census Bureau, Statistical Abstract of the United States, 2011).

Hypertension is the single largest risk factor for cardiovascular disease and heart attack among African Americans. Current statistics reveal that 39 percent of African American men and 43 percent of African American women are diagnosed with hypertension (U.S. Department of Health and Human Services, Centers for Disease Control (CDC) and Prevention National Center for Health Statistic, 2010). Compared with hypertension in other ethnic groups, hypertension among African Americans is more severe, is more resistant to treatment, begins at a younger age, and results in significantly worse target organ damage (Brewster, van Montfrans, & Kleijnen 2005; Moore, 2005). The literature suggests that the pathophysiology of hypertension in African Americans is related to volume expansion, decreased renin, and increased intracellular concentration of sodium and calcium. Genetic cardiovascular researchers have hypothesized that there might be a "hypertensive-heart failure genotype" (Moore, 2005). However, it is more likely that the etiology of hypertension among African Americans is multifaceted, including genetics, diet, lifestyle, stress, environment, and socioeconomic status (Moore, 2005; Saunders, 1997).

African American adults are 1.7 times as likely as their European American counterparts to have a stroke, while African American males are 60 percent more likely to die from a stroke when compared with European Americans. In addition, analysis from a CDC health interview survey reveals that African American stroke survivors were more likely to become disabled and have difficulty with activities of daily living than their non-Hispanic white counterparts.

African Americans also experience higher rates of diabetes. The incidence of type 2 diabetes in African Americans is among the highest in the world (Sowers, Ferdinand, Bakris, & Douglas, 2002). Compared with white adults, the risk of diagnosed diabetes was 77 percent higher among African Americans (National Diabetes Information Clearinghouse, 2011). African Americans experience double the prevalence of complications related to their diabetes. These complications include higher occurrence of lower-limb amputations, end-stage renal disease, eye disease, and higher rates of hospitalization for diabetes when compared with whites. African Americans also have a higher rate of obesity, which puts them at risk for diabetes. African Americans tend to carry upper-body obesity, an additional risk factor for diabetes (Base-Smith & Campinha-Bacote, 2003).

African Americans are 15 percent more likely to suffer from obesity than European Americans. National statistics report that 36 percent of African American men and 53 percent of African American women are obese (U.S. Department of Health and Human Services, Centers for Disease Control and Prevention, National Center for Health Statistics, 2010). More than 40 percent of African American teenagers are overweight. There are serious health implications related to obesity in African American children, including increased risk for developing heart disease, type 2 diabetes, stroke, orthopedic problems, and asthma (The HSC Foundation, 2007). In an address to the National Association for the Advancement of Colored People (NAACP), Michelle Obama, America's first African American First Lady, shared the following personal remarks regarding obesity in the African American community:

> And there's no doubt that this is a serious problem. It's one that is affecting every community across this country. But just like with so many other challenges that we face as a nation, the African American community is being hit even harder by this issue. We are living today in a time where we're decades beyond slavery, we are decades beyond Jim Crow; when one of the greatest risks to our children's future is their own health. African American children are significantly more likely to be obese than are white children. Nearly half of African American children will develop diabetes at some point in their lives. People, that's half of our children. (The White House, Office of the First Lady, 2010).

African Americans have the highest death rate and shortest survival of any racial and ethnic group in the United States for most cancers. Although the overall racial disparity in cancer death rates is decreasing, in 2007, the death rate for all cancers combined continued to be 32 percent higher in African American men and 16 percent higher in African American women than in white men and women, respectively (American Cancer Society, 2010). While African American women have a slightly lower incidence of breast cancer than that of white women, their mortality rate is 32 percent higher (Morgan et al., 2006). African American women are less likely to participate in regular breast cancer screening, which is a major factor for this disparity (Spurlock & Cullins, 2006). Unfortunately, this results in breast cancer being discovered in the later stages when it is less responsive to treatment. Once African American women are diagnosed with breast cancer, they tend to cope with the diagnosis by relying on God and seeking help from informal supportive networks such as family members and friends (Morgan et al., 2006). Health-care providers must recognize the role of spirituality and informal support systems when developing intervention strategies to have an impact on breast cancer treatment among African American women.

African American women have the highest rate of infant mortality among all ethnic groups (Mathews & MacDorman, 2010). They have 2.3 times the infant mortality rate of non-Hispanic whites and are almost 4 times as likely to die from causes related to low birth weight. African American mothers are also 2.5 times as likely as non-Hispanic white mothers to begin prenatal care in the third trimester or to not receive prenatal care at all. In addition, African American women have 1.8 times the sudden infant death syndrome (SIDS) mortality rate as non-Hispanic whites.

Because African Americans are concentrated in large inner cities, they are at risk for being victims of violence. Violence is a major cause of death among African Americans, with homicide being the leading cause of death among young African American males between the ages of 15 and 34. Brownstein (1995) indicated that young black men are murdered by other black men at 10 times the rate of white men between the ages of 20 and 29. This violence has been referred to as "black-on-black" violence. Gangs may be more prevalent in larger cities, which only increases the likelihood of the occurrence of violence in African American communities.

Living in urban industrial or substandard housing also exposes African Americans to the risk for developing diseases associated with environmental hazards. For example, the risk of asthma and allergies is increased by such environmental factors as exposure to house dust mite allergen and cockroach allergen. These allergens and respiratory tract irritants are commonly found in substandard housing, which has been related to the development of asthma in children (Asthma and Allergy Foundation, 2006).

Asthma is a top health problem for African American children. More than 3 million African Americans have asthma. African Americans go to the hospital emergency room more than whites because of asthma and are almost three times more likely to die from asthma-related causes than whites. Other causes of asthma in the African American population are exposure to secondhand tobacco smoke, poverty, lack of education, and not being able to get to a doctor (The National Women's Health Information, U.S. Department of Health and Human Resources, Office on Women's Health, 2011).

Lead exposure is another environmental threat for poorer African American communities. African American and urban children are most often exposed to this environmental hazard. Specifically, African American and low-income children suffer lead poisoning at highly disproportionate rates and are at higher risk of exposure to unsafe levels of lead in the home environment. The American Academy of Pediatrics (1998) reports that the prevalence of elevated blood lead levels for African American children ages 1 to 5 years is approximately five times higher than the prevalence among white children in the same age range. During the 1990s, high levels of lead in the blood were found in 4.4 percent of all U.S. children and in 22 percent of African American children (American Public Health Association, 2004).

In addition to the exposure to harmful environmental conditions, African Americans suffer from certain genetic conditions. Sickle cell disease is the most common genetic disorder among the African American population, affecting 1 in every 500 African Americans, and represents several hemoglobinopathies including sickle cell anemia, sickle cell hemoglobin C disease, and sickle cell thalassemia. Sickle cell disease is also found among people from geographic areas in which malaria is endemic, such as the Caribbean, the Middle East, the Mediterranean region, and Asia. In addition to sickle cell disease, glucose-6-phosphate dehydrogenase deficiency, which interferes with glucose metabolism, is another genetic disease found among African Americans.

Urethral prolapse is a rarely diagnosed condition that occurs most commonly in African American girls younger than 10 years, with an average age at presentation of 4 years (Fleisher & Ludwig, 2010). Urethral prolapse is a circular protrusion of the distal urethra through the external meatus, with vaginal bleeding being the most common presenting symptom. Because urethral prolapse is so rare, the prevalence of misdiagnosis is high. This uncommon condition in prepubescent African American girls should not be confused with other causes of vaginal bleeding, the most important being sexual abuse. Increased health-care provider awareness and recognition of urethral prolapse among African American girls will avoid misdiagnosis and unnecessary anxiety to both the patient and family.

Finally, in addition to environmental hazards and genetic conditions, AIDS contributes to lower life expectancy of African Americans when compared with European Americans. HIV/AIDS continues to be a devastating epidemic with African American communities carrying the brunt of the impact (Williams, Wyatt, & Wingood, 2010). Although African Americans make up only 13 percent of the total U.S. population, they accounted for 49 percent of HIV/AIDS cases in 2007. African Americans also continue to experience higher rates of sexually transmitted infections (STIs) than any other race/ethnicity in the United States. In a national study concerning African American views of the HIV/AIDS epidemic, African Americans were asked why they were not tested for this disease. Fifty-four percent responded that they felt they were not at risk for HIV/AIDS, and 11 percent stated that they did not know where to go to get tested (Kaiser Family Foundation, 2001). A knowledge deficit about HIV/AIDS was also revealed in this report. African Americans believed that kissing, sharing a drinking glass, or touching a toilet seat posed a risk of infection.

In summary, health conditions and health status for most African Americans are well below average. Health-care providers must provide culturally relevant health education, prevention practices, and screening aimed at improving the disparities in their health status and reducing their risks.

Variations in Drug Metabolism

Research conducted at the University of Maryland revealed that African Americans and other minorities do not always respond to drugs in the same manner as European Americans (Saunders, 1997). Examples of drugs that African Americans respond to or metabolize differently are psychotropic drugs, immunosuppressants, antihypertensives, cardiovascular drugs, and antiretroviral medications.

Glazer, Morganstern, & Douchette (1993) reported from their research that African Americans are twice as likely to develop tardive dyskinesia than their white counterparts when placed on specific neuroleptics. For example, Campinha-Bacote (1991) reported that African American psychiatric patients experience a higher incidence of extrapyramidal effects with haloperidol decanoate than that found in European Americans. African Americans are also more susceptible to tricyclic antidepressant (TCA) delirium than are European Americans. Strickland, Lin, Fu, Anderson, and Zheng (1995) reported that for a given dose of a TCA, African Americans show higher blood levels and a faster therapeutic response. As a result, African Americans experience more toxic side effects from a TCA than do European Americans. In addition, African Americans have a higher risk of lithium toxicity and side effects related to less efficient cell membrane lithium-sodium transport and increased lithium

red blood cell to plasma ratio (Herrera, Lawson, & Sramek, 1999). Some African Americans have a lower baseline leukocyte count (benign leukopenia), which puts them at risk for side effects of specific antipsychotic drugs, such as clozapine, which can cause agranulocytosis. Health-care providers must make extended efforts to observe African American patients for side effects related to TCAs and other psychotropic medications.

Dirks, Huth, Yates, and Melbohm (2004) reported ethnic differences in the pharmacokinetics of immunosuppressants among African Americans and European Americans. They found that the oral bioavailability of these drugs in African Americans was 20 and 50 percent lower than in non–African Americans. This finding suggests that there is a need for higher dose requirements in African Americans to maintain average concentrations of specific immunosuppressants. Dirk and colleagues (2004) maintained that recognition of these findings has the potential to improve posttransplant immunosuppressant therapy among African Americans.

African Americans may differ in their response to beta-blockers, angiotensin-converting enzyme (ACE) inhibitors, angiotensin receptor blocking agents, and diuretics used either alone or in combination for the treatment of hypertension (Burroughs, Mackey, & Levy, 2002). In 0.1 to 0.5 percent of patients, ACE inhibitors induce a rapid swelling in the nose, throat, larynx, mouth, glottis, lips, and/or tongue (angioedema), but African Americans have a 4.5 times greater risk of ACE inhibitor-induced angioedema (Brunton, Goodman, Blumenthal, & Buxman, 2008). Studies report that African Americans do not respond as readily to the beta-blocker propanolol as European Americans do. However, their response to the diuretic hydrochlorothiazide is greater when taken alone or with a calcium channel blocker. Diuretics, alone or in combination with another antihypertensive agent, are reported to counteract increases in salt retention noted among African Americans. Although there has been much discussion about the best type of antihypertensive drug to administer in African Americans, health-care providers must remember "There is no specific class of antihypertensive drugs that categorically should not be used based on race" (Burroughs, Mackey, & Levy, 2002, p. 18).

In 2005, the Food and Drug Administration (FDA) approved the drug BiDil (NitroMed) as adjunct standard therapy in self-identified black patients for heart failure (Ferdinand, 2006). This drug is based on the chemical nitric oxide, found naturally in the body, which dilates the blood vessels, allowing the blood to flow more easily and thus easing the burden on the heart. Although this drug was initially considered a drug failure in 2003, when the results were reexamined by race, it was found that a significant percentage of the 400 black patients in the trial seemed to respond.

It was postulated that heart failure in African Americans is somehow associated with how they produce and metabolize nitric oxide. Specifically, African Americans may produce less nitric oxide and destroy it too quickly (National Women's Health Report, 2005). The approval of BiDil for "blacks only" is a highly controversial subject. Schwartz (2001) argued that labeling a drug based on race is "racial profiling" and is of no proven value in treating an individual patient. However, Ferdinand (2006) contended, "While controversial, the FDA approval of BiDil does offer evidence that this therapy may be useful in the black population" (p. 157). An obvious question is, in a world of mixed heritages, how do health-care providers determine a person's race? Many contend that racial categories are more a societal construct than a scientific one. Health-care providers must be cautious in promoting drugs for specific ethnic groups, since it could easily lead to stereotyping and discrimination. Whereas race and ethnicity are important for public health issues, they are not true biological or genetic categories (Ferdinand, 2006). One solution is the designing of drugs that target specific genes, eliminating the need to rely on race.

Research has identified the possibility that a genetic mutation may make antiretroviral treatment less effective in Africans and African Americans (Schaeffeler et al., 2001). The P-glycoprotein (PGP) membrane protein appears to transport antiretroviral drugs out of cells, thus making the drugs less effective. A double mutation of the gene that encodes this protein (C/C genotype) leads to an increased amount of the PGP protein. Schaeffeler and colleagues (2001) examined the frequency of the C/C genotype in 537 Caucasians, 142 Ghanaians (from West Africa), 50 Japanese, and 41 African Americans. The C/C genotype was found in 83 percent of the Ghanaians and 61 percent of the African Americans, and only 34 percent of the Japanese and 26 percent of the Caucasians. It was hypothesized that certain antiretroviral drugs may not be as effective in people with the C/C genotype. Considering that African Americans account for half of the diagnosed HIV/AIDS cases, this finding has serious implications in efforts to treat the AIDS epidemic among the African American population.

Cultural factors, such as a health-care provider's personal beliefs and biases about a specific ethnic group, may lead to unequal treatment, misdiagnosis, and overmedication (Levy, 1993; Smedley et al., 2002). For example, African Americans are at a higher risk of misdiagnosis for psychiatric disorders and, therefore, may be treated inappropriately with drugs. Studies have found that African Americans are more likely to be overdiagnosed with having a psychotic disorder and more liable to be treated with antipsychotic drugs, regardless of diagnosis. DelBello and colleagues

(1999) found that in a study with adolescents, although there were no differences in psychotic symptoms (14 percent of the African Americans and 18 percent of the whites were diagnosed as having psychotic symptoms), those who were African American, despite not being more psychotic, received more antipsychotic medications. Specifically, among white patients, 43 percent received antipsychotic medications, and among nonwhite patients, 68 percent received antipsychotic medications. There are several possible explanations. DelBello and colleagues contended that one plausible explanation is that clinicians perceived African Americans to be more aggressive and, thus, more psychotic, and prescribed the antipsychotics. Studies by Lawson (1999); Strakowski, McElroy, Keck, and West, (1996); and Strickland, Ranganath, Lin, Poland, Mendoza, and Smith (1991) also found that African Americans were more likely to be diagnosed with schizophrenia and more likely to be prescribed antipsychotics.

Access to pain medication is an issue for African Americans and other minority groups. African Americans with severe pain are less likely than whites to be able to obtain commonly prescribed pain medication because pharmacies in predominantly nonwhite communities do not sufficiently stock opiates (Burroughs et al., 2002). Morrison, Wallenstein, Natale, Senzel, and Huang (2000) examined the percentage of pharmacies in New York City stocked with adequate opioid medications and found that pharmacies in predominantly minority neighborhoods were much less likely to stock opioid medications. Only 25 percent of the pharmacies in minority neighborhoods had an ample supply of opioid medications to treat severe pain, compared with 72 percent of pharmacies in predominantly white neighborhoods.

Eye color is another genetic variation related to difference in response to a specific drug. For example, light eyes dilate wider in response to mydriatic drugs than do dark eyes. This difference in response to a mydriatic drug must be taken into consideration when treating African Americans.

Malnutrition can also influence drug response. Protein, vitamin, and mineral deficiencies can hinder the function of metabolic enzymes and alter the body's ability to absorb or eliminate a psychotherapeutic drug. This may pose a problem for newly arriving refugees from Ethiopia/Eritrea and other East African countries where malnutrition is considered a major medical problem. In addition, psychotherapeutic medications, such as antidepressants, that require fat in order to be absorbed are not as effective in patients with exceptionally low body fat or differing fat metabolism (Wandler, 2003). This is a factor to consider when caring for Ghanaians, who may differ in fat metabolism as compared to Americans (Banini et al.,

2003). When there are unexplained variations in a patient's response to a medication, it is imperative for the health-care provider to assess the patient's dietary habits (Campinha-Bacote, 2007).

High-Risk Behaviors

Smoking is a serious high-risk behavior in the African American population. Compared with European Americans, African Americans are at increased risk for lung cancer even though they smoke about the same amount. Twenty-six percent of African American men and17 percent of African American women 18 years and over smoke (U.S. Department of Health and Human Services, Centers for Disease Control and Prevention National Center for Health Statistic, 2010). Other high-risk health behaviors among African Americans can be inferred from the high incidences of HIV/AIDS and other STIs, teenage pregnancy, violence, unintentional injuries, smoking, alcoholism, drug abuse, sedentary lifestyle, and delayed seeking of health care.

Community health workers can have a significant impact on these detrimental practices by providing health education at community affairs located in African American communities. The goals of health education are to change high-risk health behaviors and improve decision making (Edleman & Mandel, 1998). Examples of effective methods for changing behaviors are mutual goal setting and behavior contracts. Another strategy for changing high-risk behaviors is a teaching module using a culturally appropriate Afrocentric approach to early screening for breast and cervical cancer (Baldwin, 1996).

Efforts to change high-risk behaviors are not always successful. According to Edleman and Mandel (1998), health-care providers must understand influential factors affecting decision making regarding health behaviors. These factors include values, attitudes, beliefs, religion, previous experiences with the health-care system, and life goals.

Health-Care Practices

Because a significant proportion of African Americans are poor and live in inner cities, they tend to concentrate on day-to-day survival. Health care often takes second place to the basic needs of the family, such as food and shelter. In addition, the role of the family has an impact on the health-seeking behaviors of African Americans. African Americans have strong family ties; when an individual becomes ill, that individual is frequently taught to seek health care from the family rather than from health-care professionals. This cultural practice may contribute to the failure of African Americans to seek treatment at an early stage. Screening programs may best be initiated in community and church activities in which the entire family is present.

Nutrition
Meaning of Food

Historically, African American rites revolved around food. Eating foods identified with slavery has provided many African Americans with a sense of their identity and tradition. Special meaning is attached to the soul food diet, a southern tradition handed down from generation to generation. The term *soul food* comes from the need for African Americans to express the group feeling of soul, and as a result, soul foods are seen to nourish not only the body but also the spirit. Although African Americans have incorporated soul foods into their diets, these foods are more commonly consumed for occasions such as special events, holidays, and birthdays. Therefore, the everyday diet of African Americans may more closely resemble the "American" diet, based on convenience and cost.

Common Foods and Food Rituals

Chitterlings (pig intestines often either fried or boiled with hot peppers, onions, and spices), okra, ham hocks, corn, pork fat, and sweet potato pie are foods uniquely identified as Southern African American foods. Common ways for African Americans to prepare food include frying, barbecuing, and using gravy and sauces. African American diets are typically high in fat, cholesterol, and sodium. African Americans eat more animal fat, less fiber, and fewer fruits and vegetables than the rest of American society. Traditional breads of Southern African Americans are cornbread and biscuits, and the most popular vegetables are greens such as mustard, collard, or kale. Vegetables are preferred cooked rather than raw, with some type of fat, such as salt pork, fatback, and bacon or fat meat. Salt pork is a key ingredient in the diet of many African Americans. Salt pork is inexpensive and, therefore, more frequently purchased.

Infant feeding methods may vary among African Americans. African American parents may be encouraged by their elders to begin feeding solid foods, such as cereal, at an early age (usually before 2 months). The cereal is mixed with the formula and given to the infant in a bottle. African Americans believe that giving only formula is starving the baby and that the infant needs "real food" to sleep through the night. Cultural-specific interventions are needed to educate African American parents regarding the potential harmful effects of giving infants solid foods at an early age. Black, Siegel, Abel, and Bentley (2001) conducted a study with first-time African American adolescent mothers living in multigenerational households. The intervention focused on reducing the cultural barriers to the acceptance of the recommendations of the American Academy of Pediatrics and World Health Organization on complementary feeding. Culturally specific interventions included nonfood strategies for managing infant behavior and mother–grandmother negotiation strategies.

Dietary Practices for Health Promotion

Some African Americans believe that a healthy person is one who has a good appetite. Foods such as milk, vegetables, and meat are referred to as *strength foods*. In the African American community, individuals who are at an ideal body weight are commonly viewed as "not having enough meat on their bones" and, therefore, unhealthy. African Americans believe that it is important to carry additional weight in order to be able to afford to lose weight during times of sickness. Therefore, being slightly overweight is seen as a sign of good health.

One common belief among Southern African Americans is the concept of "high blood" and "low blood." The healthy state is when the blood is in balance—neither too high nor too low. High blood is viewed as more serious than low blood. High blood is often interchangeable with high blood pressure. High blood is believed to be a condition in which the blood expands in volume or moves higher in the body, usually to the head. Some African Americans believe that rich foods or foods red in color, especially red meat, are considered the primary cause of high blood. Some African Americans believe that the treatment of high blood is to drink vinegar or eat pickles to "thin" the blood. Garlic is also seen as a health food. Garlic water is consumed to treat hypertension as well as hyperlipidemia in the African American population. In contrast, low blood is believed to be caused by eating too many acidic foods. Low blood is believed to be the cause of anemia. Treatment is aimed at trying to thicken the blood by eating rich foods and red meats. Another treatment for anemia, as well as for malnutrition, is to drink "pot liquor," the liquid that remains after a pot of greens has been cooked.

Nutritional Deficiencies and Food Limitations

The calcium consumption in African American women is particularly low. Williams (2005) cites that the diets of older African Americans are also extremely low in calcium. The National Health and Nutrition Examination Surveys (NHANES II) reported that the intake levels for African American women 55 to 74 years of age were 460/mg, the lowest among all age and ethnic groups (Williams, 2005, p. 89). One factor that may explain the low calcium intake among African Americans is the lack of awareness of the health risks associated with this deficiency. Another factor is the high level of lactose intolerance in this population. Lactose intolerance occurs in 75 percent of the African American population. Low levels of thiamine, riboflavin, vitamins A and C, and iron are noted among African Americans and are

mostly associated with a poor diet secondary to a low socioeconomic status.

Many African Americans are Protestant and have no specific food restrictions. However, a significant number of African Americans are members of religious groups who have dietary restrictions. These may include Seventh-Day Adventists, Muslims, and Jehovah's Witnesses. For example, a Muslim *halal* diet forbids pork or pork products. Muslims also refuse pork-based insulin. They consider these products to be filthy. In addition, some African Americans, especially those from Jamaica and other parts of the Caribbean, may be Rastafarians. Their religious beliefs mandate that they follow a clear dietary restriction, which includes eating fresh foods of vegetable origin and avoiding meat, salt, and alcohol. The health-care provider must always ask about any religious or cultural prohibitions on types of food consumed.

Pregnancy and Childbearing Practices

Fertility Practices and Views Toward Pregnancy

Historically, African American families have been large, especially in rural areas. A large family was viewed as an economic necessity, and African American parents depended on their children to support them when they could no longer work. However, as families moved to cities, they soon found that large families could become an economic burden. To some extent, this shifted attention to family planning.

Although oral contraceptives may be the most popular choice of birth control among African Americans, religious beliefs also play a role in choices made. For example, African American Catholics may choose the rhythm method over other forms of birth control. African American communities also hold many views on the issue of pregnancy versus abortion. Many

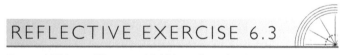

REFLECTIVE EXERCISE 6.3

Donna White, a 59-year-old African American woman, presents to her local community health clinic for a physical examination. Selected physical findings reveal that she is 5 feet, 4 inches tall; weighs 278 pounds; has a blood pressure of 160/96; and has a total cholesterol of 297.

1. What cultural factors may have contributed to her hypertension?
2. What environmental factors may have contributed to her obesity?
3. Discuss some culturally relevant interventions when rendering care for Mrs. White's hypertension, obesity, and hyperlipidemia.

African Americans who oppose abortion do so because of religious or moral beliefs. Others oppose abortion because of moral, cultural, or Afrocentric beliefs. Such beliefs may cause a delay in making a decision so that having an abortion is no longer safe.

Prescriptive, Restrictive, and Taboo Practices in the Childbearing Family

African American women usually respond to pregnancy in the same manner as women in other ethnic groups, based on their satisfaction with self, economic status, and career goals. The elders in the family provide advice and counseling about what should and should not be done during pregnancy. The African American family network guides many of the practices and beliefs of the pregnant woman, including *pica*.

Pica is the eating of nonnutritive substances such as clay, dirt (*geophagia*), sand, laundry starch, burnt matches, plastic, paint chips and plaster, lightbulbs, needles, coffee grounds, and string. Women have reported that these items reduce nausea and cause an easy birth. One theory of geophagia is that this natural craving alleviates several mineral deficiencies and that the unborn child "needs" this supplement. However, geophagia can lead to a potassium deficiency, constipation, and anemia. Although it is a common practice among many African Americans, independent of socioeconomic or educational level, some are unaware that the practice exists.

Certain practices are believed to be taboo during pregnancy. For example, some African Americans believe that pregnant women should not take pictures because it may cause a stillbirth, nor should they have their picture taken because it captures their soul. Some also believe that it is not wise to reach over their heads if they are pregnant because the umbilical cord will wrap around the baby's neck. Another taboo concerns the purchase of clothing for the infant.

Many African American women expect to experience cravings during pregnancy. Several beliefs related to the failure to satisfy this food craving exist. Some African Americans claim that if the mother does not consume the specific food craving, the child can be birthmarked, or, more seriously, it can result in a stillbirth. Caribbean food beliefs during pregnancy focus on pregnancy outcomes and eating specific food groups. For example, consuming milk, eggs, tomatoes, and green vegetables is believed to result in a large baby, whereas drinking too many liquids will drown the baby.

Snow (1993) reported several home practices related to initiating labor in pregnant African American women. Taking a ride over a bumpy road, ingesting castor oil, eating a heavy meal, or sniffing pepper are all thought to induce labor. If a baby is born with the amniotic sac (referred to as a "veil") over its head or face, the neonate is thought to have special powers. In addition, certain children are thought to have received special powers from God: those born after a set of twins, those born with a physical problem or disability, or a child who is the seventh son in a family.

The postpartum period for the African American woman can be greatly extended. Some believe that during the postpartum period, the mother is at greater risk than the baby. She is cautioned to avoid cold air and is encouraged to get adequate rest to restore the body to normal. Postpartum practices for child care can involve the use of a bellyband or a coin. When placed on top of the infant's umbilical area, these objects are believed to prevent the umbilical area from protruding outward.

Death Rituals
Death Rituals and Expectations

Death rituals for African Americans may vary owing to the diversity in their religious affiliations, geographic location, educational level, and socioeconomic background. African Americans are very family oriented, and it is important that family members and extended family stay at the bedside of the dying patient in the hospital. They desire to hold on to their loved ones for as long as possible, and as a result may avoid signing Do Not Resuscitate (DNR) orders or making preparations for death (Lobar, Youngblut, & Brooten, 2006, p. 47).

Lobar and colleagues (2006) conducted a qualitative study regarding cross-cultural beliefs, ceremonies, and rituals surrounding death of a loved one and found that African American participants described the importance of giving their loved one a "big send-off." This practice involved elaborate financial decisions concerning the type of coffin to buy and the vehicle for carrying the coffin.

Johnson, Elbert-Avila, and Tulsky (2005, p. 711) maintained that spirituality is an important part of African American culture and is often the rationale for more aggressive treatment preferences of some African Americans at the end of life. Specifically, Americans are more likely to prefer life-sustaining treatments than do other ethnic groups (Fairrow, McCallum, & Messinger-Rapport, 2004; Welch, Teno, & Mor, 2005). African Americans do not believe in rushing to bury the deceased. Therefore, it is common to see the burial service held 5 to 7 days after death. Allowing time for relatives who live far away to attend the funeral services is important. Visual display of the body is also important. Southern and rural blacks observe the custom of having the deceased's body remain in the house the evening before the funeral (Lobar et al., 2006). This practice allows the extended family time to "pay respect" to their deceased loved one.

African Americans believe that the body must be kept intact after death. For example, it is common to hear an African American say, "I came into this world with all my body parts, and I'll leave this world with all my body parts!" Based on this belief, African Americans are less likely to donate organs or consent to an autopsy. Health-care providers must be aware that talking about organ donation may be considered an insult to the family.

For most African Americans, death does not end the connection among people, especially family. They believe the deceased is in God's hands and that they will be reunited in heaven after death. Relatives communicating with the deceased's spirit is one example of this endless connection. Snow (1993) studied African American families in the southern United States and noted interesting rituals regarding spirits of the deceased. For example, if one passes an infant over the casket of the deceased who has died a sudden or violent death, this protects the infant from the deceased's "haunting spirits."

Responses to Death and Grief

Grieving and death rituals of African Americans are often influenced by religion. Descendants from the Caribbean may practice a blend of Catholicism and African religion known as *Voudoun,* also spelled *Voodoo, Vodoun,* and *Vodun.* The name has its roots in an ancient African Yoruban word for "spirit." Some African Americans believe in "voodoo death," which is a belief that illness or death may come to an individual via a supernatural force (Campinha-Bacote, 1992). Voodoo is more commonly known as "root work," "hex," "fix," "conjuring," "tricking," "mojo," "witchcraft," "spell," "black magic," or "hoodoo."

One response to hearing about a death of a family member or close member in the African American culture is "falling out," which is manifested by sudden collapse, paralysis, and the inability to see or speak. However, the individual's hearing and understanding remain intact. Health-care providers must understand the African American culture to recognize this condition as a cultural response to the death of a family member or other severe emotional shock and not as a medical condition requiring emergency intervention. Some African Americans are less likely to express grief openly and publicly. However, they do express their feelings openly during the funeral. Funeral services encourage emotional expression, such as crying, screaming, and wailing.

Several studies suggest that African Americans are less likely to complete advance directives such as DNR orders or living wills (Curriculum Ethnogeriatrics, 2001; Waters, 2000). This may be due to their feeling that if they choose DNR orders, it would give the health-care system the legal authorization to provide substandard care or give up on them. Another factor may be the role of religious beliefs. Many African Americans believe that God is in ultimate control of

the timing of death. Research has also found that African Americans use end-of-life services at a considerable lower rate than whites. Washington, Bickel-Swenson, and Stephens (2008) conducted an in-depth review of the literature regarding the underuse of hospice services by African Americans and found the following six factors:

1. Lack of awareness of hospice services
2. Mistrust of the health-care system
3. Anticipated lack of ethnic minority employees in hospice agencies
4. Personal or cultural values in conflict with hospice philosophy
5. Concerns about burdening the family
6. Economic factors

An example of a conflict with hospice philosophy focused on religious beliefs. Specifically, accepting the terminality of their loved one's life meant giving up on God's power to heal. Implications of these findings suggest a need for culturally relevant discussion and education in the African American community regarding advance directives and end-of-life services.

Spirituality
Dominant Religion and Use of Prayer

Religion and religious behavior are integral parts of the African American community. African American churches have played a major role in the development and survival of African Americans. As eloquently stated by Lincoln (1974, pp. 115–116):

> *To understand the power of the black Church, it must first be understood that there is no disjunction between the black Church and the black community. . . . Whether one is a church member or not is beside the point in any assessment of the importance and meaning of the black Church.*

REFLECTIVE EXERCISE 6.4

Rena Broadnaux, a 74-year-old African American woman, has been unexpectedly diagnosed with terminal lung cancer. She does not have any advance directives in place. The health-care team plans to discuss do not resuscitate (DNR) orders and palliative care, such as hospice, with the family. When the physician told Mrs. Broadnaux's two daughters about the pending death of their mother, one daughter suddenly collapsed and could not speak.

1. What could explain the daughter's sudden collapse and inability to communicate?
2. What are some of the cultural beliefs you might encounter when discussing DNR orders with the family?
3. What potential barriers must you consider when offering such services as hospice care to the family?

African Americans take their religion seriously, and they expect to receive a message in preaching that helps them in their daily lives. Brown and Gary (1994) found that religious involvement is associated with positive mental health. Furthermore, most African Americans expect to take an active part in religious activities. In reviewing the literature, Johnson and colleagues (2005, p. 712) found that African Americans "participate more often in organizational (attendance at religious services) and nonorganizational (prayer or religious study) religious activities and endure higher levels of intrinsic religiosity (personal religious commitment) than do Caucasians." In addition, research has noted that church attendance was an important correlate of positive health-care practices (Aaron, Levine, & Burstin 2003).

Most African American Christians are affiliated with the Baptist and Methodist denominations. In 1990, 50 percent of African Americans considered themselves Baptist. However, that percentage dropped to 45 percent by 2008 (Black Demographics.com, 2011). There is also a substantial decrease in the percentage of Methodist and Orthodox from 12 percent in 1990 to 7 percent in 2008 (Black Demographics.com, 2011). Many other denominations and distinct religious groups are also represented in African American communities in the United States. These include African Methodist, Episcopalian, Jehovah's Witnesses, Church of God in Christ, Seventh-Day Adventists, Pentecostal, Apostolic, Presbyterian, Lutheran, Roman Catholic, Nation of Islam, and Islamic sects, as well as nondenominational and evangelical churches.

African Americans strongly believe in the use of prayer for all situations they may encounter. They also pray for the sake of others who are experiencing problems. According to Roberson (1985), "Prayers reflect the trust and faith one has in God." African Americans also believe in the laying on of hands while praying. The belief is that certain individuals have the power to heal the sick by placing hands on them. African Americans may pray in a language that is not understood by anyone but the person reciting the prayer. This expression of prayer is referred to as *speaking in tongues*.

Meaning of Life and Individual Sources of Strength

Most African Americans' inner strength comes from trusting in God and maintaining a biblical worldview of health and illness. Some African Americans believe that whatever happens is "God's will." Because of this belief, African Americans may be perceived to have a fatalistic view of life. For example, Snow (1993) reported that African Americans trust in "Doctor Jesus," and some believe that sickness and pain are forms of weakness that come directly from Satan. Therefore, for African Americans, having faith in God is a major source of inner strength. Frameworks such as Campinha-Bacote's (2005) Biblically Based Model of Cultural Competence in the Delivery of Healthcare Services can provide health-care providers with strategies for implementing culturally specific interventions for African Americans who share a biblical worldview of health and illness.

Spiritual Beliefs and Health

Spiritual beliefs strongly direct many African Americans as they cope with illness and the end of life. In a review of the literature on spiritual beliefs and practices of African Americans, Johnson and colleagues (2005) noted the following recurrent themes: "spiritual beliefs and practices are a source of comfort, coping, and support and are the most effective way to influence healing; God is responsible for physical and spiritual health; and the doctor is God's instrument." African Americans consider themselves spiritual beings, and God is thought to be the supreme healer. Health-care practices center on religious and spiritual activities such as going to church, praying daily, laying on of hands, and speaking in tongues. Drayton-Brooks and White (2004) conducted a qualitative study to explore health-promoting behaviors among African American women with faith-based support. They concluded that "health beliefs, attitudes, and behaviors are not developed outside of social systems; therefore, the facilitation of healthy lifestyle behaviors may be best addressed and influenced within a context of reciprocal social interaction such as a church."

As health-care providers develop culturally specific interventions for African Americans, it is important to understand that the church community can serve as a viable support system in developing health-promoting behaviors. Underwood and Powell (2006) further added that considerable improvements can occur in the health status of African Americans if health education and outreach efforts are presented and promoted through religious, spiritual and faith-based efforts. Musgrave, Allen, and Allen (2002) cautioned public health not to "use" faith communities or the spirituality of individuals to its own end. Instead, there must be a partnership between public health and faith communities in which the central undertaking of faith is respected.

Health-Care Practices

Health-Seeking Beliefs and Behaviors

Spirituality, communalism, oral tradition, internal strength, resolve, and respect for elders are central values that guide the health-seeking beliefs and behaviors among the traditional African American culture (NMAETC, 2006). Spirituality depicts an inner strength that comes from trusting in God for good health. Communalism reflects a strong history of collective group orientation that includes personal relationships, social support systems, and shared resources over individualism in maintaining health. Oral tradition is an important tool for African Americans in sharing knowledge about health behaviors and practices. Internal strength and resolve originates from survival skills learned through challenging conditions and slavery. Respect for elders refers to African American elders who are revered for their experience and wisdom in areas concerning health and well-being.

According to Snow (1974), many African Americans are pessimistic about human relationships and believe that it is more natural to do evil than to do good. Snow concluded that some African Americans' belief systems emphasize three major themes:

1. The world is a very hostile and dangerous place to live.
2. The individual is open to attack from external forces.
3. The individual is considered to be a helpless person who has no internal resources to combat such an attack and, therefore, needs outside assistance.

Because many African Americans tend to be suspicious of health-care providers, they may see a physician or nurse only when absolutely necessary. Some older African Americans continue to use the *Farmers' Almanac* to choose what are thought to be good times for medical and dental procedures.

Some African Americans, particularly those of Haitian background, may believe in sympathetic magic. *Sympathetic magic* assumes everything is interconnected and includes the practice of imitative and contagious magic. *Contagious magic* is the belief that once an entity is physically connected to another, it can never be separated; what one does to a specific part, they also do to the whole. This type of belief is seen in the practice of voodoo. An individual will take a piece of the victim's hair or fingernail and place a hex, which they believe will cause the person to become ill (voodoo illness). *Imitative magic* is the belief that "like follows like" (Campinha-Bacote, 1992). For example, a pregnant woman may sleep with a knife under her pillow to "cut" the pains of labor. Another example is the use of a doll or a picture of an individual to inflict harm on that person. Whatever harm is done to the picture is also simultaneously done to the person.

Responsibility for Health Care

The African American population believes in natural and unnatural illnesses. *Natural illness* occurs in response to normal forces from which individuals have not protected themselves. *Unnatural illness* is the belief that harm or sickness can come to you via a person or spirit. In treating an unnatural illness, African Americans seek clergy or a folk healer or pray directly to God. In general, health is viewed as harmony with nature, whereas illness is seen as a disruption in this harmonic state owing to demons, "bad spirits," or both.

African Americans may use home remedies to maintain their health and treat specific health conditions as well as seek health care from Western health-care providers. When taking prescribed medications, African Americans commonly take the medications differently from the way prescribed. For example, in treating hypertension, African Americans may take their antihypertensive medication on an "as-needed" basis. To provide services that are effective and culturally acceptable to African Americans, health-care providers must conduct thorough cultural assessments and become partners with the African American community. Strategies such as focus groups can provide health-care providers with insight into health-care practices acceptable to African Americans.

Folk and Traditional Practices

African Americans, like most ethnic groups, engage in folk medicine. The history of African American folk medicine has its origin in slavery. Slaves had a limited range of choices in obtaining health care. Although they were expected to inform their masters immediately when they were ill, slaves were reluctant to submit themselves to the harsh prescriptions and treatments of eighteenth- and nineteenth-century European American physicians (Savitt, 1978). They preferred self-treatment or treatment by friends, older relatives, or "folk doctors." This led to a dual system: "white medicine" and "black medicine" (Savitt, 1978). Snow (1993) studied hundreds of folk practices used by African Americans. One example is the belief that drinking a mixture of an alcoholic beverage and fish blood can cure alcoholism. This is believed to give an undesirable taste and cause nausea and vomiting when subsequent alcoholic drinks are taken.

Traditionally, African Americans have practiced healing with botanicals. A botanical is a plant or plant part valued for its medicinal or therapeutic properties, flavor, and/or scent. A secondary analysis conducted of a nationally representative cross-sectional sample of 2107 adult African Americans living in the United States in 1979 and 1980 found that 69.6 percent reported that their families used home remedies and 35.4 percent reported that they used home remedies themselves (Boyd, Taylor, Shimp, & Semler, 2000). However, newer research suggests that the use of botanicals among African Americans has decreased (Gunn & Davis, 2011; Kelly, Kaufman, Kelley, Rosenberg, & Mitchell, 2006). In a study of contemporary use of herbal/natural supplements in the largest racial/ethnic groups in the United States, it was noted that use was lowest among African Americans, with a decline in recent years (Kelly et al., 2006). One possible reason cited in the literature is the continued strong belief in

God as healer and maintainer of health (Gunn & Davis, 2011).

Barriers to Health Care

Healthy People 2010 defined health literacy as "the degree to which individuals have the capacity to obtain, process, and understand basic health information and services needed to make appropriate health decisions" (U.S. Department of Health and Human Services, 2002). Research shows that health literacy is the single best predictor of health status. Low health literacy affects older people, immigrants, the impoverished, and minorities. Low health literacy affects 40 percent of African Americans and is considered a barrier to receiving optimal health care. Low health literacy is also driven by poor patient-provider communication. Health-care providers can reduce low health literacy by limiting the amount of information provided at each visit, avoiding medical jargon, using pictures or models to explain important health concepts, ensuring understanding with the "show-me" technique, and encouraging patients to ask questions.

Negative attitudes from health-care professionals can greatly affect African Americans' decision to seek medical attention (McNeil, Campinha-Bacote, Tapscott, & Vample, 2002). McNeil and colleagues maintained that the attitude of the health-care provider is one of the most significant barriers to the care of African Americans (p. 132). One study reported that 12 percent of African Americans, compared with 1 percent of whites, felt that health-care providers treated them unfairly or disrespectfully because of their race (Kaiser Family Foundation, 2001). Kennedy, Mathis, and Woods (2007) reported that African Americans feel that just receiving health care is very often a demeaning and humiliating experience.

Some African Americans may experience economic and geographic barriers to health-care services. Needed health-care services may not be accessible or affordable for African Americans in lower socioeconomic groups. Although some services may be available, accessible, and affordable for other African Americans, they may not be culturally relevant. For example, a health-care provider may prescribe a strict American Diabetic Association diet to a newly diagnosed diabetic African American patient without taking into consideration this person's dietary habits. Therefore, therapeutic interventions developed by health-care providers may be underused or ignored.

Underrepresentation of ethnic minority health-care providers is an additional barrier to health care for many minorities. In the absence of adequate representation, minority populations are less likely to access and use health-care services. Research investigated doctor–patient race concordance and its impact on predicting greater health-care utilization and satisfaction among minorities (LaVeist & Carroll, 2002;

LaVeist & Nuru-Jeter, 2002). LaVeist and Nuru-Jeter found that patients who were race-concordant with their physician reported greater satisfaction with their physician compared with respondents who were not race-concordant. These authors concluded that efforts must be made to increase the number of minority physicians, as well as improve the ability of physicians to interact with patients who are not of their own race. These findings are relevant for all health-care providers.

Another barrier that many African Americans face in obtaining health care is inadequate health insurance coverage. In 2009, 19 percent of African Americans did not have health insurance. Having access to health insurance is a critical factor in reducing the current health disparities that exit among African Americans. In an attempt to reduce these disparities, the Affordable Care Act was passed in 2010. This health insurance reform legislation includes a series of measures to guarantee that insurance companies will no longer be able to deny coverage to anyone with preexisting conditions, a significant benefit for the many African Americans who are plagued with higher rates of chronic diseases, illnesses, and comorbidity (Cord, 2010). The Affordable Care Act also expands access to preventive care, a needed service to reduce health disparities for millions of African Americans by helping to prevent many diseases that have a disproportionate impact on this group.

Cultural Responses to Health and Illness

To understand the African American responses to health and illness, it is important to first understand their worldview. The literature discusses an Afrocentric, or African-centered, worldview held by some African Americans (Carroll, 2010; Dixon, 1971). Within an Afrocentric worldview, the highest value of African Americans lies in interpersonal relationships. Therefore, it is key to establish a rapport early on in the patient–health-care provider interaction. African Americans come to knowledge affectively, or through feelings (Nichols, 1987). This worldview maintains that one can discover knowledge and truth through feelings or emotions. It is not uncommon for an African American patient to say, "It doesn't *feel* right" when asked questions regarding compliance issues. Afrocentric logic highlights seeing the union of opposites (diunital logic). For example, an African American patient may be both optimistic and pessimistic about the future at the same time and see no conflict in this view. An Afrocentric worldview asserts that one should live in harmony with nature, and spirituality must hold the most significance place in life. Cooperation, collective responsibility, and interdependence are the central values to which all should aspire. The Afrocentric worldview is a circular one, in which all events are tied together with one another. Therefore, it may be challenging for health-care providers to isolate specific health problems when taking a patient history.

African Americans often perceive pain as a sign of illness or disease. Therefore, it is possible that if they are not experiencing severe and/or immediate pain, a regimen of regularly prescribed medicine may not be followed. For example, African Americans may take their antihypertensive drugs or diuretics only when they experience head or neck pain. This cultural practice interferes with successful and effective treatment of hypertension. In other cases, some African Americans believe, as part of their spiritual and religious foundation, that suffering and pain are inevitable and must be endured, thus contributing to their high tolerance levels for pain. Prayers and the laying on of hands are thought to free the person from all suffering and pain, and people who still experience pain are considered to have little faith.

In addition to religious beliefs, low educational levels among African Americans may limit their access to information about the etiology and treatment of mental illness. Some African Americans hold a stigma against mental illness. The high frequency of misdiagnosis among African Americans contributes to their reluctance to trust mental health professionals. For example, Adebimpe (1981) reported that over the years, a major diagnostic issue has been the high frequency of the diagnosis of schizophrenia among African American patients. Specifically, African Americans are more likely to report hallucinations when suffering from an affective disorder, which may lead to the misdiagnosis of schizophrenia.

Close family and spiritual ties within the African American family allow one to enter the sick role with ease. Extended and nuclear family members willingly care for sick individuals and assume their role responsibilities without hesitation. Sickness and tragedy bring African American families together, even in the presence of family conflict.

Blood Transfusions and Organ Donation

Blood transfusions are generally accepted in the African American patient. However, some religious groups, such as Jehovah's Witnesses, do not permit this practice. In addition, Jehovah's Witnesses believe that any blood that leaves the body must be destroyed, so they do not approve of an individual storing her or his own blood for a later autologous transfusion.

A low level of organ donation among African Americans has been cited (Plawecki & Plawecki, 1992). This reluctance is associated with a lack of information about organ donation, religious fears and beliefs, distrust of health-care providers, fear that organs will be taken before the patient is dead, and concern that proper medical attention will not be given to patients if they are organ donors. However, in regard to kidney donations, it must be noted that African Americans donate in proportion to their share of the population. African Americans, for example, represent about 13 percent of the population and account for 12 percent of kidney donors. It may appear that there is a low level of kidney donation among the African American community because they are disproportionately represented (35 percent) on the kidney waiting list. Their rate of organ donation does not keep pace with the number of those needing transplants. This increased need for organ donors led the Congress of National Black Churches to make organ and tissue donation a top-priority health issue.

Health-Care Providers

Traditional Versus Biomedical Providers

Physicians are recognized as heads of the health-care team, with nurses having lesser importance. However, as nurses are becoming more educated and operating in advanced practice roles, both African American males and female are holding them in higher regard. For example, Wehbe-Alamah and colleagues (2011) found that African American men receiving primary care in a nurse-managed clinic reported that that they felt nurse practitioners (NPs) spent more time with patients and demonstrated more caring behaviors. Similar studies revealed that African Americans reported that NPs provided nonjudgmental care, showed more care than physicians, spent more time with them than physicians to explain things, were trusted more, and rendered a holistic approach to find the best treatment (Benkert & Tate, 2008; Gunn & Davis, 2011; Wehbe-Alamah, McFarland, Macklin, & Riggs, 2011). These findings suggest that some African Americans are able to develop a strong and trusting relationship with health-care providers despite their long history of distrust.

Whereas some African Americans may prefer a health-care provider of the same gender for urological and gynecological conditions, generally gender is not a major concern in the selection of health-care provider. Men and women can provide personal care to the opposite sex. On occasion, young men may prefer that another man or an older woman give personal care. With the current emphasis on women's health and the responses of women to illness and treatment regimens, some African American women prefer female primary-care providers. Health-care providers should respect these wishes when possible.

Among the African American community, traditional/folk practitioners can be spiritual leaders, grandparents, elders of the community, voodoo doctors, or priests. For example, the pastor in the African American church is noted to be "a healer of the sick" (Drayton-Brooks & White, 2004, p. 86).

Status of Health-Care Providers

Western health-care providers do not generally regard folk practitioners with high esteem. However, as homeopathic and alternative medicine increases in importance in preventive health, these practitioners are gaining more recognition, respect, and utilization. Folk practitioners are respected and valued in the African American community and frequently used by African Americans of all socioeconomic levels. Many African Americans perceive health-care providers as outsiders, and they resent them for telling them what their problems are or telling them how to solve them (Underwood, 1994). Generally, most African Americans are suspicious and cautious of health-care providers they have not heard of or do not know. Because interpersonal relationships are highly valued in this group, it is important to initially focus on developing a sound, trusting relationship.

REFERENCES

Aaron, K., Levine, D., & Burstin, H. (2003). African American church participation and health care practices. *Journal of General Internal Medicine, 18*(11), 908–913. Retrieved from http://www.ncbi.nlm.nih.gov/pmc/articles/PMC1494942/

Adebimpe, V. (1981). Overview: White norms in psychiatric diagnosis of Black American patients. *American Journal of Psychiatry, 138*(3), 279–285.

Agency for Healthcare Research and Quality (AHRQ). (2005, December). *National Healthcare Disparities Report.* AHRQ Publication No. 06-0017. Retrieved from http://www.ahrq.gov/qual/nhdr05/nhdr05.pdf

Allender, J., & Spradley, B. (2001). *Community health nursing: Concepts and practice.* Philadelphia: Lippincott.

American Academy of Pediatrics. (1998). Screening for elevated blood levels. *Pediatrics, 101*(6), 1072–1078.

American Cancer Society. (2010). *Cancer facts and figures for African Americans 2011–2012.* Retrieved from http://www.cancer.org/acs/groups/content/@epidemiologysurveilance/documents/document/acspc-027765.pdf

American Public Health Association. (1999). More research needed to guide policy on environmental justice. *Nation's Health, 29*(3), 4.

American Public Health Association. (2004). *Eliminating Disparities: Communities moving from statistics to solutions—Toolkit.* National Public Health Week, April 5–11, 2004. Washington, DC: Author. Retrieved from http://www.nphw.org/2005/toolkit/Toolkit-PHW04-LR.pdf

The Asthma and Allergy Foundation of America and the National Pharmaceutical Council. (2006). *Ethnic disparities in the burden and treatment of asthma.* Washington, DC: Author. Retrieved from http://www.scribd.com/doc/7514016/ethnic-disparities-in-the-burden-and-treatment-of-asthma

Baldwin, D. (1996). Model for describing low-income African-American women's participation in breast and cervical cancer early detection and screening. *Advances in Nursing Science 19*(2), 21–42.

Banini, A., Allen, J., Boyd, L., & Lartey, A. (2003). Fatty acids, diet, and body indices of type II diabetic American whites and blacks and Ghanaians. *Nutrition, 19*(9), 722–726.

Barbarin, O. (1983). Coping with ecological transitions by Black families: A psycho-social model. *Journal of Community Psychology, 11*(4), 308–322.

Base-Smith, V., & Campinha-Bacote, J. (2003). The culture of obesity. *Journal of the National Black Nurses Association, 14*(1), 52–56.

Bender, D. (1998). *The family: Opposing viewpoints.* San Diego, CA: Greenhaven Press.

Benkert, R., & Tate, N. (2008). Trust of nurse provider and physicians among African Americans with hypertension. *Journal of the American Academy of Nurse Provider, 20*(5), 273–280.

Bigler, R., & Averhart, C. (2003). Race and the workforce: Occupational status, aspirations, and stereotyping among African American children. *Developmental Psychology, 39*(3), 572–580.

Billingsley, A. (1968). *Black families in White America.* Upper Saddle River, NJ: Prentice Hall.

Black, M., Siegel, E., Abel, Y., & Bentley, M. (2001). Home and videotape intervention delays early complementary feeding among adolescent mothers. *Pediatrics, 107*(5). Retrieved from http://pediatrics.aappublications.org/cgi/content/full/107/5/e67

Black Demographics.com. *African American Religion.* Retrieved from http://www.blackdemographics.com/religion.html

Bland-Stewart, L. (2005). Difference or deficit in speakers of African American English. What every clinician should know. *ASHA Leader, 10*(6), 6–7, 30–31.

Blum, J., Morgan, E., Rose, W., Schlesinger, A., Stampp, K., & Woodward, C. (1981). *The national experience.* New York: Harcourt Brace Jovanovich.

Boyd, E., Taylor, S., Shimp L., & Semler, C. (2000). An assessment of home remedy use by African Americans. *Journal of the National Medical Association, 92*(7), 341–353. Retrieved from http://www.ncbi.nlm.nih.gov/pmc/articles/PMC2608585/pdf/jnma00343-0057.pdf

Braithwaite, R., Taylor, S., & Austin, J. (2000). *Building health coalitions in the black community.* Thousand Oaks, CA: Sage Publications.

Brewster, L., van Montfrans, G., & Kleijnen, J. (2005). Systematic review: Antihypertensive drug therapy in Black patients. *Annals of Internal Medicine, 14*(18), 614–627.

Brown, D., & Gary, L. (1994). Religious involvement and health status among African-American males. *Journal of the National Medical Association, 86*(11), 825–831.

Brownstein, R. (1995, November 6). Why are so many black men in jail? Numbers in debate equal a paradox. *Los Angeles Times,* p. A5.

Brunton, L., Goodman, L., Blumenthal, D., & Buxman, L. (2008). *Goodman & Gillman's manual of pharmacology and therapeutics.* New York: McGraw-Hill Companies.

Burroughs, V., Mackey, M., & Levy, R. (2002). Racial and ethnic differences in response to medicines: Towards individualized pharmaceutical treatment. *Journal of the National Medical Association, 94*(10), 1–20.

Campinha-Bacote, J. (1991). Community mental health services for the underserved: A culturally specific model. *Archives of Psychiatric Nursing, 5*(4), 29–35.

Campinha-Bacote, J. (1992). Voodoo illness. *Perspectives in Psychiatric Nursing, 28*(1), 11–19.

Campinha-Bacote, J. (1993). Soul therapy: Humor and music with African American patients. *Journal of Christian Nursing, 10*(2), 23–26.

Campinha-Bacote, J. (1997). Humor therapy for culturally diverse psychiatric patients. *Journal of Nursing Jocularity, 7*(1), 38–40.

Campinha-Bacote, J. (2005). *A biblically based model of cultural competence in the delivery of healthcare services*. Cincinnati, OH: Transcultural C.A.R.E. Associates.

Campinha-Bacote, J. (2007). *The Process of cultural competence in the delivery of healthcare services: The journey continues*. Cincinnati, OH: Transcultural C.A.R.E. Associates.

Carroll, K. (2010). A genealogical analysis of the worldview framework in African-centered psychology. *The Journal of Pan African Studies, 3*(8), 109–143.

Chin, J. (2009). Diversity in mind and action. Volume 2. Disparities and competence: Service delivery, education and employment contexts. Santa Barbara CA: Praeger/ABC-CLIO.

Clark, M.J. (1999). *Nursing in the community: Dimensions of community health nursing*. Stamford, CT: Appleton & Lange.

Cokley, K., Cooke, B., & Nobles, W. (2005, September 29). *Guidelines for providing culturally appropriate services for people of African ancestry exposed to the trauma of Hurricane Katrina*. Washington, DC: The Association of Black Psychologists. Retrieved from http://www.abpsi.org/index.php/the-news/133-guidelines-for-providing-culturally-appropriate-services

Conant, J. (1961). *Slums and suburbs*. New York: New American Library Publishers.

Cord, J. (2010). What health-care reform means for African Americans. *The Root*. Retrieved from http://www.theroot.com/views/what-health-care-reform-means-african-americans

Curriculum Ethnogeriatrics. (2001). *Core curriculum and ethnic specific modules: African American*. Retrieved from http://www.stanford.edu/group/ethnoger/

DelBello, M., Soutullo, C., Ochsner, J., McElroy, J., Keck, P., Strakowski, S., et al. (1999, May 18). Racial differences in the treatment of adolescents with bipolar disorder, *New Research 379*. Presented at the 152nd annual meeting of the American Psychiatric Association. Washington, DC.

Dirks, N., Huth, B., Yates C., & Melbohm, B. (2004). Pharmacokinetics of immunosuppressants: A perspective on ethnic difference. *International Journal of Clinical Pharmacology and Therapeutics, 42*(12), 719–723.

Dixon, V. (1971). African-oriented and Euro-American-oriented worldviews: Research methodologies and economics. *Review of Black Political Economy, 7*(2), 119–156.

Drayton-Brooks, S., & White, N. (2004). Health promoting behaviors among African American women with faith-based support. *The ABNF Journal, 15*(5), 84–90.

Edleman, C., & Mandel, C. (1998). *Health promotion throughout the lifespan* (3rd ed.). St. Louis, MO: C. V. Mosby.

Fairrow, A., McCallum, T., & Messinger-Rapport, B. (2004). Preferences of older African-Americans for long-term tube feeding at end of life. *Aging & Mental Health, 8*(6), 530–534.

Ferdinand, K. (2006). The isosorbide-hydralazine story: Is there a case for race-based cardiovascular medicine? *The Journal of Clinical Hypertension, 8*(3), 156–158.

Fleisher, G., & Ludwig, S. (2010). *Textbook of pediatric emergency medicine*. PA: Lippincott Williams & Wilkins.

Frazier, E. (1957). *Black bourgeoisie*. New York: Collier Books.

Glazer, W.M., Morganstern, H., & Doucette, J.T. (1993). Predicting the long-term risk of tardive dyskinesia in outpatients maintained on neuroleptic medications. *Journal of Clinical Psychiatry, 54*(4), 133–139.

Gloster, H. & Neal, K. (2006). Skin cancer in skin of color. *Journal of American Academy of Dermatology, 55*(5), 741–760.

Green, L. (2002). *African American English: A linguistic introduction*. United Kingdom: Cambridge University Press.

Gunn, J., & Davis, S. (2011). Beliefs, meanings, and practices of healing with botanicals re-called by elder African American women in the Mississippi Delta. *Online Journal of Cultural Care in Nursing and Healthcare, 1*(1), 37–49.

Herrera, J., Lawson, W., & Sramek, J. (1999). *Cross-cultural psychiatry*. New York: John Wiley & Sons.

Hill, R. (1997, July 7). Sociologist taught strength of black family. *Baltimore Sun Times*, p. 2B.

The HSC Foundation. (2007). *Preventing childhood obesity in lower-income communities: A focus group report of African-American and Latino families' understanding of healthy lifestyles, barriers and challenges*. Washington, DC: Author.

Institute of Medicine (IOM). (2004). *In the nation's compelling interest: Ensuring diversity in the health care workforce*. Washington, DC: Author.

Jaynes, D., & Williams, R. (1989). *A common destiny: Blacks and American society*. Washington, DC: National Academy Press.

Johnson, K., Elbert-Avila, K., & Tulsky, J. (2005). The influence of spiritual beliefs and practices on the treatment preferences of African Americans: A review of the literature. *Journal of the American Geriatrics Society, 53*(4), 711–719.

Kaiser Family Foundation. (2001). *African Americans view of the HIV/AIDS epidemic at 20 years*. Menlo Park, CA: Author.

Kelly, J., Kaufman, D., Kelley, K., Rosenberg, L., & Mitchell, A. (2006). Use of herbal/natural supplements according to racial/ethnic group. *The Journal of Alternative and Complementary Medicine, 12*(6), 555–561.

Kennedy, B., Mathis, C., & Woods, A., (2007). African Americans and their distrust of the health care system: Healthcare for diverse populations. *Journal of Cultural Diversity, 14*(2), 56–60.

Kwate, N., & Meyer, I. (2010). The myth of meritocracy and African American health. *American Journal of Public Health, 100*(10), 1831–1834.

Ladner, J., & Gourdine, R. (1992). Adolescent pregnancy in the African-American community. In R. Braithwaite & S. Taylor (Eds.), *Health issues in the black community* (pp. 206–221). San Francisco, CA: Josey-Bass.

LaVeist, T., & Carroll, T. (2002). Race of physician and satisfaction with care among African American patients. *The Journal of the National Medical Association, 94*(11), 937–943.

LaVeist, T., & Nuru-Jeter, A. (2002). Is doctor-patient concordance associated with greater satisfaction with care? *Journal of Health and Social Behavior, 43*(3), 296–306.

Lawson, W. (1999, May 19). *Ethnicity and treatment of bipolar disorder*. Presented at the 152nd annual meeting of the American Psychiatric Association. Washington, DC.

Levy, R. (1993). Ethnic and racial differences in response to medicines: Preserving individualized therapy in managed pharmaceutical programmes. *Pharmaceutical Medicine, 7*, 139–165.

Lincoln, C. (1974). *The Black church since Frazier*. New York: Schocken Books.

Lobar, S., Youngblut, J., & Brooten, D. (2006). Cross-cultural beliefs, ceremonies, and rituals surrounding death of a loved one. *Pediatric Nursing, 32*(1), 44–55.

Low-wage labor market. (2006). Retrieved from http://aspe.hhs.gov/hsp/lwlm99/henly.htm

Lowenstein, A., & Glanville, C.L. (1995). Cultural diversity and conflict in the health care workplace. *Nursing Economics, 13*(4), 203–209.

Matas, A., Sowa, M., Taylor, V., Taylor, G., Schattka, B., & Mantsch, H. (2001). Eliminating the issue of skin color in assessment of the blanch response. *Advances in Skin Wound Care, 14*, 180–8.

Mathews, T., & MacDorman, M. (2010). Infant mortality statistics from the 2006 period linked birth/infant death data set. *National Vital Statistics Report, 58*(17), 1–32. Retrieved from http://www.cdc.gov/nchs/data/nvsr/nvsr58/nvsr58_17.pdf

McNeil, J., Campinha-Bacote, J., Tapscott, E., & Vample, G. (2002). *BESAFE: National minority AIDS education and training center cultural competency model.* Washington, DC: Howard University Medical School.

Michaels, D. (1993). Occupational cancer in the black population: The health effects of job discrimination. *Journal of the National Black Medical Association, 75,* 1014–1018.

Moore, J. (2005). Hypertension: Catching the silent killer. *Nurse Provider, 30*(10), 16–18, 23–24, 26–27.

Morgan, P., Barnett, K., Perdue, B., Fogel, J., Underwood, S., Gaskins, M., & Brown-Davis, C. (2006). African American women with breast cancer and their spouses' perception of care received from physicians. *The ABNF Journal, 17*(1), 32–37.

Morrison, R., Wallenstein, S., Natale, D., Senzel, R., & Huang L. (2000). "We don't carry that"—failure of pharmacies in predominantly nonwhite neighborhoods to stock opioid analgesics. *New England Journal of Medicine, 342,* 1023–1026.

Murray, R., & Zentner, J. (2001). *Health promotion strategies through the lifespan.* Upper Saddle River, NJ: Prentice Hall.

Musgrave, C., Allen, C., & Allen, G. (2002). Rural health and women of color: Spirituality and health for women of color. *American Journal of Public Health, 92*(4), 557–560.

National Diabetes Information Clearinghouse. *National Diabetes Statistics, 2011.* Bethesda, MD: Author. Retrieved from www.diabetes.niddk.nih.gov

National Women's Health Information (2011). U.S. Department of Health and Human Resources, Office on Women's Health: *Overweight and obesity.* Retrieved from http://www.4women.gov/minority/africanamerican/obesity.cfm

National Women's Health Report. (2005). African-American women & heart health. *National Women's Health Report, 27*(10), 6.

Navarro, V. (1997). Race or class versus race and class: Mortality differentials in the U.S. In P. R. Lee & C. L. Estes (Eds.), *The nation's health* (pp. 32–36). Sudbury, MA: Jones & Barlett.

Negy, C., & Eisenman, R. (2005). A comparison of African American and white college students' affective and attitudinal reactions to lesbian, gay, and bisexual individuals: An exploratory study. *The Journal of Sex Research, 42*(4), 291–298).

Nichols, E. (1987). *Nichols' Model of the Philosophical Aspects of Cultural Difference.* Unpublished paper. Contact: Nichols and Associates, Inc.; 1523 Underwood Street, NW; Washington, DC, 20012.

NMAETC. (2006). *African American/Black fact sheet.* Washington, DC: Author.

Parks-Yancy, R. (2010). *Equal work, unequal career: African Americans in the workforce.* Boulder, CO: First Forum Press.

The Pew Forum on Religion and Public Life. (2009). *A religious portrait of African Americans.* http://pewforum.org/A-Religious-Portrait-of-African-Americans.aspx

Plawecki, H., & Plawecki, J. (1992). Improving organ donation rates in the black community. *Journal of Holistic Nursing, 10*(1), 34–46.

Queralt, M. 1996. *The social environment and human behavior: A diversity perspective.* Needham Heights, MA: Allyn & Bacon.

Rickford, J. (1999). The Ebonics controversy in my backyard: A sociologist's experiences and reflections. *Journal of Sociolinguistics, 3*(2), 267.

Ries, L., Melbert, D., Krapcho, M., Mariotto, A., Miller, B., Feuer, E., Clegg, L., Horner, M., Howlader, N., Eisner, M.,

Reichman, M, & Edwards, B. (Eds). (2008). *SEER Cancer Statistics Review, 1975–2004, National Cancer Institute.* Bethesda, Retrieved from http://seer.cancer.gov/csr/1975_2004/results_merged/sect_16_melanoma.pdf. Based on November 2006 SEER data submission.

Roberson, M. (1985). The influence of religious beliefs on health choices of Afro-Americans. *Topics in Clinical Nursing, 7*(3), 57–63.

Salcido, S. (2002). Finding a window into the skin. *Advances in Skin and Wound Care, 15*(3), 100.

Saunders, E. (1997). High blood pressure: A call to action for African-Americans. *Baltimore Sun,* p. A3.

Savitt, T. (1978). *Medicine and slavery.* Chicago: University of Illinois Press.

Schaeffeler, E., Eichelbaum, M., Brinkmann, U., Penger, A., Asante-Poku, S., Zanger, U., & Schwab, M. (2001). Frequency of C3435T polymorphism of gene in African people. *The Lancet, 358*(9279), 383–384.

Schwartz, R. (2001). Racial profiling in medical research. *New England Journal of Medicine, 344,* 1392–1393.

Smedley, B., Stith, A., & Nelson, A. (2002). Unequal treatment: Confronting racial and ethnic disparities in healthcare. Washington, DC: National Academy Press.

Snow, L. (1974). Folk medical beliefs and their implications for care of patients. *Annals of Internal Medicine, 81,* 82–96.

Snow, L. (1993). *Walkin' over medicine.* Boulder, CO: Westview Press.

Sommers, M. (2011). Color awareness: A must for patient assessment. *American Nurse Today. 6*(1). Retrieved from http://www.americannursetoday.com/Article.aspx?id=7434&fid=7360

Sommers, M., Zink, T., Fargo, J., Baker, R.B., Buschur, C., Shambley-Ebron, D.Z., & Fisher, B.S. (2008). Forensic sexual assault examination and genital injury: Is skin color a source of health disparity? *American Journal of Emergency Medicine, 26,* 857–866.

Sowa, M., Matas, A., Schattka, B., & Mantsch, H. (2002). Spectroscopic assessment of cutaneous hemodynamics in the presence of high epidermal melanin concentration. *Clinica Chimica Acta, 317,* 203–212.

Sowers, J., Ferdinand, K., Bakris, G., & Douglas, J. (2002). Hypertension-related disease in African Americans. *Postgraduate Medicine, 112*(4), 24–48.

Spurlock, W., & Cullins, L. (2006). Cancer fatalism and breast cancer screening in African American women. *The ABNF Journal, 17*(10), 38–43.

Strakowski, S., McElroy, S., Keck P., & West, S. (1996). Racial influence on diagnosis in psychotic mania. *Journal of Affect Disorders, 39*(2), 157–162.

Strickland, T.I., Lin, K.M., Fu, P., Anderson, D., & Zheng, Y. (1995). Comparison of lithium ratio between African-American and Caucasian bipolar patients. *Biological Psychiatry, 37*(5), 325–330.

Strickland, T.L., Ranganath, V., Lin, K.M., Poland, R.E., Mendoza, R., & Smith, M.W. (1991). Psychopharmacologic considerations in the treatment of black American populations. *Psychopharmacology Bulletin, 27*(4), 441–448.

Sullivan, L. (2004). *Missing persons: Minorities in the health professions: A report of the Sullivan Commission on diversity in the healthcare workforce.* Battle Creek, MI: W. K. Kellogg Foundation.

Taulbert, C. (1969). *Once upon a time when we were colored.* Tulsa, OK: Counsel Oak Books.

The White House, Office of the First Lady. (2010). *Remarks by the first lady to the NAACP national convention in Kansas City,*

Missouri. Retrieved from http://www.whitehouse.gov/the-press-office/remarks-first-lady-naacp-national-convention-kansas-city-missouri

Thompson, C., Craig, H., & Washington, J. (2004). Variable production of African American English across oral and literary contexts. *Language, Speech, and Hearing in Schools, 35*(3), 269–282.

Underwood, S. (1994). Increasing the participation of minorities and other at-risk groups in clinical trials. *Innovations in Oncology Nursing, 10*(4), 106.

Underwood, S., Buseh, A., Canales, M., Powe, B., Dockery, B, Kather, T., & Kent, N. (2005). Nursing contributions to the elimination of health disparities among African Americans: Review and critique of a decade of research (part II). *Journal of National Black Nurses Association, 16*(10), 31–47.

Underwood, S., & Powell, R. (2006). Religion and spirituality: Influence on health/risk behavior and cancer screening behavior of African Americans. *The ABNF Journal, 17*(10), 20–31.

Underwood, S., Berry, M., & Haley, S. (2009). Promoting health and wellness of African American brethren: Because we are our brother's keeper. *The ABNF, 20*(2), 53–59.

U.S. Census Bureau, Statistical Abstract of the United States: 2011. (2011). *Births, deaths, marriages, and divorces*. Retrieved from http://www.census.gov/compendia/statab/2011/tables/11s0103.pdf

U.S. Department of Commerce, Bureau of the Census. (1993). *We the American blacks*. Washington, DC: U.S. Government Printing Office.

U.S. Department of Commerce, Bureau of the Census. (2006). www.census.gov.

U.S. Department of Commerce, Bureau of the Census. (2008). *American community survey*. Retrieved from http://www.census.gov/acs/www/

U.S. Department of Commerce, Bureau of the Census. (2010). Retrieved from http://2010.census.gov/2010census/

U.S. Department of Health and Human Services. (1997). *Healthy People 2010: National health promotion and disease prevention objectives*. Washington, DC: Author.

U.S. Department of Health and Human Services. (2002). *Healthy PEOPLe 2010: Understanding and improving health* (2nd ed.). Washington, DC: Author.

U.S. Department of Health and Human Services. (2009). *Office of Minority Health: African American Profile*. Washington, DC: Author. Retrieved from http://minorityhealth.hhs.gov/templates/browse.aspx?lvl=2&lvlID=51

U.S. Department of Health and Human Services, Center for Disease Control and Prevention National Center for Health Statistics (2010). *Health, United States, 2010*. Washington, DC: Author.

U.S. Department of Justice Office of Justice Programs. (2008). Prison and jail inmates at midyear 2006. *Bureau of Justice Statistics Bulletin*. Retrieved from http://bjs.ojp.usdoj.gov/content/pub/pdf/pjim06.pdf

Wandler, K. (2003). Psychopharmacology of patients with eating disorders. *Remuda Review, 2*(1), 1–7.

Washington, K., Bickel-Swenson, D., & Stephens, N. (2008). Barriers to hospice use among African Americans: A systematic review. *Health & Social Work, 33*(4), 267–274.

Waters, C. (2000). End-of-life directives among African Americans: A need for community-centered discussion and education. *Journal of Community Health Nursing, 17*(1), 25–37.

Watts, R. (2003, January). Race consciousness and the health of African Americans. O*nline Journal of Nursing, 8*(1), Manuscript 3. Retrieved from http://www.nursingworld.org/MainMenuCategories/ANAMarketplace/ANAPeriodicals/OJIN/TableofContents/Volume82003/No1Jan2003/RaceandHealth.aspx

Wehbe-Alamah, H., McFarland, M., Belanger, B., Bender, J., Brandon, C., Gensel, B., & Ross, L. (2011). The lived experience of African American Men receiving primary care in a nurse managed clinic within an urban context. *Online Journal of Cultural Competence in Nursing and Healthcare, 1*(1), 54.

Wehbe-Alamah, H., McFarland, M., Macklin, J., & Riggs, N. (2011). The lived experiences of African American women receiving care from nurse provider leave as practitioner in an urban nurse-managed clinic. *The Online Journal in Cultural Competence in Nursing and Healthcare, 1*(1), 15–26.

Welch, L., Teno, J., & Mor, V. (2005). End-of-life care in black and white: Race matters for medical care of dying patients and their families. *Journal of the American Geriatrics Society, 53*(7), 11154–11161.

Williams, B. (2005). Older African Americans and calcium-deficient diets: What rehabilitation specialists need to know. *Topic in Geriatric Rehabilitation, 21*(1), 88–92.

Williams, J., Wyatt, G., & Wingood, G. (2010). The four Cs of HIV prevention with African Americans: Crisis, condoms, culture, and community. *Current HIV/AIDS Report, 7*(4), 185–193.

Wood, J. (2009). *Communication in our lives*. Boston, MA: Wadsworth Cengage Learning.

DavisPlus For case studies, review questions, and additional information, go to
http://davisplus.fadavis.com

Chapter 7

The Amish

Anna Frances Z. Wenger and Marion R. Wenger

Overview, Inhabited Localities, and Topography

Overview

As dusk gathers on the hospital parking lot, a man first ties his horse to the hitching rack and then helps down from the carriage a matronly figure who is wrapped in a shawl as dark as his own greatcoat. On their mother's heels, a flurry of children dressed like undersized replicas of their parents turn their wide eyes toward the fluorescent-lit glass façade of the reception area, a glimmering beacon from the world of high-technology health care. Their excitement is muted by their father's soft-spoken rebuke in a language more akin to German than English, and in a hush, the Amish family crosses a cultural threshold—into the workaday world of health-care providers.

This Amish family appears to come from another time and place. Those familiar with the health-care needs of the Amish know the profound cultural distance they have bridged in seeking professional help. Others, only marginally acquainted with Amish ways, may ask why this group dresses, acts, and talks like visitors to the North American cultural landscape of the 21st century. Amish are "different" by intention and by conviction. That is to say, for most of the ways in which they depart from the norm for contemporary American culture, they cite a reason related to their understanding of the biblical mandate to live a life separated from a world they see as unregenerate or sinful.

As noted in the variant cultural characteristics in the introduction to cultural diversity in Chapter 1, dissimilar appearance, behavior, or both may signal deeper underlying differences in the Amish culture. Noting these differences does not, of necessity, lead to better acceptance or deeper understanding of attitudes and behaviors. Appearances can be misleading. For example, the Amish family's arrival at the hospital by horse and carriage might suggest a general taboo against modern technological conveniences. In fact, most Amish homes are not furnished with electric and electronic labor-saving devices and appliances. But that does not preclude the Amish's openness to using state-of-the-art medical technology if it is perceived as necessary to promoting their health.

This minority group's exotic features of dress and language may disguise true motivations regarding health-seeking behaviors, which they share in common with the larger, or majority, culture. To enable such patients to attain their own standard of health and well-being, health-care providers need to look beyond the superficial appearance and to listen more carefully to the cues they provide.

Heritage and Residence

It is as important to locate the Amish topographically according to cultural and religious coordinates as well as to the geographical areas they inhabit. The hospital visit scene just portrayed could have taken place in any one of a number of towns spanning the American Midwest from the eastern seaboard, but the basic circumstances surrounding the interaction with professional caregivers and the cultural assumptions underlying it are basically similar. For the Amish, seeking help from health-care providers requires them to go outside their own people and, in so doing, to cross over a significant "permeable boundary" that delimits their community in cultural-geographic terms.

Today's Amish live in rural areas in a band of over 20 states stretching westward from Pennsylvania, Ohio, and Indiana as far as Montana, with some scattered settlements as far south as Florida and as far north as the province of Ontario, Canada (Huntington, 2001) as well as other parts of the United States. About 75 percent of their estimated total population of over 175,000 is concentrated in Pennsylvania, Ohio, and Indiana (Kraybill & Hostetter, 2001; C.N. Hostetter, personal communication). The **Old Order Amish**, so-called for their strict observance of traditional ways that distinguishes them from other, more progressive "plain folk," are the largest and most notable group among the Amish. As such, they constitute an ethnoreligious cultural group in modern America with roots in Reformation-era Europe.

Reasons for Migration and Associated Economic Factors

The Amish emerged after 1693 as a variant of one stream of the **Anabaptist** movement that originated in Switzerland in 1525 and spread to neighboring lands to the east, north, and northwest, especially along the Rhine River, to the Netherlands. The Amish embraced, among other essential Anabaptist tenets of faith, the baptism of adult believers as an outward sign of membership in a voluntary community with an inner commitment to live peaceably with all. The Amish parted ways with the larger Anabaptist group, now known as *Mennonites*, over the Amish propensity to strictly avoid community members whom they excluded from fellowship in their church (Hostetler, 1993). The *Amish* name is derived from the surname of Jacob Ammann, a 17th-century Anabaptist who led the Amish division from the Anabaptists in 1693 (Hüppi, 2000). Similarly, the name *Mennonite* is derived from the given name of Menno Simons, a former Catholic priest, who was a key leader of the Anabaptist movement in Europe.

Anabaptists were disenfranchised and deported, and their goods expropriated for their refusal to bear arms as a civic service and to accept the authority of the state church in matters of faith and practice. Their attempts at radical discipleship in a "free church," following the guidelines of the early church as set forth in the New Testament, resulted in conflict with Catholic and Protestant leaders. After experiencing severe persecution and martyrdom in Europe, the Amish and related groups emigrated to America in the 17th and 18th centuries. No Amish live in Europe today, the last survivors having been assimilated into other religious groups (Hostetler, 1993). As a result, the Amish, unlike many other ethnic groups in the United States, have no larger reference group in their former homeland to which their customs, language, and lifeways can be compared.

Denied the right to hold property in their homelands, the Amish sought not only religious freedom but also the opportunity to buy farmland where they could live out their beliefs in peace. In their communities, the Amish have transplanted and preserved a way of life that bears the outward dress of preindustrial European peasantry. In modern industrial America, they have persisted in social isolation based on religious principles, a paradoxically separated life of Christian altruism. Living for others entails a caring concern for members of their in-group, a community of mutuality, but it also calls them to reach out to others in need outside their immediate Amish household of faith (Hostetler, 1993).

Although the Amish value inner harmony, mutual caring, and a peaceable life in the country, it would be a mistake to see Amish society as an idyllic, pastoral folk culture, frozen in time and serenely detached from the dynamic developments all around them. Since the mid-19th century, Amish communities have experienced inner conflicts and dissension as well as outside pressures to conform and modernize. Over time, the Amish have continued to adapt and change, but at their own pace, accepting innovations selectively.

One cost of controlled, deliberate change has been the loss of some members through factional divisions over "progressive" motivations, both religious and material. The influence of revivalism led to religious reform variants, which introduced Sunday schools, missions, and worship in meetinghouses instead of homes. Others who were impatient to use modern technology, such as gasoline-powered farm machinery, telephones, electricity, electronic devices, and automobiles, also split off from the main body of the most conservative traditionalists, now called the *Old Order Amish*. Some variant groups were named after their factional leaders (e.g., Egli and Beachy Amish); some were called *Conservative Amish Mennonites*, and others *The New Order Amish*. Today, these progressives stand somewhere between the parent body, the Mennonites, and the Old Order Amish (technically Old Order Amish Mennonites), hereafter simply referred to as the Amish (Hostetler, 1993). This latter group, the (Old Order) Amish, which has been widely researched and reported on, provides the observational basis for this present culture study.

Educational Status and Occupations

The controversy over schooling of Amish children is a good example of a policy issue that attracts public attention. Amish parents assume primary responsibility for child rearing, with the constant support of the extended family and the church community to reinforce their teachings. On the family farm, parents and older siblings model work roles for younger siblings. Corporate worship and community religious practices nurture and shape their faith. Learning how to live and to prepare for death is more important in the Amish tradition than acquiring special skills or knowledge through formal education or training (Hostetler & Huntington, 1992).

The mixed-grade, one-room schoolhouses (Fig. 7-1), typical of rural America before 1945, were acceptable to the Amish because the schools were more amenable to local control. With the introduction of consolidated high schools, however, the Amish resisted secondary education, particularly compulsory schooling mandated by state and federal agencies, and raised objections both on principle and on scale. To illustrate the latter, the amount of time required by secondary education and the distances required to bus students out

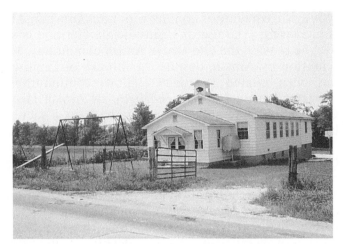

Figure 7-1 A one-room Amish schoolhouse in Indiana. *(Photograph by Joel Wenger.)*

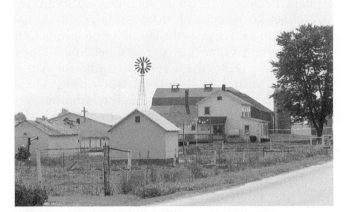

Figure 7-2 An Amish farm. The windmill in the background is used to pump water. *(Photograph by Joel Wenger.)*

of their home communities were cited as problems. But probably more crucial was the understanding that the high school promised to socialize and instruct the young in a value system that was antithetical to the Amish way of life. For example, in the high school, individual achievement and competition were promoted, rather than mutuality and caring for others in a communal spirit. On pragmatic grounds, Amish parents objected to "unnecessary" courses in science, advanced math, and computer technology, which seemed to have no place and little relevance in their tradition (Meyers, 1993).

The Amish response to this perceived threat to their culture was to build and operate their own private elementary schools. Their right to do so was litigated but finally upheld in the U.S. Supreme Court in the 1972 *Wisconsin v. Yoder* ruling. Today, school-age children are encouraged to attend only eight grades, but Amish parents actively support local private and public elementary schools.

The Amish rejection of higher learning for their children means that only the rare individual may pursue professional training and still remain Amish. Health-care providers, by definition, are seen as outsiders who mediate information on health promotion, make diagnoses, and propose therapies across cultural boundaries. To the extent that they do so with sensitivity and respect for Amish cultural ways, they are respected, in turn, and valued as an important resource by the Amish.

As the 20th century drew to a close, important changes were underway among the Amish in North America, whose principal and preferred occupations have long been agricultural work and farm-related enterprises (Fig. 7-2). They had typically settled on good farmland from their earliest immigration some 250 years ago. As cultivatable land at an affordable price became an increasingly scarce commodity near centers of Amish settlements, the trend toward other

work away from home led to a reshaping of the Amish family. Income from goods and services once delivered for internal domestic consumption came increasingly from cottage industry production for the retail market and wage-earning with nearby employers. The alternative, seeking new farmland at a distance, has led to community resettlement as far away from Pennsylvania as Montana.

Young women who have learned quantity cookery at the many church and family get-togethers may find jobs in restaurants and catering, or skills learned in household chores may be exchanged for wages in child care or housecleaning. Young men who bring skills from the farm may practice carpentry or cabinetmaking in the trades and construction industry. This, in turn, brings a change in family patterns, since "lunchbox daddies" are absent during daylight workday hours and the burden for parenting is borne more by stay-at-home mothers. The bonds of family and church have proved resilient but are clearly experiencing more tension in the current generation.

In summary, jobs away from home, an established majority culture pattern, and increased contacts with non-Amish people test the strength of sociocultural bonds that tie young people to the Amish culture. Given the enticements of the majority culture to change and to acculturate, it is noteworthy that so many young Amish find their way back to full membership in the ethnoreligious culture that nurtured them.

Communication

Dominant Languages and Dialects

Like most people, the Amish vary their language usage depending on the situation and the individuals being addressed. American English is only one of three language varieties in their repertoire. For the Amish, English is the language of school, of written and printed communications, and, above all, the language used in contacts with most non-Amish outsiders, especially business contacts. Because English serves a useful function as the contact language with the outside world, Amish schools all use English as the language of instruction, with the strong support of parents, because elementary schooling offers the best opportunity for Amish children to master the language. But within Amish homes and communities, use of English is discouraged in favor of the vernacular **Deitsch**, or Pennsylvania German. Because all Amish except preschool children are literate in their second language, American English, language usage helps to define their cultural space (Hostetler, 1993).

The first language of most Amish is *Deitsch,* an amalgamation of several upland German dialects that emerged from the interaction of immigrants from the Palatinate and Upper Rhine areas of modern France, Germany, and Switzerland. Their regional linguistic differences were resolved in an immigrant language better known in English as "Pennsylvania German" (also known as "Pennsylvania Dutch"). Amish immigrants who later moved more directly from the Swiss Jura and environs to midwestern states (with minimal mixing in transit with *Deitsch*-speakers) call their home language *Düütsch,* a related variety with marked Upper Alemannic features. Today, *Deitsch* and *Düütsch* both show a strong admixture of vocabulary borrowed from English, whereas the basic structure remains clearly nonstandard German. Both dialects have practically the same functional distribution (Meyers & Nolt, 2005; Wenger, 1970).

Deitsch is spoken in the home and in conversation with fellow Amish and relatives, especially during **visiting**, a popular social activity by which news is disseminated orally. It is important to note that *Deitsch* is primarily a spoken language. Some written material has been printed in Pennsylvania German, but Amish seldom encounter it in this form. Even Amish publications urging the use of *Deitsch* in the family circle are printed in English, by default the print replacement for the vernacular, the spoken language (What is in a language?, 1986).

Health-care providers can expect all their Amish patients of school age and older to be fluently bilingual. They can readily understand spoken and written directions and answer questions presented in English, although their own terms for some symptoms and illnesses may not have exact equivalents in *Deitsch* and English. Amish patients may be more comfortable consulting among themselves in *Deitsch,* but generally they intend no disrespect for those who do not understand their mother tongue.

Although of limited immediate relevance for health-care considerations, the third language used by the Amish deserves mention in this cultural profile to complete the scope of their linguistic repertoire. Amish proficiency in English varies according to the

type and frequency of contact with non-Amish, but it is increasing. The use of Pennsylvania German is in decline outside the Old Order Amish community. Its retention by Amish, despite the inroads of English, has been related to their religious communities' persistent recourse to *Hochdeitsch,* or Amish High German, their so-called third language, as a sacred language (Huffines, 1994).

Amish do not use Standard Modern High German, but an approximation, which gives access to texts printed in an archaic German with some regional variations. Rote memorization and recitation for certain ceremonial and devotional functions, and for selected printed texts from the Bible, from the venerable "Ausbund" hymnbook, and from devotional literature are a part of public and private prayer and worship among the Amish. Such restricted and nonproductive use of a third language hardly justifies the term "trilingual" because it does not encompass a fully developed range of discourse. However, Amish High German does provide a situational-functional complement to their other two languages (Enninger & Wandt, 1982). Its retention is one more symbol of a consciously separated way of life that reaches back to its European heritage.

Within a highly contextual subculture like the Amish, the base of shared information and experience is proportionately larger. As a result, less overt verbal communication is required than in the relatively low-contextual American culture, and more reliance is placed on implicit, often unspoken understandings. Amish children and youth may learn adult roles in their society more through modeling, for example, than through explicit teaching. The many and diverse kinds of multigenerational social activities on the family farm provide the optimal framework for this kind of enculturation. Although this may facilitate the transmission of traditional, or accepted, knowledge and values within a high-context culture, this same information network may also impede new information imparted from the outside, which entails some behavior changes. Wenger (1988; 1991c) suggested that nurses and other health-care providers should consider role modeling as a teaching strategy when working with Amish patients. Later, a brief example of the promotion of inoculation is presented to illustrate how public-health workers can use culture-appropriate information systems to achieve fuller cooperation among the Amish.

In a final note on language and the flow of verbal information, health-care providers should be aware that much of what passes for "general knowledge" in our information-rich popular culture is screened, or filtered, out of Amish awareness. The Amish have severely restricted their own access to print media, permitting only a few newspapers and periodicals. Most have also rejected the electronic media, beginning with radio and television, but also including entertainment and information applications of film and computers. Conversely, the Amish are openly curious about the world beyond their own cultural horizons, particularly regarding a variety of literature that deals with health and quality-of-life issues. They especially value the oral and written personal testimonial as a mark of the efficacy of a particular treatment or health-enhancing product or process. Wenger (1988; 1994) identified testimonials from Amish friends and relatives as a key source of information in making choices about health-care providers and products.

Cultural Communication Patterns

Fondness and love for family members are held deeply but privately. Some nurses have observed the cool, almost aloof behavior of Amish husbands who accompany their wives to maternity centers, but it would be presumptuous to think that it reflects a lack of concern. The expression of joy and suffering is not entirely subdued by dour or stoic silence, but Amish are clearly not outwardly demonstrative or exuberant. Amish children, who can be as delightfully animated as any other children at play, are taught to remain quiet throughout a worship service lasting more than two hours. They grow up in an atmosphere of restraint and respect for adults and elders. But privately, Amish are not so sober as to lack a sense of humor and appreciation of wit.

Beyond language, much of the nonverbal behavior of Amish is also symbolic. Many of the details of Amish garb and customs were once general characteristics without any particular religious significance in Europe, but in the American setting, they are closely regulated and serve to distinguish the Amish from the dominant culture as a self-consciously separate ethnoreligious group (Kraybill, 2001).

It is precisely in the domain of ideas held to be normative for the religious aspects of Amish life that they find their English vocabulary lacking. The key source texts in *Hochdeitsch* and the oral interpretation of them in *Deitsch* are crucial to an understanding of two German values, which have an important impact on Amish nonverbal behavior. *Demut*, German for "humility," is a priority value, the effects of which may be seen in details such as the height of the crown of an Amish man's hat, as well as in very general features such as the modest and unassuming bearing and demeanor usually shown by Amish people in public. This behavior is reinforced by frequent verbal warnings against its opposite, *hochmut*, which means "pride" or "arrogance," and should be avoided (Hostetler, 1993).

The second term, *gelassenheit*, is embodied in behavior more than it is verbalized. *Gelassenheit* is treasured not so much for its contemporary German connotations of passiveness, even of resignation, as it is for its earlier religious meanings, denoting quiet acceptance and reassurance, encapsulated in the biblical formula "godliness with contentment" (1 Tim. 6:5). The following Amish paradigm for the good life flows from the calm assurance found through inner yielding and forgoing one's ego for the good of others:

1. One's life rests secure in the hands of a higher power.
2. A life so divinely ordained is therefore a good gift.
3. A godly life of obedience and submission will be rewarded in the life hereafter (Kraybill, 2001).

A combination of these inner qualities; an unpretentious, quiet manner; and modest outward dress in plain colors lacking any ornament, jewelry, or cosmetics presents a striking contrast to contemporary fashions, both in clothing styles and in personal self-actualization. Amish public behavior is consequently seen as deliberate rather than rash, deferring to others instead of being assertive or aggressive, avoiding confrontational speech styles and public displays of emotion in general.

Health-care providers should greet Amish patients with a handshake and a smile. Amish use the same greeting both among themselves and with outsiders, but little touching follows the handshake. Younger children are touched and held with affection, but older adults seldom touch socially in public. Therapeutic touch, conversely, appeals to many Amish and is practiced informally by some individuals who find communal affirmation for their gift of **warm hands**. This concept is discussed further in the section on health-care practices.

In public, the avoidance of eye contact with non-Amish may be seen as an extension, on a smaller scale, of the general reserve and measured larger body movements related to a modest and humble being. But in one-on-one clinical contacts, Amish patients can be expected to express openness and candor with unhesitating eye contact.

Among their own, Amish personal space may be collapsed on occasions of crowding together for group meetings or travel. In fact, Amish are seldom found alone, and a solitary Amish person or family is the exception rather than the rule. But Amish are also pragmatic, and in larger families, physical intimacy cannot be avoided in the home, where childbearing and care of the ill and dying are accepted as normal parts of life. Once health-care providers recognize that Amish prefer to have such caregiving within the home and family circle, providers will want to protect modest Amish patients who feel exposed in the clinical setting.

Temporal Relationships

So much of current Amish life and practice has a traditional dimension reminiscent of a rural American past that it is tempting to view the Amish culture as "backward-looking." In actuality, Amish self-perception is very much grounded in the present, and historical antecedents or reasons for current consensus have often been lost to common memory. Conversely, the Amish existential expression of Christianity focused on today is clearly seen as a preparation for the afterlife. One may say that Amish are also future-oriented, at least in a metaphysical sense, although not as it relates to modern, progressive, or futuristic thought.

After generations of rural life guided by the natural rhythms of daylight and seasons, the Amish manage the demands of clock time in the dominant culture. They are generally punctual and conscientious about keeping appointments, although they may seem somewhat inconvenienced by not owning a telephone or car. These communication conveniences, deemed essential by the dominant American culture, are viewed by the most conservative Amish as technological advances that could erode the deeply held value of community, in which face-to-face contacts are easily made. Therefore, telephones and automobiles are generally owned by nearby non-Amish neighbors and used by Amish only when it is deemed essential, such as for reaching health-care facilities.

Because the predominant mode of transportation for the Amish is horse and carriage, travel to a doctor's office, a clinic, or a hospital requires the same adjustment as any other travel outside their rural community to shop, trade, or attend a wedding or funeral. The latter three reasons for travel are important means of reinforcing relationship ties, and on these occasions, the Amish may use hired or public transportation, excluding flying. Taking time out of normal routines for extended trips related to medical treatments is not uncommon, such as a visit to radioactive mines in the Rocky Mountains or to a laetrile clinic in Mexico to cope with cancer (Wenger, 1988).

Format for Names

Using first names with Amish people is appropriate, particularly because generations of intermarriage have resulted in a large number of Amish who share only a limited number of surnames. So it is preferable to use John or Mary during personal contacts rather than Mr. or Mrs. Miller, for example. In fact, within Amish communities, with so many Millers, Lapps, Yoders, and Zooks, given names like Mary and John are overused to the extent that individuals have to be identified further by nicknames, residence, a spouse's given name, or a patronymic, which may reflect three or more generations of patrilineal descent. For example, a particular John Miller may be known as "Red John," or "Gap John," or "Annie's John," or "Sam's Eli's Roman's John" (Hostetler, 1993).

During an interview with an Amish mother and her 5-year-old son, Wenger (1988) asked the child where he was going that day. The boy replied that he was going to play with Joe Elam John Dave Paul, identifying his age-mate Paul with four preceding generations. This little boy was giving useful everyday information, while at the same time, unknown to him, keeping oral history alive. The patronymics also illustrate the cultural value placed on intergenerational relationships and help to create a sense of belonging that embraces several generations and a broad consanguinity. Thus, one can see that medical record keeping can be a challenge when serving an extensive number of Amish patients.

Family Roles and Organization
Head of Household and Gender Roles

From the time of marriage, the young Amish man's role as husband is defined by the religious community to which he belongs. Titular patriarchy is derived from the Bible: Man is the head of the woman as Christ is the head of the church (I Cor. 3). This patriarchal role in Amish society is balanced or tempered by realities within the family, in which the wife is accorded high status and respect for her vital contributions to the success of the family. Practically speaking, husband and wife may share equally in decisions regarding the family farming business. In public, the wife may assume a retiring role, deferring to her husband, but in private, they are typically partners. However, it is best to listen to the voices of Amish women themselves as they reflect on their values and roles within Amish family and their shared ethnoreligious cultural community.

Traditionally, the highest priority for the parents is child rearing, an ethnoreligious expectation in the Amish culture. With a completed family averaging seven children, the Amish mother contributes physically and emotionally to the burgeoning growth in the Amish population. She also has an important role in providing family food and clothing needs, as well as a major share in child nurturing. Amish society expects the husband and father to contribute guidance, serve as a role model, and discipline the children. This shared task of parenting takes precedence over other needs, including economic or financial success in the family business. On the family farm, all must help as needed, but in general, field and barn work and animal husbandry are primarily the work of men and boys, whereas food production and preservation, clothing production and care, and management of the household are mainly the province of women.

Prescriptive, Restrictive, and Taboo Behaviors for Children and Adolescents

Children and youth represent a key to the vitality of the Amish culture. Babies are welcomed as a gift from God, and the high birth rate is one factor in their population growth. Another is the surprisingly high retention of youth, an estimated 75 percent or more, who choose as adults to remain in the Amish way. Before and during elementary school years, parents are more directive as they guide and train their children to assume responsible, productive roles in Amish society.

Young people over age 16 may be encouraged to work away from home to gain experience or because of insufficient work at home or on the family farm, but their wages are still usually sent home to the parental household because of the cultural value that the whole family contributes to the welfare of the family. Some experimentation with non-Amish dress and behavior among Amish teenagers is tolerated during this period of relative leniency, but the expectation is that an adult decision to be baptized before marriage will call young people back to the discipline of the church, as they assume adult roles.

In recent years, the media have been fascinated with this period of Amish teenage life as Americans in general have learned more about the Amish as a distinctive culture. Meyers and Nolt (2005) contended that although some Amish teenagers do experiment with behaviors that are incongruent with Amish beliefs and values, they do so in a distinctive Amish way. Amish teenagers are aware of the dominant American culture, and when they choose to participate in behaviors, some of which may involve the legal system, they do so in distinctive Amish ways, not in ways more common to American teenagers in general. For example, Amish youth will usually experiment within an Amish context and with other Amish youth, rather than with non-Amish teenagers.

Family Goals and Priorities

The Amish family pattern is referred to as the *freindschaft*, the dialectical term used for the three-generational family structure. This kinship network includes consanguine relatives consisting of the parental unit and the households of married children and their offspring. All members of the family personally know their grandparents, aunts, uncles, and cousins, with many Amish knowing their second and third cousins as well.

Individuals are identified by their family affiliation. Children and young adults may introduce themselves by giving their father's first name or both parents' names so they can be placed geographically and genealogically. Families are the units that make up church districts, and the size of a church district is measured by the number of families rather than by the number of church members. This extended family pattern has many functions. Families visit together frequently, thus learning to anticipate caring needs and preferences. Health-care information often circulates through the family network, even though families may be geographically dispersed. Wenger (1988) found that informants referred to *freindschaft* when discussing the factors influencing the selection of health-care options. "The functions of family care include maintaining *freindschaft* ties, bonding family members together

intergenerationally, and living according to God's will by fulfilling the parental mandate to prepare the family for eternal life" (Wenger, 1988, p. 134).

As grandparents turn over the primary responsibility for the family farm to their children, they continue to enjoy respected status as elders, providing valuable advice and sometimes material support and services to the younger generation. Many nuclear families live on a farm with an adjacent grandparent's cottage, which promotes frequent interactions across generations. Grandparents provide child care and help in rearing grandchildren and, in return, enjoy the respect generally paid by the next generations. This emotional and physical proximity to older adults also facilitates elder care within the family setting. In an ethnonursing study on care in an Amish community, Wenger (1988) reported that an informant discussed the reciprocal benefits of having her grandparents living in the attached **daadihaus** and her own parents living in a house across the road. Her 3-year-old daughter could go across the hall to spend time with her great-grandfather, which, the mother reported, was good for him in that he was needed, whereas the small child benefited from learning to know her great-grandfather, and the young mother gained some time to do chores. There is no set retirement age among the Amish, and grandmothers also continue in active roles as advisers and assistants to younger mothers.

Assuming full adult membership and responsibility means the willingness to put group harmony ahead of personal desire. In financial terms, it also means an obligation to help others in the brotherhood who are in need. This mutual aid commitment also provides a safety net, which allows Amish to rely on others for help in emergencies. Consequently, the Amish do not need federal pension or retirement support; they have their own informal "social security" plan. Amish of varying degrees of affluence enjoy approximately the same social status, and extremes of poverty and wealth are uncommon. Property damage or loss and unusual health-care expenses are also covered to a large extent by an informal brotherhood alternative to commercial insurance coverage. The costs of high-technology medical care present a new and severe test of the principle of mutual aid or "helping out," which is almost synonymous with the Amish way of life.

Alternative Lifestyles

There is little variation from the culturally sanctioned expectations for parents and their unmarried children to live together in the same household while maintaining frequent contact with the extended family. Unmarried children live in the parents' home until marriage, which usually takes place between the ages of 20 and 30. Some young adults may move to a different community to work and live as a boarder with another Amish family. Being single is not stigmatized, although almost all Amish do marry. Single adults are included in the social fabric of the community with the expectation that they will want to be involved in family-oriented social events.

Individuals of the same gender do not live together except in situations in which their work may make it more convenient. For example, two female schoolteachers may live together in an apartment or home close to the Amish school where they teach. There are no available statistics on the incidence of homosexuality in Amish culture. Isolated incidents of homosexual practice may come to the attention of health providers, but homosexual lifestyles do not fit with the deeply held values of Amish family life and procreation.

Pregnancy before marriage does not usually occur, and it is viewed as a situation to be avoided. When it does occur, in most Amish families, the couple would be encouraged to consider marriage. If they are not yet members of the church, they need to be baptized and to join the church before being married. Although not condoning pregnancy before marriage, the families and the Amish community support the young couple about to have a child. If the couple chooses not to marry, the young girl is encouraged to keep the baby and her family helps raise the child. Abortion is an unacceptable option. Adoption by an Amish family is an acceptable alternative.

Workforce Issues
Culture in the Workplace

In every generation except the present one, the Amish have worked almost exclusively in agriculture and farm-related tasks. Their large families were ideally suited to labor-intensive work on the family farm. As the number of family farms has been drastically reduced because of competition from agribusinesses that use mechanized and electronically controlled production methods, few options are available for Amish youth.

Traditionally, the Amish have placed a high value on hard work, with little time off for leisure or recreation. Productive employment for all is the ideal, and the intergenerational family provides work roles appropriate to the age and abilities of each person. But prospects began to narrow with the increased concentration of family farms in densely settled Amish communities as their population increased.

In addition, several cultural factors combine to limit the opportunities for young Amish to adapt to new work patterns. Amish children, who are encouraged to attend school through only eight grades, have a limited basis for vocational training in many work areas other than agriculture. Amish avoidance of compromising associations with "worldly" organizations, such as labor unions, restricts them to nonunion work, which often pays lower hourly rates. Work off the family farm, at one time a good option for unmarried youth, has become an economic necessity for some parents, although it is considered less acceptable for social reasons. Fathers who "work away," sometimes called "lunchpail daddies," have less contact with children during the workday, which in turn has an impact on the traditional father's modeling role and places more of the responsibility for child rearing on stay-at-home mothers. This shift in traditional parental roles is a source of some concern, although the effects are not yet clear.

Another concern for the Amish culture in relation to the workplace is the use of technologies that may be of concern for them. Hurst and McConnell (2010) describe survey results of Amish in Holmes County, Ohio, where 9 out of 10 persons "believe there are some technologies that are harmful to the stability and integrity of Amish culture, regardless of how they are used" (p. 210). Computers, Internet, and TV were mentioned the most. These technologies seem to be so pervasive in non-Amish lifestyles and workplaces. For the Amish, their concern is the difficulty in using these technologies in healthy ways that uphold Amish beliefs and values.

Issues Related to Autonomy

As described previously, external and internal factors have converged in the early 21st century to cause doubt about the continued viability of compact Amish farming communities. Exorbitant land prices triggered group outmigrations and resettlement in states to the west and south. The declining availability of affordable prime arable land in and around the centers of highest Amish population density is due in part to their non-Amish neighbors' land-use practices, especially in areas of suburban sprawl. A powerful internal force is at work as well in the population growth rate among the Amish, now well above the national average. So, contrary to popular notions that such a "backward" subculture is bound to die out, the Amish today are thriving.

Population growth continues even without a steady influx of new immigrants from the European homeland or significant numbers of new converts to their religion or way of life (Kraybill, 2001). The Young Center for Anabaptist and Pietist Studies at Elizabethtown College (2010) reported, "In the 20-year period from 1991 to 2010, the Amish in North America (adults and children) doubled in population, increasing from 123,500 in 1991 to 249,000 in 2010, an overall growth of 102 percent." This population growth has been attributed largely to the size of families and the retention rate of young adults.

The resulting pressures to control the changes in their way of life while maintaining its religious basis, particularly the high value placed on in-group harmony, have challenged the Amish to develop adaptive strategies. One outcome is an increasingly diversified employment base, with a trend toward cottage industries and related retail sales, as well as toward wage labor to generate cash needed for higher taxes and increasing medical costs. Another recent development includes a shift from traditional multigenerational farmsteads, as some retirees and crafts workers employed off the farm have begun to relocate to the edges of country towns. In summary, pressures to secure a livelihood within the Amish tradition have heightened awareness of the tension field within which the Amish coexist with the surrounding majority American culture.

Because English is the language of instruction in schools and is used with business contacts in the outside world, there is generally no language barrier for the Amish in the workplace. English vocabulary that is lacking in their normative ideas for religious aspects of Amish life is rarely a concern in the workplace.

Biocultural Ecology

Skin Color and Other Biological Variations

Most Amish are descendants of 18th-century Southern German and Swiss immigrants; therefore, their physical characteristics vary, as do those of most Europeans, with skin variations ranging from light to olive tones. Hair and eye colors vary accordingly. No specific health-care precautions are relevant to this group.

Diseases and Health Conditions

Since 1962, several hereditary diseases have been identified among the Amish. The major findings of the genetic studies have been published by Dr. Victor McKusick (1978) of the Johns Hopkins University. Because Amish tend to live in settlements with relatively little domiciliary mobility, and because they keep extensive genealogical and family records, genetic studies are more easily done than with more mobile cultural groups. Many years of collaboration between the Amish and a few geneticists from the Johns Hopkins Hospital have resulted in mutually beneficial projects (Hostetler, 1993). The Amish received printed community directories, and geneticists compiled computerized genealogies for the study of genetic diseases that continue to benefit society in general.

The Amish are essentially a closed population with exogamy occurring very rarely. However, they are not a singular genetically closed population. The larger and older communities are consanguineous, meaning that within the community the people are related through bloodlines by common ancestors. Several consanguine groups have been identified in which relatively little intermarriage occurs between the groups. "The separateness of these groups is supported by the history of the immigration into each area, by the uniqueness of the family names in each community, by the distribution of blood groups, and by the different hereditary diseases that occur in each of these groups" (Hostetler, 1993, p. 328). These diseases are one of the indicators of distinctiveness among the groups.

Hostetler (1993) cautioned that although inbreeding is more prevalent in Amish communities than in the general population, it does not inevitably result in hereditary defects. Through the centuries in some societies, marriages between first and second cousins were relatively common without major adverse effects. However, in the Amish gene pool are several recessive tendencies that in some cases are limited to specific Amish communities in which the consanguinity coefficient (degree of relatedness) is high for the specific genes. Of at least 12 recessive diseases, 4 should be noted here (Hostetler, 1993; McKusick, 1978; Troyer, 1994).

Dwarfism has long been recognized as obvious in several Amish communities. Ellis–van Creveld syndrome, known in Europe and named for Scottish and Dutch physicians, is especially prevalent among the Lancaster County, Pennsylvania, Amish (McKusick, Egeland, Eldridge, & Krusen, 1964). This syndrome is characterized by short stature and an extra digit on each hand, with some individuals having a congenital heart defect and nervous system involvement, resulting in a degree of mental deficiency. The Lancaster County Amish community, the second largest Amish settlement in the United States, is the only one in which Ellis–van Creveld syndrome is found. The lineage of all affected people has been traced to a single ancestor, Samuel King, who immigrated in 1744 (Troyer, 1994).

Cartilage hair hypoplasia, also a dwarfism syndrome, has been found in nearly all Amish communities in the United States and Canada and is not unique to the Amish (McKusick, Eldridge, Hostetler, Ruanquit, & Egeland, 1965). This syndrome is characterized by short stature and fine, silky hair. There is no central nervous system involvement and, therefore, no mental deficiency. However, most affected individuals have deficient cell-mediated immunity, thus increasing their susceptibility to viral infections (Troyer, 1994).

Pyruvate kinase anemia, a rare blood cell disease, was described by Bowman and Procopio in 1963. The lineage of all affected individuals can be traced to Jacob Yoder (known as "Strong Jacob"), who immigrated to Mifflin County, Pennsylvania, in 1792 (Hostetler, 1993; Troyer, 1994). This same genetic disorder was found later in the Geauga County, Ohio, Amish community. Notably, the families of all those who were affected had migrated from Mifflin County, Pennsylvania, and were from the "Strong Jacob" lineage. Symptoms usually appear soon after birth, with the presence of jaundice and anemia. Transfusions during the first few years of life and eventual removal of the spleen can be considered cures.

Hemophilia B, another blood disorder, is disproportionately high among the Amish, especially in Ohio. Ratnoff (1958) reported on an Amish man who was treated for a ruptured spleen. It was discovered that he had grandparents and 10 cousins who were hemophiliacs; 5 of the cousins had died from hemophilia. Research studies on causative mutations indicated a strong probability that a specific mutation may account for much of the mild hemophilia B in the Amish population (Ketterling, Bottema, Koberl, Setsuko, & Sommer, 1991).

Through the vigilant and astute observations of some public-health nurses known to these authors, a major health-care problem was noted in a northern Indiana Amish community. A high prevalence of phenylketonuria (PKU) was found in the Elkhart-Lagrange Amish settlement (Martin, Davis, & Askew, 1965). Those affected are unable to metabolize the amino acid phenylalanine, resulting in high blood levels of the substance and, eventually, severe brain damage if the disorder is untreated. Through epidemiological studies, the health department found that 1 in 62 Amish were affected, whereas the ratio in the general population was 1 in 25,000 at that time. Through the leadership of these nurses, the county and the state improved case funding for PKU and health-care services for affected families throughout Indiana, which was followed by improved health services in Amish communities in other states as well.

In recent years, a biochemical disorder called *glutaric aciduria* has been studied by Dr. Holmes Morton, a Harvard-educated physician who has chosen to live and work among the Amish in Lancaster County, Pennsylvania. Morton made house calls, conducted research at his own expense because funding was not forthcoming, and established a clinic in the Amish community to screen, diagnose, and educate people to care for individuals afflicted with the disease (Allen, 1989). By observing the natural history of glutaric aciduria type I, the researchers postulated that the onset or progression of neurological disease in Amish patients can be prevented by screening individuals at risk; restricting dietary protein; and thus limiting protein catabolism, dehydration, and acidosis during illness episodes.

Dr. Morton was well received in the Amish community, with many people referring friends and relatives to him. When he noted the rapid onset of the symptoms and the high incidence among the Amish, he did not wait for them to come to his office. He went to their homes and spent evenings and weekends driving from farm to farm, talking with families, running tests, and compiling genealogical information (Wolkomir & Wolkomir, 1991). In 1991, he built a clinic with the help of donations, in part the result of an article in the *Wall Street Journal* about the need for this nonprofit clinic. Hewlett-Packard donated the needed spectrometer that cost $80,000; local companies provided building materials, and an Amish couple donated the building site. Although volunteers helped to build the clinic, a local hospital provided temporary clinic space lease-free because the community recognized the very important contribution Morton was making, not only to the Amish and the advancement of medical science but also to the public health of the community.

A countywide screening program is now in place. Health-care providers are able to recognize the onset of symptoms. Research continues on this metabolic disorder, its relationship to cerebral palsy in the Amish population, and the biochemical causes and methods of preventing spastic paralysis in the general population. However, education remains a highly significant feature of any community health program. Nurses and physicians need to plan for family and community education about genetic counseling, screening of newborns, recognition of symptoms during aciduric crises in affected children, and treatment protocols. In *The New York Times Magazine* (Belkin, 2005), Dr. Morton was called "a doctor for the future'" because he practices what is now referred to as genetic medicine, which recognizes genetics as part of all medicine. But to the Amish, he is their friend who cares about their children, knows their families by name, and comes to their homes to see how they are able to cope with the manifestations of these genetically informed diseases.

Extensive studies of manic-depressive illnesses have been conducted in the Amish population. At first, there seemed to be evidence of a link between the Harvey-*ras*-1 oncogene and the insulin locus on chromosome 11. Studies on non-Amish families (Foroud, Casteluccio, Kollar, Edenberg, Miller, & Boman, 2000) and more extensive studies on Amish families have revealed new information on the genome, although the locus for the bipolar disorder has not yet been found (Ginns, Egeland, Allen, Pauls, & Falls, 1992; Kelsoe, Ginns, & Egeland, 1989; Kelsoe et al., 1993; Law, Richard, Cottingham, Lathrop, Cox, & Meyers, 1992; Myers, 1992; Pauls, Morton, & Egeland, 1992). Attempts have been made to gain knowledge about the affective response the Amish have to their ethnoreligious cultural identity and experience. Reiling (1998) studied the relationship between Amish self-identity and mental health.

The incidence of alcohol and drug abuse, which can complicate psychiatric diagnoses, is much lower among the Amish than in the general North American population, thus contributing to the importance of the Amish sample. Although the incidence of bipolar affective disorder is not found to be higher in the Amish, some large families with several affected members continue to contribute to medical science by being subjects in the genetic studies. Because the Old Order Amish descend from 30 pioneer couples whose descendants have remained genetically isolated in North America, have relatively large kindred groups with multiple living generations, and generally live in close geographic proximity, they are an ideal population for genetic studies (Kelsoe et al., 1989).

Variations in Drug Metabolism

No drug studies specifically related to the Amish were found in the literature. However, given the genetic disorders common among selected populations of Amish, this is one area in which more research needs to be conducted.

High-Risk Behaviors

Amish are traditionally agrarian and prefer a lifestyle that provides intergenerational and community support systems to promote health and mitigate against the prevalence of high-risk behaviors. Genetic studies using Amish populations are seldom confounded by the use of alcohol and other substances. However, health providers should be alert to potential alcohol and recreational drug use in some Amish communities, especially among young, unmarried men. When young adult men exhibit such behavior as straying from the Amish way of life and "sowing their wild oats" before becoming baptized church members and before marriage, it is tolerated. Although this may be considered a high-risk behavior, it is not prevalent in all communities, nor is it promoted in any. Parents confide in each other and sometimes in trusted outsiders that this errant behavior causes many heartaches, although at the same time, they try to be patient and keep contact with the youth so the latter may choose to espouse the Amish lifeways.

Another lifestyle pattern that poses potential health risks is nutrition. Amish tend to eat high-carbohydrate and high-fat foods with a relatively high intake of refined sugar. Wenger (1994) reported that in an ethnonursing study on health and health-care perceptions, informants talked about their diet being too high in "sweets and starches" and knowing they should eat more vegetables. The prevalence of obesity was found to be greater among Amish women than for women in general in the state of Ohio (Fuchs, Levinson, Stoddard, Mullet, & Jones, 1990). In this major health-risk survey of 400 Amish adults and 773 non-Amish adults in Ohio, the authors found that the pattern of obesity in Amish women begins in the 25-year-old and older cohort, with the concentration occurring between the ages of 45 and 64. An explanation for the propensity for weight gain among the Amish may be related to the central place assigned to the consumption of food in their culture and the higher rates of pregnancy throughout their childbearing years (Wenger, 1994). However, in recent studies related to eating behaviors, obesity, and diabetes, the Old Order Amish cohorts showed some significant

differences from other whites in the majority culture. Hsueh and colleagues (2002) reported in the Third National Health and Nutrition Examination Survey that the Old Order Amish sample evidenced diabetes approximately half as frequently as did other whites in the survey. Another important difference was the level of daily physical activity, which was reported to be higher among both Amish men and women than among other white cohorts (Bassett, 2004).

Health-Care Practices

Most Amish are physically active, largely owing to their chosen agrarian lifestyle and farming as a preferred occupation. Physical labor is valued, and men as well as women and children help with farmwork. Household chores and gardening, generally considered to be women's work, require physical exertion, particularly because the Amish do not choose to use electrically operated appliances in the home or machinery, such as riding lawn mowers, that conserve human energy. Nevertheless, many women do contend with a tendency to be overweight. In recent years, it is not uncommon to find Amish women seeking help for weight control from Weight Watchers® and similar weight control support groups.

Farm and traffic accidents are an increasing health concern in communities with a dense Amish population. In states such as Indiana, with relatively high concentrations of Amish who drive horse-drawn vehicles (Fig. 7-3), blinking red lights and large red triangles are required by law to be attached to their vehicles. Jones (1990) reported on a study of trauma by examining hospital records of Amish patients admitted to one hospital in mideastern Ohio. Transportation-related injuries were the largest group, with many of those involving farm animals. Falls from ladders and down hay

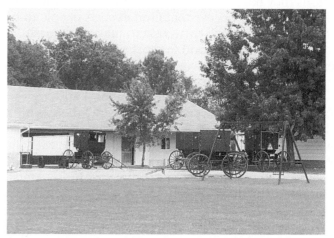

Figure 7-3 Amish buggies parked outside a home. Note the reflective safety triangle attached to the back of the rightmost buggy in the picture. These are usually required by law in areas that have large Amish populations. *(Photograph by Joel Wenger.)*

REFLECTIVE EXERCISE 7.1

In many communities, laws have been enacted that require drivers under the influence (DUI) to complete a course on safe driving and the use of alcohol and drugs. A culturally perceptive social service agency in Brightville offered a separate course for Amish offenders. The organizers first met with the Amish bishops and deacons to ask for their assistance in learning more about Amish values and beliefs, while also describing their intent to offer a separate course for the Amish. The Agency made it known that they wanted to employ a young Amish man to attend all the classes, assist with group discussions, and assist the instructors in relating with the participants in a culture congruent manner.

1. If you were one of the Agency leaders, how would you guide your organization in crossing the Amish cultural boundary?
2. How would you develop a plan to orient this young Amish employee to his new job?

holes resulted in orthopedic injuries, but no deaths. Amish families need to be encouraged to monitor their children who operate farm equipment and transportation vehicles and to teach them about safety factors. Concern about accidents is evident in Amish newsletters, many of which have a regular column reporting accidents and asking for prayers or expressing gratitude that the injuries were not more severe, that God had spared the person, or that the community had responded in caring ways (Wenger, 1988).

Nutrition

Meaning of Food

Among the Amish, food is recognized for its nutritional value. Most Amish prefer to grow their own produce for economic reasons and because for generations they have been aware of their connections with the earth. They believe that God expects people to be the caretakers of the earth and to make it flourish.

The Amish serve food in most social situations because food also has a significant social meaning. Because visiting has a highly valued cultural function, occasions occur during most weeks for Amish to visit family, neighbors, and friends, especially those within their church district. Some of these visits are planned when snacks or meals are shared, sometimes with the guests helping to provide the food. Even if guests come unexpectedly, it is customary in most Amish communities for snacks and drinks to be offered.

Common Foods and Food Rituals

Typical Amish meals include meat; potatoes, noodles, or both; a cooked vegetable; bread; something pickled (e.g., pickles, red beets); cake or pudding; and coffee. Beef is usually butchered by the family and then kept in the local commercially owned freezer for which they pay a rental storage fee. Some families also preserve beef by canning, and most families have chickens and other fowl, such as ducks or geese, which they raise for eggs and for meat. Amish families still value growing their own foods and usually have large gardens. A generation ago, this was an unquestioned way of life, but an increasing number of families living in small towns and working in factories and construction own insufficient land to plant enough food for the family's consumption.

Snacks and meals in general tend to be high in fat and carbohydrates. A common snack is large, home-baked cookies about 3 inches in diameter. Commercial non-Amish companies have recognized large, soft cookies as a marketable commodity and have advertised their commercially made products as "Amish" cookies, even though no Amish are involved in the production. Other common snacks are ice cream (purchased or homemade), pretzels, and popcorn.

When Amish gather for celebrations such as weddings, birthdays, work bees, or quiltings, the tables are usually laden with a large variety of foods. The selection, usually provided by many people, includes several casseroles, noodle dishes, white and sweet potatoes, some cooked vegetables, few salads, pickled dishes, pies, cakes, puddings, and cookies. Hostetler (1993) provided a detailed ethnographic description of the meaning and practices surrounding an Amish wedding, including the food preparation, the wedding dinner and supper, and the roles and functions of various key individuals in this most important rite of passage that includes serving food.

In communities in which tourists flock to learn about the Amish, many entrepreneurs have used the Amish love of wholesome, simple foods to market their version of Amish cookbooks, food products, and restaurants that more aptly reflect the Pennsylvania German, commonly referred to as *Pennsylvania Dutch*, influence of communities such as Lancaster County, Pennsylvania. Many of these bear little resemblance to authentic Amish foods, and some even venture to sell "Amish highballs" or "Amish sodas" (Hostetler, 1993). Some Amish families help to satisfy the public interest in their way of life by serving meals in their homes for tourists and local non-Amish. But most Amish view their foods and food preparation as commonplace and functional, not something to be displayed in magazines and newspapers. Because many Amish are wary of outsiders' undue interest, health providers need to discuss nutrition and food as a part of their lifeways to promote healthy nutritional lifestyles.

In Amish homes, a "place at the table" is symbolic of belonging (Hostetler, 1993). Seating is traditionally arranged with the father at the head and boys seated youngest to oldest to his right. The mother sits to her husband's left, with the girls also seated youngest to oldest or placed so that an older child can help a younger one. The table is the place where work, behavior, school, and other family concerns are discussed. During the busy harvesting season, preference is given to the men and boys who eat and return to the fields or barn. At mealtimes, all members of the household are expected to be present unless they are working away from home or visiting at a distance, making it difficult to return home.

Sunday church services, which for the Old Order Amish are held in their homes or barns, are followed by a simple meal for all who attended church (Fig. 7-4). The church benches, which are transported from home to home wherever the church service is to be held, are set up with long tables for serving the food. In many communities, some of the benches are built so they can quickly be converted into tables. Meals become ritualized so the focus is not on what is being served but rather on the opportunity to visit together over a simple meal. In one community, an Amish informant who had not attended services because of a complicated pregnancy told the researcher that she missed the meal, which in that community consisted of bread, butter, peanut butter mixed with marshmallow creme and honey, apple butter, pickles, pickled red beets, soft sugar cookies, and coffee (Wenger, 1988).

Pregnancy and Childbearing Practices

Fertility Practices and Views Toward Pregnancy

Children are viewed as a gift from God and are welcomed into Amish families. Estimates place the average number of live births per family at seven (Hostetler & Huntington, 1992). The Amish fertility pattern has remained constant during the past 100 years, while many others have declined. Household size varies from

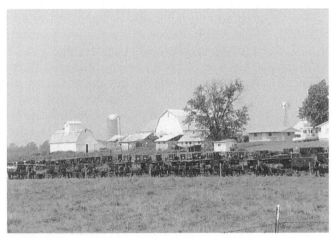

Figure 7-4 Buggies parked in a field on an Amish farm where people have gathered for a Sunday church service and noon meal. *(Photograph by Joel Wenger.)*

families with no children to couples with 15 or more children (Huntington, 1988; Meyers & Nolt, 2005). Even in large families, the birth of another child brings joy because of the core belief that children are "a heritage from the Lord," and another member of the family and community means another person to help with the chores (Hostetler, 1993).

Having children has a different meaning in Old Order Amish culture than in the dominant American culture. In a study on women's roles and family production, the authors suggested that women in Amish culture enjoy high status despite the apparent patriarchal ideology because of their childbearing role and their role as producers of food (Lipon, 1985). A large number of children benefit small labor-intensive farms, and with large families comes an apparent need for large quantities of food. Interpretation of this pragmatic view of fertility should always be moderated with recognition of the moral and ethical core cultural belief that children are a gift from God, given to a family and community to nurture in preparation for eternal life.

Scholars and researchers of long-term acquaintance with Old Order Amish agree that the pervasive Amish perception of birth control is that it interferes with God's will and thus should be avoided (Kraybill, 2001). Nevertheless, fertility control does exist, although the patterns are not well known and very few studies have been reported. Wenger (1980) discussed childbearing with two Amish couples in a group interview, and they conceded that some couples do use the rhythm method. In referring to birth control, one Amish father stated, "It is not discussed here, really. I think Amish just know they shouldn't use the pill" (Wenger, 1980, p. 5). Three physicians and three nurses were interviewed, and they reported that some Amish do ask about birth control methods, especially those with a history of difficult perinatal histories and those with large families. Some Amish women do use intrauterine devices, but this practice is uncommon. Most Amish women are reluctant to ask physicians and nurses and, therefore, should be counseled with utmost care and respect because this is a topic that generally is not discussed, even among themselves. Approaching the subject obliquely may make it possible for the Amish woman or man to sense the health provider's respect for Amish values and thus encourage discussion. "When you want to learn more about birth control, I would be glad to talk to you" is a suggested approach.

Prescriptive, Restrictive, and Taboo Practices in the Childbearing Family

Amish tend to have their first child later than do non-Amish. In a retrospective chart review examining pregnancy outcomes of 39 Amish and 145 non-Amish women at a rural hospital in southern New York, it was found that Amish had their first child an average of one year later than non-Amish couples (Lucas, O'Shea, Zielezny, Freudenheim, & Wold, 1991). The Amish had a narrower range of maternal ages and had proportionately fewer teenage pregnancies. All subjects received prenatal care, with the Amish receiving prenatal care from Amish lay midwives during the first trimester.

In some communities, Amish have been reputed to be reluctant to seek prenatal health care. Providers who gain the trust of the Amish learn that they want the best perinatal care, which fits with their view of children being a blessing (Miller, 1997). However, they may choose to use Amish and non-Amish lay midwives who promote childbearing as a natural part of the life cycle. In a study of childbearing practices as described by Amish women in Michigan, Miller (1997) learned that they prefer home births, they had "limited formal knowledge of the childbirth process" (p. 65), and health-care providers were usually consulted only when there were perceived complications. Although many may express privately their preference for perinatal care that promotes the use of nurse-midwifery and lay midwifery services, home deliveries, and limited use of high technology, they tend to use the perinatal services available in their community. In ethnographic interviews with informants, Wenger (1988) found that grandmothers and older women reported greater preference for hospital deliveries than did younger women. The younger women tend to have been influenced by the increasing general interest in childbirth as a natural part of the life cycle and the deemphasis on the medicalization of childbirth. Some Amish communities, especially those in Ohio and Pennsylvania, have a long-standing tradition of using both lay midwifery and professional obstetric services, often simultaneously.

In Ohio, the Mt. Eaton Care Center developed as a community effort in response to retirement of an Amish lay midwife known as Bill Barb (identified by her spouse's name, as discussed in the section on communication). She provided perinatal services, including labor and birth, with the collaborative services of a local Mennonite physician who believed in providing culturally congruent and safe health-care services for this Amish population. At one point in Bill Barb Hochstetler's 30-year practice, the physician moved a trailer with a telephone onto Hochstetler's farm so that he could be called in case of an emergency (Huntington, 1993). Other sympathetic physicians also delivered babies at Bill Barb's home. After state investigation, which coincided with her intended retirement, Hochstetler's practice was recognized to be in a legal gray area. The Mt. Eaton Care Center became a reality in 1985 after careful negotiation with the Amish community, Wayne County Board of

Health, Ohio Department of Health, and local physicians and nurses. Physicians and professional nurses and nurse-midwives, who are interested in Amish cultural values and health-care preferences, provide low-cost, safe, low-technology perinatal care in a homelike atmosphere. In 1997, the New Eden Care Center, modeled after the Mt. Eaton Care Center, was built in LaGrange County in northern Indiana and, in recent years, has had more than 400 births per year (Meyers & Nolt, 2005).

Because the Amish want family involvement in perinatal care, outsiders may infer that they are open in their discussion of pregnancy and childbirth. In actuality, most Amish women do not discuss their pregnancies openly and make an effort to keep others from knowing about them until physical changes are obvious. Mothers do not inform their other children of the impending birth of a sibling, preferring for the children to learn of it as "the time comes naturally" (Wenger, 1988). This fits with the Amish cultural pattern of learning through observation that assumes intergenerational involvement in life's major events. Anecdotal accounts exist of children being in the house, though not physically present, during birth. Fathers are expected to be present and involved, although some may opt to do farm chores that cannot be delayed, such as milking cows.

Amish women do participate in prenatal classes, often with their husbands. The women are interested in learning about all aspects of perinatal care but may choose not to participate in sessions when videos are used. Prenatal class instructors should inform them ahead of time when videos or films will be used so they can decide whether to attend. For some Amish in which the **Ordnung** (the set of unwritten rules prescribed for the church district) is more prescriptive and strict, the individuals may be concerned about being disobedient to the will of the community. Even though the information on the videos may be acceptable, the type of media is considered unacceptable.

Amish have no major taboos or requirements for birthing. Men may be present, and most husbands choose to be involved. However, they are likely not to be demonstrative in showing affection verbally nor physically. This does not mean they do not care; it is culturally inappropriate to show affection openly in public. The laboring woman cooperates quietly, seldom audibly expressing discomfort. Because many women tend to be stoical with pain, the health-care provider needs to assess vital signs that may indicate the need for pain medicine.

Given the Amish acceptance of a wide spectrum of health-care modalities, the nurse or physician should be aware that the woman in labor might be using herbal remedies to promote labor. Knowledge about and a respect for Amish health-care practices alert the physician or nurse to a discussion about simultaneous treatments that may be harmful or helpful. It is always better if these discussions can take place in a low-stress setting before labor and birth.

As in other hospitalizations, the family may want to spend the least allowable time in the hospital. This is generally related to the belief that birth is not a medical condition and because most Amish do not carry health insurance. In their three-generational family, and as a result of their cultural expectations for caring to take place in the community, many people are willing and able to assist the new mother during the post-partum period. Visiting families with new babies are expected and generally welcomed. Older siblings are expected to help care for the younger children and to learn how to care for the newborn. The postpartum mother resumes her family role managing, if not doing, all the housework, cooking, and child care within a few days after childbirth. For a primiparous mother, her mother often comes to stay with the new family for several days to help with care of the infant and give support to the new mother.

The day the new baby is first taken to church services is considered special. People who had not visited the baby in the family's home want to see the new member of the community. The baby is often passed among the women to hold as they become acquainted and admire the newcomer.

Death Rituals

Death Rituals and Expectations

Amish customs related to death and dying have dual dimensions. On the one hand, they may be seen as holdovers from an earlier time when, for most Americans, major life events such as birth and death occurred in the home. On the other hand, Amish retention of such largely outdated patterns is due to distinctively Amish understandings of the individual within and as an integral part of the family and community. Today, when 70 percent of elderly Americans die in hospitals and nursing homes, some still reflect nostalgically on death as it should be and as, in fact, it used to be, in the circle of family and friends, a farewell with familiarity and dignity. In Amish society today, in most cases, this is still a reality. As physical strength declines, the expectation is that the family will care for the aging and the ill in the home. Hostetler's (1993) brief observation that Amish prefer to die at home is borne out by research findings. Tripp-Reimer and Schrock (1982) reported from their comparative study of the ethnic aged that 75 percent of the Amish surveyed expressed a preference for living with family, 25 percent preferred living at home with assistance, and none would choose to live in a care facility, even if bedridden.

Clearly, these preferences are motivated by more than a wish to dwell in the past or an unwillingness to change with the times. The obligation to help others, in illness as in health, provides the social network that supports Amish practices in the passage from life to death. In effect, it is a natural extension of caregiving embraced as a social duty with religious motivation. The Amish accept literally the biblical admonition to "bear one another's burdens," and this finds expression in communal support for the individual, whether suffering, dying, or bereaved. Life's most intensely personal and private act becomes transformed into a community event.

Visiting in others' homes is, for the Amish, a normal and frequent reinforcement of the bonds that tie individuals to extended family and community. As a natural extension of this social interaction, visiting the ill takes on an added poignancy, especially during an illness believed to be terminal. Members of the immediate family are offered not only verbal condolences but many supportive acts of kindness as well. Others close to them prepare their food and take over other routine household chores to allow them to focus their attention and energy on the comfort of the ailing family member.

Responses to Death and Grief

Ties across generations, as well as across kinship and geographic lines, are reinforced around death as children witness the passing of a loved one in the intimacy of the home. Death brings many more visitors into the home of the bereaved, and the church community takes care of accommodations for visitors from a distance as well as funeral arrangements. The immediate family is thus relieved of responsibility for decision making, which otherwise may add distraction to grief. In some Amish settlements, a wake-like "sitting up" through the night provides an exception to normal visiting patterns. The verbal communication with the bereaved may be sparse, but the constant presence of supportive others is tangible proof of the Amish commitment to community. The return to normal life is eased through these visits by the resumption of conversations.

Apart from the usual number of visitors who come to pay their respects to both the deceased and the family, the funeral ceremony is as simple and unadorned as the rest of Amish life. A local Amish cabinetmaker frequently builds a plain wooden coffin. In the past, interment was in private plots on Amish farms, contrasting with the general pattern of burial in a cemetery in the churchyard of a rural church. Because Amish worship in their homes and have no church buildings, they also have no adjoining cemeteries. An emerging pattern is burial in a community cemetery, sometimes together with other Mennonites.

Grief and loss are keenly felt, although verbal expression may seem muted, as if to indicate stoic acceptance of suffering. In fact, the meaning of death as a normal transition is embedded in the meaning of life from the Amish perspective. Parents are exhorted to nurture their children's faith because life in this world is seen as a preparation for eternal life.

Spirituality

Dominant Religion and Use of Prayer

Amish religious and cultural values include honesty; order; personal responsibility; community welfare; obedience to parents, church, and God; nonresistance or nonviolence; humility; and the perception of the human body as a temple of God.

Amish settlements are subdivided into church districts similar to rural parishes with 30 to 50 families in each district. Local leaders are chosen from their own religious community and are generally untrained and unpaid. Authority patterns are congregationalist, with local consensus directed by local leadership, designated as bishops, preachers, and deacons, all of whom are male. No regional or national church hierarchy exists to govern internal church affairs, although a national committee may be convened to address external institutions of government regarding issues affecting the broader Amish population.

In addition to prayer in church services, silent prayer is always observed at the beginning of a meal, and in many families, a prayer also ends the meal. Children are taught to memorize prayers from a German prayer book for beginning and ending meals and for silent prayer. The father may say an audible "amen" or merely lift his bowed head to signal the time to begin eating.

Meaning of Life and Individual Sources of Strength

Outsiders, who are aware of the Amish detachment from the trappings of our modern materialistic culture, may be disappointed to discover in their "otherworldliness" something less than a lofty spirituality. Amish share the earthy vitality of many rural peasant cultures and a pragmatism born of immediate life experiences, not distilled from intellectual pursuits such as philosophy or theology. Amish simplicity is intentional, but even in austerity, there is a relish of life's simpler joys rather than a grim asceticism.

If death is a part of life and a portal to a better life, then individuals are well advised to consider how their lives prepare them for life after death. Amish share the general Christian view that salvation is ultimately individual, preconditioned on one's confession of faith, repentance, and baptism. These public acts are undertaken in the Amish context as part of preparing to fully assume one's adult role in a community of faith.

In contrast with the ideals of American individualism, however, the Amish surrender much of their individuality as the price of full acceptance as members of a community. In practical, everyday terms, the religiously defined community is inextricably intertwined with a social reality, which gives it its distinctive shape.

For the Amish, the importance of conformity to the will of the group can hardly be exaggerated. To maintain harmony within the group, individuals often forgo their own wishes. In terms of faith-related behavior, outsiders sometimes criticize this "going along with" the local congregational group as an expression of religiosity, rather than spirituality. The frequent practice of corporate worship, including prayer and singing, helps to build this conformity. It is regularly tested in "counsel" sessions in the congregational assembly in which each individual's commitment to the corporate religious contract is reviewed before taking communion (Kraybill, 2001).

Non-Amish occasionally are baffled at reports of the Amish response to grave injury or even loss of life at the hands of others. Owing to deeply held community values, and especially constrained by love for others, Amish often eschew retaliatory or vengeful attitudes and actions when the majority culture might justify such means. Amish are socialized to sustain such injuries, grieve, and move on without fixing blame or seeking redress or punishment for the perpetrator. The felt need to forgive is for the Amish as strong as others perceive a need to bring wrongdoers to justice. The need to forgive is considered to be "second nature" in the Amish community. It does not indicate moral superiority or a heroic strength of forbearance in the face of adversity, but flows consistently from a biblical mandate to express love, even for an apparent adversary, as a practical application of the "The Golden Rule" (Matt. 7:12). A current example, claiming both national and international attention, was the Amish response of forgiveness in the face of the Nickel Mines, Pennsylvania, tragedy when 10 Amish schoolgirls were held hostage and 5 of the girls were shot to death on October 2, 2006 (Complete Coverage of Nickel Mines Tragedy Web site at http://local.lancasteronline.com/1/91). Forgiveness in such situations may not come easily for many persons. Krabill, Nolt, and Weaver-Zercher (2007) contend that for the Amish, forgiveness is part of the Anabaptist "habits" begun in the sixteenth century that continue to undergird Old Order Amish culture even today. Amish "values incorporate a willingness to place tragedy in God's hands without demanding divine explanation for injustice" (p. 71).

Spiritual Beliefs and Health-Care Practices

As seen in earlier sections on communication among Amish and their socioreligious provenance, many symbols of Amish faith point to the separated life, which they live in accordance with God's will. Over time, they have chosen to embody their faith rather than verbalize it. As a result, they seldom proselytize among non-Amish and nurture among themselves a noncreedal, often primitive form of Christianity that emphasizes "right living." Their untrained religious leaders offer unsophisticated views of what that entails based on their interpretation of the Bible. Most members are content to submit to the congregational consensus on what right living means, with the assumption that it is based on submission to the will of a loving, benevolent God, an aspect of their spirituality that is seldom articulated (Kraybill, 2001).

Although the directives of religious leaders are normative for many types of decisions, this appears not to be the case for health-care choices (Wenger, 1991a). When choosing among health-care options, families usually seek counsel from religious leaders, friends, and extended family, but the final decision resides with the immediate family. Health-care providers need to be aware of the Amish cultural context and may need to adjust the normal routines of diagnosis and therapy to fit Amish patients' socioreligious context.

Health-Care Practices
Health-Seeking Beliefs and Behaviors

The Amish believe that the body is the temple of God and that human beings are the stewards of their bodies. This fundamental belief is based on the Genesis account of creation. Medicine and health care should always be used with the understanding that it is God who heals. Nothing in the Amish understanding of the Bible forbids them from using preventive or curative medical services. A prevalent myth among health-care providers in Amish communities is that Amish

REFLECTIVE EXERCISE 7.2

The Nickle Mines tragedy in Pennsylvania, where 10 Amish schoolgirls were held hostage in an Amish elementary school, and 5 of the girls were killed, claimed national and international attention. One of the most frequent questions asked by non-Amish was how and why did Amish forgived the perpetrator so readily. A representative group of Amish even went to visit the widow of the perpetrator and his family to express their condolences to her for the loss of her husband and to invite her to the funerals of some of the young Amish girls.

1. What have you learned about Amish ethnoreligious values and beliefs that might explain forgiveness as practiced following that tragedy?
2. Krabill, Nolt, and Weaver-Zercher (2007) spoke with many Amish following the tragedy who said that "forgiveness is hard work that never ends" (p. 113). Describe what is meant by that statement based on the Amish worldview.

are not interested in preventive services. Although it is true that many times the Amish do not use mainstream health services at the onset of recognized symptoms, they are highly involved in the practices of health promotion and illness prevention.

Although the Amish, as a people, have a reputation for honesty and forthrightness, they may withhold important medical information from medical providers by neglecting to mention folk and alternative care being pursued at the same time. When questioned, some Amish admit to being less than candid about using multiple therapies, including herbal and chiropractic remedies, because they believe that "the doctor wouldn't be interested in them." Making choices among folk, complementary, and professional health-care options does not necessarily indicate a lack of confidence or respect for the latter, but rather reflects the belief that one must be actively involved in seeking the best health care available (Wenger, 1994).

Responsibility for Health Care

The Amish believe that it is their responsibility to be personally involved in promoting health. As in most cultures, health-care knowledge is passed from one generation to the next through women. In the Amish culture, men are involved in major health-care decisions and often accompany the family to the chiropractor, physician, or hospital. Grandparents are frequently consulted about treatment options. In one situation, a scheduled consultation for a 4-year-old was postponed until the maternal grandmother was well enough after a cholecystectomy to make the three-hour automobile trip to the medical center.

A usual concern regarding responsibility for health care is payment for services. Many Amish do not carry any insurance, including health insurance. However, in most communities, there is some form of agreement for sharing losses caused by natural disasters as well as catastrophic illnesses. Some have formalized mutual aid, such as the Amish Aid Society. Wenger (1988) found that her informants were opposed to such formalized agreements and wanted to do all they could to live healthy and safe lives, which they believed would benefit their community in keeping with their Christian calling. Many hospitals have been astounded by the Amish practice of paying their bills despite financial hardship. Because of this generally positive community reputation, hospitals have been willing to set up payment plans for the larger bills.

Active participation was found to be a major theme in Wenger's (1991a; 1994; 1995) studies on cultural context, health, and care. The Amish want to be actively involved in health-care decision making, which is a part of daily living. "To do all one can to help oneself" involves seeking advice from family and friends, using herbs and other home remedies, and then choosing from a broad array of folk, alternative, and professional health-care services. One informant, who visited an Amish healer while considering her physician's recommendation that she have a computerized axial tomography (CAT) scan to provide more data on her continuing vertigo, told the researcher, "I will probably have the CAT scan, but I am not done helping myself, and this [meaning the healer's treatment] may help and it won't hurt." In this study, health-care decision making was found to be influenced by three factors: type of health problem, accessibility of health-care services, and perceived cost of the service. When the Amish use professional health-care services, they want to be partners in their health care and want to retain their right to choose from all culturally sanctioned health-care options.

Caring within the Amish culture is synonymous with being Amish. "It's the Amish way" translates into the expectation that members of the culture be aware of the needs of others and thus fulfill the biblical injunction to bear one another's burdens. Caring is a core value related to health and well-being. Care is expressed in culturally encoded expectations that they can best describe in their dialect as **abwaarde**, meaning "to minister to someone by being present and serving when someone is sick in bed." A more frequently used term for helping is *achtgewwe*, which means "to serve by becoming aware of someone's needs and then to act by doing things to help." Helping others is expressed in gender-related and age-related roles, *freindschaft* (the three-generational family), church district, community (including non-Amish), Amish settlements, and worldwide. No outsiders or health-care providers can be expected to fully understand this complex, caring network, but health-care providers can learn about it in the local setting by establishing trust in relationships with their Amish patients.

When catastrophic illness occurs, the Amish community responds by being present, helping with chores, and relieving family members so that they can be with the afflicted person in the acute care hospital. Some do opt to accept medical advice regarding the need for high-technology treatment, such as transplants or other high-cost interventions. The patient's family seeks prayers and advice from the bishop and deacons of their church and their family and friends, but the decision is generally a personal or family one.

Amish engage in self-medication. Although most Amish regularly visit physicians and use prescription drugs, as indicated previously, they also use herbs and other nonprescription remedies, often simultaneously. When discussing the meaning of health and illness, Wenger (1988; 1994) found that her Amish informants considered it their responsibility to investigate their treatment options and to stay personally involved in the treatment process rather than to relegate their care to the judgment of the professional physician or nurse. Consequently, they seek testimonials from other family members and friends about what treatments work

best. They may also seek care from Amish healers and other alternative-care practitioners, who may suggest nutritional supplements. One informant told how she would take "blue cohosh" pills with her to the hospital when she was in labor because she believed they would speed up the labor.

Because of the Amish practice of self-medication, it is essential that health-care providers inquire about the full range of remedies being used. For the Amish patient to be candid, the provider must develop a context of mutual trust and respect. Within this context, the Amish patient can feel assured that the provider wants to consider and negotiate the most advantageous yet culturally congruent care.

Folk and Traditional Practices

The Amish, like many other cultures, have an elaborate health-care belief system that includes traditional remedies passed from one generation to the next. They also use alternative health care that is shared by other Americans, though often not sanctioned by medical and other health-care providers. Although the prevalence of specific health-care beliefs and practices, such as use of chiropractic, Western medical and health-care science, reflexology, iridology, osteopathy, homeopathy, and folklore, is influenced mainly by *freindschaft* (Wenger, 1991b), variations depend on geographic region and the conservatism of the Amish community.

Herbal remedies include those handed down by successive generations of mothers and daughters. One elderly grandmother showed the researcher the cupboard where she kept some cloths soaked in a herbal remedy and shared the recipe for it. She stated that the cupboard was where she remembered her grandmother keeping those same remedies when her grandmother lived in the *daadihaus,* the grandparents' cottage attached to the family farmhouse where her daughter and son-in-law lived. She also confided that, although she prepared the herb-soaked cloths for her daughters when they married, she thought they opted for more modern treatments, such as herb pills and prescription drugs. This is a poignant example of the effect of modern health care on a highly contextual culture.

"Of all Amish folk health care, **brauche** has claimed the most interest of outsiders, who are often puzzled by its historical origins and contemporary application" (Wenger, 1991b, p. 87). *Brauche* is a folk-healing art that was practiced in Europe around the time of the Amish immigration to North America and is not unique to the Amish, but is a common healing art used among Pennsylvania Germans. As with some other European practices, the Amish have retained *brauche* in some communities. In other communities, the practice is considered suspect, and it has been the focus of some church divisions.

Brauche is sometimes referred to as sympathy curing or pow-wowing. It is unrelated to American

Indian pow-wowing, and the use of this English term to refer to the German term *brauche* is unclear. In most literary descriptions of sympathy curing, it refers to the use of words, charms, and physical manipulations for treating some human and animal maladies. In some communities, the Amish refer to *brauche* as "warm hands," the ability to feel when a person has a headache or a baby has colic. Informants describe situations in which some individuals can "take" the stomachache from the baby into their own bodies in what is described by researchers as *transference*. Wenger (1991a; 1994) stated that all informant families volunteered information about *brauche*, using that term or "warm hands" to describe folk healing. One informant asked the author if she could "feel" it, too.

A few folk illnesses have no Western scientific equivalents. The first is **abnemme**, which refers to a condition in which the child fails to thrive and appears puny. Specific treatments given to the child may include incantations. Some of the older people remember these treatments, and some informants remember having been taken to a healer for the ailment. The second is **aagwachse**, or *livergrown*, meaning "hidebound" or "grown together," once a common ailment among Pennsylvania Germans (Hostetler, 1993). Symptoms include crying and abdominal discomfort that is believed to be caused by jostling in rough buggy rides. Wenger (1988) reported accompanying an informant with her newborn baby to an Amish healer, and the woman carried the baby on a pillow because she believed the baby to be suffering from *aagwachse*. As stated previously, Amish patients are more likely to discuss folk beliefs and practices with providers if the nurse or physician gives cues that it is acceptable to do so.

Barriers to Health Care

Barriers to health care include delay in seeking professional health care at the onset of symptoms, occasional overuse of home remedies, and a prevailing perception that health-care providers are not interested in, or may disapprove of, the use of home remedies and other alternative treatment modalities. In addition, some families may live far from professional health-care services, making travel by horse and buggy difficult or inadvisable. Because in some Amish communities, such as the Old Order Amish, telephones are not permitted in the home, there may be delays in communication with Amish patients. Finally, the cost of health care without health insurance can deter early access to professional care, which could result in more complex treatment regimens.

Cultural Responses to Health and Illness

The Amish are unlikely to display pain and physical discomfort. The health-care provider may need to check changes in vital signs for pain and remind the Amish patient that medication is available for pain relief if they choose to accept it.

Community for the Amish means inclusion of people who are chronically ill or "physically or mentally different." Amish culture approaches these differences as a community responsibility. Children with mental or physical differences are sometimes referred to as "hard learners," who are expected to go to school and be incorporated into the classes with assistance from other student "scholars" and parents. A culturally congruent approach is for the family and others to help engage those with differences in work activities, rather than to leave them sitting around and getting more anxious or depressed.

Hostetler (1993) stated that "Amish themselves have developed little explicit therapeutic knowledge to deal with cases of extreme anxiety" (p. 332). They do seek help from trusted physicians, and some are admitted to mental health centers or clinics. However, the mentally ill are generally cared for at home whenever possible. Studies of clinical depression and manic-depressive illness were discussed in the section on biocultural ecology.

As previously mentioned, when individuals are sick, other family members take on additional responsibilities. Little ceremony is associated with being sick, and members know that to be healthy means to assume one's role within the family and community. Caring for the sick is highly valued, but at the same time, receiving help is accompanied by feelings of humility. Amish newsletters abound with notices of thanks from individuals who were ill. A common expression is "I am not worthy of it all." A care set identified in one research study is that "giving care involves privilege and obligation, and receiving care involves expectation and humility" (Wenger, 1991a). The sick role is mediated by very strong values related to giving and receiving care.

The Amish culture also sanctions time out for illness when the sick are relieved of their responsibilities by others who minister to their needs. A good analogy to the communal care of the ill is found in the support offered by family and church members at the time of bereavement, as noted in the section on dying. The informal social support network is an important factor in the individual's sense of well-being. An underlying expectation, however, is that healthy individuals will want to resume active work and social roles as soon as their recovery permits. With reasonable adjustments for age and physical ability, it is understood that a healthy person is actively engaged in work, worship, and social life of the family and community (Wenger, 1994). Work and rest are kept in balance, but for the Amish, the accumulation of days or weeks of free time or time off for vacation outside the framework of normal routines and social interactions is a foreign idea.

In a study of Amish women's construction of health narratives, Nelson (1999) found that the "collective descriptions [of] health included a sense of feeling well and the physical ability to complete one's daily work responsibilities" (p. vi). Women's health traditions included the use of herbal and other home remedies and consulting lay practitioners. In general, health values and beliefs are influenced by cultural group membership and personal developmental history.

Blood Transfusions and Organ Donation

No cultural or religious rules or taboos prohibit Amish from accepting blood transfusions or organ transplantation and donation. In fact, with the genetic presence of hemophilia, blood transfusion has been a necessity for some families. Anecdotal evidence is available regarding individuals who have received heart and kidney transplants, although no research reports or other written accounts were found. Thus, some Amish may opt for organ transplantation after the family seeks advice from church officials, extended family, and friends, but the patient or immediate family generally makes the final decision.

Health-Care Providers

Traditional Versus Biomedical Providers

Amish usually refer to their own healers by name rather than by title, although some say *brauch-doktor* or **braucher**. In some communities, both men and women provide these services. They may even specialize, with some being especially good with bed-wetting,

---

REFLECTIVE EXERCISE 7.3

In an ethno-nursing research study, Wenger (1991c, p. 106), described culture congruent caring among the Amish as a care set:

Giving care involves both obligation and privilege.
Receiving care involves both expectation and humility.

Explain how each of the following statements relates to the care set:

1. Amish will experience acts of caring within the Amish community throughout their lifetime.
2. Amish describe one of the benefits of caring for others as "feeling good."
3. In Amish newsletters, notices of appreciation for having received care may include the closing phrase "I'm so unworthy of it all."
4. Amish social networks expressed in various visiting patterns provide an opportunity for persons to learn about one another's caring needs.
5. Personal submission and obedience to God includes a consideration of others before oneself.

---

nervousness, women's problems, or livergrown. Some set up treatment rooms, and people come early in the morning and wait long hours to be seen. They do not charge fees but do accept donations. A few also treat non-Amish patients. In some communities, Amish folk healers use a combination of treatment modalities, including physical manipulation, massage, *brauche,* herbs and teas, and reflexology. A few have taken short courses in reflexology, iridology, and various types of therapeutic massage. In a few cases, their practice has been reported to the legal authorities by individuals in the medical profession or others who were concerned about the potential for illegal practice of medicine. Huntington (1993) chronicled several cases, including those of Solomon Wickey and Joseph Helmuth, both in Indiana. Both men continue to practice with some carefully designed restrictions.

Status of Health-Care Providers

For the Old Order Amish, health-care providers are always outsiders because, thus far, this sect has been unwilling to allow their members to attend medical, nursing, or other health-related professional schools or to seek higher education in general. Therefore, the Old Order Amish must learn to trust individuals outside their culture for health care and medically related scientific knowledge. Hostetler (1993) contended that the Amish live in a state of flux when securing health-care services. They rely on their own tradition to diagnose and sometimes treat illnesses, while simultaneously seeking technical and scientific services from health-care providers.

Most Amish consult within their community to learn about physicians, dentists, and nurses with whom they can develop trusting relationships. For more information on this practice, see the Amish informants' perceptions of caring physicians and nurses in Wenger's (1994; 1995) chapter and article on health and health-care decision making. Amish prefer health-care providers who discuss their health-care options, giving consideration to cost, need for transportation, family influences, and scientific information. They also like to discuss the efficacy of alternative methods of treatment, including folk care. When asked, many Amish, like others from diverse cultures, claim that health-care providers do not want to hear about non-traditional health-care modalities that do not reflect dominant American health-care values.

Amish hold all health-care providers in high regard. Health is integral to their religious beliefs, and care is central to their worldview. They tend to place trust in people of authority when they fit their values and beliefs. Because Amish are not sophisticated in their knowledge of physiology and scientific health care, the health-care provider who gains their trust should bear in mind that because the Amish respect authority, they may unquestioningly follow orders. Therefore, health-care providers should make sure that their patients understand instructions. Role modeling and other concrete teaching strategies are recommended to enhance understanding.

REFERENCES

Allen, F. (1989, September 20). Country doctor: How a physician solved the riddle of rare disease in children of Amish. *Wall Street Journal*, pp. 1, A16.

Bassett, D.R. (2004, January). Old-Time fitness in Old-Order Amish: Why are we less fit than our ancestors? Amish offer clues. *Medicine and Science in Sports and Exercise*, (36), 79–85.

Belkin, L. (2005, November 6). A doctor for the future. *New York Times WSJ Magazine*, 68–115.

Bowman, H.S., & Procopio, J. (1963). Hereditary non-sperocytic hemolytic anemia of the pyruvate kinase deficient type. *Annals of Internal Medicine, 58*, 561–591.

Elizabeth Town College. (2010). The Young Center for Anabaptist and Pietist Studies at Elizabethtown College. Retrieved from http://www.etown.edu/centers/young-center/

Enninger, W., & Wandt, K.-H. (1982). Pennsylvania German in the context of an Old Order Amish settlement. *Yearbook of German-American Studies, 17*, 123–143.

Foroud, T., Casteluccio, P., Kollar, D., Edenberg, H., Miller, M., & Boman, L. (2000). Suggestive evidence of a locus on chromosome 10p using the NIMH genetics initiative bipolar affective disorder pedigrees. *American Journal of Medical Genetics, 96*(1), 18–23.

Fuchs, J.A., Levinson, R., Stoddard, R., Mullet, M., & Jones, D. (1990). Health risk factors among Amish: Results of a survey. *Health Education Quarterly, 17*(2), 197–211.

Ginns, E.D., Egeland, J., Allen, C., Pauls, D., & Falls, K. (1992). Update on the search for DNA markers linked to manic-depressive illness in the Old Order Amish. *Journal of Psychiatric Research, 26*(4), 305–308.

Hostetler, J.A. (1993). *Amish society* (4th ed.). Baltimore, MD: Johns Hopkins University Press.

Hostetler, J.A., & Huntington, G.E. (1992). *Amish children: Education in the family, school, and community* (2nd ed.). Dallas, TX: Harcourt Brace Jovanovich.

Hsueh W.C., Mitchell B.D., Aburomia R., Pollin T., Sakul, H., Gelder Ehm M., Michelsen B.K., Wagner, M.J., St. Jean, P.L., Knowler, W.C., Burns, D.K., Bell, C.J., & Shuldine A.R. (2002). Diabetes in the Old Order Amish: Characterization and heritability analysis of the Amish Family Diabetes Study. *American Journal of Clinical Nutrition, 75*(6), 1098–1106.

Huffines, M.L. (1994). Amish languages. In J.R. Dow, W. Enninger, & J. Raith (Eds.), *Internal and external perspectives on Amish and Mennonite life. 4: Old and new world Anabaptist studies on the language, culture, society and health of Amish and Mennonites* (pp. 21–32). Essen, Germany: University of Essen.

Huntington, G.E. (1988). The Amish family. In C. Mindel & R. Haberstein (Eds.), *Ethnic families in America* (3rd ed.). (pp. 367–399). New York: Elsevier.

Huntington, G.E. (1993). Health care. In D.B. Kraybill (Ed.), *The Amish and the state*. Baltimore, MD: Johns Hopkins University Press.

Huntington, G.E. (2001). *Amish in Michigan*. East Lansing, MI: Michigan State University Press.

Hüppi, J. (2000). Research note: Identifying Jacob Ammann. *Mennonite Quarterly Review, 74*(10), 329–339.

Hurst, C.E., & McConnell, D.L. (2010). *An Amish paradox: Diversity and change in the world's largest Amish community*. Baltimore, MD: The Johns Hopkins University Press.

Jones, M.W. (1990). A study of trauma in an Amish community. *Journal of Trauma, 30*(7), 899–902.

Kelsoe, J.R., Ginns, E.D., & Egeland, J.A. (1989). Re-evaluation of the linkage relationship between chromosome 11p loci and the gene for bipolar affective disorder in the Old Order Amish. *Nature, 342*, 338–342.

Kelsoe, J.R., Kristobjanarson, H., Bergesch, P., Shilling, S., Attirad, S., Mirow, A., Moises, H., Gillin, J., & Egeland, J. (1993). A genetic linkage study of bipolar disorder and 13 markers on chromosome 11, including the D2 dopamine receptor. *Neuropsychopharmocology, 9*(4), 293–307.

Ketterling, R.P., Bottema, C.D., Koberl, D.D., Setsuko. I, & Sommer, S.S. (1991). T^{296}M, a common mutation causing mild hemophilia B in the Amish and others: Founder effect, variability in factor IX activity assays, and rapid carrier detection. *Human Genetics, 87*, 333–337.

Kraybill, D.B. (2001). *The riddle of Amish culture* (rev. ed.). Baltimore, MD: Johns Hopkins University Press.

Kraybill, D.B., & Hostetter, C.N. (2001). *Anabaptist World USA*. Scottdale, PA: Herald Press.

Krabill, D.B., Nolt, S.M., & Weaver-Zercher, D.L. (2007). *Amish grace: How forgiveness transcended tragedy*. San Francisco, CA: John Wiley and Sons.

Law, A., Richard, C.W., Cottingham, R.W., Lathrop, M.G., Cox, D.R., & Meyers, R.M. (1992). Genetic linkage analysis of bipolar affective disorder in an Old Order Amish pedigree. *Human Genetics, 88*, 562–568.

Lipon, T. (1985). Husband and wife work roles and the organization and operation of family farms. *Journal of Marriage and the Family, 47*(3), 759–764

Lucas, C.A., O'Shea, R.M., Zielezny, M.A., Freudenheim, J.L., & Wold, J.F. (1991). Rural medicine and the closed society. *New York State Journal of Medicine, 91*(2), 49–52.

Martin, P.H., Davis, L., & Askew, D. (1965). High incidence of phenylketonuria in an isolated Indiana community. *Journal of the Indiana State Medical Association, 56*, 997–999.

McKusick, V.A. (1978). *Medical genetics studies of the Amish: Selected papers assembled with commentary*. Baltimore, MD: Johns Hopkins University Press.

McKusick, V.A., Egeland, J.A., Eldridge, D., & Krusen, E.E. (1964). Dwarfism in the Amish I. The Ellis-van Creveld syndrome. *Bulletin of the Johns Hopkins Hospital, 115*, 306–330.

McKusick, V.A., Eldridge, D., Hostetler, J.A., Ruanquit, U., & Egeland, J.A. (1965). Dwarfism in the Amish II. Cartilage hair hypoplasia. *Bulletin of the Johns Hopkins Hospital, 116*, 285–326.

Meyers, T.J. (1993). Education and schooling. In D. Kraybill (Ed.), *The Amish and the state* (pp. 87–106). Baltimore, MD: Johns Hopkins University Press.

Meyers, T.J., & Nolt, S.M. (2005). *An Amish patchwork: Indiana's Old Orders in a modern world*. Bloomington, IN: Quarry Books, Indiana University Press.

Miller, N.L. (1997). Childbearing practices as described by Old Order Amish women. Doctoral dissertation, Michigan State University. *Dissertation Abstracts International*, UMI 1388555.

Myers, R.M. (1992). Genetic linkage analysis of bipolar affective disorder in an Old Order Amish pedigree. *Human Genetics, 88*, 562–568.

Nelson, W.A. (1999). *A study of Amish women's construction of health narratives*. Unpublished doctoral dissertation, Kent State University, Kent, Ohio.

Pauls, D.L., Morton, L.A., & Egeland, J.A. (1992). Risks of affective illness among first-degree relatives of bipolar and Old Order Amish probands. *Archives of General Psychiatry, 49*, 703–708.

Ratnoff, O.D. (1958). Hereditary defects in clotting mechanisms. *Advances in Internal Medicine, 9,* 107–179.

Reiling, D.M. (1998). An explanation of the relationship between Amish identity and depression among Old Order Amish. Doctoral dissertation, Michigan State University. *Dissertation Abstracts International*, UMI 9985454.

Tripp-Reimer, T., & Schrock, M. (1982). Residential patterns of ethnic aged: Implications for transcultural nursing. In C. Uhl & J. Uhl (Eds.), *Proceedings of the Seventh Annual Transcultural Nursing Conference* (pp. 144–153). Salt Lake City, UT: University of Utah, Transcultural Nursing Society.

Troyer, H. (1994). Medical considerations of the Amish. In J.R. Dow, W. Enninger, & J. Raith (Eds.), *Internal and external perspectives on Amish and Mennonite life 4: Old and new world Anabaptist studies on the language, culture, society and health of the Amish and Mennonites* (pp. 68–87). Essen, Germany: University of Essen.

Wenger, A.F. (1980, October). *Acceptability of perinatal services among the Amish.* Paper presented at a March of Dimes symposium, Future Directions in Perinatal Care, Baltimore, MD.

Wenger, A.F.Z. (1988). The phenomenon of care in a high-context culture: The Old Order Amish. Doctoral dissertation, Wayne State University. *Dissertation Abstracts International,* 50/02B.

Wenger, A.F.Z. (1991a). The culture care theory and the Old Order Amish. In M.M. Leininger (Ed.), *Cultural care diversity and universality: A theory of nursing* (pp. 147–178). New York: National League for Nursing.

Wenger, A.F.Z. (1991b). Culture-specific care and the Old Order Amish. *Imprint, 38*(2), 81–82, 84, 87, 93.

Wenger, A.F.Z. (1991c). The role of context in culture-specific care. In P.L. Chinn (Ed.), *Anthology of caring* (pp. 95–110). New York: National League for Nursing.

Wenger, A.F.Z. (1994). Health and health-care decision-making: The Old Order Amish. In J.R. Dow, W. Enninger, & J. Raith, (Eds.), *Internal and external perspectives on Amish and Mennonite life 4: Old and New World Anabaptists studies on the language, culture, society and health of the Amish and Mennonites* (pp. 88–110). Essen, Germany: University of Essen.

Wenger, A.F.Z. (1995). Cultural context, health and health-care decision making. *Journal of Transcultural Nursing, 7*(1), 3–14.

Wenger, M.R. (1970). *A Swiss German dialect study: Three linguistic islands in Midwestern USA.* Ann Arbor, MI: University Microfilms.

What is in a language? (1986, February). *Family Life,* p. 12.

Wolkomir, R., & Wolkomir, J. (1991, July). The doctor who conquered a killer. *Reader's Digest, 139,* 161–166.

DavisPlus *For Reflective Exercises, review questions and additional information, go to*
http://davisplus.fadavis.com

Chapter 8

People of Appalachian Heritage

Kathleen W. Huttlinger

Overview, Inhabited Localities, and Topography

Overview

Appalachia consists of that large geographic expanse in the eastern United States that is associated with the Appalachian mountain system, a 205,000-square-mile region that extends from the northeastern United States in southern New York to northern Mississippi. It includes all of West Virginia and parts of Alabama, Georgia, Kentucky, Maryland, Mississippi, New York, North Carolina, Ohio, Pennsylvania, South Carolina, Tennessee, and Virginia. This very rural area is characterized by a rolling topography with very rugged ridges and hilltops, some extending over 4000 feet high, with remote valleys between them. The surrounding valleys are often 2000 feet or more in elevation and give one a sense of isolation, peacefulness, and separateness from the lower and more heavily traveled urban areas. This isolation and rough topography have contributed to the development of secluded communities in the hills and natural hollows or narrow valleys where people, over time, have developed a strong sense of independence and family cohesiveness. These same isolated valleys and rugged mountains can present accessibility issues for those who do not have access to private transportation because public transportation is not widely available, and even then only in the larger, more urbanized areas.

Even though the Appalachian region includes several large cities, most people live in small settlements and in inaccessible hollows or "hollers" (Huttlinger, Schaller-Ayers, & Lawson, 2004a). The rugged location of many communities in Appalachia results in a population that is isolated from the mainstream of health-care services. In some areas, substandard secondary and tertiary roads, as well as limited public bus, rail, and airport facilities, prevent easy access to the area (Fig. 8-1). Difficulty in accessing the area is partially responsible for continued geographic and social isolation. In addition, the rugged terrain and secondary roads can delay ambulance response times and are deterrents to people who need emergency health care. This is one area in which telehealth innovations can and often do provide needed services (University of Virginia, 2009).

Many of the approximately 24.8 million people who live in Appalachia can trace their family roots back 150 years or more, and it is common to find whole communities comprising extended, related families (Appalachia Regional Commision (ARC), 2010). The cultural heritage of the region is rich and reflected by a distinctive music, art, and literature. Even though family roots are strong, many of the region's younger residents have left the area to pursue job opportunities and college in the larger urban cities of the North, South, and West Coast. The remaining, older population reflects a group that often has less than a high school education, is frequently unemployed, may be on welfare and/or disability, and is regularly uninsured (20.4 percent) (ARC, 2010). In fact, 80 percent of the population over age 65 is higher in Appalachia (14.3 percent) than in the rest of the United States (12.4 percent). The lack of education has often been associated with nonparticipation in health promotion activities (ARC, 2010; Graduate Medical Education Consortium [GMEC], 2001). Completion of a high school degree and matriculation to college are well below average throughout central and southern Appalachia. For example, in central Appalachia, 25 percent of the residents have attended college, compared to 50 percent for the nation (ARC, 2010). Graduation rates from high school in the year 2000 vary widely from 60.7 to 91.4 percent, with the lowest number of graduates occurring in West Virginia, southwestern Virginia, eastern Kentucky, and northeastern Tennessee (ARC, 2010; Haaga, 2004).

Heritage and Residence

Appalachians generally identify themselves by family surname. At one time an individual's country of origin—Germany, Scotland, Ireland, and so on—was also

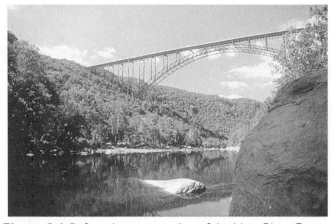

Figure 8-1 Before the construction of the New River Gorge bridge, many people were isolated from health care. *(Courtesy of West Virginia Division of Tourism and Parks.)*

included as an identification, but this tradition has generally disappeared, except for older adults who still deem this aspect an important part of their residence. Germans, Scots-Irish, Welsh, French, and British constitute the primary groups who settled the region between the 17th and 19th centuries. It is important to remember that simply taking up residence in Appalachia does not make one an "Appalachian," since a significant value is held for those whose roots are well identified within the region. Historically, the population has been predominantly white, although many maintain a strong family identity with the American Indian tribes that once populated the area (e.g., Cherokee, Choctaw) (Huttlinger, Schaller-Ayers, Kenney, & Ayers, 2004b). In addition, African Americans have been in Appalachia since the 1500s. Early Spanish and French explorers brought with them African slaves, and free persons of color were among the earliest settlers. While a plantation economy never developed in the region, many wealthy mountain people owned slaves who worked in stores and inns, logging, and mining, as well as on farms. After the Civil War, many freed African Americans bought land to farm and lived rural lifestyles very similar to those of their white neighbors (Watkins, 2011).

African American Appalachians have endured the same kinds of racial problems that exist elsewhere. While they recognize their ties to the larger African American population, they also have a unique identification with the region. Celebration of family heritage through the collection of family memorabilia and attendance at family reunions strengthens their separate identity as African American Appalachians (Watkins, 2011).

Appalachians in general cannot be distinguished from other white cultural and ethnic groups by either dress or physical appearance. However, similarities in beliefs and practices, tempered by variant cultural characteristics (see Chapter 1), give them a unique and rich ethnic identity. Like many disenfranchised groups, the people of Appalachia have been described

in stereotypically negative terms (e.g., "poor white trash") that in no way represent the people or the culture as a whole. They have also been called "mountaineers," "hillbillies," "rednecks," and "Elizabethans." During the past 60 years, the media have perpetuated the stereotypes with cartoon strips such as "Li'l Abner" and "Snuffy Smith," television programs such as the *Dukes of Hazzard*, and stories of the feuding Hatfields and McCoys and the Whites and Garrards. Interestingly, these feuds were among wealthy families over salt deposits and land and families who had high political profiles. Failure of the courts to intervene and a propensity of Appalachians to handle things themselves perpetuated the longevity of the feuds.

However, in recent times, works by popular authors such as Sharon McCrumb, James Dickey, Lee Smith, and John Ehle reflect values for deep-seated work ethics, low cost of living, and a high quality of life that permeate their Appalachian daily lives. All told, Appalachians see themselves as loyal, caring, family-oriented, religious, hardy, independent, honest, patriotic, and resourceful (Huttlinger et al., 2004a).

Other groups in the region who may identify with Appalachian culture include American Indians, African Americans, and Melungeons, who are of mixed African American, American Indian, Middle Eastern, Mediterranean, and white ethnic descent (Costello, 2000; Kennedy, 1997). Although Melungeon heritage is often denied, there is, of late, a resurgence of identification of Melungeon ancestry. In fact, annual Melungeon get-togethers are now held once a year in Appalachia (Kennedy, 1997). With the increase in immigration to the United States since the 1970s, the Appalachian region is becoming more ethnically and culturally diverse, and it is now very common to observe other ethnic groups, including those of southeast Asian, Chinese, and Hispanic heritage.

Reasons for Migration and Associated Economic Factors

Approximately 300 years ago, people came to Appalachia to seek religious freedom, land for themselves, and control over social interactions with the outside world. Over the years, mining and timber resources have become depleted, farmland has eroded, and jobs have become scarce, which has resulted in an out-migration of people, especially those of working age, to larger urban areas of the North such as Cincinnati, Cleveland, and Louisville; to the South in cities like Charlotte and Atlanta; and even to the Southwest to places like Nevada and California (ARC, 2010). This migration began after World War II and has remained constant ever since (Obermiller & Brown, 2002). Those who move to urban areas often feel alone and sometimes become depressed as they are separated from family and friends. Many families fear for their young family members and worry that they will succumb to crime, drug use, and the other perils of living in an urban environment. In spite of these concerns, many of those who have remained in urban settings have become bicultural, adapting to the culture of urban life while retaining, as much as possible, their traditional Appalachian culture.

The limited opportunities for employment in Appalachia often require wage earners to leave their families to seek work elsewhere, returning home on weekends and holidays or vacations to maintain their close ties with kinfolk. Their migration pattern is regional, where individuals from one area primarily migrate to the same urban areas as their relatives and friends—a pattern that is common with many migrants. This practice helps decrease the occurrence of depression and feelings of isolation and provides a support network of family and friends that is so important for members of the Appalachian culture.

Appalachian migration patterns reflect the economic conditions found in the area, as well as some of the cultural values of home, connection to the land, and importance of the family. Working-age individuals move from Appalachia to make their living but often return to their home hills and hollows in Appalachia to retire. Because of these patterns, Appalachia has one of the highest existing aging populations (ARC, 2010; Haaga, 2004). The pattern of returning home to retire has given rise to challenges for health-care delivery. In fact, older people were once able to rely on home care services, but severe budget cuts in 1977 left home care health service unreliable and ineffective. A study by Carter (2005) indicated that Appalachian nursing homes served resident populations with higher activities of daily living (ADL) impairment levels, had a larger proportion of residents whose stays were reimbursed by Medicaid, and had a lower proportion of residents who paid privately for their care. Carter noted that the long-term care facilities located in Appalachia were more likely to be hospital-based, reflecting hospital swing-bed policies in rural areas, and were less likely to offer specialty beds designated for the care of residents with Alzheimer's disease. Although important differences in operational and organizational characteristics were found (potential indicators of the poor quality of nursing home care), findings suggested that these did not necessarily lead to higher deficiency citation rates in Appalachia. Rather, Carter's findings indicated that facilities whose resident populations have higher levels of ADL impairment have a greater proportion of Medicaid- reimbursed stays, and a smaller proportion of privately paid days received more deficiencies than did otherwise similar facilities, holding other factors constant. Lastly, her findings indicated that after adjusting for other factors, a clear pattern of fewer deficiencies emerged across the Appalachian region that cannot be fully unexplained by either urban-rural or quality of care differences in the region, suggesting most likely that other, unexplained but regionally distributed, factors are contributing to the number and types of deficiencies found in nursing home facilities.

A recent perusal of local phone directories shows, as of 2011, many private and community-based home care services throughout the Appalachian region. In the past, older people and the chronically ill had to rely on options for short-term and expensive hospital care, nursing homes, or no care at all (Hurley & Turner, 2000), whereas now they appear to have other options.

For generations, the region has been a symbol of poverty in a land of wealth and opportunity. During the 1960s, the Appalachian Regional Commission (ARC) appropriated funds for building roads to attract industry and provided loans for residents to start their own businesses. In many areas of Central Appalachia, the unemployment rate and the number of people living in poverty have remained consistently above the national average, while the per capita income has remained below the national average. Eight of the 13 states in Appalachia have an unemployment rate higher than the national average, and the national poverty rate of 12.6 percent is exceeded by 10 of the 13 states in Appalachia. During the recent recession, Appalachia lost a disproportionate number of jobs compared with some other states (ARC, 2010). The average per capita income rate in Appalachia is $20,434. Not one Appalachian state achieves the national per capita income of $25,470. Of 410 counties in Appalachia, 77 are considered economically distressed, 81 are at risk, and 222 are transitional (ARC, 2010). Even though the cost of living in much of the area is lower than that in many other parts of the United States, costs for transportation of food, basic living supplies, and transportation fuels rise, thus creating hardships for an area that is already economically stressed (ARC, 2010).

Educational Status and Occupations

Although many of the original immigrants to this area were highly educated when they arrived, limited access to more formal education resulted in the isolation of later generations with fewer educational opportunities. Despite the value placed on education, a disparity in the number and placement of educational facilities exists throughout the region. Access to colleges and universities has improved, but there is still a lack of knowledge about life outside of Appalachia and the educational opportunities available. Examples of universities and colleges in Appalachia include, but are not limited to, West Virginia University, Appalachian State, University of Virginia's College at Wise, East Tennessee State, Shawnee State, and the University of North Alabama. A dichotomy between those who are poorly educated and those who are extremely well educated still exists today (Huttlinger et al., 2004a).

Because isolation results in a cultural lag, IQ scores of children from Appalachia are sometimes lower than those in the populations outside of Appalachia who have access to larger schools and live in urban settings. However, with television and the Internet now available throughout the area, this cultural lag has been slowly improving. In fact, U.S. representatives from many of the districts that lie in Appalachia made it a priority to have broadband and Internet connections made accessible. Factors such as improved mobility, access to better schools with qualified teachers, increased employment opportunities in some regions, and greater use of technology are responsible for improving socioeconomic conditions and better performance on standard IQ tests (ARC, 2010). However, the mountainous terrain often limits those services that require "line of sight" and may include cell phone and advanced TV technologies.

Although a value is placed on education, education beyond high school is often viewed as not as important as earning a living to help support the family. Many Appalachian parents, and especially those who belong to more conservative and secular religious sects, do not want their children influenced by mainstream middle-class American behaviors and actions. However, fewer children drop out of school today than in previous decades. One interesting fact is that several states in Appalachia have laws that grant permanent driving privileges only upon completion of high school, which has lowered dropout rates significantly.

Parents who value higher education encourage their children to seek quality education at the best institutions possible. Despite this value, the graduation rate from college is, at best, 27 percent compared with 45 percent for non-Appalachian counterparts (ARC, 2010). Unfortunately, the highly educated, including health-care workers, who return to the area are often unable to secure financially lucrative employment and soon leave to seek employment elsewhere.

Because educational levels of individuals within the Appalachian regions vary, it is essential for health-care providers to assess the health literacy and basic understanding of health and disease of individuals when providing any kind of intervention. Educational materials and explanations must be presented at literacy levels that are consistent with patients' understanding. If materials are presented at a level that is not understandable to patients, providers may be seen as being "stuck-up," "putting on airs," or "not understanding them and their ways" (Huttlinger et al., 2004b) (see Chapter 1).

Communication

Dominant Language and Dialects

The dominant language of the Appalachian region is English, with many words derived from 16th-century Saxon and Gaelic. Because the Appalachian dialect tends to be very concrete, continued exposure is necessary to avoid misunderstandings. Negative interpretations of Appalachian behaviors by non-Appalachian health-care providers can be detrimental to positive and facilitative working relationships.

Some of the more isolated groups in Appalachia speak an Elizabethan English, which has its own distinct vocabulary and syntax and can cause communication difficulties for those who are not familiar with it. Some examples of variations in pronunciation for words are *allus* for "always" and *fit* for "fight." Word meanings that may be different include *poke* or *sack* for "paper bag" and *sass* for "vegetables." The Appalachian region is also noted for its use of strong preterits such as *clum* for "climbed," *drug* for "dragged," and *swelled* for "swollen." Plural forms of monosyllabic words are formed like Chaucerian English, which adds *es* to the word—for example, "post" becomes *postes*, "beast" becomes *beastes*, "nest" becomes *nestes*, and "ghost" becomes *ghostes*. Many people, especially in the nonacademic environment, drop the *g* on words ending in *ing*. For example, "writing" becomes *writin'*, "reading" becomes *readin'*, and "spelling" becomes *spellin'*. In addition, vowels may be pronounced with a diphthong that can cause difficulty to one unfamiliar with this dialect—hence, *poosh* for "push," *boosh* for "bush," *warsh* for "wash," *hiegen* for "hygiene," *deef* for "deaf," *welks* for "welts," *whar* for "where," *hit* for "it," *hurd* for "heard," and *your'n* for "your." However, when the word is written, the meaning is apparent. Comparatives and superlatives are formed by adding a final *er* or *est*, making the word "bad" become *badder* and "preaching" become *preachin'est* (Wilson, 1989).

If health-care providers are unfamiliar with the exact meaning of a word, it is best to ask patients to explain. Otherwise, miscommunication can occur and will probably result in incorrect diagnoses and/or other poor health outcomes. A health-care provider may want to ask the person to write the words (if the person has writing skills) to help prevent errors in communication and to improve outcomes and following directions with health prescriptions and treatments.

Cultural Communication Patterns

Appalachians practice the ethic of neutrality, which helps shape communication styles, their worldview, and other aspects of the Appalachian culture. Four dominant themes affect communication patterns in the Appalachian culture: avoiding aggression and assertiveness, not interfering with others' lives unless asked to do so, avoiding dominance over others, and avoiding arguments and seeking agreement (Smith & Tessaro, 2005).

Appalachians are often accepting of others and do not want to pass judgment. This value is reflected in written and oral communications in which fewer adjectives and adverbs are used. Thus, many Appalachians may be less precise in describing their emotions, may be more concrete in conversations, and will answer questions in a more direct manner. Accordingly, a health-care provider may need to use more open-ended questions when obtaining health information and eliciting opinions and beliefs about health-care practices, such as "What do you believe might be causing your illness?" Otherwise, Appalachian providers are likely to give a yes or no answer without expanding or clarifying their answers.

In general, Appalachians are a very private people who do not want to offend others, nor do they easily trust or share their thoughts and feelings with *outsiders*. They are more likely to say what they think the listener wants to hear rather than what the listener needs to hear. In addition, because of past, and often unfavorable, experiences with large mining and timber companies, many Appalachians dislike authority figures and institutions that attempt to control their behavior. Individualism and self-reliant behavior are idealized; personalism and individualism are admired; and people are accepted on the basis of their personal achievements, qualities, and family lineage.

Appalachians' perceptions of themselves, their community, and their families influence many aspects of their communication styles. Families are more than genetic relationships and are described as including brothers, sisters, aunts, uncles, parents, grandparents, cousins, in-laws, and out-laws (those related by marriage). This perception of family and community transcends the concept of self as "I." The use of the pronoun "we" throughout speech patterns recognizes the concept of self. Thus, "we can make it," "we will survive," or "we will be there" may refer to only the person speaking.

An example of a typical interaction in an Appalachian community may be illustrated by this statement from a key informant in the Counts and Boyle (1987) Genesis Project, which took place from 1985 to 1994. Miss Ruth, a 94-year-old native Appalachian, was interviewed in the house in which she was born. In fact, she had her appendix removed in the living room of this same house by a traveling nurse. After returning from a trip to Africa (she had a doctorate and liked to travel, but always returned home), Miss Ruth described the concept of "neighboring" as a double-edged sword. The positive side is that when you are sick, everyone comes around to take care of you; however, on the negative side, when you try to do something quietly, everyone knows about it.

Appalachians may be sensitive to direct questions about personal issues. Sensitive topics are best approached with indirect questions and suggestions and without critical innuendo. Appalachians are taught to deny anger and not complain. Information should be gathered in the context of broader relationships with respect for the ethic of equality, which implies more horizontal than hierarchical relationships, allowing cordiality to precede information sharing. Starting with sensitive issues may invite ineffectiveness; thus, the health-care provider may need to "sit a spell" and "chat" before getting down to the business of collecting health information. To establish trust, the health-care provider must show interest in the community, the patient's family, and other personal matters; drop hints instead of give orders; and solicit the patient's opinions and advice. These actions increase the patient's self-worth and self-esteem and help to establish the trust needed for an effective working relationship.

Traditional Appalachians value personal physical space, so they are more likely to stand at a distance when talking with people in both social and health-care situations. This physical distancing has its origins in religious persecution endured by this group in their history and has been perpetuated by a social isolation that has encouraged family members to become the main social contact (Coyne, Demian-Popescu, & Friend, 2006). Therefore, many people may perceive direct eye contact, especially from strangers, as an aggressive or hostile act. Staring is considered bad manners.

To communicate effectively with Appalachian patients, nonverbal behaviors must be assessed within the contextual framework of the culture. Many Appalachians are comfortable with silence, and when talking with health-care providers who are outsiders, they are likely to speak without emotion, facial expression, or gestures and avoid telling unpleasant news to avoid hurting someone's feelings. Health-care providers who are unfamiliar with the culture may interpret these nonverbal communication patterns as not caring. Within this context, the health-care provider needs to allow sufficient time to develop rapport by dropping hints instead of giving orders (Coyne et al., 2006). In addition, to communicate effectively with traditional Appalachians, health-care providers must not ignore speech patterns; they must clarify any differences in word meanings, translate medical terminology into everyday language using concrete terms, explain not only what is to be done but also why, and ask patients to repeat or demonstrate instructions to ensure understanding. Adopting an attitude of respect and flexibility demonstrates interest and helps bridge barriers imposed by health-care providers' personal ideologies and cultural values. Throughout history, Appalachians have enjoyed storytelling, a practice that still continues; accordingly, some individuals may respond better to verbal instructions and education, with reinforcement from videos rather than printed communications.

Temporal Relationships

The traditional Appalachian culture is "being"-oriented (i.e., living for today) as compared with "doing"-oriented (i.e., planning for the future).

A being orientation not only opposes progress but also may mean ignoring expert advice and "accepting one's lot in life." With the potential for economic and cultural lag, other problems may be more pressing, and "just getting by" may be the most important activity. Health-care providers must realize that the emphasis on illness prevention in our current society is still relatively new for many Appalachians (GMEC, 2001). For those living in poverty and isolation, the trend is to "live for today" and to rely on more traditional approaches for those things that cannot be controlled. This worldview is common with present-oriented societies, in which some higher power is in charge of life and its outcomes, but it is a deterrent to preventive health services. With a fatalistic view in which individuals have little or no control over nature, and the time of death is "predetermined by God," one frequently hears expressions such as "I'll be there, God willing and if the crick [creek] don't rise." As communication systems such as televisions, satellite dishes, and the Internet become more commonplace, temporal relationships are becoming more future-oriented.

For the traditional Appalachian, life is unhurried and body rhythms, not the clock, control activities. One may come early or late for an appointment and still expect to be seen. If individuals are not seen because they are late for an appointment and are asked to reschedule, they are likely to not return because they may feel rejected. Many Appalachians are hesitant to make appointments because "somethin' better might come up" or they may not be sure of transportation until the last minute.

Appalachians who live outside the area usually talk about, and sometimes even dwell upon, "home" in a nostalgic way. To some, this might seem like a glorification of a past temporal orientation. However, these authors believe that it is nostalgia for "the way things used to be" as, in reality, most people do not want to return to the harshness of the life experienced by past generations.

Format for Names

Although the format for names in Appalachia follows the U.S. standard given name plus family name, individuals address nonfamily members by their last name. A common practice that denotes neighborliness with respect is to call a person by his or her first name with the title Mr. or Miss (pronounced "miz" similar to "Ms.," when referring to women, whether single or married)—for example, Miss Lillian or Mr. Bill. Miss Lillian may or may not be married. There is also a need to provide a link with both families of origin. Many times Appalachians refer to a married woman as "she was [born] a . . . ," thus linking the families and enhancing the feeling of continuity.

Family Roles and Organization
Head of Household and Gender Roles

In previous decades, gender roles for Appalachian men and women were more clearly defined. Men were supposed to do physical work, to support the family financially, and to provide transportation. Women took care of the house and assumed responsibility for child rearing. Self-made individuals and families, or those who carried out their own subsistence and depended little on outsiders, were idealized.

The traditional Appalachian household continues to be patriarchal, although many families are becoming more egalitarian in their beliefs and practices. This is especially true if the woman makes more money than the man. Women are generally the providers of emotional strength, with older women having a lot of clout in health-care matters. Older women are usually responsible for preparing herbal remedies and folk medicines and are sought out by family members and neighbors for these preparations. Older women have a higher status in the community than older men, who in turn have a higher status than younger women. With the advent of better access to education and improved transportation throughout Appalachia, more women are working outside the home, thus creating an environment in which gender roles are becoming more egalitarian.

Prescriptive, Restrictive, and Taboo Behaviors for Children and Adolescents

Children are important to the Appalachian culture (Coyne et al., 2006). Large families are common, and children are usually accepted regardless of whether the parents are married. Parents may impose strict social conformity for family members in fear of community censure and their own parental feelings of inferiority. Permissive behavior at home is unacceptable, and hands-on physical punishment, to a degree that some perceive as abuse, is common. For Appalachian children who have problems with school performance, the most effective approach to increase performance is to provide individualized attention rather than group support or attention, an approach that is congruent with the ethic of neutrality. To be effective in changing negative behavior, it is necessary to emphasize positive points.

As children progress into their teens, mischievous behavior is accepted but not condoned. Continuing formal education may not be stressed because many teens are expected to get a job to help support the family. Children are seen as being important, and to many, having a child, even at an early age (less than 18 years), means fulfillment. Motherhood increases the woman's status in the church and the community. In previous generations, it was not uncommon for teenagers to marry by the age of 15, and some as early as 13. Children, single or married, may return to their parents' home, where they are readily accepted, whenever the need arises.

Teens in Appalachia enter into a cultural dilemma when exposed to other lifestyles outside the home and family. Health-care providers can assist adolescents and their family members in working through these cultural differences by helping them resolve personal conflicts resulting from being exposed to different cultures and lifestyles. Some ways to promote a positive self-awareness that conveys a respect for their culture are discussing personal parenting practices and providing information about health promotion and wellness; disease, illness, and injury prevention; and health restoration and maintenance in a culturally congruent way.

Family Goals and Priorities

Appalachian families take great pride in being independent and doing things for themselves. Even though economics may permit paying others to do some tasks, great pride is taken in being able to do for oneself. This is an area in which the editor (L. Purnell) can still strongly relate to Appalachian roots. Even though reaching a financial position at which he can pay someone to do chores on home and farm, he continues to take pride in doing them for himself. For many, family priorities include men getting a job and making a living and, for women, bearing children. Traditionally, nuclear and extended families are important in the Appalachian culture, so family members frequently live in close proximity. Relatives are sought for advice on child rearing and most other aspects of daily living.

Elders are respected and honored in the Appalachian family. Grandparents frequently care for grandchildren, especially if both parents work. This form of child care is readily accepted and is an expectation in large extended families. Elders usually live close to or with their children when they are no longer able to care for themselves. The physical structure of the home is designed to assist aging parents. Many adult children do not consider nursing home placement because it is the equivalent of a death sentence. Migration of children out of the home area may force many older people to relocate outside their home area to be with their children. A dilemma occurs because they have an equally strong Appalachian value of attachment to place and family. As a compromise, some practice "snow birding"—leaving their home in the winter and moving in with their children, then returning to their home in the summer. It is not unusual for adult children to drive 3 to 5 hours on days off work to spend time with and help maintain their aging parents at their homes in Appalachia.

One's obligation to extended family outweighs the obligations to school or work. The nuclear family feels a personal responsibility for nieces and nephews and readily takes in relatives when the need arises. This extended family is important regardless of the socioeconomic level. Upon migration to urban areas, the nuclear family becomes dominant because the extended family is usually left behind in Appalachia. This strong sense of family, in which the family distrusts outsiders and values privacy, can be a deterrent to getting involved in community activities or joining self-help group activities.

The Appalachian family network can be a rich resource for the health-care provider when health teaching and assistance with personalized care are needed. For programs with Appalachians to be effective, support must begin with the family, specifically the grandmothers, and immediate neighborhood activities. The health-care provider must respect each person as an individual and be nonbureaucratic in nature. The family, rather than the individual, must be considered as the basic treatment unit.

Social status is gained from having the respect of family and friends. Formal education and position do not gain one respect. Respect has to be earned by proving that one is a good person and "living right." Living right is based on the ethic of neutrality and on being a good "Christian person." Having a job, regardless of what the work might be, is as important as having a prestigious position. Families are very proud of their family members and let the entire community know about their accomplishments. In some instances, migration to the city may result in mixed views toward one's status. Monetary gain does not necessarily improve one's status in the family and community. Rather, skills and character traits that allow one to achieve financial comfort are given high status.

Alternative Lifestyles

Alternative lifestyles such as single and divorced parents are usually readily accepted in the Appalachian culture. Same-sex couples and families living together are accepted and rarely discussed. Such acceptance is congruent with the ethic of neutrality, the Appalachian need for privacy, not interfering with others' lives unless asked to do so, avoiding arguments, and seeking agreement, even though agreement may be implied rather than spoken.

Workforce Issues
Culture in the Workplace

Because many Appalachians value family above all else, reporting to work may become less of a priority when a family member is ill or other family obligations are pressing. When family illnesses occur, many

Appalachian individuals willingly quit their jobs to care for family members. For some, the preferred work pattern is to work for an extended period of time, take some time off, and then return to work. Although work patterns may change, a deep-seated work ethic exists. Liberal leave policies for funerals and family emergencies are seen as a necessary part of the work environment.

Because personal space is important, many Appalachians use a greater distance when communicating in the workplace. Close, face-to-face encounters; hugs; and the like are rarely seen. A harmonious environment that fosters cooperation and agreement in decision making is valued and desired. Health-care providers who come from outside the area may have some difficulty establishing rapport in the workplace if they lack an understanding and appreciation for Appalachian workplace etiquette.

Appalachian individuals usually wish to maintain independent lifestyles and often frown upon or not engage in the latest fads of the larger macroculture. Although most people want progress, they also wish to remain isolated from the mainstream. Thus, more traditional Appalachians may be slower to assimilate the values of middle-class society into their daily work habits.

Issues Related to Autonomy

In general, a lack of leadership is not uncommon because ascribed status is more important than achieved status and because there is an attempt to keep hierarchal relationships to a minimum (Coyne et al., 2006). The Appalachian ethic of neutrality and the values of individualism and nonassertiveness, with a strong people orientation, may pose a dichotomous perception at work for outsiders who may not be familiar with the Appalachian way of life. However, when conflicts occur, mutual collaboration for seeking agreement is consistent with the ethic of neutrality. Because many Appalachians align themselves more closely with horizontal rather than hierarchical relationships, they are sometimes reluctant to take on management roles. When they do accept management roles, they take great pride in their work and in the organization as a whole.

Most middle-class Americans gain self-actualization through work and personal involvement with doing. Appalachians seek fulfillment through kinship and neighborhood activities of being. To foster positive and mutually satisfying working relationships, organizations should capitalize on individual strengths such as independence, sensitivity, and loyalty, which are recognized values in the Appalachian culture. Many Appalachians prefer to work at their own pace, devising their own work rules and methods for getting the job done. Some local factories, mines, lumber mills, and health-care facilities that hire managers and administrators from outside the region often provide educational seminars about the Appalachians' worldview, work culture, and way of life in order to foster cultural sensitivity and a general understanding of the people with whom they work.

Biocultural Ecology

Skin Color and Other Biological Variations

Since its first settlement, the Appalachian region has had a predominantly white population with little variation over time. Some individuals can trace their heritage to a mixture of white ancestry along with Cherokee, Apalachee, Choctaw, and other indigenous tribes of the region. A few blacks, a distinct minority of 3.2 percent, may identify themselves as Appalachian, and intermarriage with American Indians and white settlers was not uncommon (ARC, 2006a). The influence of American Indians and blacks can be seen in skin color along with pronounced epicanthic eye folds, high cheekbones characteristic for American Indian ancestory, and darker skin tones and black, curly hair that are characteristic in blacks.

Diseases and Health Conditions

Those Appalachians who have migrated and live in the urban centers of the north are often exposed to poor housing conditions that include inadequate sewage and plumbing systems, lack of refrigeration, and various environmental problems stemming from industrial pollution (Obermiller & Brown, 2002). Even those who have remained and live in Appalachia are often exposed to substandard housing where there is a lack of safe potable water and sewage disposal (ARC, 2010; GMEC, 2001).

Although national safety programs implemented by the Occupational Safety and Health Administration (OSHA) have been implemented throughout Appalachia, many people are still exposed to the harmful by-products of the predominant occupations in the region: farming, textile manufacturing, mining, furniture making, and timbering (ARC, 2006a). Occupational hazards include respiratory diseases such as black lung, brown lung, emphysema, and tuberculosis. The incidence of other health conditions including hypochromic anemia, otitis media, cardiovascular diseases, female obesity, non-insulin-dependent diabetes mellitus, and parasitic infections is greater than the national norm (GMEC, 2001; Huttlinger et al., 2004a). White Appalachian residents may have a 20 percent greater chance of dying from heart disease between the ages of 35 and 64 than other white Americans. This rate may be due to limited access to healthy foods, a general lack and use of recreational facilities, and a lack of access to medical care (Centers for Disease Control and Prevention (CDC), 2004; GMEC, 2001). Appalachia is one of the areas in the United States with the highest rate of disability (Hurley & Turner, 2000).

Coal mining comprises a major economic activity throughout Appalachia. Many of the coal mining areas have been linked to socioeconomic disadvantages among its residents. Appalachian areas where economic disadvantage has been most persistent over time are those characterized by low economic diversification, low employment in professional services, and low educational attainment rates. Rural economies that are dependent on sole-source resource extraction, such as mining, are vulnerable to employment declines and market fluctuations.

The health costs due to illness and premature deaths in the coal mining regions of Appalachia far outweigh the economic benefits to the area from the coal industry (Hendryx & Ahern, 2009). Hendryx and Ahern state that throughout Appalachia, "people in counties with no coal mining operations experience better health, a cleaner environment, and greater economic prosperity than counties where mining takes place (p. 541)." The authors maintain that while the coal mining industry had an $8 billion economic impact on Appalachia, the costs (in terms of health and shortened life span) ranged from $16 billion to $84 billion in 2005. In fact, Appalachian coal mining areas have almost 11,000 more deaths every year when compared with areas elsewhere in the United States, and about 2300 of those deaths were related to environmental factors such as air and water pollution worsened by coal mining. A sad fact is that "those who are falling ill and dying young are not just the coal miners. Everyone who lives near the mines or processing plants or transportation centers is affected by chronic socioeconomic weakness that takes a toll in longevity and health (p. 543)."

1. What specific illnesses might you associate with the coal mining industry?
2. How might a community's water table be affected by runoff from coal mines?
3. Many regions of Appalachia are experiencing "mountaintop removal" as a way to extract coal. What are the environmental consequences of "mountaintop removal"? Can you identifiy potential health risks involved with this approach?

Children are at greater risk for sudden infant death syndrome (SIDS), congenital malformations, and infections. The infant mortality rate throughout the Appalachian region varies greatly, with an overall rate of 7.7 per 100 live births, which is lower than the national average of 7.9. However, the states of Alabama, Mississippi, and North Carolina have an infant mortality rate that exceeds the national rate (ARC, 2006a). Only 70 percent of children are immunized, compared with 90 percent for the nation as a whole. Childhood injuries due to burns, trauma, poisoning, child neglect, and abuse are also higher than the national average (*Voices of Appalachia,* 2001).

Cancer, suicide, and accident rates in some parts of Appalachia are significantly greater than the national average. The higher rate of cancer in Appalachia prompted the National Cancer Institute in 1999 to create the Appalachian Leadership Initiative on Cancer (ALIC) to help communities challenge cancer at the grassroots level. Through ALIC, significant progress has been made on screening for cervical and breast cancer among low-income older women (CDC, 2004).

In many parts of Appalachia, tooth decay remains an unfortunate rite of childhood that may lead to a lifetime of poor oral health. For example, in West Virginia, dentists pulled an estimated 31,800 children's teeth in 2006 (from a population of 1.8 million). By age 65, about 40 percent of the state's retirees have none of their natural teeth remaining. Given the troubling scope and consequences of this largely preventable problem across Appalachia, several service organizations are attempting to more clearly define the causes of poor oral health in the region and develop practical, low-cost solutions (Center for Oral Health Research in Appalachia (COHRA), 2010). When prioritizing health and other needs of the family, dental health often falls last, and most people will simply "do without" or rely upon home remedies and/or home extraction (Fig. 8-2).

Educational information presented in a nonjudgmental manner can have a significant impact on the health of Appalachian patients. Patients generally prefer verbal rather than printed material to obtain health-related information. In fact, an effective success strategy used by ALIC is storytelling, a strong tradition in Appalachia and one in which people can relate. Thus, the presentation of health and educational material needs to include the entire family and be linked with improvement in function in order to be taken seriously.

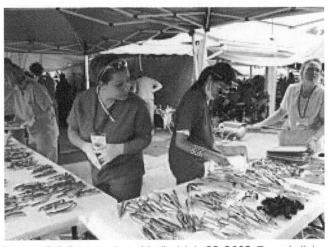

Figure 8-2 Remote Area Medical. July 23, 2003. Dental clinic. Wise, Virginia. 2003.

REFLECTIVE EXERCISE 8.1

Throughout Appalachia, general tooth decay is a problem for children and adults. Many adults who receive little or no dental care while children are faced with severe dental caries and ultimate extraction in adulthood. Some estimates indicate that by age 65, between 30 and 40 percent of the general population throughout Appalachia have none of their natural teeth remaining (National Institute of Dental and Craniofacial Research, 2011). A survey conducted by Huttlinger and colleagues in 2004 in southwestern Virginia indicated that 70 percent of the people surveyed (N = 1278) noted that they "did without" dental care and that it was not part of their overall medical priorities. In the same study, 48 percent of the people surveyed stated that they relied heavily on over-the-counter dental aids or other home treatment measures such as poultices or rubs. Extraction was seen as a final but acceptable remedy, and people who used this method performed the extraction themselves or had someone in their family do it for them. In addition, 31 percent of those surveyed related that they knew of at least one household member who had "cavities," and 26 percent noted at least one household member had lost one or more of their teeth.

All health-care providers should include a dental inspection as part of their overall health assessment. Importantly, relatively inexpensive measures such as tooth brushing and oral rinsing as a child can prevent decay, chronic pain, and the social stigma of having lost teeth throughout the lifetime.

1. What kinds of things might you observe on an oral examination of the mouth?
2. How would you respond to an individual who, during a physical examination, requests that you help him (or her) arrange to have all of her teeth pulled?
3. Identify at least three over-the-counter dental (OTC) aids that people might use to assist them with their dental problems?

Variations in Drug Metabolism

Current medical and research literature reports no studies specific to the pharmacodynamics of drug interactions among Appalachians. Given the diverse gene pool of many residents, the health-care provider needs to observe each individual for adverse drug interactions.

High-Risk Behaviors

Compared with non-Appalachians, Appalachians seem to be less concerned about their overall health and risks associated with smoking (Huttlinger et al., 2004a; 2004b). Their use of smokeless tobacco is the highest in the country, and deaths from tobacco-related uses are the highest in the nation (CDC, 2004). Underage use of tobacco and alcohol is widespread among teens.

The Appalachian definition of health encompasses three levels: body, mind, and spirit. This definition precludes viewing disease as a problem unless it interferes with one's functioning. Consequently, many conditions are denied or ignored until they progress to the point of decreasing function. (Nutrition practices are covered more extensively later in the chapter.)

OxyContin has become one of the most widely abused drugs in America. Dubbed "Hillbilly heroin," it has become the drug of choice for narcotic abusers in Appalachia. Although chronic pain sufferers are finding it increasingly difficult to obtain, elaborate OxyContin underground transportation systems have developed to sustain a lucrative drug trafficking business throughout many mountain communities (Hays, 2004; Lubell, 2006). There has been a tremendous response from lawmakers and law enforcement agencies throughout the region to curb the trafficking of OxyContin. The result is that many physicians have become increasingly unwilling to provide the drug, even to the cancer patients and chronic pain sufferers who need it (Lubell, 2006). One woman with cancer relates how she searched for seven months before she found a specialist near Cincinnati, Ohio, who would prescribe OxyContin for her (Hays, 2004).

Several states have tightened the control of OxyContin. At least nine have limited Medicaid patients' access to the drug. Virginia adopted a resolution to study the use and abuse of OxyContin, whereas Kentucky has legislation pending that would restrict distribution of the drug. In Virginia, police have provided fingerprint kits to pharmacies for customers wanting OxyContin (ARC, 2006b; Lubell, 2006).

Another high-risk behavior involves the proliferation of methamphetamine laboratories throughout Appalachia. The seclusion of mountain hollows and the number of remote and available barns and sheds have contributed to the rise in methamphetamine production. This highly addictive drug is made using common ingredients such as over-the-counter (OTC) cold medications, acetone, and rock salt. Setting up a laboratory does not require a lot of room. Unfortunately, ingredients and recipes are not hard to find. It is cooked up in homemade laboratories using items such as paint thinner, camping fuel, starter fluid, gasoline additives, mason jars, and coffee filters (U.S. Drug Enforcement Agency (DEA), 2006a).

Marijuana abuse and trafficking are serious problems throughout the region and especially in the more remote areas. Tennessee is a major supplier of domestically grown marijuana. In fact, the DEA (2006b) reported that Tennessee, along with West Virginia and Kentucky, produces the majority of the United States' supply of domestic marijuana. Prosecution of marijuana growers in the state has been extremely difficult owing to a lack of intelligence and because many of the domestic marijuana sites detected are so small that even if the owner/grower were identified, the U.S. attorney general would be reluctant to prosecute (DEA, 2006b).

Health-Care Practices

A 10-step pattern of health-seeking behaviors has been identified among Appalachians:

1. At the onset of symptoms, Appalachians typically implement self-care practices that are usually learned from mothers.
2. When the symptoms persist, they call their mother, if she is available.
3. If the mother is unavailable, they call the female in their kin network who is perceived as knowledgeable regarding health. If a nurse is available, they may seek the nurse's advice.
4. If relief is not achieved, they use OTC medicine they have seen advertised on television for symptoms that most closely match their own.
5. If that is ineffective, they use some of "Mable's medicine" (she lives down the road, had similar symptoms, and did not finish her medicine).
6. Next, they ask the local pharmacist for a recommendation; this usually marks the first encounter with a professional health provider. (Of course, they usually do not tell the pharmacist that they tried Mable's medicine.) The pharmacist may strongly suggest that they see a health-care provider; however, on their insistence, the pharmacist may recommend another OTC medication.
7. When no relief is achieved, they seek a local health-care provider or utilize local emergency- and urgent-care centers.
8. If the condition does not resolve itself, the local health-care provider refers them to a specialist in the area or to a larger urban area (e.g., Lexington, Cincinnati).
9. The specialist treats the condition to the best of her or his ability.
10. If unsuccessful, the specialist refers him or her to the closest tertiary medical center.

These 10 steps may not always follow the sequence presented here; some steps may be skipped, and not all steps are always completed. Moreover, the time frame around these 10 steps may be several years. Often by the time typical Appalachians are referred for definitive treatment, compensatory reserves have been depleted and they die at large medical centers. The story is then passed on in the "holler": "So-and-so went to [Hospital X] and died." This pattern leads to a significant mistrust of large medical centers and continued reluctance to use these facilities effectively.

Health-care providers can have a significant impact on improving a patient's health-seeking behaviors by providing information early on in the pattern of health-seeking behaviors. Nurses especially can help to reverse this pattern because they are viewed, by the clients they serve in Appalachia, as knowledgeable, nonjudgmental, and respectful of Appalachian lifestyles.

Nutrition
Meaning of Food

As with most ethnic and cultural groups, food has meaning beyond providing nutritional sustenance. To many Appalachians, wealth means having plenty of food to share with family, friends, and at social gatherings. It is generally believed that one should drink plenty of fluids and eat plenty of good food to have a strong body. A strong body is a healthy body. Food and the sharing of food have broad social implications. Appalachians love to get together with family members, friends, and neighbors for meals. Weekend meals at a family member's home are common and serve as a mechanism to share information, community events and happenings, and gossip. Church suppers are also commonplace, with members contributing favorite dishes.

Common Foods and Food Rituals

Many Appalachians, and especially those living in the more remote areas, include wild game in their diet. Muskrat, groundhog, rabbit, squirrel, duck, turkey, and venison commonly supplement "store-bought" meats. Wild game traditionally has a lower fat content than meat raised for commercial purposes. However, consistent with traditional practices from previous decades, most parts of both wild and domesticated animals are eaten. High-cholesterol organ meats such as tongue, liver, heart, lungs (called *lights*), and brains are considered delicacies. Bone marrow is used to make sauces, and stomach, intestines (chitterlings or "chitlins"), pigs' feet, tail, and ribs are also commonly eaten. Low-fat game meat is usually breaded and fried with lard or animal fat, negating the overall gains from these low-fat meat sources. Most diets include sweet prepackaged drinks, Kool-Aid with added sugar, very sweet iced tea, and soda. In fact, "sweet tea" is a year-round favorite, and most people keep a jar of it in the refrigerator or on the porch in cooler weather.

Food preparation practices may increase dietary risk factors for cardiac disease because many recipes contain lard and meats that are preserved with salt. Other common foods in particular regions of Appalachia that may be unfamiliar to nonnative Appalachians are sweet potato pie; molasses candy; apple beer; gooseberry pie; pumpkin cake; and pickled beans, fruit, corn, beets, and cabbage, all of which are high in sodium. Frying foods with bacon grease or lard was once a common practice, but recent publicity on the dangers of lard has initiated a cutback in its use in cooking (Huttlinger et al., 2004a). Fried green tomatoes, biscuits, and thick gravies are ongoing favorites.

Appalachians celebrate Thanksgiving, Christmas, other national and religious holidays, and many other occasions with food. In rural areas, people celebrate with food when game and livestock are slaughtered because this is usually an extended-family or community affair. The value of self-reliance is enhanced during the "cannin" season when foodstuffs are preserved. Canning becomes a social or family occasion and is an excellent avenue for health teaching if the health-care provider is willing to participate and learn. Additional celebrations with food occur during times of death and grieving, when friends and participants bring dishes specifically prepared for the occasion.

Dietary Practices for Health Promotion

Many Appalachians believe that good nutrition has an effect on one's health. In one study with rural Appalachians, young mothers were asked what it meant to eat well for good health. They referred to "taking fluids" and "eating right," but they were unable to describe healthy eating patterns any further (Gainor, Fitch, & Pollard, 2006). Because of health intervention programs, publicity though television, magazines, newspapers, and the Internet, residents of most Appalachian communities are aware of "good foods" and "bad foods" in terms of general health. However, a lack of money and having a meager budget that requires the use of food stamps may limit choices.

Many believe that the sooner a baby can take food other than milk, the healthier it will be. At one time, babies from the first month were fed grease, sugar, and coffee to promote hardiness, but the practice seems to have fallen by the wayside with the younger generations of mothers. The editor (L. Purnell) fondly remembers being fed teaspoons of bacon grease as a child to be sure to grow up strong and healthy. Another example is a family who saved the skin from fried chicken for him to eat to increase his body fat, because they believed that he was too thin. The Special Supplemental Nutrition Program for Women, Infants, and Children, commonly known as WIC, has done much to change some of these practices. Health-care providers have a rich opportunity to provide education in healthy eating practices. Factual information that describes health risks with early feeding of solid foods may help prevent later nutritional allergies in children.

An example of how a community intervention can work is illustrated by the decrease in the incidence of hypertension in one community. A local health-care provider participated in the "cannin'" of beans and showed the residents that the beans would remain crisp with a "tige (a pinch) of vinegar" rather than a "pile of salt." It is essential for health-care providers to assess specific food practices and food preparation practices in order to provide effective dietary counseling for health promotion and wellness. Health-care providers in clinics and school settings have an excellent opportunity to have a positive impact on the nutritional status of individuals and families. School breakfast and lunch programs, Meals on Wheels, and church-sponsored meal plans are some of the ways in which health-care providers can encourage and support families to attain better nutrition practices.

Nutritional Deficiencies and Food Limitations

A common practice for rural and urban Appalachian children is to replace meals with snacks. The most common snacks are candy, salty foods, desserts, and carbonated beverages. Many adolescents skip breakfast and lunch entirely, preferring to eat snack foods. This pattern of snacking can result in deficiencies in vitamin A, iron, and calcium.

There are no specific food limitations or enzyme deficiencies associated with the people of Appalachia. With subsistence farming and commercial farms from nearby areas, all foods for a healthy diet are readily available during the growing season. Even though the climate is ideal for growing a large variety of vegetables, broccoli, cauliflower, or asparagus are rarely seen as vegetables of choice in the mountainous regions of Appalachia.

Pregnancy and Childbearing Practices

Fertility Practices and Views Toward Pregnancy

Birth outcomes in the more rural areas of Appalachia are poorer than among middle-class white groups in rural, suburban, and urban populations. In one study that compared birth outcomes among rural, rural-adjacent, and urban women, rural women had the worst birth outcomes overall; rural-adjacent women had the best birth outcomes of the three groups, yet they were the youngest, least educated, least likely to be married, and least likely to be privately insured (Gainor et al., 2006). Contraceptive practices of Appalachians follow the general pattern of the U.S. population. Methods include birth control pills, condoms, and tubal ligation; abortion is an individual choice. A popular belief among many is that taking laxatives facilitates an abortion. As a group, a disproportionate number of teenage pregnancies occur at a younger age compared with non-Appalachians.

Fertility practices and sexual activity, both sensitive topics for many teenagers, are topics in which outsiders unknown to the family may be more effective than health-care practitioners who are known to the family. To be effective, counseling by the health-care provider must be accomplished within the cultural belief patterns of this group and must be approached in a nonhierarchical manner, preferably with a health-care provider of the same gender.

Prescriptive, Restrictive, and Taboo Practices in the Childbearing Family

Although the literature reports no specific research or studies related to prescriptive, restrictive, or taboo practices during pregnancy, the following are some of the current beliefs:

- Pregnant women subscribe to the belief that to have a healthy baby, they need to eat well and take care of themselves.
- Boys are carried higher and the mother's belly appears pointy, whereas girls are carried low.
- The expectant mother should not have her picture taken because it can cause a stillbirth.
- Reaching over one's head can cause the cord to strangle the baby.
- Wearing an opal ring during pregnancy may harm the baby.
- Being frightened by a snake or eating strawberries or citrus fruit can cause birthmarks.
- If the mother experiences a tragedy, a congenital anomaly may occur.
- If the mother craves a particular food during her pregnancy, then she should eat that food or the baby will have a birthmark resembling the craved food.

Childbearing is a family affair. The birthing mother is expected to accept childbirth as a short, intense, natural process that will bring her closer to the earth and must be endured (Gainor et al., 2006).

The literature reports no specific studies on beliefs related to postpartum practices. When a new baby is born, relatives and extended family members gather to assist the new mother with household chores until she is able to complete them herself. Some newborns wear a band around the abdomen to prevent umbilical hernias and an asafetida bag around the neck to prevent or ward off contagious diseases. The health-care professional providing pregnancy counseling to the Appalachian family needs to demonstrate an openness to discuss cultural differences.

Death Rituals
Death Rituals and Expectations

When a death is expected, family and friends may stay through the night and prepare food for the event and provide comfort for family members. Because death is such an important occasion in Appalachia, many employers give workers three days of funeral leave for deaths of extended family members. After a death, extended family and friends may spend several nights with the deceased's immediate family to prevent loneliness.

Deaths in Ohio, Michigan, and other adjoining states are frequently published in Appalachian newspapers with a notice that the individual will be returned to their mountain home for burial. Funeral services serve an important social function and are usually simple. This is a time when extended family and friends come together for services that can last for three hours or longer. The length of time for a service varies according to the age of the deceased. The service for an older person may be longer than that for a younger person. The body is displayed for hours, either in the home or at the church, so that all those who wish to view the body can do so. At the end of the service, all who wish to can view the body again, with the closest relative being the last. Many Appalachian families go to funeral homes that specialize in personal services to the Appalachian culture. Urban Appalachian areas have funeral homes that specialize in long-distance transport for burial and have become familiar with Appalachian customs to meet culturally specific requirements.

The deceased is usually buried in her or his best clothes. Some individuals have a custom-made set of clothes in which to be buried and may even design their own funeral services long before their death. A common practice is to bury the deceased with personal possessions. At the funeral home, the person's favorite chair, a picture of the deceased, or other personal items may be displayed. Flowers are more important than donations to a charity. Cremation is an acceptable practice, and disposition of the ashes is a personal decision. After the funeral services are completed, elaborate meals are served either in the home or at the church. Services are accompanied by singing before, during, and after the service. Cemeteries throughout Appalachia show frequent visitations and give a sense of place and relationship to the land. Plots are carefully tended with displays of flowers, wreaths, and flags. Other beliefs regarding burial practices include placing graveyards on hillsides for fear that graves may be flooded out in low-lying areas. If the body is exhumed and reburied, it is believed that the person might not go to heaven.

Responses to Death and Grief

Clergy help families through the grieving process by providing counseling and support to family members. Family members, fellow church members, friends, a nd community leaders often assist the bereaved. Typically, family members get together and reminisce about their deceased loved one. Friends and neighbors bring food for about a week and share memories of the "one who passed on."

Spirituality
Dominant Religion and Use of Prayer

The original inhabitants of Appalachia were mostly Protestant and Episcopalian. In the early settlement years, because central organization of churches was difficult to retain, people individualized their chosen church structure. Today, the predominant religions in the Appalachian region are Baptist, Methodist, Presbyterian, Holiness, Pentecostal, and Episcopalian. For most Appalachians, the church is the center for social and community activities. Some of the more religiously devout pray daily whether or not they formally attend church. Very often, religious beliefs are of a spiritual nature and not tied to the tenets of any singular faith and reflect the harmony of the mountains and being at one with life.

In addition to Protestant and Episcopalians, there are congregations of Roman Catholics and Jehovah's Witnesses as well as other groups who, although they call themselves Baptists, are not associated with the national church organization. These Baptist sects are quite diverse and have important central beliefs, including the belief in autonomy at the local level. As a result, many divisions have occurred within and among churches to accommodate more personal beliefs and philosophies. Regardless of the denomination, most churches in the region stress fundamentalism in religious practices and use the King James Version of the Bible.

Many small churches have lay preachers instead of trained ministers, and there is a belief that to be a preacher, a person must have a divine calling. Thus, a minister may or may not be ordained. Many of the Baptist faiths believe that baptism must be done in a river, pond, or lake so that the body can be submerged. Another practice, feet washing, is believed to demonstrate humility and occurs when men wash men's feet and women wash women's feet. Many of the more fundamentalist churches segregate women and children from men in the seating arrangement within the church; men and older boys sit on one side, and women and children sit on the opposite side. In some churches, men sit on the right side of the church to represent the "right hand of God," while women sit on the left (Huttlinger, personal communication, 2006).

Some denominations believe in divine healing, and the region is full of examples to testify to its effectiveness. Two or more weekly services are common, and revival meetings are customary. Revivals tend to be lively, allowing individuals to shout out when the spirit moves them. Some denominations speak in tongues and believe in visions. Stringed music is played in some churches.

Some freewill churches—for example, the Holiness Church—preach against attending movies, ball games, and social functions where dancing occurs. Other sects believe in handling poisonous snakes. Although the practice is rare, it is believed that the snake will not bite those who have faith. The common Bible verse "And these signs shall follow them that believe; In my name shall they cast out devils; they shall speak with new tongues; They shall take up serpents; and if they drink any deadly thing, it shall not hurt them; they shall lay hands on the sick, and they shall recover" (Mark 16:17–18) is usually associated with snake-handling practices. A few people do get bitten by snakes, and their usual course of action is to heal themselves rather than go to a hospital, even though deaths occur each year following snake-handling rituals.

Another practice, the ingestion of strychnine in small doses during religious services, is believed to increase sensory stimuli. Needless to say, this practice can precipitate convulsions if ingested in large enough amounts. Fire-handling is still practiced by some groups, again with the belief that the hot coals will not burn those who have faith.

Prayer for many Appalachians is a primary source of strength. Prayer is personally designed around specific church and religious beliefs and practices, which vary widely throughout the region and between and among churches of similar faith.

Meaning of Life and Individual Sources of Strength

Meaning in life comes from the family and "living right," which is defined by each person and usually means living right with God and in the beliefs of a chosen church. Religion tends to be less focused on institutional rituals and ceremonies and consists more of personalized beliefs in God, Christ, and church. Because life in the mountainous regions can often be harsh, religious beliefs and faith make life worth living in a grim situation. The church provides a way of coping with the hurts, pains, and disappointments of a sometimes hostile environment and becomes a source for celebration and a social outlet.

Common themes that give Appalachians strength are family, traditionalism, personalism, self-reliance, religiosity, a worldview of being, and not having undue concern about things that one cannot control, such as nature and the future. Appalachians believe that rewards come in another life, in which God repays one for kind deeds done on earth.

Spiritual Beliefs and Health-Care Practices

Within the context of **fatalism** comes the belief that what happens to the individual is largely a result of God's will. Many Appalachians may not seek health care until symptoms of illness are well advanced. This practice is described more thoroughly under "High-Risk Behaviors," earlier in this chapter. Forming partnerships between health-care providers and faith-related organizations for health promotion and illness and disease prevention has strong potential for improving the health status of Appalachians. Health-care providers who are aware of patients' religious practices and spirituality needs are in a better position to promote culturally competent health care and to incorporate nonharmful practices into patients' care plans. Health-care providers must indicate an appreciation and respect for the dignity and spiritual beliefs of Appalachians without expressing negative comments about differing religious beliefs and practices.

Health-Care Practices

Health-Seeking Beliefs and Behaviors

Beliefs that influence health-care practices for many Appalachians are derived from concepts such as family, fatalism, traditionalism, self-reliance, individualism, and the ethic of neutrality. Even though many Appalachians believe that health is God's will, the concept of self-reliance can foster good health practices through self-care. Many may not see formal biomedical health-care providers until self-medicating and folk remedies have been exhausted. At one time, Appalachians, compared with non-Appalachians, were less likely to use the emergency room or to have private physicians, but the trend has since changed, and today emergency rooms and urgent-care centers are communly used (GMEC, 2001; Obermiller & Brown, 2002).

Health information on the Appalachian patient should be gathered in the context of broader family relationships and cordiality that precedes information sharing, as the family rather than the individual is the basic unit for treatment. Because direct approaches are frowned upon, health-care providers need to learn to approach sensitive topics, such as contraception and alcohol and drug use, indirectly. Many Appalachians expect the health-care provider to establish an advocacy role and to understand and accept their cultural differences; thus, it is best to involve professionals from the same backgrounds, if they are available.

Huttlinger and colleagues (2004a) surveyed a large sample of Appalachians from southwestern Virginia and northeastern Tennessee to determine access to health care. They also addressed factors related to "good health." Over 75 percent stated that their health was "God's will," and over half stated that their families, church, and community played a vital role in their overall health and well-being.

Responsibility for Health Care

When entering the biomedical health-care arena, Appalachians might feel powerless to control their own health. They often abdicate responsibility for their own care and expect that the health-care provider will completely take over their care. Many have high expectations for their health-care provider, with an unrealistic dependence on the system and an abandonment of more self-reliance activities (Coyne et al., 2006).

One major health concern for many Appalachians is the state of the blood, which is described as being thick or thin, good or bad, and high or low; these conditions can be regulated through diet (Huttlinger, personal communication, 2006; Obermiller & Brown,

2002). Venereal disease and Rh-negative blood fall into the category of bad blood. Sour foods can also cause bad blood. Appalachian men, in general, report a greater number of backaches, with women reporting a greater number of headaches, than the rest of society (Coyne et al., 2006).

Self-care is a primary focus of health. Self-care is primarily perceived as an individual responsibility, and care is focused within the family rather than within the community. Because many Appalachians value the ability to respond to, and cope with, events of daily life, home remedies, treatments, and active consultation with family members are sought before seeking outside help (Huttlinger et al., 2004a). Good health is feeling well and being able to meet one's obligations. Care within the medical system is used when the condition is perceived as serious, does not respond to self-care, or has a high potential for death. Furthermore, because self-reliance activities and nature predominate over people, many believe that it is best to let nature heal. Health-care providers need to keep this in mind when giving explanations and instructions to make them more acceptable to patients and their families.

When older Appalachians go to a physician or another health-care provider, they usually expect immediate help. Physicians who dispense medications in their offices are seen as helpful; providing prescriptions may be interpreted as rejection. The average Appalachian patient does not understand the restrictions and limitations that are placed on physicians and nurse practitioners with respect to dispensing "sample" medications.

Health-care providers can assist Appalachian patients by reinforcing their preferred coping methods and strategies when they are ill. The five most frequently used coping methods are helping, thinking positively, worrying about the problem, trying to find out more about the problem, and trying to handle things one step at a time. Coping strategies include talking the problem over with friends, praying, thinking about the good things in life, trying to handle things one step at a time, and trying to see the good side of the situation (Hunsucker, Flannery, & Frank, 2000). When establishing rapport, a health-care provider can go a long way in achieving trust by using churches, grange halls, and other community places (e.g., libraries, schools) as meeting places for the entire family to work with Appalachian families at the community level.

Folk and Traditional Practices

A strong belief in folk medicine is a traditional part of the Appalachian culture. Using herbal medicines, poultices, and teas is common practice among individuals of all socioeconomic levels. Table 8-1 presents a reference guide for the health-care provider with the major ingredients and conditions for which the folk

IID Table 8-1 **Health Conditions and Appalachian Folk Medicine Practices**

Health Condition	Folk Medicine Practices
Arthritis	Make tea from boiling the roots of ginseng. Drink the tea or rub it on the arthritic joint.
	Mix roots of ginseng and goldenseal in liquor and drink it. Ginseng is used heavily by many Koreans and was exported to Korea in the 18th and 19th centuries.
	Eat large amounts of raw fruits and vegetables.
	Carry a buckeye around in a pocket.
	Drink tea from the stems of the barbell plant.
	Drink a mixture of honey, vinegar, and moonshine (or other liquor).
	Drink tea made from alfalfa seeds or leaves.
	Drink tea made from rhubarb and whiskey.
	Place a magnet over the joint to draw the arthritis out of the joint.
Asthma	Drink tea from the bark of wild yellow plum trees, mullein leaves, and alum. Take every 12 hours.
	Combine gin and heartwood of a pine tree. Take twice a day.
	Suck salty water up the nose.
	Smoke or sniff rabbit tobacco.
	Swallow a handful of spiderwebs.
	Smoke strong tobacco until choking occurs.
	Drink a mixture of honey, lemon juice, and whiskey.
	Inhale smoke from ginseng leaves.
Bedbugs/chiggers	Apply kerosene liberally to all parts of the body. *Caution:* Kerosene can cause significant irritation to sensitive skin, especially when exposed to sunlight.
Bleeding	Place a spiderweb across the wound. This is also used in rural Scotland.
	Put kerosene oil on the cut.
	Place soot from the fireplace into a cut. Be sure to wash out the soot after bleeding is stopped, or the area will scar.
	Apply a mixture of honey and turpentine on the bleeding wound.
	Apply a mixture of soot and lard on the wound.
	Place a cigarette paper over the wound.
	Put pine resin over the cut.
	Place kerosene oil on the wound. *Caution:* If used in large doses, kerosene will burn the skin.
Blood builders	Drink tea from the bark of a wild cherry tree.
	Combine cherry bark, yellowroot, and whiskey. Take twice each day.
	Eat fried pokeweed leaves.
Blood purifiers	Drink tea from burdock root.
	Drink tea from spice wood.
Blood tonic	Take a teaspoon of honey and a tiny amount of sulfur.
	Take a teaspoon of molasses and a tiny amount of sulfur.
	Drink tea made from bloodroot.
	Soak nails in a can of water until they become rusty. Drink the rusty water.
Boils or sores	Apply a poultice of walnut leaves or the green hulls with salt.
	Apply a poultice of the houseleek plant.
	Apply a poultice of rotten apples.
	Apply a poultice of beeswax, mutton tallow, sweet oil, oil of amber, oil of spike, and resin.
	Apply a poultice of kerosene, turpentine, petroleum jelly, and lye soap.
	Apply a poultice of heart leaves, lard, and turpentine.
	Apply a poultice of bread and milk.
	Apply a poultice of slippery elm and pork fat.
	Apply a poultice of flaxseed meal.
	Apply a poultice of beef tallow, brown sugar, salt, and turpentine.

ID Table 8-1   **Health Conditions and Appalachian Folk Medicine Practices** *Continued from page 152*

Health Condition	Folk Medicine Practices
Burns	Apply a poultice of baking soda and water. Place castor oil on the burn. Apply a poultice of egg white and castor oil. Place a potato on the burn. Wrap the burn in gauze and keep moist with salt water. Place linseed oil on the burn. Apply a poultice of lard and flour. Put axle grease on the burn. This is also a practice with some Germans in Minnesota.
Chapped hands and lips	Apply lard, grease, or tallow from pork or mutton.
Chest congestion	Apply a poultice of kerosene, turpentine, and lard to the chest. Make sure the poultice is not applied directly to the chest but rather on top of a cloth. Apply mutton tallow directly to the chest. Apply a warm poultice of onions and grease. Rub pine tar on the chest. Chew leaves and stems of peppermint. Drink a combination of ginger and sugar in hot water. Make a mixture of rock candy and whiskey. Take several teaspoons several times each day. Drink tea made from ginger, honey, and whiskey. Drink tea made from pine needles. Put goose grease on the chest. Drink red pepper tea. Eat roasted onions. Drink brine from pickles or kraut. Make tea from boneset, rosemary, and goldenrod. Make tea from butterfly weed.
Colic	Make tea from calamus root and catnip. (Calamus is a suspected carcinogen.) Tie an asafetida bag around the neck. Drink baking soda and water. Chew and swallow the juice of camel root. Massage stomach with warm castor oil. Drink ginseng tea.
Constipation	Take two tablespoons of turpentine. Combine castor oil and mayapple roots. Take castor oil or Epsom salts.
Croup	Have child wear a bib containing pine pitch and tallow. Apply cloth to the chest saturated with groundhog fat, turpentine, and lamp oil. Drink juice from a roasted onion. Apply a poultice of mutton tallow and beeswax to the back. Eat a spoonful of sugar with a drop of turpentine. Eat honey with lemon or vinegar. Eat onion juice and honey.
Diarrhea	Drink tea from the ladyslipper plant. Place soot in a glass of water, let the soot settle to the bottom of the glass, and drink the water. Drink tea made from blackberry roots. Drink tea from red oak bark. Drink blackberry or strawberry juice. Drink tea made from strawberry or blackberry leaves. Drink tea made out of willow leaves. Drink the juice from the bark of a white oak or a persimmon tree.

Continues on page 154

▋▶ Table 8-1 **Health Conditions and Appalachian Folk Medicine Practices** *Continued from page 153*

Health Condition	Folk Medicine Practices
Earache	Place lukewarm salt water in the ear.
	Put castor oil or sweet oil in the ear.
	Put sewing machine oil in the ear.
	Place a few drops of urine in the ear.
	Place cabbage juice in the ear.
	Blow smoke from tobacco in the ear.
	Place a Vicks VapoRub–soaked cotton ball in the ear.
Eye ailments	Place a few drops of castor oil in the eye.
	Drop warm, salty water in the eye.
	Drink tea made from rabbit tobacco or snakeroot.
Fever	Drink tea made from butterfly weed, wild horsemint, or feverweed.
	Mash garlic bulbs and place in a bag tied around the pulse points.
	Drink water from wild ginger.
Headache	Drink tea made of ladyslipper plants.
	Tie warm fried potatoes around the head.
	Take Epsom salts.
	Tie ginseng roots around the head.
	Place crushed onions on the head.
	Rub camphor and whiskey on the head.
Heart trouble	Drink tea made from heartleaf leaves or bleeding heart.
	Eat garlic.
High blood pressure (not to be mistaken for high blood)	Drink sarsaparilla tea.
	Drink a half cup of vinegar.
Kidney trouble	Drink tea made from peach leaves or mullein roots.
	Drink tea made from corn silk or arbutus leaves.
Liver trouble	Drink tea made from lion's tongue leaves.
	Drink tea made from the roots of the spinet plant.
Poison ivy	Urinate on the affected area.
	Take a bath in salt water and then apply petroleum jelly.
	Wash the area with bleach.
	Wash the area with the juice of the milkweed plant.
	Apply a poultice of gunpowder and buttermilk.
	Apply baking soda to wet skin.
Sore throat	Gargle with sap from a red oak tree.
	Eat honey and molasses.
	Eat honey and onions.
	Drink honey and whiskey.
	Tie a poultice of lard of cream with turpentine and Vicks VapoRub to the neck.
	Apply a poultice of cottonseed to the throat.
	Swab the throat with turpentine.

treatments are used (Fig. 8-3). These treatments can be adjusted to accommodate prescription therapies or education regarding folk treatments. Information in this table has been derived from the *Foxfire* series, the authors' backgrounds and experiences, and health-care providers who practice in the area. Note that specific amounts are not given, and in many cases, the amounts vary from person to person, according to the geographic region and local family practices. Local names are given rather than scientific names because this is how the residents identify them. Folk and traditional practices were learned from the Cherokee and Apalachee Indians living in the region and have been passed down from generation to generation. Although many of these home remedies are not harmful, some may have a deleterious effect when used to the exclusion

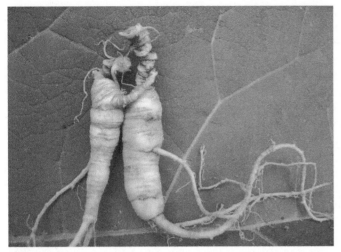

Figure 8-3 American ginseng root.

of, or in combination with, prescription medications. This should be evident from the 10-step pattern health-seeking behaviors among Appalachians presented in the section on health-care practices.

Because ingredients in some of these herbal medicines can have serious side effects, especially if taken in large quantities, health-care providers must become familiar with folk medicines used by Appalachians as part of patient assessments. Health-care providers must ascertain whether individuals intend to use folk medicines simultaneously with prescription medications and treatment regimens so that these remedies can be incorporated into the plan of care and that dialogue can be undertaken to prevent adverse effects. Health-care providers who integrate folk medicine into allopathic prescriptions have a greater chance of improving patients' compliance with health prescriptions and interventions. Health-care providers must remember that today's scientific medicine may be traditional or folk medicine to the next generation.

Barriers to Health Care

Barriers to health care for Appalachians are numerous and center on accessibility, affordability, adaptability, acceptability, appropriateness, and awareness. Bureaucratic, written forms foster fear and suspicion of health-care providers, which can lead to confusion, distrust, and negative stereotyping by both parties. Some individuals fear "being cut on" or "going under the knife" and feel that a hospital is a place where you go only to give birth or die.

As noted earlier, the rugged terrain and distance to health-care facilities and service is a deterrent to accessing services. Even though the ARC has sponsored road-building campaigns in the mountainous regions of Appalachia since 1965, transportation problems continue to exist in parts of the region (see Fig. 8-1). The high rate of unemployment in Appalachia means

REFLECTIVE EXERCISE 8.2

American ginseng (*Panax Quinquefolius*) is a therapeutic root found throughout Appalachia. Known for its strong medicinal value, ginseng (or locally known as "SANG") is grown in "patches" that are highly coveted and fiercely protected. The American species of ginseng was discovered in the Appalachia hills in the 1700s, and a significant trade for the root with China was begun. An estimated 750,000 pounds or more of wild ginseng roots were exported in 1822 (Pokladnik, 2009) and at that time sold for 2 cents per pound. Today's rates for ginseng vary from $200 to $1500 per dry pound. By the early 1900s, it was recognized that unless the ginseng root was protected, Appalachia would soon become depleted of this valuable product. Wild ginseng root is currently protected under Appendix II of the Convention of International Trade of Endangered Species, and the ginseng trade is closely monitored by the U.S. Fish and Wildlife Services (Pokladnik, 2009).

Ginseng root is sold in health food stores throughout the United States and is used to boost energy, relieve stress, improve concentration, and enhance physical or cognitive performance. Ginseng is also believed to act as a general restorative or tonic, which have strengthening properties that restore the body's balance, enhance stamina, and increase resistance to stress and disease. When compared to the Chinese variety of ginseng, the American ginseng is thought to have a more cooling or calming quality, as opposed to the Asian ginseng which is thought to have more heating or stimulating properties. According to Traditional Chinese Medical (TCM) theory, American ginseng is used to calm the ailing respiratory or digestive systems and as therapy for diabetes or "thirsty" syndromes. It also seems to be preferred by people who live in warmer climates. Native Americans traditionally employed American ginseng to help with childbirth and fertility and to strengthen mental powers, and for a variety of ailments such as respiratory disorders, headaches, and fevers.

1. How do you think the ginseng root is prepared for consumption?
2. Go to a health food store and identify the ways in which ginseng is prepared for sale (i.e., tablets, as a mixture with other plants, etc.).
3. A patient wants to include ginseng with prescriptive medication. What is your advice?

that many people cannot afford basic health care. A disproportionate number of Appalachians, especially those who are self-employed, unemployed, or underemployed, do not have health insurance. For some who do not believe in owing money, seeing a health-care provider may be postponed until the condition is severe or until they have the money. If services can be offered on a sliding scale, more people may be willing to access them.

Health-care facilities are closing in some areas of Appalachia. Most often, the closings are related to decreasing availability of health-care providers and the ability to pay competitive salaries, especially for registered nurses (Huttlinger, personal communication, 2006). These changes have resulted in the relocation of highly educated and trained professionals of all professions.

Recent studies have demonstrated that there is not a lack of primary-care providers in Appalachia (Huttlinger et al., 2004a); however, a large portion of health-care being provided by nurse practitioners is readily evident. There is, however, an acute shortage of specialty providers and especially those for respiratory and pulmonary diseases, oncology, dental services, and ophthalmology. Those physicians who settle in the region quickly learn that flexible fee schedules, patience, and hands-on treatment approaches work best. Referral to specialty care in the larger urban centers must be made with consideration of travel and other expenses. For example, a referral to a pulmonologist in Charlottesville, Virginia, for a person who lives in Wise might require a 3-day trip because 2 days are needed just to travel each way. Add to this the expense of gasoline, a relative taking off work to drive the person, and two nights in a motel, and it becomes something many Appalachians cannot afford.

Preventive health services have not been stressed in the past and are not perceived as important by many (GMEC, 2001). Even when services are available, people may feel they are not delivered in an appropriate manner. Outsider health-care providers may be seen as disrespectful of Appalachian ways and self-care practices, and patients may see the health-care providers' advice as criticism. If the health-care provider uses language that the patient does not understand, the health-care provider may be perceived as "stuck up." Many Appalachians do not like the impersonal care delivered in large clinics and, therefore, shop around and ask friends and family for suggestions for a private health-care provider. "Sittin' for a spell and engagin' in small talk" with the patient before an examination or treatment will help ensure return visits for follow-up care.

When health-care facilities have limited hours or are not adaptable, patients may not return for scheduled appointments. For example, a mother may bring her child in for an immunization. If the mother has a health problem and perhaps needs a Pap smear, she may be willing to have the test performed while having the child examined. However, if she is given an appointment to return at a later date, she may not keep the appointment because it is too far to travel for a problem she sees as nonurgent. If services are not available during evening hours, people may be afraid of taking time off during regular work hours for fear of losing their job.

Cultural Responses to Health and Illnesses

Appalachians take care of their own and accept a person as a "whole individual." Thus, those with mental impairments or physical handicaps are generally accepted into their communities and not turned away. People with a mental handicap are not seen as "crazy" but are seen as having "bad nerves," "quite turned," or "odd turned." Appalachians may label certain behaviors as "lazy," "mean," "immoral," "criminal," or "psychic" and will either recommend punishment by either the social group or the legal system or tolerate these behaviors (Obermiller & Brown, 2002).

Traditional Appalachians believe that disability is a natural and inevitable part of the aging process. Their culture of being discourages the use of rehabilitation as an option. To establish trust and rapport when working with Appalachian patients with chronic diseases, health-care providers must avoid assumptions regarding health beliefs and provide health maintenance interventions within the scope of cultural customs and beliefs.

Individual responses to pain cannot be classified among Appalachians. The Appalachian background is too varied, and no studies regarding cultural beliefs about pain could be found in the literature. For many Appalachians, pain is something that is to be endured and accepted stoically. However, when a person becomes ill or has pain, personal space collapses inward, and the person expects to be waited on and to be cared for by others. A belief among many is that if one places a knife or axe under the bed or mattress of a person in pain, the knife will help cut the pain. This practice occurs with childbearing and other conditions that cause pain. The editor (L. Purnell) is aware of an Appalachian woman who requested to have a knife or axe placed under the bed or mattress postoperatively to help cut (or decrease) the pain associated with surgery. He offered a small pocketknife or butter knife to place under the bed. Both were unacceptable as the pocketknife was too small and the butter knife was too dull to be of use. A sharp meat-cutting knife from the kitchen was deemed appropriate because it was both large enough and sharp enough to help cut the pain.

Blood Transfusions and Organ Donation

Appalachians generally do not have any specific rules or taboos about receiving blood, donating organs, or undergoing organ transplantation. These decisions are largely one's own, but advice is usually sought from family and friends.

Health-Care Providers
Traditional Versus Biomedical Providers

For decades, both lay and trained nurses have provided significant health-care services, including obstetrics. Granny midwives and more formally trained midwives have provided obstetric services throughout the history of Appalachia. Although many practitioners and herbalists are older women, men may also become healers. Grannies and herb doctors are trusted and known to the individual and the community for giving more personalized care.

The entire Appalachian area has a shortage of health personnel even though recent years have evidenced a good supply of primary-care providers, thanks to government incentives for medical school loans. As a result, nurse practitioners have delivered the bulk of health care to some areas of Appalachia (Huttlinger et al., 2004a; 2004b).

The Frontier Nursing Service, started by Mary Breckenridge, is one of the oldest and most well-known nurse-run clinics in the United States and is a notable example of nurses, midwives, and nurse practitioners taking the initiative to provide health care in Appalachia. It was started in one of the most rural areas of Appalachia in response to a lack of physicians and the high birth and child mortality rates in the area (Dawley, 2003; Jesse & Blue, 2004). Many Appalachians prefer to go to *insider* health-care professionals, especially in the more rural areas, because the system of payment for services is accepted on a sliding scale, and in some communities, even an exchange of goods for health services exists. One nurse practitioner in private practice states that the only time she locks her car is when the zucchini are "in." If she does not, when she gets in her car after a clinic session, she has no room to drive because of all the "presents" of the large vegetable.

Locally respected Appalachians are engaged to facilitate acceptance of outside programs and of the staff who participate at the grassroots level in planning and initiating programs. For Appalachian patients to become more accepting of biomedical care, it is important for health-care providers to approach individuals in an unhurried manner consistent with their relaxed lifestyle, to engage patients in decision making and care planning, and to use locally trained support staff whenever possible.

Status of Health-Care Providers

Most herbal and folk practitioners are highly respected for their treatments, mostly because they are well known to their people and trusted by those who need health care. Physicians and other health-care providers are frequently seen as outsiders to the Appalachian population and are, therefore, mistrusted. This initial mistrust is rooted in outsider behaviors that exploited the Appalachian people and took their land for timbering and coal mining in earlier generations. Trust for an outsider is gained slowly. Once the person gets to know and trust the health-care provider, the provider is given much respect. Trust and respect for health-care providers depend more on personal characteristics and personal behavior than on knowledge.

In terms of provider care, Appalachians seem to prefer home-based nurses, health-care workers, and social workers. To obtain full cooperation, the health-care provider needs to ask clients what they consider to be the problem before devising a plan of care. If the provider begins with an immediate diagnosis without considering the patient's explanation, there is a good chance that the provider's treatment or recommendation will be ignored. Lastly, it is important to decrease language barriers by decoding the jargon of the health-care environment.

REFERENCES

Appalachian Regional Commission (ARC). (2006a). Contains various articles on economics, population statistics, health-care delivery, education, and general life in Appalachia. http://www.arc.gov/

Appalachian Regional Commission (ARC). (2006b). *Twenty-six communities awarded seed grants to battle substance abuse in Appalachia.* News Brief. http://arc.gov/

Appalachian RegionalCommission (2010). The Appalachian Region. http://www.arc.gov/appalachian_region/TheAppalachian-Region.asp

Carter, M. (2005). *Nursing home quality of care in Appalachia.* Report to the Regional Research Institute. Morgantown, WV: Regional Research Institute (West Virginia University).

Center for Oral Health Research in Appalachia. (2010). *A Look at oral health disparities in Appalachia.* University of Pittsburgh. Center for Oral Health Research.

Centers for Disease Control and Prevention (CDC). (2004). *CDC report shows cancer death rates in Applachia higher than national.* https://www.scienceblog.com/community

Costello, C. (2000, May 30). Beneath myth, Melungeons find roots of oppression: Appalachian descendants embrace heritage. *The Washington Post*, p. A4.

Counts, M. M., & Boyle, J. S. (1987). Nursing, health, and policy within a community context. *Advances in Nursing Science, 9*(3), 12–23.

Coyne, C., Demian-Popescu, C., & Friend, D. (2006). Social and cultural factors influencing health in southern West Virginia: A qualitative study. *Preventing Chronic Disease, 3*(4), A. 124.

Dawley, K. (2003). Origins of nurse-midwifery in the United States and its expansion in the 1940s. *Journal of Midwifery and Womens' Health, 48*(2), 86–95.

Gainor, R., Fitch, C., & Pollard, C. (2006). Maternal diabetes and perinatal outcomes in West Virginia Medicaid enrollees. *West Virginia Medical Journal, 102*(1), 314–316.

Graduate Medical Education Consortium (GMEC). (2001, August). *Report to the board.* Wise, VA: Graduate Medical Education Consortium.

Haaga, J. (2004). *The aging of Appalachia: Demographic and socioeconomic change in Appalachia.* Washington, DC: Appalachian Regional Commission.

Hays, J. (2004). A profile of oxycontin addiction. *Journal of Addictive Disorders, 23*(4), 1–9.

Hendryx, M., & Ahern, M. (2009). Mortality in Appalachian coal mining regions: The value of statistical life lost. *Public Health Reports, 124*(4), 541–546.

Hunsucker, S., Flannery, J., & Frank, D. (2000). Coping strategies of rural families of critically ill patients. *Journal of the American Academy of Nurse Practitioners, 12*(4), 123–127.

Hurley, J., & Turner, H.S. (2000). Development of a health service at a rural community college in Appalachia. *Journal of American College Health, 48*(4), 181–189.

Huttlinger, K., Schaller-Ayers, J., & Lawson, T. (2004a). Health care in Appalachia: A population-based approach. *Public Health Nursing, 21*(2), 103–110.

Huttlinger, K., Schaller-Ayers, J., Kenny, B., & Ayers, J. (2004b). Rural, community health nursing, research and collaboration. *Online Journal of Rural Nursing and Health Care, 4*(1). www.rno.org

Jesse, D., & Blue, C. (2004). Mary Breckinridge meets *Healthy People 2010*: A teaching strategy for visioning and building healthy communities. *Journal of Midwifery & Womens' Health, 49*(2), 126–131.

Kennedy, N. (1997). *Melungeons.* Macon, GA: Mercer University Press.

Lubell, J. (2006). Virginia doctors report controlled substances. Program targets substances with high potential for abuse. *Modern Healthcare, 36*(26), 32.

National Institute of Dental and Craniofacial Research. (2010). *A look at oral health disparities in Appalachia.* http://www.nidcr.nih.gov/Research/ResearchResults/InterviewsOHR/COHRA.htm Obermiller, P., & Brown, M. (2002, February). *Appalachian health status in greater Cincinnati: A research overview.* Urban Council Working Paper No. 18. Cincinnati, OH: Urban Appalachian Council.

Pokladnik, R. (2009). *Preserving an Appalachian treasure—American ginseng.* http://www.ecowatch.org/pubs/aug09/ginseng.htm

Smith, S., & Tessaro, I. (2005). Cultural perspectives on diabetes in an Appalachian population. *American Journal of Health Behavior, 29*(4), 291–301.

University of Virginia. (2009). *Health Appalachia: Improving cancer control through telehealth in Southwestern Virginia.* http://www.virginiacpac.org/PDFs/HealthyAppalachia_0909.pdf

U.S. Drug Enforcement Agency (DEA). (2006a, September 9). *DEA briefs and backgound drugs and drug abuse, drug descriptions.* News Release. Washington, DC: Drug Enforcement Agency.

U.S. Drug Enforcement Agency (DEA). (2006b, November 29). *National methamphetamine awareness day events represent largest single-day education effort in the dangers of methamphetamine.* News Release. Washington, DC: Drug Enforcement Agency.

Voices of Appalachia Health Start Project. (2001). Whitley County Public Health Department. http://www.wcphd.com

Watkins, C. (2011). *Blacks in Appalachia.* Retrieved from http://www.museum.appstate.edu/exhibits/blacks/pages/blacks.shtml

Wilson, C.M. (1989). Elizabethan America. In W.K. Neil (Ed.), *Appalachian images in folk and popular cultures* (pp. 205–216). London: UMI Press.

DavisPlus *For reflective exercises, review questions, and additional information, go to*

http://davisplus.fadavis.com

Chapter 9

People of Arab Heritage

Anahid Dervartanian Kulwicki and Suha Ballout

Overview

Overview, Inhabited Localities, and Topography

Arabs trace their ancestry and traditions to the nomadic desert tribes of the Arabian Peninsula. They share a common language, **Arabic**, and most are united by **Islam**, a major world religion that originated in 7th-century Arabia. Despite these common bonds, Arab residents of a single Arab country are often characterized by diversity in thoughts, attitudes, and behaviors. Indeed, cultural variations may be significant within and across countries and regions. For example, a poor tradition-bound farmer from rural Yemen may appear to have little in common with an educated professional from cosmopolitan Beirut. Immigrant Arab populations may exhibit great cultural differences based on such additional factors as religion, country of origin, refugee status, time since arrival, ethnic identity, education, economic status, employment status, social support, and English language skills.

Since the September 11, 2001, terrorist attack on the United States, there has been an observable increase in hostility toward Arabs and Arab Americans. Health-care providers need to understand that few Arab Americans support the terrorist attacks and that individuals must not be stereotyped by their cultural background. A study conducted by Kulwicki and colleagues (2008) on the effects of 9/11 on Arab American nurses in Detroit revealed that Muslims and Arabs were discriminated against by being called names, intimidation, and verbal attacks about their appearance and religion. They were also subject to suspicious questioning, and the media supported this.

The diversity among Arabs makes presenting a representative account of Arab Americans a formidable task because of the variant cultural characteristics (see Chapter 1) and the limited research literature on Arabs in the Americas. The earliest Arab immigrants arrived as part of the great wave of immigrants at the end of the 19th century and the beginning of the 20th century. They were predominantly Christians from the region that is present-day Lebanon and Syria and, like most newcomers of the period, they valued assimilation and were rather easily absorbed into mainstream U.S. society. Arab Americans tend to disappear in national studies because they are counted as white in census data rather than as a separate ethnic group. Therefore, to portray Arab Americans as fully as possible, including the large numbers of new arrivals since 1965, literature that describes Arabs in their home countries is used to supplement research completed by groups studying Arab Americans residing in Michigan, Illinois, New York, Ohio, and the San Francisco Bay area of California. An underlying assumption is that the attitudes and behaviors of first-generation immigrants are similar in some aspects to those of their counterparts in the Arab world.

Islamic doctrines and practices are included because most post-1965 Arab American immigrants are **Muslims**. Religion, whether Islam, Christianity, or minority faiths, is an integral part of everyday Arab life. In addition, Islam is the official religion in most Arab countries, Lebanon being a notable exception, and Islamic law is identified as the source of national laws and regulations. Consequently, knowledge of religion is critical to understanding the Arab American patient's cultural frame of reference and for providing care that considers specific religious beliefs.

Heritage and Residence

Arab Americans are defined as immigrants from the 22 Arab countries of North Africa and Southwest Asia: Algeria, Bahrain, Comoros, Djibouti, Egypt, Iraq, Jordan, Kuwait, Lebanon, Libya, Mauritania, Morocco, Oman, Palestine, Qatar, Saudi Arabia, Somalia, Sudan, Syria, Tunisia, United Arab Emirates, and Yemen. Some Arabs may originate from neighboring states such as Chad and Iran. The Arab American Institute (2010) estimates that 3.5 million Arab Americans live in the United States, with approximately 94 percent living in metropolitan areas. The largest concentrations are in Los Angeles County, California; Wayne County, Michigan; and Kings County, New York. However,

Zogby International (2011) estimates the number of Arab Americans as three times greater than estimates from the Arab American Institute.

Reasons for Migration and Associated Economic Factors

First-wave immigrants came to the United States between 1887 and 1913 seeking economic opportunity and perhaps the financial means to return home and buy land or set up a shop in their ancestral villages. Most first-wave Arab Americans worked in unskilled jobs, were male and illiterate (44 percent), and were from mountain or rural areas (Naff, 1980). Today, 32 percent of Arab Americans are from Lebanon, and 11 percent come from Egypt (Arab American Institute, 2010).

Second-wave immigrants entered the United States after World War II; the numbers increased dramatically after the Palestinian-Israeli conflict erupted and the passage of the Immigration Act of 1965 (Naff, 1980). Unlike the more economically motivated Lebanese-Syrian Christians, most second-wave immigrants are refugees from nations beset by war and political instability—chiefly, occupied Palestine, Jordan, Iraq, Yemen, Lebanon, and Syria. Included in this group are a large number of professionals and individuals seeking educational degrees who have subsequently remained in the United States. Of the current Arab American population, 57 percent are male, 25 percent are age 18 years or younger, and 9 percent are age 65 years or older; their median age is 33 years (Arab American Institute, 2010).

Educational Status and Occupations

Because Arabs favor professional occupations, education, as a prerequisite to white-collar work, is valued. Not surprisingly, both U.S. and foreign-born Arab Americans are more educated than the average American. Over 89 percent of Arab Americans have a high school education, compared with all Americans at 81 percent, and 46 percent have a college education, compared with 28 percent of the total population (U.S. Census Bureau, 2005).

In comparison with European Americans, Arab Americans are more likely to be self-employed and much more likely to be in managerial and professional specialty occupations (U.S. Census Bureau, 2005). Nearly 44 percent are employed in managerial and professional positions, 29 percent in sales, and 11.7 percent in retail trade. Few Arab Americans are employed in farming, forestry, fishing, precision production, crafts, or work as operators and fabricators (U.S. Census Bureau, 2005). Arab American households in the United States have a mean annual income of $59,012, compared with $52,029 for all households (Arab American Institute, 2010).

Communication

Dominant Language and Dialects

Arabic is the official language of the Arab world. Modern or classical Arabic is a universal form of Arabic used for all writing and formal situations ranging from radio newscasts to lectures. Dialectal or colloquial Arabic, of which each community has a variety, is used for everyday spoken communication. Arabs often mix Modern Standard Arabic and colloquial Arabic according to the complexity of the subject and the formality of the occasion. The presence of numerous dialects with differences in accent, inflection, and vocabulary may create difficulties in communication between Arab immigrants from Syria and Lebanon and, for example, Arab immigrants from Iraq and Yemen.

An Arab person's speech is likely to be characterized by repetition and gesturing, particularly when involved in serious discussions. Arabs may be loud and expressive when involved in serious discussions to stress their commitment and their sincerity in the subject matter. Observers witnessing such impassioned communication may assume that Arabs are argumentative, confrontational, or aggressive.

English is a common second language in Egypt, Jordan, Lebanon, Yemen, Iraq, and Kuwait; French is a common second language in Algeria and Morocco. In contrast, literacy rates among adults in the Arab world vary from 70 percent for men and 30 percent for women (*CIA World Factbook*, 2011a, b, c) in Yemen; 93 percent for men and 82 percent for women in Lebanon; and 95 percent for men and 85 percent for women in Jordan. More than half speak a language other than English at home, although many have a good command of the English language (Arab American Institute, 2010). Despite this, ample evidence indicates that language and communication pose formidable problems in American health-care settings. For example, Kulwicki and Miller (1999) reported that 66 percent of respondents using a community-based health clinic spoke Arabic at home, and only 30.2 percent spoke both English and Arabic. Even English-speaking Arab Americans report difficulty in expressing their needs and understanding health-care providers.

Health-care providers have cited numerous interpersonal and communication problems including erroneous assessments of patient complaints, delayed or failed appointments, reluctance to disclose personal and family health information, and in some cases adherence to medical treatments (Kulwicki, 1996; Kulwicki, Miller, & Schim, 2000), as well as a tendency to exaggerate when describing complaints (Sullivan, 1993). This has been shown to create a barrier to access (Kulwicki, Aswad, Carmona, & Ballout, 2010).

Cultural Communication Patterns

Arab communication has been described as highly nuanced, with more communication contained in the context of the situation than in the actual words spoken. Arabs value privacy and resist disclosure of personal information to strangers, especially when it relates to familial disease conditions. Conversely, among friends and relatives, Arabs express feelings freely. These patterns of communication become more comprehensible when interpreted within the Arab cultural frame of reference. Many personal needs may be anticipated without the individual having to verbalize them because of close family relationships. The family may rely more on unspoken expectations and nonverbal cues than overt verbal exchange.

Arabs need to develop personal relationships with health-care providers before sharing personal information. Because meaning may be attached to both compliments and indifference, manner and tone are as important as what is said. Arabs are sensitive to the courtesy and respect they are accorded, and good manners are important in evaluating a person's character. Therefore, greetings, inquiries about well-being, pleasantries, and a cup of tea or coffee precede business. Conversants stand close to one another, maintain steady eye contact, and touch (only between members of the same sex) the other's hand or shoulder. Sitting and standing properly is critical, because doing otherwise is taken as a lack of respect. Within the context of personal relationships, verbal agreements are considered more important than written contracts. Keeping promises is considered a matter of honor.

Substantial efforts are directed at maintaining pleasant relationships and preserving dignity and honor. Hostility in response to perceived wrongdoing is warded off by an attitude of **maalesh**: "Never mind; it doesn't matter." Individuals are protected from bad news for as long as possible and are then informed as gently as possible. For example, they may be protected from being informed about a cancer diagnosis. When disputes arise, Arabs hint at their disagreement or simply fail to follow through. Alternatively, an intermediary, someone with influence, may be used to intervene in disputes or present requests to the person in charge. Mediation saves face if a conflict is not settled in one's favor and reassures the petitioner that maximum influence has been employed (Nydell, 1987).

Guidelines for communicating with Arab Americans include the following:

1. Health-care providers should employ an approach that combines expertise with warmth. They should minimize status differences, because Arab Americans report feeling uncomfortable and self-conscious in the presence of authority figures. Also, health-care providers should pay special attention to the person's feelings. Arab Americans perceive themselves as sensitive, with the potential for being easily hurt, belittled, and slighted (Reizian & Meleis, 1987).

2. Nurses and other health-care providers should take time to get acquainted before delving into business. If sincere interest in the person's home country and adjustment to American life is expressed, he or she is likely to enjoy relating such information, much of which is essential to assessing risk for traumatic immigration experience (see Barriers to Health Care, later in this chapter) and understanding the person's cultural frame of reference. Sharing a cup of tea does much to give an initial visit a positive beginning (Kulwicki, 1996).

3. Nurses may need to clarify role responsibilities regarding history taking, performing physical examinations, and providing health information for newer immigrants. Although some recent Arab American immigrants may now recognize the higher status of nurses in the United States, they are still accustomed to nurses functioning as medical assistants and housekeepers (see Status of Health-Care Providers, later in this chapter).

4. Nurses will need to perform a comprehensive assessment and explain the relationship of the information needed for physical complaints.

5. Health-care providers should interpret family members' communication patterns within a cultural context. Care providers should recognize that a spokesperson may answer questions directed to the patient and that the family members may edit some information that they feel is inappropriate (Kulwicki, 1996). Family members can also be expected to act as the patient's advocates; they may attempt to resolve problems by taking appeals "to the top" or by seeking the help of an influential intermediary.

6. Health-care providers need to convey hope and optimism. The concept of "false hope" is not meaningful to Arabs because they regard God's power to cure as infinite. The amount and type of information given should be carefully considered.

7. It is important to be mindful of the patient's modesty and dignity. Islamic teachings forbid unnecessary touch (including shaking hands) between unrelated adults of opposite sexes (al-Shahri, 2002). Observation of this teaching is expressed most commonly by female patients with male health-care providers and may cause the patient to be shy or hesitant in allowing the health-care provider to do physical assessments. Health-care providers must make concerted efforts to understand the patient's feelings and to take them into consideration.

Temporal Relationships

First-generation Arab immigrants may believe in predestination—that is, God has predetermined the events of one's life. Accordingly, individuals are expected to make the best of life while acknowledging that God has ultimate control over all that happens. Consequently, plans and intentions are qualified with the phrase ***inshallah***—"if God wills"—and blessings and misfortunes are attributed to God rather than to the actions of individuals.

Throughout the Arab world, there is nonchalance about punctuality except in cases of business or professional meetings; otherwise, the pace of life is more leisurely than in the West. Social events and appointments tend not to have a fixed beginning or end. Although certain individuals may arrive on time for appointments, the tendency is to be somewhat late. However, for most Arab Americans who belong to professional occupations or who are in the business field, punctuality and respecting deadlines and appointments are considered important (Kulwicki, 2001).

Format for Names

Etiquette requires shaking hands on arrival and departure. However, when an Arab man is introduced to an Arab woman, the man waits for the woman to extend her hand. Traditional Muslims may not shake hands with the opposite sex. Women and men put their hand on their chest as a gesture to replace shaking hands.

Titles are important and are used in combination with the person's first name (e.g., Mr. Khalil or Dr. Ali). Some may prefer to be addressed as mother (*Um*) or father (*Abu*) of the eldest son (e.g., Abu Khalil, "father of Khalil"). Married women usually retain their maiden names.

Family Roles and Organization

Head of Household and Gender Roles

Arab Muslim families are characterized by a strong patrilineal tradition (Aswad, 1999). Women are subordinate to men, and young people are subordinate to older people. Consequently, within his immediate family, the man is the head of the family and his influence is overt. In public, a wife's interactions with her husband are formal and respectful. However, behind the scenes, she typically wields tremendous influence, particularly in matters pertaining to the home and children. A wife may sometimes be required to hide her power from her husband and children to preserve the husband's view of himself as head of the family.

Within the larger extended family, the older male figure assumes the role of decision maker. Women attain power and status in advancing years, particularly when they have adult children. The bond between mothers and sons is typically strong, and most men make every effort to obey their mother's wishes, and even her whims (Nydell, 1987).

Gender roles are clearly defined and regarded as a complementary division of labor. Men are breadwinners, protectors, and decision makers, whereas women are responsible for the care and education of children and for maintenance of a successful marriage by tending to their husbands' needs. Although women in more urbanized Arab countries such as Lebanon, Syria, Jordan, and Egypt often have professional careers, with some women advocating for women's liberation, the family and marriage remain primary commitments for the majority. Most educated women still consider caring for their children as their primary role after marriage. The authority structure and division of labor within Arab families are often interpreted in the West as creating a subservient role for women, fueling common stereotypes of the overly dominant Arab male and the passive and oppressed Arab female. Thus, by extension, conservative Arab Americans perceive the stereotypical understanding of the subordinate role of women as a criticism of Arab culture and family values (Kulwicki, 2000).

Arabs value modesty among both men and women and typically will cover the extremities and avoid revealing garb. Many Muslim women view the ***hijab***—"covering the body except for one's face and hands"—as offering them protection in situations in which the sexes mix, because it is a recognized symbol of Muslim identity and good moral character. Ironically, many Americans associate the *hijab* with oppression rather than protection. The *hijab* is not universal, and one may find women within the same family choosing to wear or not wear it as a matter of personal choice. Even if Muslim women don't wear the *hijab* during the day, they wear it during prayer and while reading the Quran.

Prescriptive, Restrictive, and Taboo Behaviors for Children and Adolescents

In the traditional Arab family, the roles of the father and mother as they relate to the children are quite distinct. Typically, the father is the disciplinarian, whereas the mother is an ally and mediator, an unfailing source of love and kindness. Although some fathers feel that it is advantageous to maintain a degree of fear, family relationships are usually characterized by affection and sentimentality. Children are dearly loved, indulged, and included in all family activities.

Among Arabs, raising children so they reflect well on the family is an extremely important responsibility. A child's character and successes (or failures) in life are attributed to upbringing and parental influence. Because of the emphasis on collective familism rather than individualism within the Arab culture, conformity to adult rules is favored. Correspondingly, child-rearing methods are oriented toward accommodation and cooperation. Family reputation is important; children are expected to behave in an honorable manner and not bring shame to the family. Child-rearing patterns also include great respect toward parents and elders. Children are raised to not question elders and to be obedient to older brothers and sisters (Kulwicki, 1996). Methods of discipline include physical punishment and shaming. Children are made to feel ashamed because others have seen them misbehave, rather than to experience guilt arising from self-criticism and inward regret.

Whereas adolescence in the West is centered on acquiring a personal identity and completing the separation process from family, Arab adolescents are expected to remain enmeshed in the family system. Family interests and opinions often influence career and marriage decisions. Arab adolescents are pressed to succeed academically, in part because of the connections between professional careers and social status. Conversely, behaviors that would bring family dishonor, such as academic failure, sexual activity, illicit drug use, and juvenile delinquency, are avoided. For girls in particular, chastity and decency are required. Adolescence in North America may provide more opportunities for academic success and more freedom in making career choices than can be accessed by their counterparts in the Arab countries. Cultural conflicts between American values and Arab values often cause significant conflicts for Arab American families. Arab American parents cite a variety of concerns related to conflicting values regarding dating, after-school activities, drinking, and drug use (Zogby, 2002).

Family Goals and Priorities

The family is the central socioeconomic unit in Arab society. Family members cooperate to secure livelihood, rear children, and maintain standing and influence within the community. Family members live nearby, sometimes intermarry (first cousins), and expect a great deal from one another regardless of practicality or ability to help. Loyalty to one's family takes precedence over personal needs. Maintenance of family honor is paramount.

Within the hierarchical family structure, older family members are accorded great respect. Children, sons in particular, are held responsible for supporting elderly parents. Therefore, regardless of the sacrifices involved, the elderly parents are almost always cared for within the home, typically until death.

Responsibility for family members rests with the older men of the family. In the absence of the father, brothers are responsible for unmarried sisters. In the event of a husband's death, his family provides for his widow and children. In general, family leaders are expected to use influence and render special services and favors to kinsmen.

Although educational accomplishments (doctoral degrees), certain occupations (medicine, engineering, law), and acquired wealth contribute to social status, family origin is the primary determinant. Certain character traits such as piety, generosity, hospitality, and good manners may also enhance social standing.

Alternative Lifestyles

Most adults marry. Although the Islamic right to marry up to four wives is sometimes exercised, particularly if the first wife is chronically ill or infertile, most marriages are monogamous and for life. Recent studies have reported that 2 to 5 percent of Arab Muslim marriages are polygamous (Kulwicki, 2000). Whereas homosexuality occurs in all cultures to some extent, it is stigmatized among Arab cultures. In Michigan, 46 percent of the Arab HIV/AIDS cases were men having sex with men (Michigan Department of Community Health, 2010). In some Arab countries, it is considered a crime. Fearing family disgrace and ostracism, gays and lesbians remain closeted (*Global Gayz*, 2006). However, in recent years, Arab American gays and lesbians have been active in gay and lesbian organizations, and some have been outspoken and publicly active in raising community awareness about

REFLECTIVE EXERCISE 9.1

Mr. and Mrs. AbulMuna presented to the clinic with Samah, their 17-year-old daughter, who is not married. Samah was complaining of nausea and a metallic aftertaste. Mrs. AbulMuna also told the nurse that she noticed Samah was pale and seemed weak during that period. Samah also told the nurse that she was having breast tenderness for the past 2 weeks but did not get her menstrual period yet. Mr. and Mrs. AbulMuna were worried because they did not want Samah to be sick for her final exams. During the assessment, the nurse asked Samah if she was sexually active and if she could be pregnant. Mr. and Mrs. AbulMuna were angry and thought the nurse's questions were inappropriate. They argued that because Samah was unmarried, it was inappropriate for the nurse to ask her about sexual activity and pregnancy. After he left the room, the nurse could hear Mr. and Mrs. AbulMuna furiously asking Samah why the nurse would ask her such a question. Samah insisted that she believes her symptoms were related to something she ate and that she cannot possibly be pregnant. Mr. AbulMuna told the nurse they were going to take their daughter to another facility.

1. How should the nurse deal with this situation?
2. Identify culturally appropriate strategies that may be effective in addressing the needs of the AbulMuna family.
3. How might the nurse ensure that the best care is provided to Samah?
4. Should the nurse ask Samah if she might be pregnant while her parents are out of the room?

gay and lesbian rights in Arab American communities. Recently, some Arab countries like Lebanon have gay organizations that support the rights of this population and are working toward decreasing or removing the legal and cultural barriers to homosexuality. In the United States, several gay and lesbian Arab organizations are actively involved in educating the Arab communities on the rights of gay and lesbian populations, aiming at removing cultural stereotypes and stigma associated with being gay or lesbian.

Workforce Issues

Culture in the Workplace

Cultural differences that may have an impact on work life include beliefs regarding family, gender roles, one's ability to control life events, maintaining pleasant personal relationships, guarding dignity and honor, and the importance placed on maintaining one's reputation. Arabs and Americans may also differ in attitudes toward time, instructional methods, patterns of thinking, and the amount of emphasis placed on objectivity. However, because many second-wave professionals were educated in the United States, and thereby socialized to some extent, differences are probably more characteristic of less-educated, first-generation Arab Americans.

Stress is a common denominator in recent studies of first-generation immigrants. Sources of stress include separation from family members, difficulty adjusting to American life, marital tension, and intergenerational conflict, specifically coping with adolescents socialized in American values through school activities (Seikaly, 1999). Issues related to discrimination have been reported as a major source of stress among Arab Americans in their work environment. In a recent study exploring the perceptions and experiences of Arab American nurses in the aftermath of 9/11, the majority of nurses did not experience major episodes of discrimination at work such as termination and physical assaults. However, some did experience other types of discrimination such as intimidation, being treated suspiciously, negative comments about their religious practices, and refusal by some patients to be treated by them (Kulwicki & Khalifa, 2008). Arab Americans are keenly aware of the misperceptions Americans hold about Arabs, such as notions that Arabs are inferior, backward, sinister, and violent. In addition, the American public's ignorance of mainstream Islam and the stereotyping of Muslims as fanatics, extremist, and confrontational burden Muslim Arab Americans. Muslim Arab Americans face a variety of challenges as they practice their faith in a secular American society. For example, Islamic and American civil law differ on matters such as marriage, divorce, banking, and inheritance. Individuals who wish to attend Friday prayer services and observe religious holidays frequently encounter job-related conflicts. Children are often torn between fulfilling Islamic obligations regarding prayer, dietary restrictions, and dress and hiding their religious identity in order to fit into the American public school culture.

Issues Related to Autonomy

Whereas American workplaces tend to be dominated by deadlines, profit margins, and maintaining one's competitive edge, a more relaxed, cordial, and relationship-oriented atmosphere prevails in the Arab world. Friendship and business are mixed over cups of sweet tea to the extent that it is unclear where socializing ends and work begins. Managers promote optimal performance by using personal influence and persuasion, and performance evaluations are based on personality and social behavior as well as job skills.

Significant differences also exist in workplace norms. In the United States, position is usually earned, laws are applied equally, work takes precedence over family, honesty is an absolute value, facts and logic prevail, and direct and critical appraisal is regarded as valuable feedback. In the Arab world, position is often attained through one's family and connections, rules are bent, family obligations take precedence over the demands of the job, subjective perceptions often dictate actions, and criticism is often taken personally as an affront to dignity and family honor (Nydell, 1987). In Arab offices, supervisors and managers are expected to praise their employees to assure them that their work is noticed and appreciated. Whereas such direct praise may be somewhat embarrassing for Americans, Arabs expect and want praise when they feel they have earned it (Nydell, 1987).

Biocultural Ecology

Skin Color and Other Biological Variations

Although Arabs are uniformly perceived as swarthy, and whereas many do, in fact, have dark or olive skin, they may also have blonde or auburn hair, blue eyes, and fair complexions. Arabs from North Africa, such as Egypt, Morocco, and Tunis, may be black and have African features. Because color changes are more difficult to assess in dark-skinned people, pallor and cyanosis are best detected by examination of the oral mucosa and conjunctiva.

Diseases and Health Conditions

The major public health concerns in the Arab world include trauma related to motor vehicle accidents, maternal-child health, and control of communicable diseases. The incidence of infectious diseases such as tuberculosis, malaria, trachoma, typhus, hepatitis, typhoid fever, dysentery, and parasitic infestations varies between urban and rural areas and from country to country. For example, disease risks are relatively low in modern urban centers of the Arab world, but are quite high in the countryside, where animals such as goats and sheep virtually share living quarters, open toilets are commonplace, and running water is not available. Schistosomiasis (also called bilharzia), with which about one-fifth of Egyptians are infected, has been called Egypt's number-one health problem. Its prevalence is related to an entrenched social habit of using the Nile River for washing, drinking, and urinating. Similarly, outbreaks of cholera and meningitis are continuous concerns in Saudi Arabia during the Muslim pilgrimage season. In Jordan, where contagious diseases have declined sharply, emphasis has shifted to preventing accidental death and controlling noncommunicable diseases such as cancer and heart disease. Correspondingly, seat belt use, smoking habits, and pesticide residues in locally grown produce are major issues. Campaigns directed at improving children's and young adults' health include smoking prevention, hepatitis B vaccinations, and dental health programs.

Glucose-6-phosphate dehydrogenase (G-6-PD) deficiency, sickle cell anemia, and the thalassemias are extremely common in the eastern Mediterranean region, probably because carriers enjoy an increased resistance to malaria (Hamamy & Alwan, 1994). High consanguinity rates—roughly 30 percent of marriages in Iraq, Jordan, Kuwait, and Saudi Arabia are between first cousins—and the trend of bearing children up to menopause also contribute to the prevalence of genetically determined disorders in Arab countries (Hamamy & Alwan, 1994).

With modernization and increased life expectancy, multifactorial disorders—hypertension, diabetes, and coronary heart disease—have also emerged as major problems in eastern Mediterranean countries (Kulwicki, 2001). In many countries, cardiovascular disease is a major cause of death. In Lebanon, the increased frequency of familial hypercholesterolemia is a contributing factor. Individuals of Arabic ancestry are also more likely to inherit familial Mediterranean fever, a disorder characterized by recurrent episodes of fever, peritonitis, or pleurisies, either alone or in some combination.

The extent to which these conditions affect the health of Arab Americans is little understood, most notably because epidemiological studies have primarily originated from southeast Michigan, home of the highest concentration of Arab Americans in the United States. A Wayne County Health Department (1994) project, which conducted telephone surveys with Arabs residing in the Detroit, Michigan, area, identified cardiovascular disease as one of two specific risks, based on the high prevalence of cigarette smoking, high-cholesterol diets, obesity, and sedentary lifestyles. Although the prevalence of hypertension was lower in the Arab community than in the rest of Wayne County, Arab respondents were less likely to report having their blood pressure checked. In fact, lower rates for appropriate testing and screening, such as cholesterol testing, colorectal cancer screening, and uterine cancer screening, were considered a major risk for this group of Arab Americans. In recent years, the rate of mammography has increased dramatically. The Institute of Medicine's report *Unequal Treatment: Confronting Racial and Ethnic Disparities in Health Care* (2002) indicated that death rates for Arab females, compared with those of other white groups, was higher from heart disease and cancer but lower from strokes. However, the death rate for Arab males from coronary heart disease is higher when compared with that of white males. Metabolic syndrome is also highly prevalent and increased with age in both male and female Arab Americans (Jaber, Brown, Hammad, Zhu, & Herman, 2004). Lung and colorectal cancer are the two leading causes of death among Arab Americans. For Arab American men, lung cancer is the leading cause of death; breast cancer is the leading cause of death in Arab American women (Schwartz, Darwish-Yassine, & Wing, 2005).

The rate of infant mortality in the Arab world is very high, ranging from 24 per 1000 births in Syria to 108 per 1000 births in Iraq. In Bahrain, the infant mortality is low: 8.5 per 1000 births (World Health Organization [WHO], 2006). Although overall infant mortality rates for Arab Americans are the same as for white infants, figures for Michigan show a lower infant mortality rate for Arab Americans (6.2 per 1000 births) than for white infants (7.8 per 1000 births).

Variations in Drug Metabolism

Information describing drug disposition and sensitivity in Arabs is limited. Between 1 and 1.4 percent of Arabs are known to have difficulty metabolizing debrisoquine and substances that are metabolized similarly, such as antiarrhythmics, antidepressants, beta-blockers, neuroleptics, and opioid agents. Consequently, a small number of Arab Americans may experience elevated blood levels and adverse effects when customary dosages of antidepressants are prescribed. Conversely, typical codeine dosages may prove inadequate because some individuals cannot metabolize codeine to morphine to promote an optimal analgesic effect (Levy, 1993).

High-Risk Behaviors

Despite Islamic beliefs discouraging tobacco use, smoking remains deeply ingrained in Arab culture. For many Arabs, offering cigarettes is a sign of hospitality. Consistent with their cultural heritage, Arab Americans are characterized by higher smoking rates and lower quitting rates than European Americans

(Darwish-Yassine & Wang, 2005; Rice & Kulwicki, 1992). Besides smoking cigarettes, smoking tobacco through a water pipe, commonly known as a hookah, shisha, or narghile, is a common practice among both adults and youths.

According to the *2001–2002 Special Cancer Behavioral Risk Factor Survey*, Arab Americans who are 50 years and older have the highest smoking rates compared with other populations in Michigan. Smoking rates for Arab women in the same age group are considerably lower (39.9 versus 10.9 percent) (Michigan Department of Community Health and Michigan Department of Public Health Institute, 2003). Preliminary research results related to tobacco use among Arab Americans suggest that the rates of tobacco smoking among Arab American youth are considerably lower than those among non-Arab youth in Michigan, with only 16 percent of Arab youths smoking versus 34 percent of non-Arabs (Templin, Rice, Gadelrab, Weglicki, Hammad, & Kulwicki, 2003). Most recently, level of acculturation was found to influence nicotine dependence, with less-assimilated Arab Americans smoking more than other Arab Americans who primarily socialized with Americans or behaved like them (Al-Omari & Scheibmeir, 2010).

Limited information is available on alcohol use among Arab Americans. However, Islamic prohibitions do appear to influence patterns of alcohol consumption and attitudes toward drug use. In a study of publicly funded treatment centers in Michigan, Arfken, Kubiak, and Koch (2007) indicated that the number of Arab Americans admitted for substance abuse treatment centers was lower for Arab Americans than others and that most abusers were concentrated in the metropolitan Detroit area. Most common drugs used were alcohol (34.8 percent), marijuana (17.9 percent), heroin (17.4 percent), and crack cocaine (15.6 percent). The majority of patients admitted to treatment centers were male (76.3 percent), mostly unemployed (62.1 percent), and more than half were involved in the criminal justice system (58 percent). Ninety percent of the Arab respondents in the survey reported that they abstain from drinking alcohol. None reported heavy drinking, with a limited number reporting binge drinking (2.2 percent) and driving under the influence of alcohol (1.4 percent). All respondents believed that occasional use of cocaine entails "great" risk, with most saying the same about occasional use of marijuana.

The actual risk for, and incidence of, HIV infection and AIDS in Arab countries and among Arab Americans is low. However, an increase in the rate of infection has been noticed among many Arab countries and among Arab Americans (Centers for Disease Control and Prevention [CDC], 2006). The reported number of individuals having AIDS in the Arab countries varies and may not be an accurate reflection of the real incidence owing to restrictions placed on HIV/AIDS research by some Arab countries. The largest number of AIDS cases is seen in Djibouti (214); the lowest numbers of individuals reported as having AIDS are found in Palestine (1), Kuwait (11), Syria (18), Lebanon (24), Yemen (45), and Egypt (63) (WHO, 2004).

Despite the reported low rate of HIV/AIDS among Arab Americans, 4 percent of the Arab American respondents surveyed by Kulwicki and Cass in 1994 reported that they were at high risk for AIDS. In addition, the sample demonstrated less knowledge of primary routes of transmission and more misconceptions regarding unlikely modes of transmission than other populations surveyed. In 2010, the Michigan Department of Community Health [MDCH] stated that only 110 Arab Americans have ever been diagnosed with HIV and reported in Michigan. Of these, 83 are living, and 54 percent have progressed to AIDS (MDCH, 2010).

Cultural norms of modesty for Arab women are also a significant risk related to reproductive health among Arab Americans. For example, the rate of breast cancer screening among Arab women was 50.8 percent, compared with 71.2 percent for other women in Michigan. The rate of cervical Pap smears was 59.9 percent, and the rate of mammogram screenings was 51.2 percent (Kulwicki, 2000). Arab American women, especially new immigrants, may be at a higher risk for domestic violence because of the higher rates of stress, poverty, poor spiritual and social support, and isolation from family members owing to immigration (Kulwicki et al., 2010).

A systematic review of the health status of Arabs living in the United States reports the following: (1) little consensus on the rates of cardiovascular disease among Arab Americans; (2) the prevalence of hypertension is comparable to non-Hispanic whites at 13 to 30 percent; (3) the prevalence of smoking among adults is comparable to other Americans, but Arab American youths have higher smoking rates; and (4) the prevalence of diabetes mellitus is similar to other Americans (El Sayed & Galea, 2009).

Many Arab Americans are refugees fleeing war and political and religious conflicts, placing them at greater risk for psychological distress, depression, and other psychiatric illnesses (Hikmet, Hakim-Larson, Farrag, & Jamil, 2002; Kinzie, Boehnlein, Riley, & Sparr, 2002; Kira, Smith, Lewandoski, Templin, 2010). Psychological distress was also documented among immigrants who themselves were not victims of war and conflict but who worried over family members that were in areas of conflict. Studies conducted with Iraqi refugees and victims of torture in the United States identified higher prevalence of post-traumatic stress disorder and depression (Kinzie et al., 2002; Kulwicki, 2010). However, Kira and colleagues

(2006) found that although tortured Arab immigrants have multilateral trauma experiences and, thus, a significantly higher trauma dose, they have more post-traumatic growth, they are more resilient, and they practice their religion more.

Health-Care Practices

According to the Wayne County Health Department (1994), Arab Americans' risk in terms of safety is mixed. Factors enhancing safety include low rates of gun ownership and high recognition of the risks associated with having guns in the house. Conversely, lower rates of fire escape planning and seat belt usage for adults and older children (car seats are generally used for younger children), as well as higher rates of physical assaults, threaten their safety.

In most health areas surveyed in Michigan, education and income were important determinants of risk for people of Arab descent. Socioeconomic status was also a strong indicator in accessing health-care services. The Wayne County Health Department (1994) indicated that 20.5 percent of the adult Arab respondents were not covered by health insurance and 18.8 percent were on Medicaid. Use of health-care services for prenatal care was, however, higher among Arab American females than other ethnic groups in Michigan (Michigan Department of Community Health, 2009). Physical or mental disability among Arab Americans in Michigan was almost equal to that of white Americans.

Nutrition

Meaning of Food

Sharing meals with family and friends is a favorite pastime. Offering food is also a way of expressing love and friendship, hospitality, and generosity. For the traditional Arab woman, whose primary role is caring for her husband and children, the preparation and presentation of an elaborate midday meal is taken as an indication of her love and caring. Similarly, in entertaining friends, the types and quantity of food served, often several entrees, are indicators of the level of hospitality and esteem for one's guests. Honor and reputation are based on the manner in which guests are received. In return, family members and guests express appreciation by eating heartily.

Common Foods and Food Rituals

Although cooking and national dishes vary from country to country, and seasoning from family to family, Arabic cooking shares many general characteristics. Familiar spices and herbs such as cinnamon, allspice, cloves, ginger, cumin, mint, parsley, bay leaves, garlic, and onions are used frequently along with nutmeg, cardamom, marjoram, thyme, and rosemary. Skewer cooking and slow simmering are typical modes of preparation. Yogurt is used in cooking or served plain. All countries have rice and wheat dishes, stuffed vegetables, nut-filled pastries, and fritters soaked in syrup. Dishes are garnished with raisins, pine nuts, pistachios, and almonds. It is also popular to prepare hot drinks from several herbs such as chamomile.

Favorite fruits and vegetables include dates, figs, apricots, guavas, mangos, melons, apples, papayas, bananas, citrus fruits, carrots, tomatoes, cucumbers, parsley, mint, spinach, and grape leaves. Grains are also an important part of the diet such as fava beans, chickpeas, peas, corn, lentils, kidney beans, and white beans. Lamb and chicken are the most popular meats. Muslims are prohibited from eating pork and pork products (e.g., lard). Arab Christians may eat pork, but few of them do. Similarly, because the consumption of blood is forbidden, Muslims are required to cook meats and poultry until well done. Bread accompanies every meal and is viewed as a gift from God. In many respects, the traditional Arab diet is representative of the U.S. Department of Agriculture's food pyramid. Bread is a mainstay, grains and legumes are often substituted for meats, fresh fruit and juices are especially popular, and olive oil is widely used. In addition, because foods are prepared "from scratch," consumption of preservatives and additives is limited.

Lunch is the main meal in Arab households. However, this practice is changing in the United States, where the main meal is becoming more common for dinner. Encouraging guests to eat is the host's duty. Guests often begin with a ritual refusal and then succumb to the host's insistence. Food is eaten with the right hand because it is regarded as clean. Beverages may not be served until after the meal because some Arabs consider it unhealthy to eat and drink at the same time. Similar concerns may exist regarding mixing hot and cold foods.

Health-care providers should also understand **Ramadan**, the Muslim month of fasting. The fast, which is meant to remind Muslims of their dependence on God and the poor who experience involuntary fasting, involves abstinence from eating, drinking (including water), smoking, and marital intercourse during daylight hours. Although the sick are not required to fast, many pious Muslims insist on fasting while hospitalized, necessitating adjustments in meal times and medications, including medications given by nonoral routes. In outpatient settings, health-care providers need to be alert to potential nonadherence to treatment. Patients may omit or adjust the timing of medications. Of particular concern are medications requiring constant blood levels, adequate hydration, or both (e.g., antibiotics that may crystallize in the kidneys). Health-care providers may need to provide appointment times after sunset during Ramadan for individuals requiring injections (e.g., allergy shots).

Dietary Practices for Health Promotion

Arabs associate good health with eating properly, consuming nutritious foods, and fasting to cure disease. For some, concerns about amounts and balance among food types (hot, cold, dry, moist) may be traced to the prophet Mohammed, who taught that "the stomach is the house of every disease, and abstinence is the head of every remedy" (Al-Akili, 1993, p. 7). Within this framework, illness is related to excessive eating, eating before a previously eaten meal is digested, eating nutritionally deficient food, mixing opposing types of foods, and consuming elaborately prepared foods. Conversely, abstinence allows the body to expel disease.

The condition of the alimentary tract has priority over all other body systems in the Arab perception of health (Meleis, 2005). Gastrointestinal complaints are often the reason Arab Americans seek care (Meleis, 2005). Obesity is a problem for second-generation Arab American women and children, most of whom report eating American snacks that are high in fat and calories. Most women try to lose weight by reducing caloric intake (Wayne County Health Department, 1994).

Nutritional Deficiencies and Food Limitations

In Arab countries, diet is influenced by income, government subsidies for certain foods (e.g., bread, sugar, oil), and seasonal availability. Arab Americans most at risk for nutritional deficiencies include newly arrived immigrants from Yemen and Iraq (Ahmad, 2004) and Arab American households below the poverty level. Lactose intolerance sometimes occurs in this population. However, the practice of eating yogurt and cheese, rather than drinking milk, probably limits symptoms in sensitive people.

Many of the most common foods are available in American markets. Some Muslims may refuse to eat meat that is not **halal**—"slaughtered in an Islamic manner." *Halal* meat can be obtained in Arabic grocery stores and through Islamic centers or **mosques**.

Islamic prohibitions against the consumption of alcohol and pork have implications for American healthcare providers. Conscientious Muslims are often wary of eating outside the home and may ask many questions about ingredients used in meal preparation: Are the beans vegetarian? Was wine used in the meat sauce or lard in the pastry crust? Muslims are equally concerned about the ingredients and origins of mouthwashes, toothpastes, and medicines (e.g., alcohol-based syrups and elixirs), as well as insulin and capsules (gelatin coating) derived from pigs. However, if no substitutes are available, Muslims are permitted to use these preparations.

REFLECTIVE EXERCISE 9.2

Rida is a 42-year-old man diagnosed with pancreatic cancer who is receiving chemotherapy. As a side effect of his cytotoxic medications, Rida is constantly nauseated with decreased appetite. Some days, Rida would not touch any of the food on his tray. The nurse realizes that Rida is not eating his food and requests that the dietician visit him and follow up with his dietary preferences. Rida tells the dietician that he is not eating his soup and most of the food because it had meat in it, and he was not sure if the meat was *halal*. The nurse tries to explain that the food was brought based on his agreement with the dietician. Rida is uncomfortable that the nurse cannot reassure him that the meat is *halal*. Rida also doesnot believe that the food is nutritious because it does not have vegetables and salads. The nurse tries to explain that having raw vegetables is not appropriate for his neutropenia. Rida continues to express his discomfort with his dietary management.

1. Based on your readings about the Arab culture, what measures should the nurse have taken?
2. How can the nurse and the dietician enhance Rida's food intake?
3. How can the nurse prevent similar instances from taking place?

Pregnancy and Childbearing Practices

Fertility Practices and Views Toward Pregnancy

Fertility rates in the countries from which most Arab Americans emigrate range from 1.8 in Tunisia and Lebanon, to 2.4 in Morocco, to 5.2 in Yemen (UNICEF, 2008). Fertility practices of Arabs are influenced by traditional Bedouin values supporting tribal dominance, popular beliefs that "God decides family size," and "God provides," and Islamic rulings regarding birth control, treatment of infertility, and abortion.

High fertility rates are favored. Procreation is regarded as the purpose of marriage and the means of enhancing family strength. Accordingly, Islamic jurists have ruled that the use of "reversible" forms of birth control is "undesirable but not forbidden." These should be employed only in certain situations, listed in decreasing order of legitimacy, such as threat to the mother's life, too frequent childbearing, risk of transmitting genetic disease, and financial hardship. Moreover, irreversible forms of birth control such as vasectomy and tubal ligation are *haram*—"absolutely unlawful." Muslims regard abortion as *haram* except when the mother's health is compromised by pregnancy-induced disease or her life is threatened (Ebrahim, 1989). Therefore, unwanted pregnancies are dealt with by hoping one miscarries "by an act of God" or by covertly arranging for an abortion. Recently, great decline in fertility rates has occurred in Arab countries and among Arab Americans. According to Michigan's birth registration data, fertility rates among Arab Americans are highest when compared with those of the total population (Office of Minority Health, 2001).

Among Jordanian husbands, religion and the fatalistic belief that "God decides family size" were most often given as reasons why contraceptives were not used. Contraceptives were used by 27 percent of the husbands, typically urbanites of high socioeconomic status. Although the intrauterine device (IUD) and the pill were most widely favored, 4.9 percent of females used sterilization despite religious prohibitions (Hashemite Kingdom of Jordan, 1985). A survey of a random sample of 295 Arab American women in Michigan indicated that 29.1 percent of the surveyed women did not use any birth control methods because of their desire to have children, 4.3 percent did not use any form of contraceptives because of their husband's disapproval, and 6 percent did not use contraceptive methods because of religious reasons. The use of birth control pills was the highest (33.2 percent) among the users of contraceptive methods, followed by tubal ligation (12.9 percent) and IUD (10.7 percent) (Kulwicki, 2000).

Indeed, among Arab women in particular, fertility may be more of a concern than contraception because sterility in a woman could lead to rejection and divorce. Islam condones treatment for infertility, as Allah provides progeny as well as a cure for every disease. However, approved methods for treating infertility are mostly limited to artificial insemination using the husband's sperm and in vitro fertilization involving the fertilization of the wife's ovum by the husband's sperm.

Prescriptive, Restrictive, and Taboo Practices in the Childbearing Family

Because of the emphasis on fertility and the bearing of sons, pregnancy traditionally occurs at a younger age, and the fertility rate among women in the Arab world was higher than among Arab American women. However, as educational and economic conditions for Arab women have improved both in the Arab world and in the United States, fertility has fallen.

The pregnant woman is indulged and her cravings satisfied, lest she develop a birthmark in the shape of the particular food she craves. Because of the preference for male offspring, the sex of the child can be a stressor for mothers without sons. Friends and family often note how the mother is "carrying" the baby as an indicator of the baby's sex (i.e., high for a girl and low for a boy). Although pregnant women are excused from fasting during Ramadan, some Muslim women may be determined to fast and thus suffer potential consequences for glucose metabolism and hydration.

Labor and delivery are women's affairs. In Arab countries, home delivery, with the assistance of *dayahs* ("midwives") or neighbors was common because of limited access to hospitals, "shyness," and financial constraints. However, recently, the practice of home delivery has decreased dramatically in Arab countries, and hospital deliveries have become common. During labor, women openly express pain through facial expressions, verbalizations, and body movements. Nurses and medical staff may mistakenly diagnose Arab women as needing medical intervention and administer pain medications more liberally to alleviate the pain.

Care for the infant includes wrapping the stomach at birth, or as soon thereafter as possible, to prevent cold or wind from entering the baby's body (Luna, 1994). The call to prayer is recited in the Muslim newborn's ear. Male circumcision is almost a universal practice, and for Muslims, it is a religious requirement. Female circumcision is practiced in some Arab countries like Egypt.

Folk beliefs influence bathing and breastfeeding. Arab mothers may be reluctant to bathe postpartum because of beliefs that air gets into the mother and causes illness (Luna, 1994) and washing the breasts "thins the milk" (Cline, Abuirmeileh, & Roberts, 1986).

Breastfeeding is often delayed until the second or third day after birth because of beliefs that the mother requires rest, that nursing at birth causes "colic" pain for the mother, and that "colostrum makes the baby dumb" (Cline et al., 1986). Postpartum care also includes special foods such as lentil soup to increase

REFLECTIVE EXERCISE 9.3

Mrs. Khairallah is a 32-year-old pregnant woman who arrives at the delivery suite with contractions. While the nurses are getting Mrs. Khairallah to her bed, her husband calls the nurse and tells her that he demands that no man be allowed to enter his wife's room. He insists that all nurses, doctors, and other staff be female. He also does not want any male person to enter the room during the night because his wife will have her veil removed while she is sleeping. The nurse is conflicted because the doctor in the delivery suite is a male, and Mrs. Khairallah is fully dilated and ready to deliver at any time. The nurse puts a note next to the Khairallah family's room saying that males are not allowed in the room based on patient preference.

1. Based on your nursing training, evaluate the response of this nurse.
2. Explain the cultural connotations of Mr. Khairallah's behavior.
3. What can the nurse do in this situation?

milk production and tea to flush and cleanse the body. The 40 days after delivery are valued for women to rest. Mothers, in-laws, and other female members of the extended family may step in to help. The newly delivered woman expects to receive guests to congratulate her for the birth of the child from all family and friends.

A Michigan study with 2755 Arab Americans reported the experiences of Arab American mothers and infants as fairly comparable with their white counterparts with regard to adequacy of prenatal care, maternal complications, infant mortality, and birth complications. In addition, fewer Arab American mothers smoke, drink alcohol, or gain too little weight (Kulwicki, Smiley, & Devine, 2007). Although these statewide statistics are quite favorable, it is important to mention that earlier studies revealed an alarming rate of infant mortality among Arab American mothers in Dearborn, Michigan, a particularly disadvantaged community of new immigrants with high rates of unemployment. Factors contributing to poor pregnancy outcomes include poverty; lower levels of educational attainment; inability to communicate in English; personal, family, and cultural stressors; cigarette smoking; and early or closely spaced pregnancies. Fear of being ridiculed by American health-care providers and a limited number of bilingual providers limit access to health-care information.

Death Rituals

Death Rituals and Expectations

Although Arabs insist on maintaining hope regardless of prognosis, death is accepted as God's will. According to Muslim beliefs, death is foreordained and worldly life is but a preparation for eternal life. Hence, from the Qur'an, Surrah III, v. 185:

> *Every soul will taste of death. And ye will be paid on the Day of Resurrection only that which ye have fairly earned. Whoso is removed from the Fire and is made to enter Paradise, he indeed is triumphant. The life of this world is but comfort of illusion. (Pickthall, 1977, p. 70)*

Muslim death rituals include turning the patient's bed to face the holy city of Mecca and reading from the Qur'an, particularly verses stressing hope and acceptance. After death, the deceased is washed three times by a Muslim of the same sex. The body is then wrapped, preferably in white material, and buried underground as soon as possible, usually the day of or the day after death, in a brick- or cement-lined grave facing Mecca. Prayers for the deceased are recited at home, at the mosque, or at the cemetery. Women dress in black but do not ordinarily attend the burial unless the deceased is a close relative or husband. Instead, they gather at the deceased's home and read the Qur'an. Similar memorials are planned one week and 40 days after the death. Cremation is not practiced.

Family members do not generally approve of autopsy because of respect for the dead and feelings that the body should not be mutilated. Islam allows forensic autopsy and autopsy for the sake of medical research and instruction.

Death rituals for Arab Christians are similar to Christian practices in the rest of the world. Arab American Christians may have a Bible next to the patient, expect a visit from the priest, and expect medical means to prolong life if possible. Organ donations and autopsies are acceptable. Wearing black during the mourning period is also common. Widows may wear black for the remainder of their lives. For both Christians and Muslims, patients, especially children, are not told about terminal illness. The family spokesperson is usually the person who should be informed about the impending death. The spokesperson will then communicate news to family members.

Responses to Death and Grief

Mourning periods and practices may vary among Muslims and Christians emigrating from different Arab countries. Extended mourning periods may be practiced if the deceased is a young man, a woman, or a child. However, in some cases, Muslims may perceive extended periods of mourning as defiance of the will of God. Family members are asked to endure with patience and good faith in Allah what befalls them, including death. Whereas friends and relatives are to restrict mourning to 3 days, a wife may mourn for 4 months, and in some special cases, mourning can extend to 1 year. Although weeping is allowed, beating the cheeks or tearing garments is prohibited. For women, wearing black is considered appropriate for the entire period of mourning.

Spirituality

Religious Practices and Use of Prayer

Not all Arab Americans are Muslims. Prominent Christian groups include the Copts in Egypt, the Chaldeans in Iraq, and the Maronites in Lebanon (Kulwicki & Kridli, 2001). Despite their distinctive practices and liturgies, Christians and Muslims share certain beliefs because of Islam's origin in Judaism and Christianity. Muslims and Christians believe in the same God and many of the same prophets, the Day of Judgment, Satan, heaven, hell, and an afterlife. One major difference from Catholicism and Christian Orthodoxy is that Islam has no priesthood. Islamic scholars or religious **sheikhs**, the most learned individuals in an Islamic community, assume the role of *imam*, or "leader of the prayer." The imam also performs marriage ceremonies and funeral prayers and acts as a spiritual counselor or reference on Islamic teachings. Obtaining the opinion of the local imam may be a helpful intervention for Arab American Muslims struggling with health-care decisions.

As with any religion, observance of religious practices varies among Muslims. Some nominally practice their religion, whereas others are devout. However, because Islam is the state religion of most Arab countries and, in Islam, there is no separation of church and state, a certain degree of religious participation is obligatory.

To illustrate, consider a few examples of Islam's impact on Jordanian life. Because of Islamic law, abortion is investigated as a crime, and foster parenting is encouraged, whereas adoption is forbidden. The infertility treatments available are those approved by Islamic jurists. Islamic law courts rule on family matters such as marriage, divorce, guardianship, and inheritance employing *shariah*, or Islamic law. Public schools have classes on Islam and prayer rooms. School and work schedules revolve around Islamic holidays and the weekly prayer. During Ramadan, restaurants remain closed during daylight hours and workdays are shortened to facilitate fasting. Because Muslims gather for communal prayer on Friday afternoons, the workweek runs from Saturday through Thursday. Finally, because of Islamic tradition that adherents of other monotheistic religions be accorded tolerance and protection, Jordan's Christians have separate religious courts and schools, and non-Muslims attending public schools are not required to participate in religious activities. Similar arrangements exist in other Arab countries. In Saudi Arabia, the practice of other religions is officially banned.

For Arab American Christians, church is an important part of everyday life. Most celebrate Catholic and Orthodox Christian holidays with fasting and ceremonial church services. They may display or wear Christian symbols such as a cross or a picture of the Virgin Mary. There are also schools that offer classes on Christianity.

Meaning of Life and Individual Sources of Strength

For Muslims, adherents of the world's second largest religion, Islam means "submission to Allah." Life centers on worshipping Allah and preparing for one's afterlife by fulfilling religious duties as described in the Qur'an and the **hadith**, the putative sayings of the Prophet Muhammad. The five major pillars, or duties, of Islam are declaration of faith, prayer five times daily, almsgiving, fasting during Ramadan, and completion of a pilgrimage to Mecca.

Despite the dominance of familism in Arab life, religious faith is often regarded as more important. Whether Muslim or Christian, Arabs identify strongly with their respective religious groups, and religious affiliation is as much a part of their identity as family name. God and his power are acknowledged in everyday life.

Spiritual Beliefs and Health-Care Practices

Many Muslims believe in combining spiritual medicine, performance of daily prayers, and reading or listening to the Qur'an with conventional medical treatment. The devout patient may request that her or his chair or bed be turned to face Mecca and that a basin of water be provided for ritual washing or ablution before praying. Providing for cleanliness is particularly important because the Muslim's prayer is not acceptable unless the body, clothing, and place of prayer are clean.

Islamic teachings urge Muslims to eat wholesome food; abstain from pork, alcohol, and illicit drugs; practice moderation in all activities; be conscious of hygiene; and face adversity with faith in Allah's mercy and compassion, hope, and acceptance. Muslims are also advised to care for the needs of the community by visiting and assisting the sick and providing for needy Muslims.

Sometimes, illness is considered punishment for one's sins. Correspondingly, by providing cures, Allah manifests mercy and compassion and supplies a vehicle for repentance and gratitude (Al-Akili, 1993). Some emphasize that sickness should not be viewed as punishment, but as a trial or ordeal that brings about expiation of sins and that may strengthen character (Ebrahim, 1989). Common responses to illness include patience and endurance of suffering because it has a purpose known only to Allah, unfailing hope that even "irreversible" conditions might be cured "if it be Allah's will," and acceptance of one's fate. Suffering by some devout Muslims may be viewed as a means for greater reward in the afterlife (Lovering, 2006). Because of the belief in the sanctity of life, euthanasia and assisted suicide are forbidden (Lawrence & Rozmus, 2001).

Arab American Christians have spiritual beliefs related to health care that are similar or the same as Orthodox or Catholic Christians. Caring for the body and burial practices are similar. A priest is always expected to visit the patient; if the patient is Catholic, a priest administers the sacrament of the sick.

Health-Care Practices
Health-Seeking Beliefs and Behaviors

Good health is seen as the ability to fulfill one's roles. Diseases are attributed to a variety of factors such as inadequate diet, hot and cold shifts, and exposure of one's stomach during sleep, emotional or spiritual distress, and envy or the evil eye. Arabs are expected to express and acknowledge their ailments when ill. Muslims often mention that the Prophet urged physicians to perform research and the ill to seek treatment because "Allah has not created a disease without providing a cure for it" (Ebrahim, 1989, p. 5), except for the problem of old age

Despite beliefs that one should care for health and seek treatment when ill, some Arab women are often reluctant to seek care. Because of the cultural emphasis placed on modesty, some women express shyness about disrobing for examination. Similarly, some families object to female family members being examined by male physicians. Because of the fear that a diagnosed illness, such as cancer or psychiatric illness, may bring shame and influence the marriage ability of the woman and her female relatives, delays in seeking medical care may be common.

Evidence also suggests that the cultural preference for male offspring influences the health care that low-income parents provide for female children. In poor communities in Jordan, boys were better nourished, more likely to be immunized, and more apt to receive prompt medical attention for illnesses (West, 1987). Delay in seeking treatment was noted by a local health-care provider who diagnosed "failure to thrive" in a young Iraqi female infant when her refugee parents sought medical attention for a feverish male sibling.

Whereas Arab Americans readily seek care for actual symptoms, preventive care is not generally sought (Kulwicki, 1996; Kulwicki et al., 2000). Similarly, pediatric clinics are used primarily for illness and injury rather than for well-child visits (Lipson, Reizian, & Meleis, 1987). Laffrey, Meleis, Lipson, Solomon, and Omidian (1989) attributed these patterns to Arabs' present orientation and reluctance to plan and to the meaning that Arab Americans attach to preventive care. Whereas American health-care providers focus on screening and managing risks and complications, Arab Americans value information that aids in coping with stress, illness, or treatment protocols. Arab Americans' failure to use preventive care services may be related to other factors such as insurance coverage, the availability of female physicians who accept Medicaid patients, and the novelty of the concept of preventive care for immigrants from developing countries.

Responsibility for Health Care

Dichotomous views regarding individual responsibility and one's control over life's events often cause misunderstanding between Arab Americans and health-care providers (Abu Gharbieh, 1993). For example, individualism and an activist approach to life are the underpinnings of the American health-care system. Accordingly, practices such as informed consent, self-care, advance directives, risk management, and preventive care are valued. Patients are expected to use information seeking and problem solving in preference to faith in God, patience, and acceptance of one's fate as primary coping mechanisms. Similarly, American health-care providers expect that the patient's hope be "realistic" in accordance with medical science.

However, in the Arab culture, quite different values, familism, and reliance on God's will influence health care and responses to illness. For Arabs, the family is the context within which health care is delivered (Lipson et al., 1987). Rather than engage in self-care and decision making, patients often allow family members to oversee care. Family members indulge the individual and assume the ill person's responsibilities. Although the patient may seem overly dependent and the family overly protective by American standards, family members' vigilance and "demanding behavior" should be interpreted as a measure of concern. For Muslims, care is a religious obligation associated with individual and collective meanings of honor (Luna, 1994). Individuals are seen as expressing care through the performance of gender-specific role responsibilities as delineated in the Qur'an.

Although most American health-care providers consider full disclosure an ethical obligation, most Arab physicians do not believe that it is necessary for a patient to know a serious diagnosis or full details of a surgical procedure. In fact, communicating a grave diagnosis is often viewed as cruel and tactless because it deprives patients of hope. Similarly, preoperative instructions are believed to cause needless anxiety, hypochondriasis, and complications. In Lebanon, a qualitative study revealed that communication with the physician was a means of relieving stress among cancer patients (Doumit & Abu-Saad, 2008). However, some patients still prefer the traditional nondisclosure approach, and thus it is best to ask patients what they want to know about their illness. Apart from the educated, most patients are not interested in actively participating in decision making (Abu Gharbieh, 1993). Most Arabs expect physicians, because of their expertise, to select treatments. The patient's role is to cooperate. The authority of physicians is seldom challenged or questioned. When treatment is successful, the physician's skill is recognized; adverse outcomes are attributed to God's will unless there is evidence of blatant malpractice (Sullivan, 1993).

Not all Arabs may be familiar with the American concept of health insurance. Traditionally, the family unit, through its communal resources, provides insurance. Certain Arab countries, such as Saudi Arabia, Syria, and Kuwait, provide free medical care, whereas in other countries many citizens are government employees and are entitled to low-cost care in government-sector facilities. Private physicians and hospitals are preferred because of the belief that the private sector offers the best care.

Because many medications requiring a prescription in the United States are available over the counter in Arab countries, Arabs are accustomed to seeking medical advice from pharmacists. In comparison with other Americans in Wayne County, Arab Americans were less likely to take prescription medications, but when they did, they were more likely to use medications as directed (Wayne County Health Department, 1994).

Folk Practices

Although Islam disapproves of superstition, witchcraft, and magic, concerns about the powers of jealous people, the evil eye, and certain supernatural agents such as the devil and **jinn** are part of the folk beliefs. Those who envy the wealth, success, or beauty of others are believed to cause adversity by a gaze, which brings misfortune to the victim. Beautiful women, healthy-looking babies, and the rich are believed to be particularly susceptible to the evil eye, and expressions of congratulations may be interpreted as envy. Protection from the evil eye is afforded by wearing amulets, such as blue beads or figures involving the number 5; reciting the Qur'an; or invoking the name of Allah (Kulwicki, 1996). Barren women, the poor, and the unfortunate are usually suspects for casting the evil eye. Mental or emotional illnesses may be attributed to possession by evil *jinn*, or demons. Some believe that insanity or jinaan ("possession by the jinn") may also be caused by the evil wishes of jealous individuals.

Traditional Islamic medicine is based on the theory of four humors and the spiritual and physical remedies prescribed by the Prophet. Because illness is viewed as an imbalance between the humors— black bile, blood, phlegm, and yellow bile—and the primary attributes of dryness, heat, cold, and moisture, therapy involves treating with the disease's opposite: hot disease, cold remedy. Although methods such as cupping, cautery, and phlebotomy (bloodletting) may be employed, treating with special prayers or simple foods such as dates, honey, salt, and olive oil is preferred (Al-Akili, 1993). Yemeni or Saudi Arabian patients may apply heat (cupping, moxibustion) or use cautery in combination with modern medical technology.

Barriers to Health Care

Newly arrived and unskilled refugees from poorer parts of the Arab world are at particular risk for both increased exposure to ill health and inadequate access to health care. Factors such as refugee status, recency of arrival, differences in cultural values and norms, inability to pay for health-care services, and inability to speak English add to the stresses of immigration (Kulwicki, 2000; Kulwicki et al., 2010) and affect both health status and responses to health problems. Moreover, these immigrants are less likely to receive adequate health care because of cultural and language barriers, lack of transportation, limited health insurance, poverty, a lack of awareness of existing services, and poor coordination of services (Kulwicki, 1996; 2000; 2010).

Although a lack of insurance coverage is a factor for a significant number of Wayne County Health Department respondents (Wayne County Health Department, 1994), other studies suggest that Arab Americans regard other barriers and services as more significant. For instance, language and communication remain serious barriers for recent Arab American immigrants (Kulwicki, 2000; 2010). Transportation to health-care facilities and culturally competent service providers also adds to the problems of accessing health-care services.

Cultural Responses to Health and Illness

Arabs regard pain as unpleasant and something to be controlled (Reizian & Meleis, 1986). Because of their confidence in medical science, Arabs anticipate immediate postoperative relief from their symptoms. This expectation, in combination with a belief in conserving energy for recovery, often contributes to a reluctance to comply with typical postoperative routines such as frequent ambulation. Although expressive, emotional, and vocal responses to pain are usually reserved for the immediate family, under certain circumstances, such as childbirth and illnesses accompanied by spasms, Arabs express pain more freely (Reizian & Meleis, 1986). The tendency of Arabs to be more expressive with their family and more restrained in the presence of health-care providers may lead to conflicting perceptions regarding the adequacy of pain relief. Whereas the nurse may assess pain relief as adequate, family members may demand that their relative receive additional analgesia.

The attitude that mental illness is a major social stigma is particularly pervasive. Psychiatric symptoms may be denied, attributed to "bad nerves" (Hattar-Pollara, Meleis, & Nagib, 2001), or blamed on evil spirits (Kulwicki, 1996). Underrecognition of signs and symptoms may occur because of the somatic orientation of Arab patients and physicians, patients' tolerance of emotional suffering, and relatives' tolerance of behavioral disturbances (El-Islam, 1994). Indeed, home management with standard but crucial adjustments within the family may abort or control symptoms until remission occurs. For example, female family members manage the mother's postpartum depression by assuming care of the newborn and/or by telling the mother she needs more help or more rest. Islamic legal prohibitions further confound attempts to estimate the incidence of problems such as alcoholism and suicide, resulting in underreporting of these conditions because of potential for social stigma.

When individuals suffering from mental distress seek medical care, they are likely to present with a variety of vague complaints, such as abdominal pain, lassitude, anorexia, and shortness of breath. Patients often expect and may insist on somatic treatment, at least "vitamins and tonics" (El-Islam, 1994). When mental illness is accepted as a diagnosis, treatment by medications rather than by counseling is preferred. In a sample of United Arab Emirates subjects, the main treatment adopted for psychiatric illness was prayer, herbal ingredients, or both, while counseling by a psychiatrist was preferred the least due to stigma (Salem, Saleh, Yousef, & Sabri, 2009). Hospitalization is resisted because such placement is viewed as abandonment (Budman, Lipson, & Meleis, 1992). Although Arab Americans report family and marital stress as well as various mental health symptoms, they often seek family counseling or social services rather than a psychiatrist (Aswad & Gray, 1996). A study in 2007 suggested that immigrant Muslim women in the United States are at an increased risk for experiencing anxiety and depressive symptoms, as well as stressors such as acculturative stress, discrimination, and trauma (Hassouneh & Kulwicki, 2007).

Yousef (1993) described the Arab public's attitude toward the disabled as generally negative, with low expectations for education and rehabilitation. Yousef also related misconceptions about mental retardation to the dearth of Arab literature about disability and the public's lack of experience with the disabled. Because of social stigma, the disabled are often kept from public view. Similarly, although there is a trend toward educating some children with mild mental retardation in regular schools, special education programs are generally institutionally based.

Reiter, Mar'i, and Rosenberg (1986) found that parents who were most intimately involved with the developmentally disabled held rather positive attitudes. More tolerant views were expressed among Arab-Israeli parents, Muslims, the less educated, and residents of smaller villages than among Christians, the educated, and residents of larger villages with mixed populations. Reiter and colleagues (1986) linked the less positive attitudes of the latter groups to the process of modernization, which affects a drive toward status and a weakening of family structures and traditions. Traditions include regarding the handicapped as coming from God, accepting the disabled person's dependency, and providing care within the home.

Dependency is accepted. Family members assume the ill person's responsibilities. The ill person is cared for and indulged. From an American frame of reference, the patient may seem overly dependent and the family overly protective.

Blood Transfusions and Organ Donation

Although blood transfusions and organ transplants are widely accepted, organ donation is a controversial issue among Arabs and Arab Americans. Practices of organ donation may vary among Arab Muslims and non-Muslims based on their religious beliefs about death and dying, reincarnation, or their personal feelings about helping others by donating their organs to others or for scientific purposes (Kulwicki, 2001). Health-care providers should be sensitive to personal, family, or religious practices toward organ donation among Arab Americans and should not make any assumptions about organ donation unless family members are asked.

Health-Care Providers
Traditional Versus Biomedical Providers

Although Arab Americans combine traditional and biomedical care practices, they are very cognizant of the effective medical treatments in the West and consider themselves privileged to be able to use the American health-care system (Kulwicki, 1996). Because of their profound respect for medicine, Arab Americans seek treatments for physical disorders or ailments. Medical treatments that require surgery, removal of causative agents, or eradicating by intravenous treatments are valued more than therapies aimed at health promotion or disease prevention. Although most Arab Americans have high regard for medicine related to physical disorders, many do not have the same respect or trust for mental or psychological/psychiatric treatment. A pervasive feeling among many Arab Americans is that psychiatric services or therapies related to mental disorders are not effective and are required only for individuals who have severe mental disorders or who are considered "crazy." Psychiatric services are, therefore, underutilized among Arab Americans despite greater need for such services among distressed immigrant populations.

Gender and, to a lesser extent, age are considerations in matching Arab patients and health-care providers. In Arab societies, unrelated males and females are not accustomed to interacting. Shyness in women is appreciated, and Muslim men may ignore women out of politeness. Health-care settings, patient units, and sometimes waiting rooms are segregated by sex. Male nurses never care for female patients.

Given this background, many Arab Americans may find interacting with a health-care provider of the opposite sex quite embarrassing and stressful. Discomfort may be expressed by refusal to discuss personal information and a reluctance to disrobe for physical assessments and hygiene. Arab American women may refuse to be seen by male American health-care providers, excluding or denying men the opportunity to interact or appropriately diagnose health conditions for high-risk Arab American females.

Status of Health-Care Providers

Arab Americans have great respect for science and medicine. Most Arab Americans are aware of the historical contributions of Arabs in the field of medicine and are proud of their accomplishments. Knowledge held by a doctor is believed to convey authority and power. When ill, most Arab American patients who lack English communication skills prefer to see Arabic-speaking doctors because of their feelings of cultural and linguistic affinity toward Arab American doctors. Many Arabic-speaking patients also feel that Arab American doctors understand them better, and they feel more at ease speaking with someone from their own culture. However, patients who are able to communicate in English do not usually show preferences for seeing Arab doctors over American doctors. In some cases, these patients prefer to be seen by American doctors because they view American doctors as more professional and more respectful to patients than their Arab American counterparts.

Although medicine is perhaps the most respected prestigious profession in Arab society, nursing is viewed as a menial profession that conflicts with societal norms proscribing certain female behavior. In this conservative culture, in which contact between unrelated males and females is often discouraged, nursing is considered particularly undesirable as an occupation because it requires close contact between the sexes and work during evening and night hours (Abu Gharbieh, 1993). American nurses are regarded more favorably because of their education, expertise, and performance of roles ascribed solely to Arab physicians (e.g., performing physical examinations). However, younger immigrants, and especially immigrants who come from Lebanon, Iraq, and Jordan, have more favorable perceptions about nursing as a profession than the older generation of Arab American immigrants (Kulwicki & Kridli, 2001).

Perhaps because Arab physicians tend to be older males and Arab nurses are typically young females, the status and roles of physicians and nurses mirror the hierarchical family structure of Arab society. Physicians require that nurses "know their place" and leave the interpretation of data, decision making, and disclosure of information to them. Nurses conform to the role expectations of physicians and the public, and they function as medical assistants and housekeepers rather than as critical thinkers and health educators. Recently, nursing has established professional organizations in many Arab countries that resemble the American Nurses Association.

REFERENCES

Abu Gharbieh, P. (1993). Culture shock. Cultural norms influencing nursing in Jordan. *Nursing and Health Care, 14*(10), 534–540.

Ahmad, N.M. (2004). Arab-American culture and health care. Retrieved from http://www.case.edu/med/epidbio/mphp439/Arab-Americans.html

Al-Akili, M. (1993). *Natural healing with the medicine of the prophet.* Philadelphia, PA: Pearl Publishing House.

Al-Omari, H., & Scheibmeir, M. (2010). Arab Americans' acculturation and tobacco smoking. *Journal of Transcultural Nursing, 20*(2), 227–233.

Al-Shahri, M.Z. (2002). Culturally sensitive caring for Saudi patients, *Journal of Transcultural Nursing, 13*(2), 133–138.

Arab American Institute. (2010). *Demographics.* Retrieved from http://www.aaiusa.org/arab-americans/22/demographics

Arab human development report. (2000). Retrieved from http://www.UNESCO.org/education

Arfken, C.L., Kubiak, S.P., & Koch, A.L. (2007). Health issues in the Arab American community. Arab Americans in publicly financed substance abuse treatment. *Ethnicity Disease, 17*(2 Suppl 3), S3-72–S3-76.

Aswad, B. (1999). Arabs in America: Building a new future. In M.W. Suleiman (Ed.), *Attitudes of Arab immigrants toward welfare* (pp. 177–191). Philadelphia: Temple University Press.

Aswad, B.C., & Gray, N. (1996). Challenges to the Arab-American family and ACCESS (Arab Community Center for Economic and Social Services). In B.C. Aswad & B. Bilgé (Eds.), *Family and gender among American Muslims: Issues facing Middle Eastern immigrants and their descendants* (pp. 223–240). Philadelphia: Temple University Press.

Budman, C., Lipson, J., & Meleis, A. (1992). The cultural consultant in mental health care: The case of an Arab adolescent. *American Journal of Orthopsychiatry, 62*(3), 359–370.

Centers for Disease Control and Prevention (CDC). (2012). *Complete HIV/AIDS resource.* Retrieved from www.cdc.gov/hiv/

CIA World Factbook. (2011a). *Jordan.* Retrieved from https://www.cia.gov/library/publications/the-world-factbook/geos/jo.html

CIA World Factbook. (2011b). *Lebanon.* Retrieved from https://www.cia.gov/library/publications/the-world-factbook/geos/le.html

CIA World Factbook. (2011c). *Yemen.* Retrieved from https://www.cia.gov/library/publications/the-world-factbook/geos/ym.html

Cline, S., Abuirmeileh, N., & Roberts, A. (1986). *Woman's life cycle. Fundamentals of health education* (pp. 48–77). Yarmouk, Jordan: Yarmouk University.

Darwish-Yassine, M., & Wang, D. (2005). Cancer epidemiology in Arab Americans and Arabs outside the Middle East. *Ethnicity and Disease, 15,* S1–S8.

Doumit, M.A., & Abu-Saad, H.H. (2008). Lebanese cancer patients: Communication and truth-telling preferences. *Contemporary Nurse, 28,* 74–82

Ebrahim, A. (1989). *Abortion, birth control and surrogate parenting. An Islamic perspective.* Indianapolis, IN: American Trust Publications.

El-Islam, M. (1994). Cultural aspects of morbid fears in Qatari women. *Social Psychiatry Psychiatric Epidemiology, 29,* 137–140.

El Sayed, A.M., & Galea, S. (2009). Health of Arab Americans living in the United States: A systematic review of the literature. *BMC Public Health, 9.* Retrieved from http://www.biomedcentral.com/

Global Gayz: Muslims. (2006). Retrieved from http://www.global-gayz.com/art-index.html#middleeast

Hamamy, H., & Alwan, A. (1994). Hereditary disorders in the Eastern Mediterranean region. *Bulletin of the World Health Organization, 72*(1), 145–154.

Hashemite Kingdom of Jordan, Department of Statistics. (1985). *Jordan's husbands' fertility survey.* Amman, Jordan: Author, in collaboration with Division of Reproductive Health, Centers for Disease Control and Prevention, Atlanta, GA.

Hassouneh, D.M., & Kulwicki, A. (2007). Mental health, discrimination, and trauma in Arab Muslim women living in the U.S.: A pilot study. *Mental Health, Religion & Culture, 10*(3), 257–262.

Hattar-Pollara, M., Meleis, A.I., & Nagib, H. (2001). A study of spousal role of Egyptian women in clerical jobs. *Health Care for Women International, 21*(4), 305–517.

Hikmet, J., Hakim-Larson, J., Farrag, M., & Jamil, L. (2002). A retrospective study of Arab American mental health clients: Trauma and the Iraqi refugees. *American Journal of Orthopsychiatry, 72,* 355–361.

Institute of Medicine (2002).*Unequal treatment: Confronting racial and ethnic disparities in health care.* Retrieved from http://www.iom.edu/?id=4475

Jaber, L.A., Brown, M.B., Hammad, A., Nowak, S.N., Zhu, Q., Ghafoor, A., & Herman, W.H. (2003). Epidemiology of diabetes among Arab Americans. *Diabetes Care, 26*(2), 308–313.

Jaber, L.A., Brown, M.B., Hammad, A., Zhu, Q., & Herman, W.H. (2004). The prevalence of the metabolic syndrome among Arab Americans. *Diabetes Care, 27,* 234–238.

Kinzie, J., Boehnlein J.K., Riley, C., & Sparr, L. (2002). The effects of September 11 on traumatized refugees: Reactivation of posttraumatic stress disorder. *Journal of Nervous and Mental Disease, 190,* 437–441.

Kira, I., Smith, I, Lewandoski, L., & Templin, T. (2010). The effects of gender discrimination on refugee torture survivors: A cross-cultural traumatology perspective. *Journal of American Psychiatric Nurses Association, 16,* 299–306.

Kira, I., Templin, T., Lewandoski, L., Clifford, D., Wieneck, P., Hammad, A., et al. (2006). The effects of torture: Two community studies. *Peace and Conflict: Journal of Peace Psychology, 12*(3), 205–228.

Kulwicki, A. (1996). Health issues among Arab Muslim families. In B.C. Aswad & B. Bilgé (Eds.), *Family and gender among American Muslims: Issues facing Middle Eastern immigrants and their descendants* (pp. 187–207). Philadelphia: Temple University Press.

Kulwicki, A. (2000). Arab women. In M. Julia (Ed.), *Constructing gender: Multicultural perspectives in working with women* (pp. 89–98). Nelson, BC, Canada: Brooks/Cole.

Kulwicki, A. (Ed.). (2001). *Ethnic resource guide.* Dearborn, MI: Henry Ford Hospital.

Kulwicki, A., Aswad, B., Carmona, T., & Ballout, S. (2010). Barriers in the utilization of domestic violence services among Arab immigrant women: Perceptions of professionals, service providers & community leaders. *Journal of Family Violence, 25*(8), 727–735.

Kulwicki, A., & Cass, P. (1994). An assessment of Arab-American knowledge, attitudes, and beliefs about AIDS.*IMAGE: Journal of Nursing Scholarship, 26*(1), 13–17.

Kulwicki, A., & Khalifa, R. (2008). The impact of September 11, 2001, on Arab American nurses in Michigan. *Journal of Transcultural Nursing, 19*(2), 134–139.

Kulwicki, A., & Kridli, S. (2001). *Health-care perceptions and experiences of Chaldean, Arab Muslim, Arab Christian, and Armenian women in the metropolitan area of Detroit.* Unpublished manuscript.

Kulwicki, A., & Miller, J. (1999). Domestic violence in the Arab American population: Transforming environmental conditions through community education. *Issues in Mental Health Nursing, 20*(3) 199–215.

Kulwicki, A., Miller, J., & Schim, S. (2000). Collaborative partnership for culture care: Enhancing health services for the Arab community. *Journal of Transcultural Nursing, 11*(1), 31–39.

Kulwicki, A., Smiley, K., & Devine, S. (2007). Smoking behavior in pregnant Arab Americans. *The American Journal of Maternal/Child Nursing, 32*(6), 363–367.

Laffrey, S., Meleis, A., Lipson, J., Solomon, M., & Omidian, P. (1989). Assessing Arab-American health care needs. *Social Science and Medicine, 29*(7), 877–883.

Lawrence, P., & Rozmus, C. (2001). Culturally sensitive care of the Muslim patient. *Journal of Transcultural Nursing, 12,* 228–233.

Levy, R. (1993). Ethnic and racial differences in response to medicines: Preserving individualized therapy in managed pharmaceutical programmes. *Pharmaceutical Medicine, 7,* 139–165.

Lipson, J., Reizian, A., & Meleis, A. (1987). Arab-American patients: A medical record review. *Social Science and Medicine, 24*(2), 101–107.

Lovering, S. (2006). Cultural attitudes and beliefs about pain. *Journal of Transcultural Nursing, 17*(4), 389–395.

Luna, L. (1994). Care and cultural context of Lebanese Muslim immigrants: Using Leininger's theory. *Journal of Transcultural Nursing, 5*(2), 12–20.

Meleis, A. (2005). Arabs. In J. Lipson & S. Dibble (Eds.), *Culture and clinical care* (pp. 42–57). San Francisco, CA: The Regents, University of California.

Michigan Department of Community Health. (2009). National Trends and Deterrent Strategies for Prescription and OTC Drug Abuse. Retrieved from www.deadiversion.usdoj.gov/pubs/presentations/stermidcpgov09.pdf

Michigan Department of Community Health. (2010). *2010 Profile of HIV/AIDS in Michigan—Special populations: Arab-Americans.* Retrieved from http://www.michigan.gov/documents/mdch/21 arab_335588_7.pdf

Michigan Department of Community Health. (2010). *Michigan Department of Community Health 2009 health disparities report.* Lansing, MI: Author.

Michigan Department of Public Health. (1994). *Health profiles of Michigan populations.* Lansing, MI: Author.

Michigan Department of Community Health and Michigan Public Health Institute. (2003). *2001–2002 special cancer behavioral risk factor survey.* Lansing, MI: Author.

Naff, A. (1980). *Arabs in America: A historical overview* (pp. 128–136). Boston: Harvard Encyclopedia of American Ethnic Groups.

Nydell, M. (1987). *Understanding Arabs. A guide for Westerners.* Yarmouth, ME: Intercultural Press.

Office of Minority Health (OMH). (2001). *Health facts.* Retrieved from http://www.mdch.state.mi.us/pha/omh/aram-ch.htm

Pickthall, M. (1977). *The meaning of the glorious Qur'an.* Mecca, Saudi Arabia: Muslim World League.

Reiter, S., Mar'i, S., & Rosenberg, Y. (1986). Parental attitudes toward the developmentally disabled among Arab communities in Israel: A cross-cultural study. *International Journal of Rehabilitation Research, 9*(4), 335–362.

Reizian, A., & Meleis, A. (1986). Arab-Americans' perceptions of and responses to pain. *Critical Care Nurse, 6*(6), 30–37.

Reizian, A., & Meleis, A. (1987). Symptoms reported by Arab-American patients on the Cornell Medical Index (CMI). *Western Journal of Nursing Research, 9*(3), 368–384.

Rice, V., & Kulwicki, A. (1992). Cigarette use among Arab Americans in the Detroit metropolitan area. *Public Health Reports, 107*(5), 589–594.

Salem, M.O., Saleh, B., Yousef, S., & Sabri, S. (2009). Help-seeking behavior of patients attending the psychiatric service in a sample of United Arab Emirates population. *International Journal of Social Psychiatry, 55*(2), 141–148.

Schwartz, S., Darwish-Yassine, M., & Wing, D. (2005). Cancer diagnosis in Arab Americans and Arabs outside the United States. *Ethnicity and Disease, 15,* 1–8.

Seikaly, M. (1999). Arabs in America: Building a new future. In M.W. Suleiman (Ed.), *Attachment and identity: The Palestinian community of Detroit* (pp. 25–38). Philadelphia: Temple University Press.

Sullivan, S. (1993). The patient behind the veil: Medical culture shock in Saudi Arabia. *Canadian Medical Association Journal, 148*(3), 444–446.

Templin, T., Rice, H., Gadelrab, H., Weglicki, L., Hammad, A., & Kulwicki, A. (2003). Michigan Trends in tobacco use among Arab/Arab American adolescents: Preliminary findings. *Ethnicity and Disease, 15*(1), S-65–S-69.

UNICEF. (2008). United Nations Population Division. Retrieved from http://www.unicef.org/infobycountry/index.html

U.S. Census Bureau. (2005). Special Report. We the People of Arab Ancestry in the United States. Retrieved from http://www.census.gov/prod/2005pubs/censr-21.pdf

Wayne County Health Department. (1994). *Arab community in Wayne County, Michigan: Behavior risk factor survey (BRFS)*. East Lansing, MI: Michigan State University, Institute for Public Policy and Social Research.

West, M. (1987, April 29). Surveys indicate girls face discrimination in provision of nutrition and health care. *Jordan Times.*

World Health Organization (WHO). (2004). *Regional database on HIV/AIDS*, WHO Regional Office for the Eastern Mediterranean. Retrieved from http://www.emro.who.int/asd/

World Health Organization (WHO). (2006). *Country and selection for infant deaths*. Retrieved from www.who.int/whosis/database/mort/table2.cfm

Yousef, J. (1993). Education of children with mental retardation in Arab countries. *Mental Retardation, 31*(2), 117–121.

Zogby, J. (2002). *What Arabs think: Values, beliefs and concerns*. Retrieved from http://www.zogby.com/News/ReadNews.dbm?ID=629

Zogby International. (2011). Retrieved from www.ibopezogby.com/

DavisPlus *For case studies, review questions, and additional information, go to*
http://davisplus.fadavis.com

Chapter 10

People of Chinese Heritage

Hsiu-Min Tsai

Overview, Inhabited Localities, and Topography

Overview

Although some Western health-care providers, including some research, categorize all Asians into aggregate data as if they were one group, each nationality is very different. Cultural values differ even among Chinese according to their geographic location within China—north, south, east, west; rural versus urban; interior versus port city—as well as other variant cultural characteristics (see Chapter 1). Chinese immigrants to Western countries are even more diverse, with a mixture of traditional and Western values and beliefs. These differences must be acknowledged and appreciated.

Han Chinese are the principal ethnic group of China, constituting about 91.5 percent of the population of mainland China, especially as distinguished from Manchus, Mongols, Huis, and other minority nationalities. The remaining 8.5 percent are a mixture of 56 different nationalities, religions, and ethnic groups (*CIA World Factbook*, 2011). Substantial genetic, linguistic, cultural, and social differences exist among these subgroups. Because of the complexity of their values, it is critical to consider social and cultural contexts to develop appropriate interventions and provide culturally competent care for multiethnic Chinese patients. The information included in this chapter is only a beginning point for understanding the Chinese people; it is not meant to be a definitive profile.

Children born to Chinese parents in Western countries tend to adopt the Western culture easily, whereas their parents and grandparents tend to maintain their traditional Chinese culture in varying degrees. Chinese who live in the "Chinatowns" of North America and other places outside of China maintain many of their cultural and social beliefs and values and insist that health-care providers respect these values and beliefs with their prescribed interventions.

Heritage and Residence

The Chinese culture is one of the oldest in recorded human history, beginning with the Xia dynasty, dating from 2200 B.C., to the present-day People's Republic of China (PRC). The Chinese name for their country is ***Zhong guo***, which means "middle kingdom" or "center of the earth." Many of the current values and beliefs of the Chinese remain grounded in their history; many believe that the Chinese culture is superior to other Asian cultures. Ideals based on the teachings of Confucius (551–479 B.C.) continue to play an important part in the values and beliefs of the Chinese. These ideals emphasize the importance of accountability to family and neighbors and reinforce the idea that all relationships embody power and rule. Although industrialization, urbanization, and interaction with Western society have affected some Chinese, the ideas and behavioral patterns related to Confucianism are still deep-seated.

During early Communist rule, an attempt was made to break down the values grounded in Confucianism and substitute values consistent with equal social responsibility. This was initially achieved, and rank in society was no longer seen as important. During the People's Revolution, feudal rank frequently meant loss of social importance, physical punishment, imprisonment, and even death. Later, during the Cultural Revolution, the young were held responsible for the deaths of many previously esteemed older adults and educated Chinese. Today, many of the Confucian values have reasserted themselves. Families, older adults, and highly educated individuals are again considered important. Research completed by the Chinese Culture Connection, a group of Chinese sociologists, lists 40 important values in modern China, including filial piety, industry, patriotism, paying deference to those in hierarchical status positions, tolerance of others, loyalty to superiors, respect for rites and social rituals, knowledge, benevolent authority, thrift, patience, courtesy, and respect for tradition (Hu & Grove, 1991).

Since China's economic reforms social development in the late 1990s, the Chinese society has been on the stage of full transformation. According to Chinese sociologists, the main social values consist of richness, democracy, harmony, and innovation (Chen, 2009).

The population of China is 1.37 billion people, with 7.1 million in Hong Kong, over 550,000 in Macau, and over 23.1 million in Taiwan (National Bureau of Statistics of China, 2011). According to 2010 National statistics, 50.32 percent live in rural communities, a decrease of approximate 133.2 million persons since the 2000 census. In other words, urban residents increased by 13.46 percentage points compared with the 2000 population census (Wang, 2011a). The higher level of urbanization is a result of economic and social development.

China is over 9.6 million square kilometers (3.7 million square miles), with 23 provinces; 5 regions, including Tibet, Hong Kong, and Taiwan; and 4 municipalities. Each province, region, and municipality functions independently and in many different ways. The Chinese consider each region as part of greater China and predict that the day will come when all of China is reunited. Tibet has already been reassimilated, Hong Kong returned to Chinese control in 1997, and Macau in 1999 (*CIA World Factbook*, 2011).

The largest communities of Chinese Americans are in California, New York, Florida, and Texas. Chinese Americans compose the largest subgroup among Asians/Pacific Islanders (APIs), exceeding 3.6 million people (U.S. Census Bureau, 2006).

Reasons for Migration and Associated Economic Factors

Chinese immigrated to the United States in three different waves: in the 1800s, in the 1950s, and in the past several years. Chinese immigration was initially fueled by economic needs. Over 100,000 male peasants from Guangdong and Fujian came to the United States without their families in the early 1830s to make their fortune on the transcontinental railroad. This immigration continued through the Gold Rush of 1849. Many believed that they could make money in the United States to help their families and later return to China. Unfortunately, most found that opportunities were limited to hard labor and other vocations not desired by European Americans. Their culture and physical features made them readily identifiable in the predominantly white American society. They could not simply change their names and blend in with other, primarily European immigrant populations. The Chinese had few rights and were barred from becoming U.S. citizens. Racial violence and prejudice against them were common, and the courts did not punish the violators. Compared with other ethnic groups, their immigration numbers were small until 1952, when the McCarran-Walters Bill relaxed immigration laws and permitted more Chinese to enter the country (U.S. Citizenship and Immigration Services, 2011).

The most recent immigrants from Taiwan, Hong Kong, and mainland China are strikingly different from earlier Chinese immigrants in that they are more diverse. In addition, whereas many emigrated to reunite with their families, students, scholars, and professionals flocked to the United States to pursue higher education or research. For their safety and the maintenance of their cultural values, most Chinese settled in closed communities.

Educational Status and Occupations

Influenced by the Confucian principles, the Chinese people believe that "to be a scholar is to be at the top of society" (Ho & Lee, 2010). In Chinese society, academic achievement is highly valued for increasing one's own career benefits and enhancing a family's reputation and position. Chinese parents are much more willing to provide their children with the best possible education and invest huge sums of money in supplementary education.

Education is compulsory in China, and most children receive the equivalent of a ninth-grade education. Middle school students must complete a state examination to determine their eligibility to enter a general high school, to go to a preparatory high school before entering technical school or college, or to begin their lives as employees. Those who complete either the general or the preparatory high school experience compete academically to continue their education at college and university levels. The Chinese educational system is complex and is not presented here in its entirety; further study is encouraged.

A university education is highly valued; however, few have the opportunity to achieve this life goal because enrollments in better educational institutions are limited. Because competition for top universities is keen, many families select less valued universities to ensure that their child is accepted into a university rather than slated for a technical school education. After their undergraduate or graduate programs, many young adults come to Western countries to attend universities to seek more advanced education or research. A foreign education is considered prestigious in Chinese society.

In the West, initially the Chinese tend to be either highly or poorly educated. This dichotomy may result in health-care providers categorizing patients in a similar manner. Many people believe that Chinese occupations are limited to restaurant work, service employment, and the garment industry. However, this phenomenon has changed since the 1980s. A significant number of Chinese students and scholars from the PRC and Taiwan come to the United States to study every year. Because of the competitive educational system in mainland China and Taiwan, where only the brightest students go to a university, Chinese immigrants with a college education are often very well educated. Student immigrants are expected to return to China or Taiwan when their education and research are completed. However, many do not return but elect to remain in Western countries, having obtained graduate degrees in the United States, and many find employment in high-technology companies or educational and research institutes.

Another group of Chinese immigrants are professionals from Hong Kong who moved to North America and other Western countries to avoid repatriation in 1997. These immigrants usually have family connections or close friends who are highly educated and skilled in Western countries. A third group of immigrants consists of uneducated individuals with diverse manual labor skills. Finding employment opportunities for this group may be more difficult. They often settle with family members who are not skilled or highly educated. This arrangement drains family resources for many years until they obtain financial security, learn the language, and become acculturated in other ways.

Communication

The Chinese speak a variety of different languages and dialects. The official language of China is *Mandarin* (**pu tong hua**), which means "common speech" (Cheung, Nelson, Advincula, Young, & Canham, 2005) spoken by about 70 percent of the population, primarily in northern China, but there are 10 major, distinct dialects, including Cantonese, Fujianese, Shanghainese, Toishanese, and Hunanese. For example, *pu tong hua* is spoken in Beijing, the capital of China in the north, and Shanghainese is spoken in Shanghai. The two cities are only 1462 kilometers (about 665 miles) apart, but because the dialects are so different, the two groups cannot understand one another verbally. Even though people from one part of China cannot understand those from other regions, the written language is the same throughout the country and consists of over 50,000 characters (about 5000 common ones); thus, most children are at least 10 to 12 years old before they can read the newspaper.

Most Chinese people tend to be more passive and less sharing when explaining or discussing something, whereas Americans appreciate more direct and clear explanations. Many Americans might not understand these communication practices and become upset because they consider Chinese communication to be indirect and offensive. In addition, the Chinese are less likely to tell the other party things that may upset him or her (O'Keefe & O'Keefe, 1997). Because of this communication style, the Chinese might avoid sharing a health concern such as a mental illness, a chronic disease, or cancer when consulting with unfamiliar health-care providers about a specific health issue. To prevent misunderstanding, American health-care providers have to be aware of these differences.

Although many times the Chinese sound loud when talking with other Chinese, they generally speak in a moderate to low voice. Americans are considered loud to most Chinese, and health-care providers must be cautious about their voice volume when interacting with Chinese patients in English so intentions are not misinterpreted.

When possible, health-care providers should use the Chinese language to communicate (Table 10-1 lists some common phrases), being careful to avoid jargon and to use the simplest terms. Many times, verbs can be omitted because the Chinese language has only a limited number of verbs. The Chinese appreciate any attempt to use their language. They do not mind mistakes and will correct speakers when they believe it will not cause embarrassment. When asked whether they understand what was just said, the Chinese invariably answer yes, even when they do not understand because admitting it is embarrassing to them. Thus, it is better to have Chinese patients repeat the instructions they have been given or ask them to give a demonstration.

Negative queries are difficult for the Chinese to understand. For example, do not say, "You know how to do that, don't you?" Instead say, "Do you know how to do that?" Also, it is easier for them to understand instructions placed in a specific order, such as the following:

1. At 9 o'clock every morning, get the medicine bottle.
2. Take two tablets out of the bottle.
3. Get your hot water.
4. Swallow the pills with the water.

Do not use complex sentences with *ands* and *buts*. The Chinese have difficulty deciding what to respond to first when the speaker uses compound or complex sentences.

Cultural Communication Patterns

There is a very obvious difference between traditional Chinese communication patterns and American communication patterns. The Chinese have a reputation for not openly displaying emotion. They tend not to discuss their concerns with health-care providers, while most Americans are willing to openly give and accept comments with others. The Chinese often consider their concerns to be personal and to be shared only with the family, friends, and relatives. They might share information freely with health-care providers once a trusting relationship has developed. This is not always easy, because Western health-care providers may not have the patience or time to develop such

Ⅲ Table 10-1 | **Frequently Used Words and Phrases**

English Word or Phrase	Chinese Pinyin	Phonetic Pronunciation
Hello	Nǐ hǎo	Nee how (note tones to be used*)
Good-bye	Zài jiàn	Dzai jee en
How are you?	Nǐ hǎo mā	Nee how mah
Please	Qing	Ching
Thank you	Xīe xie	Shee eh shee eh
I don't understand	Wǒ bù dǒng	Wah boo doong
Yes	Shì de or duì	Shur da or doee (no real yes or no comparable saying—this means I agree or okay)
No	Bú shì de or bu hǎo	Boo shur or boo how
My name is	Wǒ jiào	Wah djeeow
Very good	Hen hǎo	Hun hao
Hurt	Téng	Tung
I, you, he/she/it	Wo, nǐ, tā	Wah, nee, tah
Hot	Rè	Ruh
Cold	Leng	Lung
Happy	Gāo xi ngu	Gow shing
Where	Nǎ li	Na lee
Not have	MeiYou	May yo
Doctor	Yī shēng	Yee shung
Nurse	Hù shi	Who shur

*Each *pu tong hua* Chinese word is pronounced with five different tones: First tone is high and even across the word (–); Second tone starts low and goes high (–`);Third tone starts neutral, goes low, and then goes high (˘); Fourth tone is curt and goes low (·`); Fifth tone is neutral and pronounced very slowly.

relationships. In situations in which Chinese people perceive that health-care providers or other people of authority may lose face or be embarrassed, they may choose not to be totally truthful. As a result, they may always give a "no" response when unfamiliar health-care providers ask them questions.

Touching between health-care providers and Chinese patients should be kept to a minimum. Most Chinese maintain a formal distance with one another, which is a form of respect. Some are uncomfortable with face-to-face communications, especially when there is direct eye contact. Because they prefer to sit next to others, the health-care providers may need to rearrange seating to promote positive communication. When touching is necessary, the health-care provider should provide explanations to Chinese patients.

Facial expressions are used extensively among family and friends. The Chinese love to joke and laugh. They use and appreciate smiles when talking with others. However, if the situation is formal, smiles may be limited. In most greeting and communication situations, shaking hands is common; hugs are limited. The health-care provider should watch for cues from their Chinese patients.

Format for Names

Among the Chinese, introductions, either by name card or verbally, are different from those in Western countries. For example, the family name is stated first and then the given name. Calling individuals by any name except their family name is impolite unless they are close friends or relatives. If a person's family name is Li and the given name is Ruiming, then the proper form of address is Li Ruiming. Men are addressed by their family name, such as *Ma*, and a title such as *Ma xian sheng* ("Mister Ma"), *lao Ma* ("respected older Ma"), or *xiao Ma* ("young Ma"). Titles are important to the Chinese people, so, when possible, identify the person's title and use it.

Women in China do not use their husband's last name after they get married and retain their own family last name. Therefore, unless the woman is from Hong Kong or Taiwan, or has lived in a Western country for a long time, do not assume that her last name is the same as her husband's. Her family name comes first, followed by her given names, and finally by her title. Many Chinese living in Western countries take an English name as an additional given name because their name is difficult for Westerners to pronounce. Their English name can be used in many settings. Addressing them as "Miss Millie" or "Mr. Jonathan" rather than simply by their English name is better. Even though they have adopted an English name, some Chinese may give permission to use only the English name. In addition, some Chinese switch the order of their names to be the same as Westerners, with their family name last.

REFLECTIVE EXERCISE 10.1

Mr. Wang is a 75-year-old first-generation Chinese American and lives with his 70-year-old Chinese wife. Mr. Wang speaks very limited English, while his wife speaks only Chinese. Mr. Wang visited a clinic, where he was told by his physician that he had lung cancer. The physician wanted Mr. Wang to be hospitalized for further treatment and chemotherapy. Mr. Wang gave no response.

1. What barriers might exist for Mr. Wang in deciding to accept hospitalization and seek treatment?
2. What concerns might the nurse have regarding a support system for Mr. Wang if he decides to have his lung cancer treated?
3. With the limited English-language ability of Mr. Wang and his wife, how can a health-care professional ensure effective communication?
4. If Mr. Wang prefers traditional Chinese medical treatment, how might the nurse respond?

This practice can be confusing; therefore, health-care providers should address Chinese patients by their whole name or by their family name and title, and then ask them how they wish to be addressed.

Family Roles and Organization
Head of Household and Gender Roles

Kinship traditionally has been organized around the male lineage. Fathers, sons, and uncles are the important, recognized relationships between and among families in politics and in business. Each family maintains a recognized head who has great authority and assumes all major responsibilities for the family. A common and desirable domestic traditional structure is to have four generations under one roof. However, with the improvement in the standards of living and other changes, families have gradually gotten smaller. The first generation of one-child families appeared in the 1970s when China introduced a policy of family planning. This phenomenon led to the nuclear family of three (parents and one child) gradually becoming the mainstream family structure in cities. In 2010, of 401.52 million family households in China, the average number of people in each household was 3.10, or 0.34 persons fewer as compared with the 3.44 persons in the 2000 population census (Wang, 2011a). The shrinking household size might be caused by the decline of fertility, the increase of migration, and the independent living arrangement of young couples after marriage (Wang, 2011a).

Family life takes on various faces and follows new trends. Because young people face greater and greater pressure from work and want a higher standard of living and spiritual life, the traditional concept of raising children has faded, and more couples are choosing the "double income, no kids" (DINK) way of life.

Because increasing numbers of young people leave home to work in other parts of the country or to study abroad, the number of households consisting of older couples is also rising. Improvements in housing conditions make it possible for the younger generations to move out of the house and live apart from senior members of the family. Longer life spans have resulted in more seniors living alone and those who have lost their spouse living by themselves in one-person households. "Empty nests" will become the norm for seniors as parents of the first generation of single-child families get older. That, in turn, means a switch from an old system in which children looked after their parents to one in which seniors are cared for by society in general through benefits.

Another traditional practice in many rural Chinese families is the submissive role of the daughter-in-law to the mother-in-law. Often the mother-in-law is demanding and hostile to the daughter-in-law and may treat her worse than the servants. This relationship has changed significantly since modern culture was introduced to Chinese society. However, such relationships may continue to influence some Chinese families today to some extent, or mothers-in-law and daughters-in-law may simply not get along with each other. Overseas, Chinese are quite different. The involvement of parents, especially the husband's parents, in the new family's life may have a great impact on families.

A Confucian cosmology of gender roles permeates Chinese society. A woman is characterized as a *yin* union, while a man is a *yang* union (Shim, 2001). As *yang*, man is superior, and as *yin*, woman is inferior (Li, 2000). Thus, a woman is expected to be obedient and dependent on a man (Shrestha & Weber, 1994). Because of stereotypical roles of men and women, men are largely in control of the country. However, since the founding of the PRC, this has been changing somewhat. In 1949, the Communist Party stated that "women hold up half the sky" and are legally equal to men.

Almost half of the workforce in China are women. Favored professions are education, culture and arts, broadcasting, television and film, finance and insurance, public health, welfare, sports, and social services. In trades requiring higher technical skills and knowledge such as computer science, telecommunications, environmental protection, aviation, engineering design, real estate development, finance and insurance, and the law are preferred. To promote Chinese women's employment, the Chinese government declared "The Program for the Development of Chinese Women" in 2001 (Huangjuan, 2009). Since then, the number of women employed increased from 291 million in 1990 to 337 million in 2003. In 2006, there were 41.56 million employed women in China urban areas, accounting for 38 percent of the total employees in urban sites (Women of China, 2006a).

In patriarchal Confucianism, the roles of Chinese women are referred to as *nei* (the internal), while the roles of Chinese men are referred to as *wai* (the external) (Li, 2000). In other words, women are socialized to assume domestic roles and are expected to be responsible for household tasks (Chang, 2004; Chen, 2009). The traditional gender roles of women are changing, but a sense remains that a woman's responsibility is to maintain a happy and efficient home life, especially in rural China. Recently, some Chinese men have begun to include housework, cooking, and cleaning as their responsibilities when their spouses work. Most Chinese believe that the family is most important, and thus each family member assumes changes in roles to achieve this harmony.

Prescriptive, Restrictive, and Taboo Behaviors for Children and Adolescents

Children are highly valued among the Chinese. China's one-child rule is still in effect (Center for Reproductive

Rights, 2002; Zhuhong, 2006). Because of overpopulation in China, the government has mandated that each married couple may have only one child; however, in some specific situations, family plans for a second child may be allowed. For instance, in rural areas, if the firstborn child is female or if the only child of a couple is disabled or killed in an accident, the couple might be permitted to have a second child (Zhuhong, 2006). Families often wait many years, until they are financially secure, to have a child. After the child is born, many family resources are lavished on the child. Families may be able to afford only to live with relatives in a two-room apartment, but if the family believes that the child will benefit by having a piano, then the resources will be found to provide a piano. Children are well dressed and kept clean and well fed.

In China, the child is protected from birth, and independence is not fostered. The entire family makes decisions for the child, even into young adulthood. Children usually depend on the family for everything. Few teens earn money because they are expected to study hard and to help the family with daily chores rather than to seek employment. Children are pressured to succeed and improve the future of the family and the country. Their common goal is to score well on the national examinations when they reach age 18. Most Chinese children and adolescents value studying over playing and peer relationships. They recognize that they are constantly evaluated on having healthy bodies and minds and achieving excellent marks in school.

With the traditional structure of a patriarchal family, girls are valued less than boys in Chinese society. In rural communities, male children are more valued than female children because they continue the family lineage and provide labor. In urban areas, however, female children are valued as highly as male children. Children in China are taught to curb their expression of feelings because individuals who do not stand out are successful. However, this is changing. The young in China today frequently think that their parents are too cautious. The children are becoming even more outspoken as they read more and watch more television and movies.

From elementary school to university, students take courses in Marxist politics and learn not to question the doctrine of the country. If they do, they may be interrogated and ridiculed for their radical thoughts. Nationalism is important to Chinese children, and they want to help their country continue to be the center of the world. Children are also expected to help their parents in the home. Many times in the cities when children get home from school before their parents, they are expected to do their homework immediately and then do their household chores. They exhibit their independence not so much by expressing their individual views but by performing chores on their own. However, because of China's one-child rule and high competition for enrollment to colleges, parents and grandparents spoil most children. The children are expected to earn good grades, and household chores are not encouraged; this is exhibited in overseas Chinese families as well. Lin and Fu (1990) studied 138 children—44 Chinese, 46 Chinese Americans, and 48 white Americans—in kindergarten through second grade and found that both Chinese and Chinese American parents expected increased achievement and parental control over their children. One surprising finding was the high expectation for independence in Chinese and Chinese American children.

Boys and girls play together when they are young, but as they get older, they do not because their roles and the corresponding expectations are predetermined by Chinese society. Girls and boys both study hard. Boys are more active and take pride in physical fitness. Girls are not nearly as interested in fitness as boys, preferring reading, art, and music.

Adolescents are expected to determine who they are and what they want to do with their lives. Adolescents maintain their respect for older people even when they disagree with them. Although they may argue with their parents and teachers, they have learned that it seldom does any good. Teens value a strong and happy family life and seldom do things that jeopardize that unanimity. Adolescents question affairs of life and make great efforts to see at least two sides of every issue. They enjoy exploring different views with their peers, and they try to explore them with their parents as well.

Teenage pregnancy is becoming a common issue among the Chinese. According to a government survey, more than 70 percent of 5000 students from 10 universities in Beijing have participated in a one-night stand (Huangjuan, 2009). More female teens are willing to have sex to show their affection for their boyfriends, and most of them do not use any contraception, which leads to a high rate of pregnancy among teenage females (Zhuhong, 2009a). Young men and women enter the workforce immediately after high school if they are unable to continue their education. Many continue to live with their parents and contribute to the family, even after marriage, into their 20s and, if they have a child, into their 30s.

Family Goals and Priorities

The Chinese perception of family is through the concept of relationships. In Confucian principles, hierarchical relationships exist between father and son, ruler and ruled, husband and wife, elder brother and younger brother, and friend and friend (Cheung et al., 2005). Each person identifies himself or herself in relation to others in the family. The individual is not lost, just defined differently from individuals in Western cultures. Personal independence is not valued; rather, Confucian teachings state that true value is in the relationships a person has with others, especially the family.

Older children who experienced the Cultural Revolution may feel some discomfort with their traditional parents. During the Cultural Revolution, the young were encouraged to inform on older people and peers who did not espouse the doctrine of the time. Most of those who were reported were sent to "reeducation camps," where they did hard labor and were "taught the correct way to think." As a result, many families have been permanently separated.

Extended families are important to the Chinese and function by providing ways to get ahead. Often, children live with their grandparents or aunts and uncles so individual family members can obtain a better education or reduce financial burdens. Relatives are expected to help one another through connections, called *guanxi*, which the Chinese society uses in a manner similar to the way other cultures use money. Such connections are perceived as obligations and are placed in a mental bank with deposits and withdrawals. These commitments may remain in the "bank" for years or generations until they are used to get jobs, housing, business contacts, gifts, medical care, or anything that demands a payback.

Filial loyalty to the family is extended to other Chinese. When Chinese immigrants need additional assistance, health-care providers may be able to call on local Chinese organizations to obtain help for patients.

Older people in China are venerated just as they were in earlier years. Chinese government leaders are often older and remain in power until they are in their 70s, 80s, and older. Traditional Chinese people view older people as very wise, a view that communism has not changed. Chinese children are expected to care for their parents, and in China, this is mandated by law.

Younger Chinese who adopt Western ideas and values may find that the expectations of older people are too demanding. Even though younger Chinese Americans do not live with their older relatives, they maintain respect and visit them frequently. Older Chinese mothers are viewed as central to family feelings, and older fathers retain their roles as leaders. As generations live in areas removed from China and families become more Westernized, family relationships need to be assessed on an individual basis. An extended-family pattern is common and has existed for over 2000 years. The traditional marriage still remains nuclear. Historically in China, marriage was used to strengthen positions of families in society.

Kinship relationships are based on the concept of loyalty, and the young experience pressure to improve the family's standing. Many parents give up items of daily living to provide more for their children, thereby increasing opportunities for them to get ahead.

Maintaining reputation is very important to the Chinese and is accomplished by adhering to the rules of society. Because power and control are important to Chinese society, rank is very important. True equality does not exist in the Chinese mind; their history has demonstrated that equality cannot exist. If more than one person is in power, then consensus is important. If the person in power is not present at decision-making meetings, barriers are raised, and any decisions made are negated unless the person in power agrees. Even after negotiations have been concluded and contracts signed, the Chinese continue to negotiate.

The Chinese concept of privacy is even more important than recognized social status, corresponding values, and beliefs. The Chinese word for "privacy" has a negative connotation and means something underhanded, secret, and furtive. People grow up in crowded conditions, they live and work in small areas, and their value of group support does not place a high value on privacy. The Chinese may ask many personal questions about salary, life at home, age, and children. Refusal to answer personal questions is accepted as long as it is done with care and feeling. The one subject that is taboo is sex and anything related to sex. This may create a barrier for a Western health-care provider who is trying to assess a Chinese patient with sexual concerns. The patient may feel uncomfortable discussing or answering questions about sex with honesty. Privacy is also limited by territorial boundaries. Some Chinese may enter rooms without knocking or invade privacy by not allowing a person to be alone. The need to be alone is viewed as "not good" to some Chinese, and they may not understand when a Westerner wants to be alone. A mutual understanding of these beliefs is necessary for harmonious working relationships.

Alternative Lifestyles

In Chinese society, people have very little acceptance of gays and lesbians. In many provinces, homosexuality is illegal and punishable by death. Divorce is legal but is not encouraged; Although it is evident that divorce is a growing trend in China (Women of China, 2006b)—approaching 30 percent in 2006 Alexander & Marget, 2006)—the reasons are multifaceted. First, society is going through a transitional period, which is greatly affecting the stability of marriages. Second, as living standards improve, people have higher expectations toward marriage and love. Third, the simplification of marriage and divorce procedures has made getting a divorce much easier (Women of China, 2006b).

Tradition, consideration for children's feelings, and difficulty in remarrying are some of the reasons many Chinese families would rather stay in an unhealthy marriage than divorce. Remarriage is encouraged, but some difficult relationships may occur in the blended family, especially remarriage with children from previous marriages.

Workforce Issues
Culture in the Workplace

China is becoming more Westernized with high technology and increased knowledge. The Communist Party is responsible for establishing the ***dan wei***—local Chinese work units—that are responsible for jobs, homes, health, enforcement of governmental regulations, and problem solving for families. Although recent immigrants know that the culture in the workplace is different in the United States, they adapt to it quickly. The Chinese acculturate by learning as much as possible about their new culture in the workplace. They observe people from the culture and listen closely for nuances in language and interpersonal connections. They frequently call on other Chinese people to teach them and to discuss how to fit into the new culture more quickly. Chinese Americans support one another in new settings and help one another find resources and learn to live effectively and efficiently in the new culture. They also watch television, listen to music, and go to movies to learn about Western ways of life. They read about the new culture in magazines, books, newspapers, and on the Internet. They love to travel, and when an opportunity arises to see different aspects of the new culture, they do not hesitate to do so.

The Chinese are accustomed to giving coworkers small gifts of appreciation for helping them acculturate and adapt to the American workforce. Often, Americans seek opportunities to reciprocate with a gift, such as at a birthday party, farewell party, or other occasion. Whereas a wide variety of gifts is appropriate, some gifts are not. For example, giving an umbrella means that one wishes to have the recipient's family dispersed; giving a gift that is white in color or wrapped in white could be interpreted as meaning the giver wants the recipient to die; and giving a clock could be interpreted as never wanting to see the person again or wishing the person's life to end (Smith, 2002).

On the surface, Chinese Americans form classic external networks, including groupings by family surname, locality of origin in China, dialect or subdialect spoken, craft practiced, and trust from prior experience or recommendation. Therefore, Chinese Americans approximate external networks with some characteristic of internal networks (Haley, Tan, & Haley, 1998). *Guanxi* is a Mandarin term with no exact English translation. This term includes the concept of trust and presenting uprightness to build close relationships and connections. It definitely helps to build networks. This *Guanxi* network can be used in the work-related, decision-making process and is also used with family, friends, and community-related issues in the Chinese American community.

Issues Related to Autonomy

Historically, the Chinese have been autonomous. They had to exhibit this characteristic to survive through difficult times. However, their autonomy is limited and is based on functioning for the good of the group. When a new situation arises that requires independent decision making, many times the Chinese know what should be done but do not take action until the leader or superior gives permission. Because of deferring to authority, Chinese people tend to avoid conflict and will not challenge anyone whom they regard as a leader or expert. For example, if a doctor prescribes an incorrect medication, Chinese people might accept the doctor's prescription without saying anything. However, the Western workforce expects independence, and some Chinese may need to be taught that true autonomy is necessary to advance. Health-care providers should be aware, however, that the training might not be successful because it is foreign to Chinese cultural values. A demonstration is the best alternative, leaving it up to the individuals to determine whether assertiveness can be a part of their lives. After acculturation takes place, Chinese Americans do not differ significantly in assertiveness.

Language may be a barrier for Chinese immigrants seeking assimilation into the Western workforce. Western languages and Chinese have many differences, among them sentence structure and the use of intonation. The Chinese language does not have verbs that denote tense, as in Western languages. Whereas the ordering of the words in a sentence is basically the same, with the subject first and then the verb, the Chinese language places descriptive adjectives in different orders. Intonation in Chinese is in the words themselves rather than in the sentence. Chinese people who have taken English lessons can usually read and write English competently, but they may have difficulty understanding and speaking it. Research has reported that the ability to speak English is a significant factor among Chinese people in accessing health care (Cheung et al., 2005).

Biocultural Ecology
Skin Color and Other Biological Variations

The skin color of Chinese is varied. Many have skin color similar to that of Westerners, with pink undertones. Some have a yellow tone, whereas others are very dark. Mongolian spots, dark bluish spots over the lower back and buttocks, are present in about 80 percent of infants. Bilirubin levels are usually higher in Chinese newborns, with the highest levels occurring on the 5th or 6th day after birth.

Although Chinese are distinctly Mongolian, their Asian characteristics have many variations. China is very large and includes people from many different backgrounds, including Mongols and Tibetans. Generally, men and women are shorter than Westerners, but some Chinese are over 6 feet tall. Differences in bone structure are evidenced in the ulna, which is longer than the radius. Hip measurements are significantly smaller: Females are 4.14 cm shorter, and males 7.6 cm shorter than Westerners (Seidel, Ball, Dains, & Benedict, 1994). Not only is overall bone length shorter, but bone density is also less. Chinese have a high hard palate, which may cause them problems with Western dentures. Their hair is generally black and straight, but some have naturally curly hair. Most Chinese men do not have much facial or chest hair. The Rh-negative blood group is rare, and twins are not common in Chinese families, but they are greatly valued, especially since the emergence of China's one-child law.

Diseases and Health Conditions

Many Chinese who come to the United States settle in large cities like San Francisco and New York, so they are at risk for the same problems and diseases experienced by other inner-city populations. For example, crowding in large cities often results in poor sanitation and increases the incidence of infectious diseases, air pollution, and violence.

Noninfectious chronic diseases have become the major threat to Chinese people, claiming 85 percent of deaths in China (Zhang, 2011). The Chinese Ministry of Health (2009) reports that cerebrovascular disease, cancer, respiratory disease, and heart disease are the four principal causes of death in China.

In 1949, the average life expectancy was only 35 years (*People's Daily*, 2002). According to the *CIA World Factbook* (2011), in 2011, the overall Chinese average life expectancy was 74.68 years—72.68 years for men and 76.94 years for women. The life expectancy in China has dramatically increased due to the improvement of living conditions and medical facilities, as well as a nationwide fitness campaign. Disease incidence has decreased as well, but major problems still exist in rural China, where perinatal deaths and deaths from infectious diseases remain high. Tobacco use is a major problem and results in an increased incidence of lung disease. Health-care providers must screen newer immigrants from China for these health-related conditions and provide interventions in a culturally congruent manner.

Many Chinese immigrants have an increased incidence of hepatitis B and tuberculosis. Poor living conditions and overcrowding in some areas of China enhance the development of these diseases, which persist after immigrants settle in other countries.

According to the Office of Minority Health (2007), Chinese American women have a 20 percent higher rate of pancreatic cancer and higher rates of suicide after the age of 45 years, and all Chinese have higher death rates owing to diabetes. The incidence of different types of cancer, including cervical, liver, lung, stomach, multiple myeloma, esophageal, pancreatic, and nasopharyngeal cancers, is higher among Chinese Americans (Office of Minority Health, 2007). Overall, the incidence of disease in this population has not been studied sufficiently, and continuing research is desperately needed.

Variations in Drug Metabolism

Studies outlining problems with drug metabolism and sensitivity have been conducted among the Chinese. Results suggest a poor metabolism of mephenytoin (e.g., diazepam) in 15 to 20 percent of Chinese; sensitivity to beta-blockers, such as propranolol, as evidenced by a decrease in the overall blood levels accompanied by a seemingly more profound response; atropine sensitivity, as evidenced by an increased heart rate; and increased responses to antidepressants and neuroleptics given at lower doses. Analgesics have been found to cause increased gastrointestinal side effects, despite a decreased sensitivity to them. In addition, the Chinese have an increased sensitivity to the effects of alcohol (Levy, 1993).

Delineating specific variations in drug metabolism among the Chinese is difficult because various studies tend to group them in aggregate as Asians. Much more research needs to be completed to determine variations between Westerners and Asians, as well as among Asians. The same thing is true of Hispanics/Latinos

High-Risk Behaviors

High-risk behaviors are difficult to determine with accuracy among the Chinese in the United States because most of the data on the Chinese are included in the aggregate called *Asian Americans*. Smoking is a high-risk behavior for many Chinese men and teenagers. Smoking-related diseases kill roughly 1.2 million Chinese people every year, and the death rate is expected to keep climbing in the coming decades (Yang, 2011).

Yu, Edwin, Chen, Kim, and Sawsan (2002) reported that the male prevalence of smoking in Chicago is higher than that reported in California and exceeds the rate for African Americans aged 18 years and older. Most Chinese women do not smoke, but recently, the numbers for women are increasing, especially after immigration to the United States. Travelers in China see more cigarette street vendors than any other type. The decrease in smoking in the United States made cigarette manufacturers target China as a good market in which to sell their product.

Alcohol consumption has increased significantly in China. In two random samples of 2327 and 2613 people, it was found that 90 percent of men and 55 percent of women drank alcohol in 2005 (Zhang, Casswell, & Cai, 2008). The greatest increase in alcohol consumption occurred in 18- and 19-year-olds and among older women (Zhang et al., 2008).

Nutrition

Meaning of Food

Food habits are important to the Chinese, who offer food to their guests at any time of the day or night. Most celebrations with family and business events focus on food. Foods served at Chinese meals have a specific order, with the focus on a balance for a healthy body. The importance of food is demonstrated daily in its use to promote good health and to combat disease and injury. Traditional Chinese medicine frequently uses food and food derivatives to prevent and cure diseases and illnesses and to increase the strength of weak and older people.

Common Foods and Food Rituals

The typical Chinese diet is difficult to describe because each region in China has its own traditional foods. Peanuts and soybeans are popular. Common grains include wheat, sorghum, and maize. Rice is usually steamed but can be fried with eggs, vegetables, and meats. Many Chinese eat beans or noodles instead of rice. The Chinese eat steamed and fried rice noodles, which are usually prepared with a broth base and include vegetables and meats. Meat choices include pork (the most common), chicken, beef, duck, shrimp, fish, scallops, and mussels. Tofu, an excellent source of protein, is a staple of the Chinese diet and can be fried or boiled or eaten cold like ice cream. Bean products are another source of protein, and many of the desserts or sweets in Chinese diets are prepared with red beans.

At celebrations, before-dinner toasts are usually made to family and business colleagues. The toasts may be interspersed with speeches, or the speeches may be incorporated into the toasts. Cold appetizers often include peanuts and seasonal fruits. Chopsticks, a chopstick holder, a small plate, and a glass are part of the table setting. If the foods are messy, like Beijing duck, then a finger towel may be available. The Chinese use ceramic or porcelain spoons for soup. Knives are unnecessary because the food is usually served in bite-sized pieces. Eating with chopsticks may be difficult for some at first, but the Chinese are good-natured and are pleased by any attempt to use them. Chopsticks should never be stuck in the food upright because that is considered bad luck (Smith, 2002). Westerners soon learn that slurping, burping, and other noises are not considered offensive, but are appreciated. The Chinese are very relaxed at meals and commonly rest their elbows on the table.

Fruits and vegetables may be peeled or eaten raw. Some vegetables commonly eaten raw by Westerners are usually cooked by the Chinese. Unpeeled raw fruits and vegetables are sources of contamination owing to unsanitary conditions in China. The Chinese enjoy their vegetables lightly stir-fried in oil with salt and spices. Salt, oil, and oil products are important parts of the Chinese diet.

Drinks with dinner include tea, soft drinks, juice, and beer. Foreign-born Chinese and older Chinese may not like ice in their drinks. They may just not like anything cold while eating or may believe it is damaging to their body and shocks the body systems out of balance. Conversely, hot drinks are enjoyed and believed to be safe for the body. This "goodness" of hot drinks may stem from tradition in which the only safe drinks were made from boiled water. All food is put in the center of the table, arriving all at one time, but usually multiple courses are served. The host either serves the most important guests first or signals everyone to start.

Dietary Practices for Health Promotion

For the Chinese, food is important in maintaining their health. Foods that are considered *yin* and *yang* prevent sudden imbalances and indigestion. A balanced diet is considered essential for physical and emotional harmony. Health-care providers need to provide special instructions regarding risk factors associated with diets that are high in fats and salt. For example, the Chinese may need education regarding the use of salty fish and condiments, which increase the risk for nasopharyngeal, esophageal, and stomach cancers.

Nutritional Deficiencies and Food Limitations

Little information is available about dietary deficiencies in the Chinese diet. The life span of the Chinese is long enough to suggest that severe dietary deficiencies are not common as long as food is available. Periodically, some deficiencies, such as rickets and goiters, have occurred. The Chinese government added iodine to water supplies, and fish, which is rich in iron, is encouraged to enhance the diets of people with goiters. Native Chinese generally do not drink milk or eat milk products because of a genetic tendency for lactose intolerance. Their healthy selection of green vegetables limits the incidence of calcium deficiencies. Health-care providers may need to screen newer Chinese immigrants for these deficiencies and assist them in planning an adequate diet.

Most Chinese do not eat desserts with a high sugar content. Their desserts are usually peeled or sliced fruits or desserts made of bean and bean curd. The higher death rate from diabetes in Western countries mentioned earlier in this chapter may be due to a change from the typical Chinese diet with few sweets to a Western diet with many sweets.

Pregnancy and Childbearing Practices

Fertility Practices and Views Toward Pregnancy

China continues to make efforts to slow the rate of population growth by enforcing a one-child law. The most popular form of birth control is the intrauterine device. Sterilization is common even though oral contraception is available. Contraception is free in China. Abortion is fairly common, with 13 million abortions performed in China every year (Zhuhong, 2009b). Health-care providers working in women's health need to be aware of the abortion issues among newly arrived Chinese immigrants, as well as among Chinese Americans who may still adhere to premigration practices. It is critical for women's health to reduce the abortion issue among Chinese women.

Most Chinese families see pregnancy as positive and important in the immediate and extended family. Many couples wait a long time to have their first and only child. If a woman does become pregnant before the couple is ready to start a family, she may have an abortion. When the pregnancy is desired, the nuclear and extended families rejoice in the new family member. Overall, pregnancy is seen as a woman's business, although the Chinese men are beginning to demonstrate an active interest in pregnancy and the welfare of the mother and baby.

China has 80 million one-child families. The gender imbalance has become a serious issue in recent years because many families, especially those in rural areas, prefer boys to girls. China has 119 boys born for every 100 girls, whereas the global ratio is 103 to 107 boys for every 100 girls. In China, the "Care for Girls" program was initiated in 2003 to promote the social status of women, and attempts are being made to decrease gender identification abortions without a medical purpose and the abandonment of newborn girls. Political action is through professional organizations but it is mostly sub rosa (XinHua News Agency, 2006). As a result, the sex ratio declined from 106.74 in 2000 to 105.20 in 2010 (National Bureau of Statistics of China, 2011). However, as of 2011, the reported male to female ratio was 1.133 (*CIA World Factbook*, 2011). Of the population enumerated in the 2010 census, males accounted for 51.27 percent, while females accounted for 48.73 percent (Wang, 2011c).

Prescriptive, Restrictive, and Taboo Practices in the Childbearing Family

Because Chinese women are very modest, many women insist on a female midwife or obstetrician. Some agree to use a male physician only when an emergency arises. Pregnant women usually add more meat to their diets because their blood needs to be stronger for the fetus. Many women increase the amount of organ meat in their diet, and even during times of severe food shortages, the Chinese government has tried to ensure that pregnant women receive adequate nutrition. These traditions are also reflected in Chinese families living in the West.

Other dietary restrictions and prescriptions may be practiced by pregnant women, such as avoiding shellfish during the first trimester because it causes allergies. Some mothers may be unwilling to take iron because they believe that it makes the delivery more difficult.

The Chinese government is proud of the fact that since the People's Revolution in 1949, infant mortality has been significantly reduced. In 2001, the mortality rates for infants and children under age 5 were reduced to 30 per 1000 from 35.9 per 1000 (Women of China, 2006d). This has been accomplished by providing a three-level system of care for pregnant women in rural and urban populations. Over 90 percent of childbirths take place under sterile conditions by qualified personnel. The infant mortality rate dropped from 20.3 per thousand in 2005 to 14.1 per thousand in 2009 (Wang, 2011c). Therefore, most Chinese who have immigrated to Western countries are familiar with modern sterile deliveries.

In China, a woman stays in the hospital for a few days after delivery to recover her strength and body balance. Traditional postpartum care includes 1 month of recovery, with the mother eating cooked and warm foods that decrease the *yin* (cold) energy. The Chinese government supports this 1-month recuperation period through labor laws that entitle the mother from 56 days to 6 months of maternity leave with full pay (Ministry of Public Health, 1992). Women who return to work are allowed time off for breastfeeding, and in many cases, factories provide a special lounge for the women to breastfeed. Families who come to Western societies expect the same importance to be placed on motherhood and may be surprised to find that many Western countries do not provide similar benefits.

Traditional prescriptive and restrictive practices continue among many Chinese women during the postpartum period. Drinking and touching cold water are taboo for women in the postpartum period. Raw fruits and vegetables are avoided because they are considered "cold" foods. They must be cooked and be warm. Mothers eat five to six meals a day with high nutritional ingredients, including rice, soups, and seven to eight eggs. Brown sugar is commonly used because it helps rebuild blood loss. Drinking rice wine is encouraged to increase the mother's breast milk production, but mothers need to be cautioned that it may also prolong the bleeding time. Many mothers do not expose themselves to the cold air and do not go outside or bathe for the first month postpartum because the cold air can enter the body and cause health problems, especially for older women. Some women wear many layers of clothes and are covered from head to toe, even in the summer, to keep the air away from their bodies. However, this practice has changed among some young women who live in Western cultures for a long period of time and when there are no older Chinese parents around during the postpartum period.

Adopted Chinese children display a similar pattern of growth and developmental delays and medical problems as seen in other groups of internationally adopted children. An exception is the increased incidence of elevated lead levels (overall 14 percent). Although serious medical and developmental issues were found among Chinese children, overall their health was better than expected based on recent publicity about conditions in the Chinese orphanages. The long-term outcome of these children remains unknown (Miller, 2000). Many children adopted from China have antibody titers that do not correlate with those expected from their medical records. These children, unlike children adopted from other countries, have documented evidence of adequate vaccinations. However, they should be tested for antibody concentrations and reimmunized as necessary (Schulpen, 2001).

REFLECTIVE EXERCISE 10.2

Mrs. Huang, a 32-year-old woman from China, lives with her husband and his parents. She delivered a healthy baby girl yesterday. This morning, Mrs. Huang says she is constipated. The physician told Mrs. Huang that constipation was a common problem after delivery. The nurse suggested that she eat more fresh fruits and vegetables to facilitate a bowel movement. However, Mrs. Huang rejected fruits and vegetables and stated that a woman was characterized as a *yin* union and eating too much cold food was not good for a postpartum woman. Later in the day, Mrs. Huang told the nurse that she did not think she wanted to experience childbirth again. When the nurse approached Mrs. Huang about possible contraception, she said that her parents-in-law wanted her be become pregnant very soon in the hopes of having a male child.

1. According to Chinese perspectives, foods are divided into *yin* and *yang* categories. What information does the nurse need before discussing Mrs. Huang's concerns about constipation?
2. What other culturally congruent dietary instructions might the nurse recommend to resolve Mrs. Huang's concerns with constipation?
3. As a daughter-in-law in a traditional Chinese family, Mrs. Huang's autonomy to make decisions seems to be limited. What concerns might the nurse have when discussing contraception?
4. Describe some traditional postpartum Chinese practices.

Death Rituals
Death Rituals and Expectations

Chinese death and bereavement traditions are centered on ancestor worship. Ancestor worship is frequently misunderstood; it is not a religion, but rather a form of paying respect. Many Chinese believe that their spirits can never rest unless living descendants provide care for the grave and worship the memory of the deceased. These practices were so important to early Chinese that Chinese pioneers to the West had statements written into their work contract that their ashes or bones be returned to China (Halporn, 1992).

The belief that the Chinese greet death with stoicism and fatalism is a myth. In fact, most Chinese fear death, avoid references to it, and teach their children this avoidance. The number 4 is considered unlucky by many Chinese because it is pronounced like the Chinese word for death; this is similar to the bad luck associated with the number 13 in many Western societies. Huang (1992) wrote:

> At a very young age, a child is taught to be very careful with words that are remotely associated with the "misfortune" of death. The word "death" and its synonyms are strictly forbidden on happy occasions, especially during holidays. People's uneasiness about death often is reflected in their emphasis on longevity and everlasting life. . . . In daily life, the character "Long Life" appears on almost everything: jewelry, clothing, furniture, and so forth. It would be a terrible mistake to give a clock as a gift, simply because the pronunciation of the word "clock" is the same as that of the word "ending." Recently, many people in Taiwan decided to avoid using the number "four" because the number has a similar pronunciation to the word "death." (p. 1)

Many Chinese are hesitant to purchase life insurance because of their fear that it is inviting death. The color white is associated with death and is considered bad luck. Black is also a bad luck color.

Many Chinese believe in ghosts, and the fear of death is extended to the fear of ghosts. Some ghosts are good and some are bad, but all have great power. Communism discourages this thinking and sees it as a hindrance to future growth and development of the society, but the ever-pragmatic Chinese believe it is better not to invite trouble with ghosts just in case they might exist.

The dead may be viewed in the hospital or in the family home. Extended family members and friends come together to mourn. The dead are honored by placing objects around the coffin that signify the life of the dead: food, money designated for the dead person's spirit, and other articles made of paper. In China, cremation is preferred by the state because of a lack of wood for coffins and a limited space for burial. The ashes are placed in an urn and then in a vault. As cities grow, even the space for vaults is limited. In rural areas, many families prefer traditional burial and have family burial plots. It is preferable to burying an intact body in a coffin.

Responses to Death and Grief

The Chinese react to death in various ways. Death is viewed as a part of the natural cycle of life, and some believe that something good happens to them after they die. These beliefs foster the impression that Chinese are stoic. In fact, they feel similar emotions to Westerners but do not overtly express those emotions to strangers. During bereavement, a person does not have to go to work, but instead can use this mourning time for remembering the dead and planning for the future. Bereavement time in the larger cities is 1 day to 1 week, depending on the policy of the government agency and the relationship of family members to the deceased. Mourners are recognized by black armbands on their left arm and white strips of cloth tied around their heads.

Spirituality

Dominant Religion and Use of Prayer

In mainland China, the practice of formal religious services is minimal. The ideals and values of the different religions are practiced alone rather than with people coming together to participate in a formal religious service. In recent years, in some parts of China, religion is becoming more popular. The main formal religions in China are Taoism, Buddhism, Christianity (3 to 4 percent), and Islam (1 to 2 percent) (*CIA World Factbook*, 2011).

As immigration from China increases, Chinese people who practice Christian religions have become more visible on the American landscape. Chinese immigrants from the People's Republic of China may express perspectives on religious beliefs different from those of the Chinese from other countries, or from Hong Kong and Taiwan, where they have been permitted to practice Christianity. At first, they may go to a church attended by other Chinese people; eventually some are baptized, and others continue to attend Bible studies. In cities in the United States, churches are playing a very important role in the local Chinese community in terms of providing support and services to Chinese immigrants, students, scholars, and their families. An understanding of this concept is essential when the health-care provider attempts to obtain religious counseling services for Chinese patients.

Prayer is generally a source of comfort. Some Chinese do not acknowledge a religion such as Buddhism, but if they go to a shrine, they burn incense and offer prayers.

Meaning of Life and Individual Sources of Strength

The Chinese view life in terms of cycles and interrelationships, believing that life gets meaning from the context in which it is lived. Life cannot be broken into simple parts and examined because the parts are interrelated. When the Chinese attempt to explain life and what it means, they speak about what happened to them, what happened to others, and the importance and interrelatedness of those events. They speak not only of the importance of the current phenomena but also about the importance of what occurred many years, maybe even centuries, before their lives. They live and believe in a true systems framework.

"Life forces" are sources of strength to the Chinese. These forces come from within the individual, the environment, the past and future of the individual, and society. Chinese use these forces when they need strength. If one usual source of strength is unsuccessful, they try another. The individual may use many different techniques such as meditation, exercise, massage, and prayer. Drugs, herbs, food, good air, and artistic expression may also be used. Good luck charms are cherished, and traditional and nontraditional medicines are used.

The family is usually one source of strength. Individuals draw on family resources and are expected to return resources to strengthen the family. Resources may be financial, emotional, physical, mental, or spiritual. Calling on ancestors to provide strength as a resource requires giving back to the ancestors when necessary. The interconnectedness of life provides a source of strength for individuals from before birth to death and beyond.

Health-care providers need to understand this multidimensional manner of thinking and believing. Assessments, goal setting, interventions, and evaluations may be different for Chinese patients than for American patients. The context of client problems is the emphasis, and the physical, mental, and spiritual aspects of the person's life are the focal points.

Health-Care Practices

Health-Seeking Beliefs and Behaviors

Health care in China is provided for most citizens. Every work unit and neighborhood has its own clinic and hospital. Traditional Chinese medicine shops abound (Fig. 10-1). Even department stores and supermarkets have Western medicines and traditional Chinese medicines and herbs.

The focus of health has not changed over the centuries, and it includes having a healthy body, a healthy mind, and a healthy spirit. Preventive health-care practices are a major focus in China today. An additional focus is placed on infectious diseases such as schistosomiasis, tuberculosis, childhood diseases, and

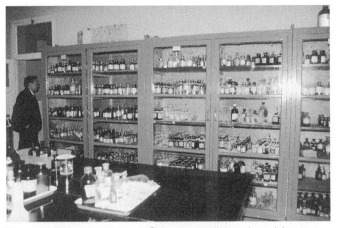

Figure 10-1 A traditional Chinese medicine shop. Many Chinese practice traditional Chinese medicine, either alone or in conjunction with Western medicine.

malaria; cancer; heart diseases; and maternal–infant care. Chinese Ministry of Health statistics indicate that China had 840,000 HIV-infected people in 2004 (Chinese Ministry of Health, 2004; *CIA World Factbook*, 2011). That means that China had the 14th highest number of HIV-infected people in the world and the second highest in Asia. Between 2000 and 2005, the percentage of people infected with HIV rose from 19.4 percent to 28.1 percent (Women of China, 2006c). The *CIA World Factbook* gives similar figures for 2011. China claimed that the country had no HIV cases, but in 2004, it was revealed that a huge number of Chinese contracted HIV from blood transfusions. China now faces a critical period in the fight to curb the spread, and ultimately the cure, of HIV and AIDS. The World Health Organization (WHO) has predicted that if China fails to control the disease's spread, there will be 10 million people with AIDS by 2010 (Gu, 2006).

A regulation on AIDS prevention and control (effective January 1, 2007) spells out the plan to administer the free test in areas of the province where the AIDS situation is "grave." HIV carriers and AIDS patients will be asked to inform their spouses or sex partners of the results, or the local disease prevention authorities will do so (Women of China, 2006c).

Whereas many Chinese have made the transition to Western medicine, others maintain their roots in traditional Chinese medicine, and still others practice both types. The Chinese are similar to other nationalities in seeking the most effective cure available. Younger Chinese people usually do not hesitate to seek health-care providers when necessary. They generally practice Western medicine unless they feel that it does not work for them; then they use traditional Chinese medicine. Conversely, older people may try traditional Chinese medicine first and only seek Western medicine when traditional medicine does not seem to work.

Among Chinese Americans, these health-seeking beliefs, practices, and patterns remain the same as the ones in China. This results in sicker older people seeking care from Western health-care providers. Even after seeking Western medical care, many older Chinese continue to practice traditional Chinese medicine in some form. However, some Chinese patients may not tell health-care providers about other forms of treatment they have been using because they are conscious of saving face. Health-care providers need to understand this practice and include it in their care. Members of the health-care team need to develop a trusting relationship with Chinese patients so all information can be disclosed. Health-care providers must impress upon patients the importance of disclosing all treatments because some may have antagonistic effects.

Responsibility for Health Care

Chinese people often self-medicate when they think they know what is wrong or if they have been successfully treated by their traditional medicine or herbs in the past. They share their knowledge about treatments and their medicines with friends and family members. This often happens among Chinese Americans as well because of the belief that occasional illness can be ameliorated through the use of nonprescription drugs. Many consider seeing Western health-care providers as a waste of time and money. Health-care providers need to recognize that self-medication and sharing medications are accepted practices among the Chinese. Thus, health-care providers should inquire about this practice when making assessments, setting goals, and evaluating the results of treatments. A trusting relationship between members of the health-care team and the patient and family is necessary to enhance the disclosure of all treatments.

Traditional Chinese Medicine Practices

Traditional Chinese medicine is practiced widely, with concrete reasons for the preparation of medications, taking medicine, and the expected outcomes. Western medicine needs to be explained to Chinese patients in equally concrete terms.

Traditional Chinese medicine has many facets, including the five basic substances (*qi*, energy; *xue*, blood; *jing*, essence; *shen*, spirit; and *jing ye*, body fluids); the pulses and vessels for the flow of energetic forces (*mai*); the energy pathways (*jing*); the channels and collaterals, including the 14 meridians for acupuncture, moxibustion, and massage (*jing luo*); the organ systems (*zang fu*); and the tissues of the bones, tendons, flesh, blood vessels, and skin. The scope of traditional Chinese medicine is vast and should be studied carefully by professionals who provide health care to Chinese patients.

Acupuncture and moxibustion are used in many of the treatments. Acupuncture is the insertion of needles into precise points along the channel system of flow of the *qi* called the 14 meridians. The system has over 400 points. Many of the same points can be used in applying pressure and massage to achieve relief from imbalances in the system. The same systems approach is used to produce localized anesthesia.

Moxibustion is the application of heat from different sources to various points. For example, one source, such as garlic, is placed on the distal end of the needle after it is inserted through the skin, and the garlic is set on fire. Sometimes, the substance is burned directly over the point without a needle insertion. Localized erythema occurs with the heat from the burning substance, and the medicine is absorbed through the skin. Cupping is another common practice. A heated cup or glass jar is put on the skin, creating a vacuum, which causes the skin to be drawn into the cup. The heat generated is used to treat joint pain.

The Chinese believe that health and a happy life can be maintained if the two forces, the *yang* and the *yin*, are balanced. This balance is called the **dao**. Heaven is *yang*, and Earth is *yin*; man is *yang*, and woman is *yin*; the sun is *yang*, and the moon is *yin*; the hollow organs (bladder, intestines, stomach, gallbladder), head, face, back, and lateral parts of the body are *yang*, and the solid viscera (heart, lung, liver, spleen, kidney, and pericardium), abdomen, chest, and the inner parts of the body are *yin*. The *yang* is hot, and the *yin* is cold. Health-care providers need to be aware that the functions of life and the interplay of these functions, rather than the structures, are important to the Chinese people.

Central to traditional medicine is the concept of the **qi**. It is considered the vital force of life; includes air, breath, or wind; and is present in all living organisms. Some of the *qi* is inherited, and other parts come from the environment, such as in food. The *qi* circulates through the 14 meridians and organs of the body to give the body nourishment. The channels of flow are also responsible for eliminating the bad *qi*. All channels, the meridians and organs, are interconnected. The results resemble a system in which a change in one part of the system results in a change in other parts, and one part of the system can assist other parts in their total functioning.

Diagnosis is made through close inspection of the outward appearance of the body, the vitality of the person, the color of the person, the appearance of the tongue, and the person's senses. The health-care provider uses listening, smelling, and questioning techniques in the assessment. Palpation is used by feeling the 12 pulses and different parts of the body. Treatments are based on the imbalances that occur. Many are directly related to the obvious problem, but many more are related through the interconnectedness of the body systems. Many of the treatments not only "cure" the problem but are also used to "strengthen" the entire human being. Traditional Chinese medicine cannot be learned quickly because of the interplay of symptoms and diagnoses. Health-care providers take many years to become adept in all phases of diagnosis and treatment.

T'ai chi, practiced by many Chinese, has its roots in the 12th century. This type of exercise is suitable for all age groups, even the very old. *T'ai chi* involves different forms of exercise, some of which can be used for self-defense. The major focus of the movements is mind and body control. The concepts of *yin* and *yang* are included in the movements, with a *yin* movement following a *yang* movement. Total concentration and controlled breathing are necessary to enable the smoothness and rhythmic quality of movement. The movements resemble a slow-motion battle, with the participant both attacking and retreating. Movements are practiced at least twice a day to bring the internal body, the external body, and the environment into balance (Mayo Clinic, 2010). Yoga is also a fashionable exercise among women. Yoga incorporates meditation, relaxation, imagery, controlled breathing, stretching, and other physical movements. Yoga has become increasingly popular in Western cultures as a means of exercise and fitness training. Yoga needs to be better recognized by the health-care community as a complement to conventional medical care.

Herbal therapy is integral to traditional Chinese medicine and is even more difficult to learn than acupuncture and moxibustion. Herbs fall into four categories of energy (cold, hot, warm, and cool), five categories of taste (sour, bitter, sweet, pungent, and salty), and a neutral category. Different methods are used to administer the herbs, including drinking and eating, applying topically, and wearing on the body. Each treatment is specific to the underlying problem or a desire to increase strength and resistance.

Barriers to Health Care

In China, the government is primarily responsible for providing basic health care within a multilevel system. Native Chinese are accustomed to the neighborhood work units called *dan wei*, where they get answers to their questions and health-care services are provided. After transition to the United States, Chinese patients face many of the same barriers to health care faced by Westerners, yet they have other special concerns and difficulties that prevent them from accessing health-care services. Ma (2000) summarized these barriers as the following:

- *Language barriers:* This is one of the major reasons that Chinese Americans do not want to see Western health-care providers. They feel uncomfortable and frustrated with not being able to communicate with them freely and not being able to adequately express their pains, concerns, or health problems. Even highly educated Chinese Americans, who have limited knowledge in the medical field and are unfamiliar with medical terminology, have difficulty complying with recommended procedures and health prescriptions.

- *Cultural barriers:* Lack of culturally appropriate and competent health-care services is another key obstacle to health-care service utilization. Many Chinese Americans have different cultural responses to health and illness. Although they respect and accept the Western health-care provider's prescription drugs, they tend to alternate between Western and traditional Chinese physicians.
- *Socioeconomic barriers:* Being unable to afford medical expenses is another barrier to accessing health-care services for some Chinese Americans. However, having health insurance does not always ensure the utilization of the health-care system or the benefits of health insurance. There may be a sense of distrust between patients and health-care providers or between patients and insurance companies. In addition, many do not know the cost of the service when they enter a clinic or hospital. They are frustrated with being caught in the battle between health insurance companies and the clinic or hospital.
- *Systemic barriers:* Not understanding the Western health-care system and feeling inconvenienced by managed-care regulations deter many from seeking Western health-care providers unless they are seriously ill. The complexity of the rules and regulations of public agencies and medical assistance programs such as Medicaid and Medicare blocks their effective use.

Tan (1992), in a different perspective, summarized barriers for Chinese immigrants seeking health care:

- Many Chinese Americans have great difficulty facing a diagnosis of cancer because families are the main source of support for patients, and many family members are still in China.
- Because many Chinese Americans do not have medical insurance, any serious illness will lead to heavy financial burdens on the family.
- Once the patient responds to initial treatment, the family tends to stop treatment and the patient does not receive follow-up care or becomes nonadherent. Chinese American families may be reluctant to allow autopsies because of their fear of being "cut up."
- The most difficult barrier is frequently the reluctance to disclose the diagnosis to the patient or the family.

In recent years, clinics of Chinese medicine and health-care providers who are originally from China have been significantly visible in the United States, especially in the larger cities. These provide opportunities or options for those Chinese Americans who prefer to seek traditional Chinese treatment for certain illness.

Cultural Responses to Health and Illness

Chinese people express their pain in ways similar to those of Americans, but their description of pain differs. A study by Moore (1990) included not only the expression of pain but also common treatments used by the Chinese. The Chinese tend to describe their pain in terms of more diverse body symptoms, whereas Westerners tend to describe pain locally. The Western description includes words like "stabbing" and "localized," whereas the Chinese describe pain as "dull" and more "diffuse." They tend to use explanations of pain from the traditional Chinese influence of imbalances in the *yang* and *yin* combined with location and cause. The study determined that the Chinese cope with pain by using externally applied methods, such as oils and massage. They also use warmth, sleeping on the area of pain, relaxation, and aspirin.

The balance between *yin* and *yang* is used to explain mental as well as physical health. This belief, coupled with the influence of Russian theorists such as Pavlov, influence the Chinese view of mental illness. Mental illness results more from metabolic imbalances and organic problems. The effect of social situations, such as stress and crises, on a person's mental well-being is considered inconsequential, but physical imbalances from genetics are the important factors. Because a stigma is associated with having a family member who is mentally ill, many families initially seek the help of a folk healer. Many use a combination of traditional and Western medicine. Many mentally ill clients are treated as outpatients and remain in the home.

Although the Chinese do not readily seek assistance for emotional and nervous disorders, a study of 143 Chinese Americans found that younger, lower socioeconomic, and married Chinese with better language ability seek help more frequently (Ying & Miller, 1992). The researchers recommended that new immigrants be taught that help is available when needed for mental disorders within the mental health-care system.

Chinese people in larger cities are becoming more supportive of people with disabilities, but for the most part, support services are popular. Because the focus has been on improving the overall economic growth of the country, the needs of the disabled have not had priority. The son of Deng Xiaoping was crippled in the Cultural Revolution and has been active in making the country more aware of the needs of the disabled. The Beijing Paralympic Games were held on September 6–17, 2008, and opened 12 days after the 29th Olympic Games. A successful Paralympics in Beijing promoted the cause of disabled persons in Beijing as well as throughout China. The Games urged the whole of society to pay more attention to this special segment of our population and reinforced the importance of building accessible facilities for the disabled and thus enhance efforts to construct a harmonious society in China (Nan, 2006). Overall, the Chinese still view mental and physical disabilities as a part of life that should be hidden.

The expression of the sick role depends on the level of education of the patient. Educated Chinese people who have been exposed to Western ideas and culture are more likely to assume a sick role similar to that of Westerners. However, the highly educated and acculturated may exhibit some of the traditional roles associated with illness. Each patient needs to be assessed individually for responses to illness and for expectations of care. Traditionally, the Chinese ill person is viewed to be passive and accepting of illness. To the Chinese, illness is expected as a part of the life cycle. However, they do try to avoid danger and to live as healthy a life as possible. To the Chinese, all of life is interconnected; therefore, they seek explanations and connections for illness and injury in all aspects of life. Their explanations to health-care providers may not make sense, but the health-care provider should try to determine those connections so they can be incorporated into treatment regimens. The Chinese believe that because the illness or injury is caused from an imbalance, there should be a medicine or treatment that can restore the balance. If the medicine or treatment does not seem to do this, they may refuse to use it.

Native Chinese and Chinese Americans like treatments that are comfortable and do not hurt. Treatments that hurt are physically stressful and drain their energy. Health-care providers who have been ill themselves can appreciate this way of thinking, because sometimes the cure seems worse than the illness. Treatments will be more successful if they are explained in ways that are consistent with the Chinese way of thinking. The Chinese depend on their families and sometimes on their friends to help them while they are sick. These people provide much of the direct care; health-care providers are expected to manage the care. The family may seem to take over the life of the sick person, and the sick person is very passive in allowing them the control. One or two primary people assume this responsibility, usually a spouse. Health-care providers need to include the family members in the plan of care and, in many instances, in the actual delivery of care.

Blood Transfusions and Organ Donation

Modern-day Chinese accept blood transfusions, organ donations, and organ transplants when absolutely essential, as long as they are safe and effective. Chinese Americans have the same concerns as Americans about blood transfusion because of the perceived high incidence of HIV and hepatitis B. No overall ethnic or religious practices prohibit the use of blood transfusions, organ donations, or organ transplants. Of course, some individuals may have religious or personal reasons for denying their use.

Health Care Providers

Traditional Versus Biomedical Providers

China uses two health-care systems. One is grounded in Western medical care, and the other is anchored in traditional Chinese medicine. The educational preparation of physicians, nurses, and pharmacists is similar to Western health-care education. Ancillary workers have responsibility in the health-care system, and the practice of midwifery is widely accepted by the Chinese. Physicians in Chinese medicine are trained in universities, and traditional Chinese pharmacies remain an integral part of health care.

Status of Health-Care Providers

Traditional Chinese medicine providers are shown great respect by the Chinese. In many instances, they are shown equal, if not more, respect than Western health-care providers. The Chinese may distrust Western health-care providers because of the pain and invasiveness of their treatments. The hierarchy among Chinese health-care providers is similar to that of Chinese society. Older health-care providers receive respect from the younger providers. Men usually receive more respect than women, but that is beginning to change. Physicians receive the highest respect, followed closely by nurses with a university education. Other nurses with limited education are next in the hierarchy, followed by ancillary personnel.

Health-care providers are usually given the same respect as older people in the family. Chinese children

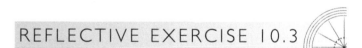

REFLECTIVE EXERCISE 10.3

Mrs. Cheng brought her 4-year-old son, Justin, to the emergency department early one morning. She stated that her son has had a high fever for 4 days. Her mother-in-law used traditional herbal medicine, but it was ineffective. The advanced practice nurse diagnosed a pulmonary infection and prescribed liquid antibiotics.

1. From a traditional Chinese medical perspective, how might the nurse incorporate Western medical prescriptions while respecting Mrs. Cheng's family, who wishes to continue Chinese herbal treatments?
2. What additional cultural and socioeconomic barriers should the nurse assess to provide culturally competent health-care and nursing services to Justin?
3. Identify and describe traditional, nonherbal Chinese medical practices that are used to treat pulmonary disorders?
4. Describe from the traditional Chinese individual the ideal health-care provider.

recognize them as authority figures. Physicians and nurses are viewed as individuals who can be trusted with the health of a family member. Nurses are generally perceived as caring individuals who perform treatments and procedures as ordered by the physician. Nursing assistants provide basic care to patients. Adult Chinese respond to health-care providers with respect, but if they disagree with the health-care provider, they may not follow instructions. They may not verbally confront the health-care provider because they fear that either they or the provider will suffer a loss of face.

The Chinese respect their bodies and are very modest when it comes to touch. Most Chinese women feel uncomfortable being touched by male health-care providers, and most seek female health-care providers.

REFERENCES

Alexander, R.M., & Marg, A.M. (2006). Chinese women local leaders exchange realities with WEI. *Women and Environments, 74,* 17–19.

Center for Reproductive Rights. (2002). *China turns one child policy into law.* Retrieved from http://www.crlp.org/ww_asia_1child.html

Chang, J.S. (2004). Refashioning womanhood in 1990s Taiwan: An analysis of Taiwanese edition of cosmopolitan magazine. *Modern China, 30,* 361–397.

Chen, S.E. (2009). Mother of the culture: Founding a Taiwanese feminist theology. *Feminist Theology, 27,* 81–88.

Cheung, R., Nelson, W., Advincula, L., Young, C.V., & Canham, D.L. (2005). Understanding the culture of Chinese children and families. *The Journal of School Nursing, 21*(1), 3–9.

Chinese Ministry of Health. (2004). *An about face on AIDS prevention.* Retrieved from http://www.highbeam.com/doc/pi-103213525.htm

Chinese Ministry of Health. (2009). *Chinese factfile.* Retrieved from http://english.gov.cn/about.htm

CIA World Factbook. (2011). *China.* Retrieved from https://www.cia.gov/library/publications/the-world-factbook/geos/ch.html

Gu, W. (2006). *Women of China: The human face of HIV/AIDS.* Retrieved from http://www.womenofchina.cn

Haley, G., Tan, C., & Haley, U. (1998). *New Asian emperors: The overseas Chinese, their strategies and competitive advantages.* Woburn, MA: Butterworth-Heinemann.

Halporn, R. (1992). Introduction. In C.L. Chen, W.C. Lowe, D. Ryan, A.H. Kutscher, R. Halporn, & H. Wang (Eds.), *Chinese Americans in loss and separation* (pp. v–xii). New York: Foundation of Thanatology.

Ho, H.F., & Lee, H.L. (2010). Great expectations: Family educational expenditure in Taiwan vs China. *European Journal of Social Sciences, 17*(4), 628–637.

Hu, W., & Grove, C.L. (1991). *Encountering the Chinese.* Yarmouth, MA: Intercultural Press.

Huang, W. (1992). Attitudes toward death: Chinese perspectives from the past. In C.L. Chen, W.C. Lowe, D. Ryan, A.H. Kutscher, R. Halporn, & H. Wang (Eds.), *Chinese Americans in loss and separation* (pp. 1–5). New York: Foundation of Thanatology.

Huangjuan. (2009). *One-night stands accepted, few practice.* Retrieved from http://www.womenofchina.cn/html/node/104673-1.htm

Levy, R.A. (1993). Ethnic and racial differences in response to medicines: Preserving individualized therapy in managed pharmaceutical programmes. *Pharmaceutical Medicine, 7,* 139–165.

Li, C. (2000). Confucianism and feminist concerns: Overcoming the Confucian "Gender complex". *Journal of Chinese Philosophy, 27,* 187–199.

Lin, C.C., & Fu, V.R. (1990). A comparison of child-rearing practices among Chinese, immigrant Chinese, and Caucasian-American parents. *Child Development, 61,* 429–433.

Ma, G.X. (2000). Barriers to the use of health services by Chinese Americans. *Journal of Allied Health, 29*(2), 64–70.

Mayo Clinic. (2010). *Tai chi: Discover the many possible health benefits.* Retrieved from http://www.mayoclinic.com/health/tai-chi/SA00087

Miller, L.C. (2000). Health of children adopted from China. *Pediatrics, 105*(6), 76.

Ministry of Health of the People's Republic of China. (2011). *Center for statistics information Ministry of Health, P. R. China.* Retrieved from http://www.moh.gov.cn/publicfiles/business/htmlfiles/mohwsbwstjxxzx/s7967/201104/51512.htm

Ministry of Public Health. (1992). *A brief introduction to China's medical and health services.* Beijing, People's Republic of China: Author.

Moore, R. (1990). Ethnographic assessment of pain coping perceptions. *Psychosomatic Medicine, 52,* 171–181.

Nan, C. (2006). *Beijing gears up for 2008 Paralympic Games.* Retrieved from http://www.btmbeijing.com

National Bureau of Statistics of China. (2011). *The sixth national population census.* Retrieved from http://www.stats.gov.cn/zgrkpc/dlc/yw/index.htm

Office of Minority Health. (2007). *Asian American profiles.* Retrieved from http://www.omhrc.gov/templates/browse.aspx?lvl=2&lvlID=32

O'Keefe, H., & O'Keefe, W. (1997). Chinese and Western behavioral differences: Understanding the gaps. *International Journal of Social Economics, 24,* 190–197.

People's Daily. (2002). *China's life expectancy averaged 71.8 year.* Retrieved from http://english.peopledaily.com.cn

Schulpen, T. (2001). Immunization status of children adopted from China. *The Lancet, 358,* 2131–2132.

Seidel, H., Ball, J., Dains, J., & Benedict, W. (1994). *Quick reference to cultural assessment.* St. Louis, MO: Mosby.

Shim, Y.H. (2001). Feminism and the discourse of sexuality in Korea: Continuities and changes. *Human Study, 24,* 133–148.

Shrestha, M., & Weber, K.E. (1994). Reflection of Confucianism, Hinduism, and Buddhism on gender relations and gender specific occupation in Thai society. *Journal of Population and Social Studies, 5*(1–2), 31–54.

Smith, C.S. (2002, April 30). Beware of cross-cultural faux pas in China. *New York Times.*

Tan, C.M. (1992). Treating life-threatening illness in children. In C.L. Chen, W.C. Lowe, D. Ryan, A.H. Kutscher, R. Halporn, & H. Wang (Eds.), *Chinese Americans in loss and separation* (pp. 26–33). New York: Foundation of Thanatology.

USAID. (2010). *HIV/AIDS health profile.* Retrieved from http://www.usaid.gov/our work/global health/aids/countries/asia/china_05.pdf

U.S. Census Bureau. (2006). *Selected population profile in the United States.* Retrieved from http://factfinder.census.gov/

U.S. Citizenship and Immigration Services. (2011). *Immigration and Nationality Act.* Retrieved from http://www.uscis.gov/

Wang, Y. (2011a). *Press release on major figures of the 2010 National Population Census.* Retrieved from http://www.womenofchina.cn

Wang, Y. (2011b). *AIDS deaths hit "peak" as 7,700 die.* Retrieved from http://www.womenofchina.cn

Wang, Y. (2011c). *Maternal, infant death rates drop in China's remote count.* Retrieved from http://www.womenofchina.cn/html/report/124973-1.htm

Women of China. (2006a). *Employment status of women.* Retrieved from http://www.womenofchina.cn

Women of China. (2006b). *Survey of divorce rates in different countries.* Retrieved from http://www.womenofchina.cn

Women of China. (2006c). *HIV test mandatory.* Retrieved from http://www.womenofchina.cn

Women of China. (2006d). *Women and children's health care services.* Retrieved from http://www.womenofchina.cn

XinHua News Agency. (2006). *Official calls for more efforts to curb gender imbalance.* Retrieved from http://english.peopledaily.com.cn

Yang, Z. (2011). *Chinese smokers not prepared to face hasty smoking ban.* Retrieved from http://www.womenofchina.cn/html/node/129421-1.htm

Ying, Y., & Miller, L.S. (1992). Help-seeking behavior and attitude of Chinese Americans regarding psychological problems. *American Journal of Community Psychology 20*(4), 549–556.

Yu, E.S., Edwin, H., Chen, K., Kim, K., & Sawsan, A. (2002). Smoking among Chinese Americans: Behavior, knowledge, and beliefs. *American Journal of Public Health*, 92(6), 1007–1013.

Zhang, J., Casswell, S., & Cai, H. (2008). Increased drinking in a metropolitan city in China: A study of alcohol consumption patterns and changes. *Addiction, 103*(3), 416–423.

Zhang, S. (2011). *Non-infectious chronic diseases become major health threat, claiming 85% of deaths in China.* Retrieved from http://www.womenofchina.cn/html/report/130433-1.htm

Zhuhong, A. (2006). *Population and family planning law of the People's Republic of China.* Retrieved from http://www.womenofchina.cn

Zhuhong, A. (2009a). *Survey shows more teens have sexual experience.* Retrieved from http://www.womenofchina.cn/html/node/102669-1.htm

Zhuhong, A. (2009b). *Abortion issue causes for concern.* Retrieved from http://www.womenofchina.cn/html/node/102775-1.htm

DavisPlus For case studies, review questions, and additional information, go to
http://davisplus.fadavis.com

Chapter 11

People of Cuban Heritage

Larry D. Purnell and Jorge Gil

Overview, Inhabited Localities, and Topography

Overview

The Republic of Cuba, with a population of over 11 million people, is located 90 miles south of Key West, Florida (*CIA World Factbook*, 2011). Approximately the size of Pennsylvania, it is the largest island in the West Indies. The capital, Havana, is the largest city. Fidel Castro was president of this communist country from 1959 until 2008, at which time he resigned due to health problems. Major agricultural products and industries include sugar, petroleum, tobacco, textiles, nickel, copper, cement, and fertilizer. Cuba is a multiracial society, with a population of primarily Spanish and African origins; other significant ethnic groups include Chinese, Haitians, and Eastern Europeans (*CIA World Factbook*, 2011).

Over 1.6 million Cuban Americans live in the United States, representing the third largest Hispanic group, after Mexican Americans and Puerto Ricans (U.S. Census Bureau, 2009). Cubans in Miami-Dade County, Florida—the dominant center of Cuban settlement—are credited with the area's socioeconomic transformation (Boswell, 2002). In this ethnic enclave, Cubans have created businesses and rejuvenated the economy, leading some to speak of the "great Cuban miracle." The distinctive Cuban culture is evidenced by their music, dance, and art. Cubans have made a number of dances popular, including the rumba, the cha-cha, the guaracha, the bolero, and the conga. The classical ballerina, Alicia Alonso, was a Cuban dancer famous for, among other things, her portrayal in the ballet *Carmen*. The film *Fresa y Chocolate* (*Strawberries and Chocolate*) won the Silver Bear Award at the Berlin Film Festival in February 1995 (Cultural Orientation Resource Center, 2002).

The experience of Cubans in their homeland and in the United States is distinct from that of other Hispanic groups. The history and culture of Cuba and the Cuban people have been heavily influenced by Spain, the United States, the Soviet Union, and, through the slave trade in Cuba's sugar industry, West African groups such as the Yoruba.

Cuba was under Spanish control from 1511 until 1898, making it one of Spain's last colonies in the New World. Control of the sugar industry by Spanish *peninsulares* (individuals born in Spain) was challenged by the growing class of *criollo* landowners (individuals of Spanish ancestry born in Cuba) and the *independentista* movement. This absentee ownership created political turmoil and social imbalances that gave rise to the Cuban national character. The mistrust of government reinforced a strong personalistic tradition, a sense of national identity evolving from family and interpersonal relationships (Szapocznik & Hernandez, 1988).

Unlike most other immigrant groups, under the Cuban Adjustment Act of 1966, Cubans were welcomed by the U.S. government and were provided with support from the Cuban Refugee Program begun by the Kennedy administration. Cubans engaged in a wide range of entrepreneurial activity, in both sales and services, within the shelter of the Cuban community. Consequently, newer Cuban immigrants found networks of support and were somewhat protected from the difficulties associated with a competitive labor market. There is a common feeling of thankfulness and appreciation among newer Cuban generations in the United States and also from the first cohort of Cuban immigrants who arrived in the early 1960s. Cubans in the United States are a strong presence, not only economically but also politically. An exile ideology, a preoccupation with events in Cuba, and militant opposition to the regime of Fidel Castro characterize their predominant political stance. Overwhelmingly, Cuban Americans tend to be conservative, Republican, and anti-Communist. They have demonstrated high voter turnout and tend to vote in blocs during local and national elections (National Council of la Raza, 2011).

Cubans have managed to adjust to mainstream American culture while remaining close to their Cuban roots. However, young adults and adolescents who were educated in Cuba with strict Communist ideation and who emigrated with their parents may find the clash in values between Cuba and their new country confusing and negative. The bicultural Cuban American population can help in their adjustment. Many Cubans outside Cuba possess a strong ethnic identity, speak Spanish, and adhere to traditional Cuban values and practices at home while working in the dominant culture of their new homeland.

Cuban Economy

From the late 1800s to mid-1900s, Cuba was considered one of the most prosperous countries in Latin America. The economy was based on treaties mainly with United States, France, and Spain. Taxes were collected from people at a high rates compared with those of countries from the "first world." At the same time, construction of new buildings and roads increased. Since the 1959 Communist Revolution of Castro, the island has based its economy on subsidies from communist countries such as the former Soviet Union and China. With *perestroika* (literally translated, "restructuring") in 1988 by ex-president Mikhail Gorbachev, Cuba tried without success to implement changes in the economy.

Cuban economy today is primarily based on tourism and gastronomy. Recently, the government established taxes for so-called "private businesses," but because Cuba has no experience with a capitalist economy, its government does not know how to implement the taxation system. The general population cannot pay these excessively high taxes and continue to depend on their families *en el extranjero*: those who reside outside Cuba.

Heritage and Residence

Ethnically, Cubans are 61.1 percent white, 24.8 percent mulatto or *mestizo*, and 10.1 percent black (*CIA World Factbook*, 2011). The native Arawak Indian population that inhabited the island when Columbus landed in 1492 died from diseases brought by Spanish settlers. Cubans have a rich historical heritage. Spain launched its conquest of Mexico from Cuba in 1519. During the Spanish colonial period (1511–1898), Spanish boats stopped in Havana on their way to Mexico and Central America. In the 19th century, the Monroe Doctrine led to a special relationship between Cuba and the United States. The U.S. military controlled the island from 1898 to 1902. In 1902, Cuba was a politically independent capitalist state. In 1959, Fidel Castro led a revolution to free Cuba of the U.S.-backed dictator Fulgencio Batista and subsequently established a totalitarian Communist government, which still controls the country through the sole party, the Cuban Communist Party (PCC).

Most Cuban Americans reside in four states: Florida, New Jersey, California, and New York. The largest proportion live in Florida, especially in Miami-Dade County. The Cuban American population is aging, with a median age of 43.6 years and more than 20 percent over 65 years old. By comparison, Mexicans, Puerto Ricans, and Central and South Americans living in the United States have median ages between 11 to 16 years younger than the average for Cuban Americans. The higher median age is explained by lower fertility rates of Cuban American women and the older age of those who immigrate from Cuba (Boswell, 2002; Martinez, 2002).

About two-thirds of Cuban Americans residing in the United States were born in Cuba, making this group a largely immigrant population as compared with other Hispanic groups. To illustrate, only 32 percent of Cuban Americans were born in the United States, compared with 64 percent for Mexican Americans and 60 percent for Puerto Ricans (Boswell, 2002).

Based on the 2010 U.S. Census, the total estimated Cuban population in the United States is almost 1.6 million, which is the third largest Hispanic population in this country (U.S. Census Bureau, 2010). The largest is the Mexican population with a total of almost 30 million people, followed by Puerto Ricans with over 4 million. The major concentration of Cubans is located in Miami-Dade County, Florida, with 778,389 (U.S. Census Bureau, 2010)—almost half of the total estimated number of Cuban Americans. The second concentration of Cubans is located in New York City with a total of 42,414, followed by Texas with 36,945. (U.S. Census Bureau, 2010). Places like South Dakota and Alaska have smaller Cuban populations with 134 and 740, respectively (U.S. Census Bureau, 2010).

Reasons for Migration and Associated Economic Factors

Approximately 1 million Cubans immigrated to the United States between 1959 and 1980; fewer than 200,000 arrived between 1990 and 2000. In the first 2 decades of the earlier period, most arrived on the U.S. mainland after the 1959 revolution that brought Fidel Castro to power and changed the social, economic, and political landscape of Cuba. Although the American government has defined the exodus as a political rather than an economic migration, a combination of these factors provided the motivation for migration. The desire for personal freedom, the hope of refuge and political exile, and the promise of economic opportunities have been the main reasons for Cuban immigration.

Portes and Bach (1985) identified six stages of Cuban immigration to the United States:

1. *First stage*: Departures from January 1959 to October 1962. When Fidel Castro overthrew the government of Fulgencio Batista in January 1959, approximately 250,000 landowners, industrialists,

professionals, and merchants left on commercial flights from Havana for the United States.

Operation Pedro Pan. In the early 1960s, some 14,000 Cuban children and teens were flown to the United States without their parents through *Operation Pedro Pan.* Triggered by fears that their children would be made wards of the state and forced to participate in counterrevolutionary activities, Cuban parents sent their children to the United States. The *Pedro Pan* children were placed with foster families and relocated to different parts of the country; some never saw their parents again (Conde, 1999). Although a number of children were eventually reunited with their parents, many suffered years of isolation and estrangement from their families.

2. *Second stage*: Departures from November 1962 to September 1965. The confrontation between Cuba and the United States over Russian missiles in Cuba ended all direct flights from Cuba to the United States. At this time, about 56,000 people left on small boats and rafts because no direct transportation was available.

3. *Third stage*: Departures from October 1965 to April 1973. Cuba and the United States reached an understanding in which an airlift was allowed from Varadero Beach, Cuba, to Miami. These "freedom flights" or "family reunification flights" provided the opportunity for about 297,000 people to immigrate.

4. *Fourth stage*: Departures from May 1973 to September 1978. The Cuban government unilaterally ended the airlift. Travel to Spain, Mexico, and Jamaica became the only means of leaving Cuba. About 39,000 people arrived in the United States on commercial flights by way of these countries.

5. *Fifth stage*: Departures from October 1978 to March 1980. Fidel Castro allowed political prisoners from Cuban jails to leave with their families. About 10,000 people arrived in this manner on airplane flights, boats, and rafts.

6. *Sixth stage*: Departures from April to September 1980. The Cuban government again allowed a massive boatlift from the Mariel Harbor in Cuba to Key West, Florida. Approximately 125,000 people arrived (known as the *Marielitos*), including people with criminal records, homosexuals, deaf-mutes, lepers, and patients from mental institutions. About 5000, or 4 percent, of these were hard-core criminals, causing an increase in the levels of violent crime in the metropolitan Miami and New York areas.

In the decade from 1990 to 2000, a total of 191,506 Cuban immigrants entered the United States (U.S. Immigration and Naturalization Service, 2000). Skaine (2004) characterized two significant groups in this period:

Balseros: The term *balseros* was derived from *balsa* (raft), denoting the arrival of Cubans in the 1990s using homemade rafts. This wave of migration was preceded by deteriorating living conditions in Cuba, with long electric power outages and chronic shortages of food and basic necessities. Of 35,000 *balseros* who were allowed by the Castro government to leave in 1994, only 30,000 were estimated to have arrived in the United States. Many did not survive the crossing because of dehydration or boats that capsized. The most-celebrated case was that of 5-year-old Elian Gonzalez, who was rescued floating on an inner tube after his mother and others perished when their boat capsized (Skaine, 2004).

Immigrating through other countries: From 2001 until the present, increasing numbers of Cubans have been immigrating by land through Mexico, Canada, Spain, or other countries (Skaine, 2004).

Two immigration accords signed by the United States and Cuba set a limit of 20,000 visas annually for Cuban immigrants and stipulated that any illegal immigrants will be repatriated. At present, U.S. law enforces the wet-foot/dry-foot policy with Cuban refugees. This means that if a Cuban refugee reaches dry land in the United States, that individual will be awarded legal immigrant status. This policy has generated some resentment from other immigrant groups such as Mexicans and Haitians, who are not awarded similar status even if they manage to arrive on dry land in the United States (Skaine, 2004).

In the 3 decades of Cuban immigration, significant change has been observed in the waves of immigrants, from the elite classes of the first stage, called the *golden exiles*, to the **Marielitos** of the sixth stage and the *balseros* of the 1990s. Each wave is distinct: The earliest waves of immigrants represented higher educational and economic status in Cuba than subsequent waves; the later groups were more representative of the Cuban population. The motivation for immigration also changed from the desire to escape political and religious persecution in the earlier waves to the hope for economic improvement in the later waves (Skaine, 2004).

Educational Status and Occupations

The level of educational attainment of Cuban Americans is higher than that of other Hispanic groups. About 22 percent of Cuban Americans are college graduates, compared with 7 percent for Mexican Americans, 12 percent for Puerto Ricans, and 16 percent for Central and South Americans. The educational preparation of Cuban Americans is reflected in their median income, which is also higher than that of other Hispanic groups. The median household income for Cubans is $38,000, higher than for other Hispanics ($36,000) but lower than for non-Hispanic whites ($48,000). Native-born Cubans have a higher median income than non-Hispanic whites ($50,000 vs. $48,000). Among foreign-born Cubans, those who arrived before 1980 have the highest median income ($38,000). However, those who arrived between 1980 and 1990 have a lower median income compared with those who arrived in 1990 or later ($30,000 vs. $33,000). Cubans living outside Florida have a higher median income than those living in Florida ($44,000 vs. $36,000) (Pew Hispanic Center, 2006). Relatively high proportions of Cubans work in wholesale and retail trade, banking and credit agencies, insurance, real estate, and finance. A larger proportion of Cuban Americans are found in higher-paying managerial and professional jobs (24 percent), compared with Mexican Americans (12 percent), Puerto Ricans (17 percent), and Central and South Americans (15 percent). Conversely, in lower-paying jobs as operators, fabricators, handlers, and farmers, Cuban Americans have a smaller proportion (18 percent) than that of Mexican Americans (18 percent), Puerto Ricans (21 percent), and Central and South Americans (24 percent) (Boswell, 2002).

Communication

Dominant Language and Dialects

Language is often used as an index of assimilation of an immigrant group into the dominant culture. Virtually all first-generation Cubans in the United States speak Spanish as their first language, although Cuban Spanish varies somewhat in choice of words and pronunciation from the Spanish spoken in Spain and Central and South America.

Some Cuban Americans consider English to be their dominant language, others consider Spanish to be their dominant language, and yet others are completely bilingual. Because many Cubans live and transact business in Spanish-speaking ethnic enclaves, they have little need or motivation to learn English and are less likely to acculturate. Many, like one of the authors, speak **Spanglish**, a mixture of Spanish and English with phrases such as *Have a buen dia; Hola, donde va today?* (Have a good day; Hello, where are you going?). The large number and variety of Spanish-language media, including newspapers, magazines, and radio programs, also reflect some Cuban immigrants' preference for Spanish over English. A stroll through Little Havana in Miami or Little Havana North along New Jersey's Union City–west New York corridor, as well as other places in the United States, reveals that Spanish is reflected in billboard and poster advertisements. Signs announcing *joyeria* (jewelry store), *carniceria* (butcher shop), *muebleria* (furniture store), *farmacia* (drugstore), or *zapateria* (shoe store) are quite commonplace. In addition, Cubans in the United States have incorporated into their everyday Spanish many English words, such as *futbol, rosbif, coctel, sueter, frigidaire,* and *bridge*. For Cuban Americans, Spanglish becomes a reflection of both their Cuban and their American heritages.

Cultural Communication Patterns

Like other Hispanic groups, Cubans value **simpatia** and **personalismo** in their interactions with others. *Simpatia* refers to the need for smooth interpersonal relationships and is characterized by courtesy, respect, and the absence of harsh criticism or confrontation. *Personalismo* emphasizes intimate interpersonal relationships over impersonal bureaucratic relationships. **Choteo**, a lighthearted attitude with teasing, bantering, and exaggerating, may often be observed in the way Cubans communicate with one another (Bernal, 1994).

Conversations among Cubans are characterized by animated facial expressions, direct eye contact, hand gestures, and gesticulations. Voices tend to be loud and the rate of speech faster than may be observed with non-Cuban groups. Linguistically, the use of the second-person form *usted* to address older people and authority figures has fallen into disuse, replaced by the familiar form *tu*, although some older people prefer the formal use of language, especially in hierarchal relationships such as with health professionals. The use of *tu* in interpersonal situations serves to reduce distance and promotes *personalismo*. Touching, in the form of handshakes or hugs, is acceptable among family, friends, and acquaintances. In the health-care setting, patients and family members may hug or kiss the health-care provider to express gratitude and appreciation.

Cubans feel a sense of "specialness" about themselves and their culture that may be conveyed in communication with others. This sense of specialness arises from pride in their unique culture, a fusion of European and African; the geopolitical importance of Cuba in relation to powerful countries in history; and the exceptional success they have achieved in adapting to their new environment. This sense of specialness, combined with the fast rate and loud volume of speech, may sometimes be interpreted as arrogance or grandiosity in a non-Cuban cultural context (Bernal, 1994).

Temporal Relationships

Cubans tend to be present oriented compared with future-oriented European Americans. A greater emphasis is paid to current issues and problems than on projections into the future. In the clinical setting, health-care providers must realize that Cuban patients tend to be motivated to seek help in response to crisis situations. Hence, visits to health-care providers for resolution of a crisis must be used

REFLECTIVE EXERCISE 11.1

Pedro is a 12-year-old child who arrived from Cuba 6 months ago. He flew from the island with his parents and a 4-year-old sister. He lives now with his paternal grandparents in the Coral Gables area of Miami. He started school one week after he came from Cuba in a local public school. "Pedrito," as he is called by his family and close friends, used to do very well in school. He had received several accommodations from his teachers, always had good grades, was very friendly and active socially, was always a team player, and had several awards in different sports.

For the past 4 or 5 months, he appears to be lonely and quiet. His mother approached him once and asked him what changed his attitude. Pedrito told her that he does not understand English, the teachers talk too fast, and when he asks questions, several children in the classroom laugh at him. He told his mother that he wants to go back to Cuba, hates his new country, and will no longer go to school.

1. Do you think Pedrito's behavior is a common pattern in all immigrant kids during the process of acculturation? Explain your answer.
2. What is the best action for the parents to take?
3. Describe three consequences of Pedrito's behavior for his future professional and personal development if his parents do not take early measures to try to help him.

as opportunities for teaching and promotion of personal growth.

Hora cubana (Cuban time) refers to a flexible time period that stretches from 1 to 2 hours beyond the designated clock time. A Cuban understands that when a party starts at 8 p.m., the socially acceptable time to arrive is between 9 and 10 p.m. However, families who have acculturated to American values may adhere to a more rigid clock time. When setting up appointments for clinic visits, the health-care provider must determine the patient's level of acculturation with respect to time and make arrangements for flexible scheduling, if necessary.

Format for Names

Modeled after Spanish and other Latin American societies, Cubans use two surnames, representing the mother's and the father's sides of the family. For example, a woman may use the name Regina Morales Colon, indicating that her patrilineal surname is Morales and her matrilineal surname is Colon. When a Cuban woman marries, she adds *de* and her husband's name after her father's surname and drops her mother's surname. In the previous example, if Regina marries Mr. Ordonez, her name will be Regina Morales de Ordonez (Skaine, 2004). When addressing Cuban patients, especially the elderly, the health-care provider should use the formal rather than the familiar form, unless told otherwise. In the previous example, the appropriate appellation would be Señora Morales, or Mrs. Morales, instead of Regina.

Cubans translate English, Russian, or any other language in their own "Cuban way," and this is true for names as well. Some examples of common terms that have been adapted from other languages are *Naivy* (like U.S. Navy), *Yusimi* (You see me), and *Yeneisy* (Yeah, nein—German for "no" and "see").

Family Roles and Organization
Head Of Household And Gender Roles

As among most Hispanic/Latino populations, family is the most important social unit among Cubans and Cuban Americans. The traditional Cuban family structure is patriarchal, characterized by a dominant and aggressive male and a passive, dependent female, although the more acculturated families in the United States have become more egalitarian. *La casa*, the house, is considered the province of the woman, and *la calle*, the street, the domain of the man. *La calle* includes everything outside the home, which is considered a proper testing ground for masculinity but dangerous and inappropriate for women. Traditionally, Cuban wives are expected to stay at home, manage the household, and care for the children. Husbands are expected to work, provide, and make major decisions for the family. However, with acculturation and more women working outside the home, egalitarian decision making prevails in the United States.

Cultural values acquired through 4 centuries of Spanish domination influence the behavior of Cuban men and women toward one another. The concept of **honor** is described as personal goodness or virtue, which can be lost or diminished by an immoral or unworthy act. Honor is maintained mainly by fulfilling family obligations and by treating others with **respeto** (respect). Verguenza, a consciousness of public opinion and the judgment of the entire community, is considered more important for women than men. **Machismo** dictates that men display physical strength, bravery, and virility.

In Cuba, the transition from an agricultural to an industrial economy, the rising educational attainment of women, the increased participation of women in the workforce, and the passage of the Family Code of 1975 resulted in more gender equality and parity beween men and women with respect to marriage, divorce, property relations, and sharing of household responsibilities (Skaine, 2004).

Since the massive migration from Cuba to the United States in 1959, the traditional Cuban family has undergone a transition to a less male-dominated, less segregated, and more egalitarian structure. Cuban women who arrived in the United States were frequently the first in the family to find jobs and contribute to the survival of the family. According to

Gallagher (1980), Cuban immigrant women were more receptive to life in the United States, more flexible, and more readily hired for jobs than men. Eventually, as their contributions to the family's economic well-being increased, the women's power to make decisions was enhanced. Cuban American women have the highest rate of labor participation when compared with all other groups of women in the United States (Suarez, 1993). Thus, contemporary Cuban families from the 1980s to the present may demonstrate greater gender equality in decision making for the family.

Prescriptive, Restrictive, and Taboo Practices for Children and Adolescents

Cuban parents tend to pamper and overprotect their children, showering them with love and attention. Among Cubans, the expectation is that children study and respect their parents and older people. Children are encouraged to acquire knowledge and learning *porque eso no te lo puede quitar nadie* (because no one can take that away from you) (Bernal, 1994).

When a Cuban daughter reaches the age of 15 years, a *quince*, or 15th birthday party, is typically held to celebrate this rite of passage. Socially, the *quince* is indicative of the young woman's readiness for courting by a *novio* (boyfriend). In Cuba, as among many families in the United States, the *quince* is celebrated with food, music, and dancing among family and friends. In Miami's Cuban enclave, as well as in other cities, the *quince* is a major social event. Parents may save up for years to prepare for a daughter's *quince*, which has today evolved into a large, extravagant party.

Many Cuban adolescents may undergo an identity crisis, not knowing whether they are fully Cuban or American. During this time, they may reject traditional cultural values, and parents may feel threatened when their authority is being challenged. The opposing values and demands of their Cuban heritage and American society create a potential for tension and conflict between Cuban adolescents and their parents. Some examples are the Cuban practice of chaperoning unmarried couples when they date. Unmarried daughters are expected to live at home with the family until they marry.

Family Goals and Priorities

Cubans have tightly knit nuclear families that allow for inclusion of relatives and *padrinos* (godparents). *La familia* (the family) is the most important source of emotional and physical support for its members. Extended, multigenerational households are common, with grandparents often being part of the nuclear family. Compared with other Hispanic ethnic or cultural groups, Cubans have the lowest proportion of families with children. Cubans also have the highest proportion of people aged 65 and older who live with

their relatives. The high proportion of older people living with family members has led to the typical three-generation Cuban family (Perez, 2002).

A system of personal relationships known as *compadrazgo* is also typical. A set of godparents, or *compadres*, is selected for each child who is baptized and confirmed. *Compadres* tend to be close friends or relatives of the child's natural parents and may be counted on for moral or financial assistance. *Compadres* are usually considered part of the Cuban family, whether or not a true blood relationship exists.

In recent years, as Cubans have become more acculturated to American society, and as the children of Cuban immigrants have become more Americanized and more economically successful than their parents, family dynamics, expectations, and behaviors are changing. Multigenerational living arrangements are markedly declining, with increased numbers of older adults becoming more independent and living alone. Despite these trends, the need and desire for frequent family contact through daily telephone calls and frequent visits are still predominant. Although more likely now to be living alone, older Cuban adults have close interactions not only with their children but also with grandchildren, siblings, cousins, and other relatives (Martinez, 2002).

Alternative Lifestyles

There is a high proportion of divorced women among Cuban Americans compared with other Hispanic and non-Hispanic groups in the United States. In spite of this, Cubans have the highest percentage of children under 18 years living with both parents, a low percentage of families headed by women with no husbands present, and the lowest rate of mothers and children living within a larger family unit. One explanation for these patterns may be that divorced Cuban women return to their parents' home, but because they typically have fewer children, they do not tend to be accompanied by children (Perez, 2002).

In dealing with some Cuban Americans, healthcare providers may hear the term *Marielito* used in a derogatory manner to refer to the estimated 4 percent of the 125,000 Cubans who arrived during the Mariel boatlift. Because some of the *Marielitos* were hard-core criminals released from Cuban jails, the increased levels of crime in metropolitan Miami and New York have been attributed in part to their arrival. Although very few of them were criminals, unfortunately, the negative attitudes toward them have been extended to Cuban Americans as a group. The *Marielitos* were predominantly single, black, working-class Cuban males, in contrast to the professional and managerial workers of earlier waves of migration.

Little or no data are available on the occurrence of homosexuality among Cuban Americans, although the gay lifestyle would be contradictory to the prevailing *machismo* orientation of Cuban culture. Same-sex

REFLECTIVE EXERCISE 11.2

Alberto Gonzaga is a 43-year-old Cuban American male. He migrated 18 years ago with his wife and 3-year-old son, Alberto. Before he emigrated to the United States, Mr. Gonzaga was imprisoned in Cuba for political reasons. He did not complete the 20-year sentence imposed by the Castro regime and was released from jail after 12 years for good behavior. He was immediately granted a U.S. visa for himself and his family. Since his arrival, he has been an active member of the Republican Party and has participated in the local Miami area in the anticommunist movement. His son is now 21, and he still lives with his parents, helping them financially. He works full-time and pursues a law degree in a local college. There have been several confrontations between Mr. Gonzaga and his son. The new, more liberal "open" era has brought Cuban musicians from the island to perform in public concerts in Miami. Mr. Gonzaga is totally opposed to this. He claims that "these Communist musicians will take our money and our taxes and give it to Castro" and prohibits his son from going to the concerts. Alberto states that music has nothing to do with politics and that many of these musicians are opposed to the regime, but this is a way to travel outside Cuba and earn some money. He confronts his father, telling him that he is an adult and he will go to the concerts, despite his father's opposition.

1. How different is the Cuban population that migrated 20 years ago compared with those who arrived 5 or 6 years ago?
2. Are the children of the Cubans who arrived in the 1980s maintaining their traditions? Is their way of thinking the same as their parents'?
3. What could be the consequences of the confrontations between Mr. Gonzaga and his son?
4. Is the Castro government still separating the family even outside Cuba, or is this situation just a matter of character?

couples living together may be alienated from their families, especially among first-generation Cubans who adhere closely to traditional gender roles and family values. Undoubtedly, gay and lesbian films such as *Gay Cuba*, *Strawberry and Chocolate*, and *La Carne de Rey* and the Miami Gay and Lesbian Film Festival are attempts at making alternative lifestyles more acceptable. Given the stigma associated with homosexuality in this culture, a matter-of-fact, nonjudgmental approach must be used by health-care providers when questioning Cuban patients regarding sexual orientation or sexual practices.

Workforce Issues

Culture in the Workplace

Cubans have enjoyed enormous economic success in the United States. Twenty percent of first-generation Cuban Americans and 43 percent of second-generation Cuban Americans are college graduates. The high educational achievement is reflected in the large proportions—53 percent for first-generation Cuban Americans and 75 percent for second-generation Cuban Americans—who are employed in managerial and technical jobs, the two highest-paying occupational categories (Boswell, 2002). Cuban families also have proportionately more people participating in the labor force and earning a higher median income than Mexican, Puerto Rican, or Central and South American families (Boswell, 2002). Their strong entrepreneurial abilities tend to be concentrated in construction, transportation, textiles, wholesale, and retail trades. The existence of several Cuban ethnic enclaves with a familiar language and culture has created numerous employment opportunities for recent Cuban immigrants.

A frequent source of tension in the workplace is the tendency of Cubans to speak Spanish with other Cuban or Hispanic coworkers. Speaking the same language allows them to form a common bond, relieve anxieties at work, and feel comfortable with one another. In Blank and Slipp's (1994) study, one Cuban supervisor asserted, "Others should know that we tend to go back and forth in language—Spanish when we're talking personally and English when it's professional."

Issues Related to Autonomy

Traditional Cubans tend to be hierarchical in their relationships, recognizing supervisors or superiors as authority figures and treating them with respect and deference. In mainstream American culture, collegial relationships, in which workers can exercise initiative, question the supervisor, and participate in decision making, may make Cubans uncomfortable. Cubans value a structure characterized by *personalismo*—that is, one that is oriented around people rather than around concepts or ideas. For Cubans, personal relationships at work are considered an extension of family relationships. Cuban workers may function best in a working environment that is warm and friendly and fosters *personalismo*. Because of the emphasis on the job or task in the American workplace, many Cubans view this workplace as being too individualistic, business-like, and detached. In the past, the language barrier may have insulated Cuban Americans from the dominant culture, retarded acculturation, and fostered some interethnic tensions; as the ability to speak English and acculturation increases, Cuban Americans have fewer interethnic tensions.

Biocultural Ecology

Skin Color and Other Biological Variations

Most Cuban Americans are white. Because of their predominantly European ancestry, Cuban Americans have skin, hair, and eye colors that vary from light to dark. A minority, who are of African Cuban extraction, are dark-skinned and may have physical features similar to those of African Americans.

REFLECTIVE EXERCISE 11.3

Pablo Perez is a 42-year-old Cuban immigrant. He arrived in the United States 2 years ago with his wife and a 10-year-old daughter. He was a successful physician in Cuba and was selected to travel outside the island in 1991 to Spain to assist in an international congress. He also was chosen to provide medical services in Senegal in 2002. Both times, he returned to Cuba—the first time because his mother was in bad health (she died a short time later), and the second time because he had a wife and daughter waiting for him. In 2006, he and his wife were selected to go to Venezuela. After 2 years there, where he demonstrated an excellent professional and communist attitude, the consulate allowed their daughter to join them.

This was the chance Dr. Perez was waiting for. He and his family immediately headed north, crossed the Mexican border into the United States, and settled in Las Vegas. Both Dr. and Mrs. Perez each have two full-time jobs. They have had problems learning the language. Dr. Perez has taken the medical boards twice, but he failed both times. He has told his wife that if they moved to Miami, it will be better for them because there are more Hispanic people there, the weather is better, and the support system is greater. Do you think that Dr. and Mrs. Perez's behavior in Venezuela is a common pattern among Cuban professionals who are trying to get into the United States?

1. How different is the Cuban health system compared to that of the United States?
2. Explain the options that Dr. and Mrs. Perez have for joining the health-care field again in the United States?
3. Do you think that moving to Miami will solve Dr. and Mrs. Perez's problems?

Diseases and Health Conditions

Nath's (2005) analysis of data from the Hispanic Health and Nutrition Examination Survey (HHANES) reported that, among Cuban Americans, major health conditions are a high prevalence of coronary heart disease, hypertension, overweight or obesity, type 2 diabetes mellitus, and depression. Twenty-nine percent of Cuban American men and 34 percent of Cuban American women are overweight, compared with 25 percent and 37 percent of Puerto Rican males and females, respectively, and 30 percent and 39 percent of Mexican American males and females, respectively. The same study found that 16 percent of Cuban Americans aged 45 to 74 had diabetes mellitus, compared with 26 percent of Puerto Ricans and 24 percent of Mexican Americans.

In a comparison of hypertension-related mortality among Hispanic groups, Cuban Americans were found to have the lowest death rate and Puerto Ricans had the highest death rate. In addition, age-standardized hypertension-related mortality rates in Cuban Americans were 39 percent lower than those for non-Hispanic whites (Centers for Disease Control and Prevention, 2006).

Variations in Drug Metabolism

Although some studies have reported differences in drug metabolism among Hispanics, little or no data specific to Cuban Americans are available.

High-Risk Behaviors

Devieux and colleagues (2005) at Florida International University conducted an assessment of HIV risk behaviors of adolescents participating in an HIV risk-reduction intervention. Of the 137 participants in the interview assessment, 81 were African American teens and 57 were Cuban American teens. Cuban American teens reported more unprotected sex acts and more anal sex acts in the 6 months prior to the interview than did African American teens. The groups were similar on the total number of sexual partners and sex acts reported. Regarding drug use, a greater proportion of Cuban American teens reported using drugs in the 6 months prior than did African American teens, and more Cuban American teens reported engaging in unprotected sex while using drugs than did African American teens. The authors speculate that higher acculturation of Cuban American teens, and accompanying family conflict, may account for the relatively more risky behaviors among Cuban American teens. More research is needed to clarify the processes leading teens of different backgrounds to initiate and maintain risky behaviors and to identify the most effective ways to intervene to reduce risk (Devieux et al., 2005).

The HHANES findings also revealed that drinking alcohol was significantly more common among Cuban males than females and among younger versus older Cuban groups, a pattern that was similar to that in Mexicans and Puerto Ricans. Among middle-aged and older Cuban males, who tend to be relatively well educated and have higher incomes compared with the younger, more recent Cuban immigrants, control of intoxication is important. Among Cuban women, the proportion of lifelong abstainers increased significantly from the younger to the older groups (Black & Markides, 1994).

Smoking is responsible for 87 percent of the lung cancer deaths in the United States. Overall, lung cancer is the leading cause of cancer deaths among Hispanics. Lung cancer deaths are about three times higher for Hispanic men (23.1 per 100,000) than for Hispanic women (7.7 per 100,000). The rates of lung cancer deaths per 100,000 were higher among Cuban American men (33.7) than among Puerto Rican (28.3) and Mexican American (21.9) men (Centers for Disease Control and Prevention, 2011).

Health-Care Practices

An obstacle to good nutritional practices is the Cuban cultural perspective of the "healthy body." A healthy and beautiful Cuban infant is fat. Even among adults, a little heaviness is considered attractive. *Que gordo* estas! (How fat you are!) is considered a compliment. The traditional Cuban diet—high in calories, starches, and saturated fats—predisposes individuals to the development of obesity. In Cuba, health care is viewed as a basic human right and occupies a prominent place in the Cuban government's domestic and foreign policies. Polyclinics in communities are the basic unit of health care. Physician–nurse teams attend patients in these polyclinics, as well as in the home, school, day-care center, and workplace.

In the United States, Cubans exhibit high levels of preventive health behaviors, as evidenced by routine physical examinations within the last 2 years. The utilization of preventive services was usually associated with accessibility, which, in turn, was significantly influenced by education, annual income, and age (Solis, Marks, Garcia, & Shelton, 1990).

Lopez and Masse (1993) found that unmarried Cuban American women who had little recreational activity tended to have a higher mean weight. In addition, in contrast to Mexican American and Puerto Rican women, body fatness in Cuban American women was not significantly associated with income (Lopez & Masse, 1993).

Nutrition

Meaning of Food

Besides satisfying hunger, food has a powerful social meaning among Cuban Americans, allowing families to reaffirm kinship ties, promote a sense of community, and perpetuate their customs and heritage. To grasp this fully, one needs only to observe multigenerational families assembled for dinner on a Saturday or Sunday evening in a Cuban restaurant in Miami's Little Havana or Cuban friends sharing a cup of *cafe cubano* and *pastelitos* at a stand-up sidewalk counter. In Miami alone, the demand for Cuban food and food products has resulted in the establishment of about 400 Latin restaurants, mostly Cuban, and some 700 *bodegas*, or grocery stores. Other Cuban enclaves paint a similar picture.

Common Foods and Food Rituals

Cuban foods reflect the environmental influences of Cuba's tropical climate and agriculture, the historical influences of Spanish colonial rule, the African slave trade, and the Arawak Indians' cultivation methods. Typical staple foods are root crops like yams, yucca, malanga, and boniato; plantains; and grains. Traditional Spanish dishes like *arroz con pollo* and *paella* are frequently served. Many dishes are prepared with olive oil, garlic, tomato sauce, vinegar, wine, lime juice (called *sofrito*), and spices. Meat is usually marinated in lemon, lime, sour orange, or grapefruit juice before cooking (Kittler & Sucher, 2008).

The main course in Cuban meals is meat, usually pork or chicken. Some popular entrees are roast pork (*lechon*), fried pork chunks (*masas de puerco*), sirloin steak (*palomilla*), shredded beef (*ropa vieja*), pot roast (*boliche*), and roasted chicken (*pollo asado*). A roasted suckling pig is traditionally served on Christmas Eve, New Year's Day, and other festive celebrations. Black beans are prepared with a sauce containing fat, pork, and spices. Ripe plantains (*platanos maduros*) or green plantains (*platanos verdes*) are served fried. Fried green plantains (*tostones* or *mariquita*) may also be smashed between a brown paper bag and the fist (*un cartucho y el puno*), giving them the familiar name *platanos a punetazo*. Desserts are rich and very sweet, such as custard (*flan*), egg pudding (*natilla*), rice pudding (*arroz con leche*), coconut pudding (*pudin de coco*), or bread pudding (*pudin de pan*) (Kittler & Sucher, 2008).

Beverages may include sugar cane juice (*guarapo*), iced coconut milk (*coco frio*), milkshakes (*batidos*), Cuban soft drinks such as Iron Beer or Materva, sangria, or beer. The strong and bittersweet coffee called *cafe cubano* is a standard drink after meals and throughout the day, whether at home, in restaurants, or in other social situations. In the United States, Cubans may drink the *cafe cubano* as *cortadito* or with a dash of milk to cut the strength and bittersweet taste. A traditional Cuban meal includes a generous helping of white rice with black beans or black bean soup, fried plantains, roasted pork or fried chicken, a tuber such as malanga or yucca, followed by dessert and espresso. Thus, the typical diet is high in calories, starches, and saturated fats. As in Spain and other Hispanic countries, a leisurely noon meal (*almuerzo*) and a late evening dinner (*comida*), sometimes as late as 10 or 11 p.m., are customary.

Nutritional Deficiencies and Food Limitations

As seen in Figure 11-1, the major food groups are well represented in the Cuban diet; however, leafy green vegetables may be lacking in the average Cuban meal. Therefore, when assessing the nutritional adequacy of a Cuban patient's diet, the health-care provider must ensure sufficient fiber content.

Pregnancy and Childbearing Practices

Fertility Practices and Views Toward Pregnancy

The low fertility rate of Cuban women, which is consistent in every maternal age group, has been attributed to three factors (Perez, 2002):

1. Cuban American women have a high rate of labor force participation.
2. Before the revolution, Cuba had the lowest birth rate in Latin America.
3. Cuba's current reproductive rate is among the lowest in the developing world.

In an analysis of HHANES data, Stroup-Benham and Trevino (1991) found that only 9 percent of Cuban

American women took oral contraceptives, compared with 11 percent among Puerto Ricans and 20 percent among Mexican Americans. In the same study, hysterectomies, oophorectomies, and tubal ligations were found to be less common among Cuban American women than among either Mexican American or Puerto Rican women. Based on these data, Cuban American women appear to be at greatest risk for unintended pregnancies. Paradoxically, they have the lowest birth rate among the three groups of Hispanic women (Stroup-Benham & Trevino, 1991). A possible explanation for this inconsistency may be the high divorce rate and the high labor force participation rate among Cuban American women. No more recent data on Cuban American women could be found.

Many Cuban folk beliefs and practices surround pregnancy. For example, some Cuban women believe that they have to eat for two during the pregnancy and end up gaining excessive weight. Some believe that morning sickness is cured by eating coffee grounds, that eating a lot of fruit ensures that the baby will be born with a smooth complexion, and that wearing necklaces during pregnancy causes the umbilical cord to be wrapped around the baby's neck.

Among Cuban Americans, childbirth is a time for celebration. Family members and friends congregate in the hospital, awaiting the delivery of the baby. Although traditionally it was not acceptable for Cuban men to attend the birth of their children, the younger and more acculturated Cuban fathers tend to be present to support their wives during labor and delivery. In the postpartum period, it is believed that ambulation, exposure to cold, and going barefoot place the mother at risk for infection. Because of this, family members and relatives often care for the mother and baby for about 4 weeks postpartum.

Prescriptive, Restrictive, and Taboo Practices in the Childbearing Family

Cuban Americans participate in prenatal care if it is affordable. Rest is encouraged, and abstaining from strenuous activities and loud noises is recommended. Fresh fruits are encouraged for the health of the mother and the fetus. More acculturated fathers participate in prenatal classes and support the mother in the delivery room. Breastfeeding among Cuban American women is becoming more popular than in the past. Most do a combination of breast- and bottle-feeding (Varela, 2005).

Thomas and DeSantis (1995) related the early introduction of solid foods and prolonged bottle-feeding of Cuban children to the traditional Cuban beliefs that "a fat child is a healthy child" and that breastfeeding may contribute to a deformity or asymmetry of the breasts. In the same study, 97 percent of Cuban mothers indicated that they administer vitamin preparations to promote the healthy development of their children.

Cuban mothers also used advice about child health given by their spouses, mothers, mothers-in-law, and clerks and pharmacists who sold them over-the-counter drugs (Thomas & DeSantis, 1995).

Traditionally, postpartum mothers and their infants are not supposed to leave the house for 41 days. This initial postpartum period is a time for mothers to rest and devote their energies to caring for the baby. The new mother's immediate family—mother and sisters—help care for the new mother and baby. The mother is sheltered from bad news and any stress that could harm her or her baby. She is also encouraged to eat more to foster milk production (Varela, 2005).

Death Rituals
Death Rituals And Expectations

In death, as in life, the support of the extended family network is important. Whether in the hospital or at home, the dying person is typically surrounded by a large gathering of relatives and friends. In Catholic families, individual and group prayers are offered for the dying to provide a peaceful passage to the hereafter. Religious artifacts such as rosary beads, crucifixes, and *estampitas* (little statues of saints) are placed in the dying person's room.

Depending on the dying person's religious beliefs, a Catholic priest, a Protestant minister, a rabbi, or a **santero** may be summoned to the deathbed to perform appropriate death rites. For adherents of **Santería**, death rites may include animal sacrifice, chants, and ceremonial gestures. Health-care providers need to be open-minded and responsive to both the physical and the psychosocial needs of the dying and the bereaved and, regardless of religious beliefs, accord them the utmost respect and privacy.

After a person's death, candles are lighted to illuminate the path of the spirit to the afterlife. A wake, or *velorio*, is usually held at a funeral parlor, where friends and relatives gather to support the bereaved family. The wake lasts for 2 to 3 days until the funeral. Burial in a cemetery is the common practice for Cuban Catholics, although some may choose cremation.

Responses to Death and Grief

Bereavement is expressed openly among Cuban Americans, with loud crying and other physical manifestations of grief considered socially acceptable. Death is an occasion for relatives living far away to visit and commiserate with the bereaved family. Women from the immediate family usually dress in black during the period of mourning. Visitors make offerings of candles and floral wreaths (*coronas*), provide assistance with household chores, and attend to visitors or funeral arrangements. Cuban Americans customarily remember and honor the deceased on their birthdays or death anniversaries by lighting candles, offering prayers or masses, bringing flowers to the grave, or gathering with family members at the grave site.

Spirituality

Dominant Religion and Use of Prayer

Approximately 85 percent of Cuban Americans are Roman Catholics, with the remaining 15 percent being Protestants, Jews, and believers in the African Cuban practice of *Santería*. The original habitants in Cuba were the Guanatayabes Indians, located mainly in the center-west area of the island, and the Taino Indians, mainly in the east side. When Spaniards arrived, they not only abused and killed the Indians, but they also imposed their Catholic religion. This religion continued in Cuba for many years and was combined with some Christian practices during the colonization period.

The Roman Catholic Church has been an important source of support, especially for first-generation Cuban immigrants. A number of predominantly Cuban parishes with Cuban clergy are located in Florida and New Jersey, where large Cuban populations reside. The Roman Catholic Church has exerted an important influence on Cuban families by providing educational opportunities in Catholic schools. Many Cuban parents, especially the upper middle class, prefer to have their children educated in private Catholic schools.

Roman Catholicism as practiced by Cubans is personal rather than institutional in nature. The religious practice of Cuban Catholics is characterized by devotion and intimate, confiding relationships with the Virgin Mary, Jesus, and the saints.

Some families may have shrines dedicated to *La Caridad del Cobre* (the patron saint of Cuba) or other saints at the entrance to their homes, in their yards, or in commercial establishments. The three favorite saints that are enshrined are Santa Barbara, San Lazaro, and *La Caridad del Cobre*. Inside the home, crucifixes and pictures or statues depicting images of saints may be found. When someone is ill, small pictures of saints, called *estampitas*, may be placed under the pillow or at the sick person's bedside.

Significant religious holidays for Cuban families include Christmas, *Los Tres Reyes Magos* (Three Kings' Day), and the festivals of the *La Caridad del Cobre* and Santa Barbara. The Cuban community usually celebrates the feast of *La Caridad del Cobre* (September 8) by transporting the statue of the patron saint on a boat to a specific location, where a mass is held in her honor. Cuban families also celebrate Christmas Eve (*Noche Buena*) with a traditional Cuban meal. Typically, a pig is cooked all day in a wooden box lined in metal (*una caja china*) and set in the backyard. The pig is placed at the bottom of the box and is covered with charcoal. The meat is served with black beans and rice, yucca, and *turones* (Spanish dessert). The evening concludes with the family attending Midnight Mass (*Misa de Gallo*).

With the arrival of slaves from Africa in the late 1700s and early 1800s, a new type of religious practice emerged in Cuba. One group from the Bantu tribe in the Congo were called *palos* (sticks) by the Spaniards because they used sticks for their religious practices. Today, the *paleros* (plural for people who practice the religion with sticks and who perform black magic) are viewed in a negative way, representing a "bad" type of African Cuban religion. Another group of slaves came from the Carabali tribe from South Nigeria (also known as the Abakua tribe). They still exist today, but they do not have a negative reputation like the *paleros*. In addition, other groups of slaves mixed with the *criollos* (native Cubans born from Spaniards and Indians), Spaniards, French, and other ethnicities who were already residing in Cuba in the mid-1800s. Because of this extensive mixture of races and ethnicities, Cubans say that *en Cuba el que no tiene de Congo tiene de Carabali* (in Cuba if you don't have it from Congo, you will have it from Carabali), denoting that wonderful combination of cultures.

Another African Cuban religion is the *Yoruba/ Lucumi*. Yoruba is an African dialect also known as Lucumi. The minister is known as "Olorisha" or owner of Orisa or Orisha, the saints. The different types of Orishas are Eleggua, Ogun, Oshun, Babalu-Aye, Chango, Oya, Obatala, Yemaya, and Orula. When this priest initiates other priests, they are known as *babalorishas* (the father of Orishas) or *Iyalorishas* (the mother of Orishas). The Supreme Priest is known as *Ifa*, the Father who knows the secret. *Ifas* are commonly known among the general population as *Babalaos* or, correctly said, *Babalawo*. They are the most widely seen *santeros* in Cuba and the ones from whom people seek help with their health or a better economy.

Santeria, or *Regla de Ocha*, is a 300-year-old African Cuban religious system that combines elements of Roman Catholicism with ancient Yoruba tribal beliefs and practices. *Santeria* originated among the Yoruba people of Nigeria, who brought their beliefs with them when they arrived in the New World as slaves. As a condition of their entry into the West Indies, slaves were required to be baptized as Roman Catholics (Perez y Pena, 1998). In the process of adapting to their new non-African environment, the slaves altered their beliefs to incorporate those of their predominantly Catholic masters. *Santeria* evolved from two main cultural antecedents: the worship of the *orishas* among the Yoruba tribe of Nigeria and the cult of saints from the Roman Catholicism of Spain. Through their exposure to the Catholic religion, the slaves came to associate their African gods, called *orishas*, with the Roman Catholic saints, or *santos*. The worship of the *orishas* and the associated beliefs, rituals, incantations, magic, and spirit possession are central to *Santeria*.

Table 11-1 displays the seven African powers, or main *orishas* (Martinez & Wetli, 1982). The Yoruba deity of fire and thunder, called *Chango*, became identified with Santa Barbara, the patron saint of the Spanish artillery, who appeared in Catholic lithographs in red, the color of the *orisha* (Sandoval, 1979). *Chango*, the most popular god in *Santeria*, controls thunder, violent storms, lightning, and fire. The six other *orishas*, the Catholic saints with whom they are identified, and their corresponding functions and powers are also shown in Table 11-1.

When people decide to practice *Santeria*, their *orishas* become known to them and must be worshipped throughout their lives. Followers of *Santeria* believe in the magical and medicinal properties of flowers, herbs, weeds, twigs, and leaves. Sweet herbs such as *manzanilla*, *verbena*, and *mejorana* are used for attracting good luck, love, money, and prosperity. Bitter herbs such as *apasote*, *zarzaparilla*, and *yerba bruja* are used to banish evil and negative energies.

Adherents of *Santeria* also believe in the power of consecrated objects such as stones (*otanes*) in which the *orishas* reside. Necklaces, bracelets, and charms may be given by *santeros* to their patients to protect them from evil and strengthen their well-being.

Sacrifice, or *ebo* (pronounced "egbo" or "igbo"), is a central ritual in *Santeria*. The main purpose of *ebo* is to establish communication between the spirits and human beings. The initiation of a *santero* involves the sacrifice of a four-legged animal and a series of rites lasting 7 days. Transition through major life events such as birth, death, and marriage requires ritual sacrifices to appease the gods and solicit their support.

Sacrificial objects in *Santeria* include plants, foods, and animals. Plants and foods include plantains, malanga, yam, okra, flour, gourds, and ground black-eyed peas wrapped in plantain leaves. Animals used for sacrifice, such as hens, birds, lambs, or goats, are killed by wringing the head or severing the carotid arteries with a knife. The animal's blood is offered as a type of communion with the deities. In 1993, the Supreme Court struck down anti–animal sacrifice laws in Hialeah, Florida, and recognized the right of a *Santeria* sanctuary, the Church of Chango Eyife, to offer an animal sacrifice as a religious sacrament (Gonzalez, 1995).

Santeria, viewed as a link to the past, is used among Cubans and other Hispanic groups to cope with physical and emotional problems. When someone is sick, that person's physical complaints may be diagnosed and treated by a physician, but the *santero* may be summoned to assist in balancing and neutralizing the

ⅠⅡⅤ Table 11-1 Seven African Powers or Main *Orishas*

Orisha	Christian Saint	Function/Power	Punishment	Propitiation
Eleggua	Holy Child of Atocha	Guardian of entrances, roads, and paths; Trickster	Blindness, paralysis, and birth deformities	Blood of goats; black rooster; smoked fish; smoked junia; yams; sugar cane
Obatala	Our Lady of Mercy	Father of all human beings; gives advice; is source of energy, wisdom, purity, and peace	Death, suicide by fire	White pigeons; white canaries; female goat; plums; yam puree
Chango	Saint Barbara	Warrior deity; controls thunder and violent storms, lightning, and fire	Abdominal distress, social and domestic strife	Roosters; goats; lambs; apples; bananas
Oshun	Our Lady of Charity	Deity that controls money and love, makes marriages, protects genitals	Respiratory distress	Female goat; white chickens; sheep; honey
Yemaya	Our Lady of Regla	Primary mother of the santos, protects womanhood, owns seas	Leprosy, gangrene, skin diseases	Ducks; lambs; female goats; watermelons; black-eyed peas
Babaluaye	Saint Lazarus	Patron of the sick, especially diseases of the skin	Violent death (such as an automobile accident)	Spotted rooster; snakes; cigars; pennies; glasses of water
Ogun	Saint Peter	Warrior deity, owns all metals and weapons		Blood and feathers; young bulls; roosters; steel knife; railroad tracks

Source: Adapted from Martinez, R., & Wetli, C. (1982). Santeria: A magicoreligious system of Afro-Cuban origin. *American Journal of Social Psychiatry*, 2(3), 34, with permission.

various aspects of the illness. *Santeria* is actively practiced in Miami, New York, New Jersey, and California where Cubans and Haitians reside.

In eliciting a complete history from patients, health-care providers must include information regarding the type of religion being practiced, if any. Patients' religious beliefs and practices must be viewed in an open, sincere, and nonjudgmental manner. In the hospital setting, maintenance of privacy is important if patients and families need to perform certain rituals or prayers. A visit from a priest, rabbi, or *santero* may provide a sense of psychological support and spiritual well-being. At times, *santeros* have been known to make sacrificial offerings at the patient's hospital bedside. As long as standards of safety and sanitation are maintained, families must be allowed space and privacy to be able to engage in specific religious ceremonies .

In Cuba today, 4 decades of Fidel Castro's revolution have significantly affected religious beliefs and practices. Only about 30 to 40 percent of Cubans are Catholic, whereas *Santeria* has about 55 to 60 percent adherents. The multiple groups that follow syncretic *Santeria* practices include *Abakua*, *Yoruba*, *Regla Conga*, *Regla Ocha*, *Regla Arara*, *Regla Arada*, and *Yebbe*. Thus, compared with their peers from previous migration waves, recent Cuban immigrants may be less likely to be Catholic. Further, large numbers of Cubans consider themselves adherents of Catholicism and *Santeria* simultaneously (Ramos, 2002).

Meaning of Life and Individual Sources of Strength

As in other Latin American communities, the family is the most important source of strength, identity, and emotional security. Cubans usually rely on a network of family members and relatives for assistance in times of need. The sense of specialness Cubans feel, stemming from pride in their culture and their remarkable success in adapting to their new country, is, likewise, a source of self-esteem and self-identity. For many Cubans, deeply held religious beliefs have provided guidance and strength during the long and difficult process of migration and adaptation and continue to play an important role in their day-to-day lives.

Spiritual Beliefs and Health-Care Practices

Many Cubans tend to be fatalistic, feeling that they lack control over circumstances influencing their lives. The belief in a higher power is evident in a variety of practices—such as using magical herbs, special prayers or chants, ritual cleansing, and sacrificial offerings—that Cubans may engage in for the purpose of maintaining health and well-being or curing illness.

When Cuban patients consult health-care providers, in all likelihood they have already tried some folk remedies advised by older women in their family or obtained from a *botanica*. Most folk remedies are harmless and do not interfere with biomedical treatment. In most cases, patients may be encouraged to continue using these remedies, such as herbal teas. Encourage patients to report the use of specific teas and herbs. For example, chamomile tea may increase bleeding time, while jaborandi may decrease bleeding time. Other teas and herbs may increase or decrease glucose metabolism. Health-care providers should be alert to the frequent practice of sharing prescription medications in families and among relatives. A family member who found an antibiotic effective in curing an ailment may share the medication with another relative suffering from the same symptoms. The health history must always include assessment of past or present medication use, whether traditional, over-the-counter, or prescription. Appropriate explanations must be given regarding the actions and adverse effects of drugs and the reasons why they cannot be shared with other family members.

Health-Care Practices
Health-Seeking Beliefs and Behaviors

As in other Latin American societies, Cubans rely on the family as the primary source of health advice. Typically, the older women in the family are sought out for information, such as traditional home remedies for common ailments. Herbal teas or mixtures may be prepared to relieve mild or moderate symptoms. Concurrently or alternatively, a *santero* may be consulted, or a trip to the botanica may be warranted to obtain treatment.

Socialized into a strong health ideology and successful primary-care system in Cuba, Cubans are able to use biomedical services as primary or secondary sources of care. Cuba has a regionalized, hierarchically organized, national health system that provides universal coverage and standardization of services. An innovative family practice program assigns physicians and nurses to city blocks and remote communities to promote physical fitness, detect risk factors for disease, and cure disease. In the United States, many Cuban clinics have evolved into health maintenance organizations (HMOs).

Responsibility for Health Care

Most Cuban Americans access the health-care system for preventive care and health screenings. Cubans with a more recent history of immigration to the United States are accustomed to preventive health activities as part of the Cuban governmental services under Castro. Practices for healthy living, including avoiding stress and bad news and avoiding extremes of hot and cold, are important for health maintenance. Most take full advantage of vaccinations.

Folk and Traditional Practices

Cubans may use traditional medicinal plants in the form of teas, potions, salves, or poultices. As noted above, in Cuban communities like Little Havana in Miami, stores called **botanicas** sell a variety of herbs, ointments, oils, powders, incenses, and religious figurines to relieve maladies, bring luck, drive away evil spirits, or break curses. In addition, *Santeria* necklaces and animals used for ritual sacrifice are available at botanicas (Fig. 11-1).

Herbal teas that may be used to treat common ailments include the following:

Cosimiento de anis (anise): to relieve stomachaches, flatulence, and baby colic; also to calm nerves.
Cosimiento de limon con miel de abeja (lemon and honey): to relieve cough and respiratory congestion.
Cosimiento de apasote (pumpkin seed): to treat gastrointestinal worms.
Cosimiento de canela (cinnamon): to relieve cough, respiratory congestion, and menstrual cramps.
Cosimiento de manzanilla (chamomile): to relieve stomachaches.
Cosimiento de naranja agria (sour orange): to relieve cough and respiratory congestion.
Cosimiento de savila (aloe vera): to relieve stomachaches.

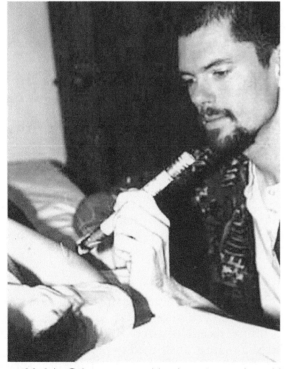

Figure 11-1 In Cuban communities, *botanicas* such as this one sell herbs, ointments, oils, powders, incenses, and religious figurines to relieve maladies, bring luck, or drive away evil spirits.

Cosimiento de tilo (linden leaves): to calm nerves.
Cosimiento de yerba buena (spearmint leaves): to relieve stomachaches and calm nerves.
Chamomile tea: to calm nerves and calm babies with colic.

Fruits and vegetables, abundant in the natural tropical environment of Cuba, may include the following:

Chayote (vegetable): to calm nerves.
Zanaoria (carrots): to help problems with vision.
Toronja y ajo (grapefruit and garlic): to lower blood pressure.
Papaya y toronja y pina (papaya, grapefruit, and pineapple): to eliminate gastrointestinal parasites.
Remolacha (beets): to treat influenza and anemia.
Cascara de mandarina (fruit): to relieve cough.

Other home remedies may include the following:

Agua con sal (salt water): to relieve sore throat.
Agua de coco (coconut water): to relieve kidney problems and infections.
Agua raja (turpentine): to relieve pain in sore muscles and joints.
Bicarbonato, limon, y agua (baking soda, lemon, and water): to relieve stomach upset or heartburn.
Cebo de carnero (fat of lamb): to treat contusions and swelling; applied directly on the skin.
Mantequilla (butter): to soothe pain; applied directly on burns.
Clara de huevos (egg white): to promote hair growth; applied directly over scalp.

Cuban families may use an *azabache*, *la manito de coral*, or *ojitos de Santa Lucia* for various protective purposes. The *azabache* is a black stone placed on infants and children as a bracelet or pin to protect them from the evil eye. *La manito de coral*, symbolic of the hand of God protecting a person, may also be worn as a necklace or bracelet. *Los ojitos de Santa Lucia*, or the eyes of Saint Lucy, may be hung on a bracelet or necklace for prevention of blindness and protection from the evil eye.

Barriers to Health Care

Poverty and lack of financial resources may be a barrier to health care for Cuban families. Other barriers include language, time lag, and transportation, especially if they do not live in an urban environment. Others indicate that the red tape and paperwork required by health-care facilities are deterrents to accessing care, especially preventive care and health wellness checkups. For some, overdependence on family and folk practices may also be a barrier to accessing care.

Cultural Responses to Health and Illness

Because of the many losses they experienced in leaving their homeland and the difficulties associated with adaptation to a new culture and environment, Cuban immigrants may suffer from loneliness, depression, anger, anxiety, insecurity, and health problems. In evaluating Cuban families, Bernal (1994) suggested that health-care providers assess the following:

1. *Migration phase associated with the family.* It is important to know how long the family has lived in the United States and the reasons for migration. Information about political and social pressures that prompted the move should be elicited. Because family members acculturate at different rates, the level of acculturation should also be determined.
2. *Degree of connectedness to the culture of origin.* Conflicts in value orientations must be identified when assessing Cuban families. For example, the varying expectations between mainstream American and Cuban cultures with respect to dependence and independence may give rise to tension and conflict.
3. *Differentiation between stresses of migration, differences in cultural values, and family developmental conflicts.* In a clinical situation, health-care providers must be able to recognize whether the patients' responses are due to migration-related problems, value orientation conflicts, or dysfunctional family development.

Among Cuban Americans, dependency is a culturally acceptable sick role. Sick family members are showered with attention and support. Frequently, a hospitalized Cuban patient will have a room full of flower arrangements and visitors. Favorite dishes may be brought to the hospital from home. The extended family network is relied on to temporarily assume the household chores and other tasks usually performed by the sick person. Family members are consulted and typically participate in decision making relative to the patient's treatment.

Cuban Americans tend to seek help in response to crisis situations. The experience of pain constitutes a signal of a physical disturbance that warrants consultation with a traditional or a biomedical healer. Similar to other Hispanic patients, Cuban Americans tend to express their pain and discomfort. Verbal complaints, moaning, crying, and groaning are culturally appropriate ways of dealing with pain. The expression of pain itself may serve a pain-relieving function and may not necessarily signify a need for administration of pain medication.

African Cubans may seek biomedical care for organic diseases but consult a *santero* for spiritual or emotional crises. Conditions such as **decensos** (fainting spells) or **barrenillos** (obsessions) may be treated

REFLECTIVE EXERCISE 11.4

Consuegro Luna is a retired 72-year-old Cuban American. She arrived in the United States in the early 1960s after Castro's Cuban Revolution. Her entire family lives in Miami, and she has no family connections in Cuba. However, she has deep emotional roots to her beloved island. Lately, she has become depressed because she is afraid she will die without ever seeing Cuba again. She sees her primary physician, but apparently is not adherent to the therapy.

1. What would be her primary physician's best approach for Mrs. Luna?
2. Based on her Cuban cultural background, how would you involve Mrs. Luna's family in her treatment?
3. Besides her nutrition and prescribed/over-the-counter medications, what other information could be relevant for the treatment of Mrs. Luna?

solely by a *santero* or simultaneously with a physician. The trance state achieved through *Santeria* enables the patient to act out emotional problems in a manner that is nonthreatening to the person's self-esteem.

Blood Transfusions and Organ Donation

Receiving blood transfusions and organ donations is usually acceptable for Cubans. This is probably due to their experience with the sophisticated, high-technology medical-care system in Cuba.

Health-Care Providers
Traditional Versus Biomedical Providers

As with many other cultural groups, Cubans use both traditional and biomedical care. Initially, folk remedies may be used at home to treat an ailment or illness. If the condition persists, folk practitioners such as *santeros* and biomedical practitioners may be used either simultaneously or successively. When seeing Cuban patients, health-care providers must always ask about the use of folk remedies and consultations with folk practitioners to prevent conflicting therapeutic regimens.

Although *Santeria* was once associated with the lower, uneducated classes in Cuba, it has emerged as a viable and dynamic religious and health system among middle-class Cubans in the United States. The *santero* may prescribe treatment or perform the appropriate rituals or ceremonies to enable ill people to recover. The *santero* may invoke various types of supernatural deities to intervene in their lives and make them well. Often, the *santero* is seen simultaneously with allopathic practitioners, sometimes without the knowledge of the other one.

Many Cubans consult a family physician for primary care. Before the revolution, Cuba had an organized, government-supported health program that provided medical care to most citizens. Since the 1959 revolution, the Cuban government has articulated a fundamental principle that health care is a right of all and a responsibility of the state. Thus, a national health-care system provides universal coverage, equitable geographic distribution of health-care facilities, and standardization of health services.

Cuban families in Miami gained access to primary health-care services predominantly through private health practitioners and private clinics, whereas in Union City, the main sources of health care were private health practitioners. An extensive network of privately owned and operated health clinics exist in Dade County, mainly located in Miami's Cuban ethnic enclaves: Little Havana and Hialeah. The private health clinics are believed to be popular among the Cubans because they provide services that are culturally sensitive to Cuban needs, such as emphasis on the family, use of the Spanish language, focus on preventive health-care behaviors, and low cost.

Status of Health-Care Providers

Although Hispanics, including Cubans, represent 13 percent of the U.S. population, they are seriously underrepresented in the health occupations. In the National Sample Survey of Registered Nurses (RNs) (U.S. Department of Health and Human Services, 2008), of over 3 million registered nurses, only 3.6 percent are Hispanic. Cubans generally have respect for all health professionals, including nurses. Respect and trust are increased if the nurse know some Spanish.

REFERENCES

Batista, C. (December 20, 2010) *Cubans are skeptic from speech of Castro.* Retrieved from http://www.elnuevoherald.com/2010/12/19/856593/cubanos-escepticos-ante-discurso.html

Bernal, G. (1994). Cuban families. In M. Uriarte-Gaston & J. Canas-Martinez (Eds.). *Cubans in the United States* (pp. 135–156). Boston: Center for the Study of the Cuban Community.

Black, S.A., & Markides, K.S. (1994). Aging and generational patterns of alcohol consumption among Mexican Americans, Cuban Americans and mainland Puerto Ricans. *International Aging and Human Development, 39*(2), 97–103.

Blank, R., & Slipp, S. (1994). *Voices of diversity* (pp. 63–64). New York: American Management Association.

Boswell, T.D. (2002). *A demographic profile of Cuban Americans.* Miami, FL: Cuban American National Council.

Centers for Disease Control and Prevention. (2006). Hypertension-related mortality among Hispanic subpoopulations—United States, 1995–2002. *MMWR Morbidity and Mortality Weekly Report, 55*(7), 177–180.

Centers for Disease Control and Prevention. (2011). *Smoking and tobacco use.* Retrieved from http://www.cdc.gov/search.do?queryText=smoking+cuban+hispanic&action=search&searchButton.x=15&searchButton.y=4

CIA World FactBook. (2011). Retrieved from https://www.cia.gov/library/publications/the-world-factbook/geos/cu.html

Conde, Y.M. (1999). Operation Pedro Pan: The untold exodus of 14,048 Cuban children. New York: Routledge.

Cultural Orientation Resource Center. (2002). *The Cubans: Their history and culture.* Retrieved from http://www.culturalorientation.net.cubans/index.htm

Devieux, J.G., Malow, R.M., Ergon-Perez, E., Samuels, D., Rojas, P., Kushal, S.R., & Jean-Gilles, M. (2005). Research findings—Research on behavioral and combined treatments for drug abuse. *Journal of Social Work Practices in Addiction, 2*(1), 69–83.

Gallagher, P.L. (1980). *The Cuban exile: A socio-political analysis.* New York: Arno Press.

Gonzalez, A.M. (1995, June 11). Santeria still shrouded in secrecy. *The Miami Herald,* pp. 1B–5B.

Kittler, P., & Sucher, K. (2008). *Food and culture in America* (3rd ed.). Belmont, CA: Wadsworth Publishing Co.

Lopez, L.M., & Masse, B.R. (1993). Income, body fatness, and fat patterns in Hispanic women from the Hispanic Health and Nutrition Examination Survey. *Health Care for Women International, 14,* 117–128.

Martinez, I L. (2002). The elder in the Cuban family. Making sense of the real and ideal. *Journal of Comparative Family Studies, 33*(3), 359–375.

Martinez, R., & Wetli, C. (1982). Santeria: A magico-religious system of Afro-Cuban origin. *The American Journal of Social Psychiatry, 2*(3), 496–503.

Nath, S.D. (2005). Coronary heart disease risk factors among Cuban Americans. *Ethnicity and Disease, 15,* 607–614.

National Council of la Raza. (2011) Retrieved from http://www.nclr.org/

Perez, L. (2002). Cuban families in the United States. In R.L. Taylor (Ed.), *Minority families in the United States: A multicultural perspective* (pp. 95–112). Englewood Cliffs, NJ: Prentice Hall.

Perez y Pena, A. (1998). Cuban Santeria, Haitian Vodun, Puerto Rican spiritualism: A multiculturalist inquiry into syncretism. *Journal for the Scientific Study of Religion, 37*(1), 15–27.

Pew Hispanic Center. (2006). *Cubans in the United States.* Retrieved from http://pewhispanic.org/files/factsheets/23.pdf

Portes, A., & Bach, R.L. (1985). *Latin journey: Cuban and Mexican immigrants in the United States.* Berkeley: University of California Press.

Ramos, M.A. (2002). Religion and religiosity in Cuba: Past, present, and future. *Cuba Occasional Paper Series.* Washington, DC: Trinity College.

Sandoval, M. (1979). Santeria as a mental health care system: An historical overview. *Social Science and Medicine, 13,* 137–151.

Skaine, R. (2004). The Cuban family. Custom and change in an era of hardship. Jefferson, NC: McFarland & Co.

Solis, J.M., Marks, G., Garcia, M., & Shelton, D. (1990). Acculturation, access to care, and use of preventive services by Hispanics: Findings from HHANES 1982–84. *American Journal of Public Health, 80*(Suppl.), 11–19.

Stroup-Benham, C.A., & Trevino, F.M. (1991). Reproductive characteristics of Mexican-American, mainland Puerto Rican, and Cuban-American women. *Journal of the American Medical Association, 265*(2), 222–226.

Suarez, Z.E. (1993). Cuban Americans. From golden exiles to social undesirables. In H.P. McAdoo (Ed.), *Family ethnicity: Strength in diversity* (pp. 164–176). Newbury Park, CA: Sage Publications.

Szapocznik, J., & Hernandez, R. (1988). The Cuban American family. In C.H. Mindel, R.W. Habenstein, & R. Wright (Eds.), *Ethnic families in America* (3rd ed., pp. 160–172). New York: Elsevier.

Thomas, J.T., & DeSantis, L. (1995). Feeding and weaning practices of Cuban and Haitian immigrant mothers. *Journal of Transcultural Nursing, 6*(2), 34–42.

U.S. Census Bureau. (2010). Hispanic or Latino origin by specific origin. Retrieved from http://factfinder.census.gov/servlet/DTTable?_bm=y&-geo_id=01000US&-ds_name=ACS_2009_5YR_G00_&-mt_name=ACS_2009_5YR_G2000_B03001

U.S. Department of Health and Human Services. (2008). *The registered nurse population: National sample survey of registered nurses.* Washington, DC: U.S. Government Printing Office.

U.S. Immigration and Naturalization Service. (2000). Immigrants, fiscal year 2000. In *Statistical yearbook of the INS* (pp. 1–67).

Varela, L. (2005). Cubans. In J. Lipson & S.L. Dibble (Eds.), *Culture and clinical care* (2nd ed., pp. 121–131).

DavisPlus *For reflective exercises, review questions, and additional information, go to*
http://davisplus.fadavis.com

Chapter 12

People of European American Heritage

Larry D. Purnell

This chapter presents the dominant European American cultural values, practices, and beliefs. The European American culture is a blended culture resulting from early immigrants in the United States, primarily Caucasians from Europe, who adapted to and adopted one another's cultures and, over time, have formed their own distinct, new cultures. Many other groups have assimilated and now self-identify with the European American culture as well. Although Canada and Mexico are part of North America, *American,* as used in this chapter, refers to the dominant middle-class values of citizens of mainland United States, and the term *European American* is shortened to American. Due to space limitations, this chapter deals not with the objective culture—arts, literature, humanities, and so on—but rather with the subjective culture. Many Americans are not aware of the subjective culture because they identify differences as individual personality traits and disregard political and social origins of culture. Many view culture as something that belongs only to foreigners or disadvantaged groups, although this is not unique to Americans. When Americans travel abroad, many times their host country inhabitants stereotypically identify them as Americans because of their values, beliefs, attitudes, behaviors, speech patterns, and mannerisms. Some feel that Americans are "fun lovers" and that, for some Americans, violence is a way of life. This may be due to the fact that American media coverage may be better than other countries, thereby giving the impression that the United States is more violent than it actually is. Accordingly, these stereotypes are not always accurate. However, "the right to bear arms" is guaranteed by the Constitution. Most likely, the United States is not any more violent than, or even as violent as, many other societies.

Overview, Inhabited Localities, and Topography

Overview

For most Americans, dominant cultural values and beliefs include individualism, free speech, rights of choice, independence and self-reliance, confidence, "doing" rather than "being," egalitarian relationships, nonhierarchical status of individuals, achievement status over ascribed status, "volunteerism," friendliness, openness, futuristic temporality, ability to control the environment, and an emphasis on material things and physical comfort.

Given the size, population density, and diversity of the United States, one cannot generalize too much about American culture. Every generalization in this chapter is subject to exceptions, although most people will agree with the descriptions to some degree and on some level. Moreover, the descriptions about the dominant American culture are aggregate data for white middle-class European Americans who hold the majority of prestigious positions in the United States. The degree to which people conform to or agree with the European American culture depends on their variant cultural characteristics as discussed in Chapter 1, as well as individual personality differences. Many foreigners believe that all Americans are rich, everyone lives in fancy apartments or houses, crime is rampant, everyone drives expensive gasoline-inefficient cars, and there is little or no poverty. For the most part, these misconceptions come from the media and Americans who travel overseas.

Heritage and Residence

The United States comprises 3.5 million square miles and a population of 308,745,538 people, making it the world's third most populous country (U.S. Census

Bureau, 2010). The United States is mostly temperate but tropical in Hawaii and Florida, arctic in Alaska, semiarid in the Great Plains west of the Mississippi River, and arid in the Great Basin of the southwest. Low winter temperatures in the northwest are ameliorated in January and February by warm Chinook winds from the eastern slopes of the Rocky Mountains. There is a vast central plain; mountains in the west; hills and low mountains in the east; rugged mountains and broad river valleys in Alaska; and rugged, volcanic topography in Hawaii (*CIA World Factbook*, 2011).

When Europeans began settling the United States in the 16th century, approximately 2 million American Indians, who mostly lived in geographically isolated tribes, populated the land. The first permanent European settlement in the United States was St. Augustine, Florida, which was settled by the Spanish in 1565. The first English settlement was Jamestown, Virginia, in 1607 (*Information Please Almanac*, 2009). By 1610, the nonnative population in the United States amounted to 350 people. By 1700, the population increased to 250,900; by 1800, to 5.3 million; and by 1900, to 75.9 million (Information Please Almanac: United States, 2009). From 1607 until 1890, most immigrants to the United States came from Europe and essentially shared a common European culture. Britain's American colonies broke with the mother country in 1776 and were recognized as the new nation of the United States of America following the Treaty of Paris in 1783.

During the 19th and 20th centuries, 37 new states were added to the original 13 as the nation expanded across the North American continent and acquired a number of overseas possessions. The two most traumatic experiences in the nation's history were the Civil War (1861–1865), in which a northern Union of states defeated a secessionist Confederacy of 11 southern slave states, and the Great Depression of the 1930s, an economic downturn during which about a quarter of the labor force lost its jobs. Buoyed by victories in World Wars I and II and the end of the Cold War in 1991, the United States remains the world's most powerful nation state. Over a span of more than 5 decades, the economy has achieved steady growth, low unemployment and inflation, and rapid advances in technology (*CIA World Factbook*, 2011)

The Constitution of the United States was ratified in 1789 and included seven articles, which laid the foundation for an independent nation. The Bill of Rights, the first 10 amendments to the Constitution, guarantees freedom of religion, speech, and the press; the right to petition; the right to bear arms; and the right to a speedy trial. Only 17 additional amendments have been made to the Constitution. The 13th Amendment in 1865 prohibited slavery; the 14th Amendment in 1868 defined citizenship and privileges of citizens; the 15th Amendment in 1870 gave suffrage rights regardless of race or color; and the 19th Amendment in 1920 gave women the right to vote.

The United States is the world's oldest constitutional democracy with three branches of government: the executive branch, which includes the Office of the President and the administrative departments; the legislative branch, Congress, which includes both the Senate and the House of Representatives; and the judicial branch, which includes the Supreme Court and the lesser federal courts. The Supreme Court has nine members appointed by the president and approved by Congress. The justices serve a life term if they so choose. The president serves a 4-year term and can be reelected only one time. The president is the commander in chief of the armed forces and oversees the executive departments. The members of the House of Representatives are divided among the states based on the population of each state. Members of the House of Representatives serve 2-year terms. Each state has two senators, regardless of the population of the state. Senators serve 6-year terms. Each of the 50 states has its own constitution establishing, for the most part, a parallel structure to the federal government, with the executive branch headed by a governor, a state congress with representatives and senators, and a state court system.

No limitations were placed on immigrants from Europe until the late 1800s. From 1892 to 1952, most European immigrants to America came through Ellis Island, New York, where they had to prove to officials that they were financially independent. More severe restrictions were placed on other immigrant groups, particularly those from Asia. In the 1960s, immigration policy changed to allow immigrants from all parts of the world without favoritism to or restrictions on ethnicity. Today, the United States includes immigrants or descendants from immigrants from almost every nation and culture of the world and is the world's premier international nation. The United States admitted over 62,000 refugees during fiscal year 2004–2005, including more than 10,000 from Somalia, over 8500 from Laos, over 6600 from Russia, 6500 from Cuba, and 3100 from Haiti (*CIA World Factbook*, 2011).

The United States has the largest and most technologically powerful economy in the world, with a per capita gross domestic product (GDP) of $41,061 (U.S. Census Bureau, 2011). In this market-oriented economy, private individuals and business firms make most of the decisions, and the federal and state governments buy needed goods and services predominantly in the private marketplace. U.S. firms are at or near the forefront in technological advances, especially in computer technology and in medical, aerospace, and military equipment; their advantage has narrowed since the end of World War II. The on-rush of technology largely explains the gradual development of a "two-tier labor market," in which those at the bottom lack the education and the professional/technical skills of those at the top and, more and more, fail to get comparable pay raises, health insurance coverage, and other benefits. People have been attracted to the United States because of its vast resources and economic and personal freedoms, particularly the dogma that "all men are created equal." Immigrants and their descendants achieved enormous material success, which further encouraged immigration.

Reasons for Migration and Associated Economic Factors

The United States has a very large middle-class population and a small, but growing, wealthy population. Approximately 13.4 percent of the population lives in poverty, with higher rates among children, older persons, blacks, and nonwhite Hispanics (U.S. Census Bureau, 2010).

The earlier settlers in the United States came for better economic opportunities because of religious and political oppression; environmental disasters, such as earthquakes and hurricanes in their home countries; and by forced relocation, such as with slaves and indentured servants. Others have immigrated for educational opportunities and personal ideologies or a combination of factors. Most people immigrate in the hope of a better life; however, the individual or group personally defines this ideology.

Educational Status and Occupations

In the United States, preparation in elementary and secondary education varies widely. There is no national curriculum that each school is expected to follow, although there is standardized testing at a national level, which is used in the selection process for admission to institutions of higher education. Most states require children to attend school until the age of 16, although the child can drop out of school at a younger age with parents' signed permission. Overall, the United States has the goal of producing a well-rounded individual with a variety of courses and 100 percent literacy. Theoretically, people have the freedom to choose a profession, regardless of gender and background. The American educational system stresses application of content over theory. The United States' dominant system places a high value on the student's ability to categorize information using linear, sequential thought processes, which is common in individualistic cultures.

Communication

Dominant Language and Dialects

Over 82 percent of the U.S. population speaks English (*CIA World Factbook*, 2011), mostly *American English,* which differs somewhat in its pronunciation, spelling, and choice of words from English spoken in Great Britain, Australia, and other English-speaking countries. Within the United States, several dialects exist, but generally the differences do not cause a major concern with communications. Aside from people with foreign accents, in certain areas of the United States, people speak with a dialect; these include the South and Northeast, in addition to local dialects such as "Elizabethan English" and "western drawl." In such cases, dialects that vary widely may pose substantial problems for health-care providers and interpreters in performing health assessments and in obtaining accurate health data, in turn increasing the difficulty of making accurate diagnoses.

American English is a monochromic, low-contextual language in which most of the message is in the verbal mode, and verbal communication is frequently seen as being more important than nonverbal communication. Other common languages spoken in the United States include Spanish (10 percent), other Indo-European languages (3.8 percent), Asian and Pacific Islander languages (2.7 percent), and other (0.7 percent) (*CIA World Factbook*, 2011). In addition, the speed at which people speak varies by region; for example, in parts of Appalachia and the South, people speak more slowly than do people in the northeastern part of the United States. Americans may be perceived as being loud and boisterous because their volume carries to those nearby.

Cultural Communication Patterns

Many Americans are willing to disclose very personal information about themselves, including information about sex, drugs, and family problems. In fact, personal sharing is encouraged in a wide variety of topics, but not religion. In the United States, having well-developed verbal skills is seen as important.

For the most part, America is a low-touch society, which has recently been reinforced by sexual harassment guidelines and policies. For many, even casual touching may be seen as a sexual overture and should be avoided whenever possible until people get to know each other. People of the same sex (especially men) or opposite sex do not generally touch each other unless they are close friends.

American conversants tend to place at least 18 inches of space between themselves and the person with whom they are talking. Clients may interpret American health-care providers as being cold because they stand so far away. An understanding of personal space and distancing characteristics can enhance the quality of communication among individuals.

Regardless of class or social standing of the conversants, Americans are expected to maintain direct eye contact without staring. A person who does not maintain eye contact may be perceived as not listening, not being trustworthy, not caring, or being less than truthful.

Most Americans gesture moderately when conversing and smile easily as a sign of pleasantness or happiness, although one can smile as a sign of sarcasm. A lack of gesturing can mean that the person is too stiff, too formal, or too polite. However, when gesturing to make, emphasize, or clarify a point, one should not raise one's elbows above the head unless saying hello or good-bye.

For American men and women in business, the practice is to extend the right hand with a firm handshake when greeting someone for the first time. Confidence and competence are associated with a relaxed posture. Although many people consider it impolite or offensive to point with one's finger, many Americans do so, and do not see it as impolite.

Temporal Relationships

The American culture is future oriented, and people are encouraged to sacrifice for today and work to save and invest in the future. The future is important in that people can influence it. Americans generally see fatalism, the belief that powers greater than humans are in control, as negative; to many others, however, it is seen as a fact of life not to be judged. However, for many, temporality is balanced among past, present, and future in the sense of respecting the past, valuing and enjoying the present, and saving for the future.

Americans see time as a highly valued resource and do not like to be delayed because it "wastes time." When visiting friends or meeting for strictly social engagements, punctuality is less important, but one is still expected to appear within a "reasonable" time frame. In the health-care setting, if an appointment is made for 8 a.m., the person is expected to be there at 7:45 a.m. so she or he is ready for the appointment and does not delay the health-care provider. Some organizations refuse to see the patient if he or she is more than 15 to 30 minutes late for an appointment; a few charge a fee, even though the patient was not seen, giving the impression that money is more important than the person.

Format for Names

The American name David Thomas Jones denotes a man whose first name is David, middle name is Thomas, and family surname is Jones. Friends would call him by his first name, David. In the formal setting, he would be called Mr. Jones. In addition, he could also have a nickname that would be used by family and close friends—for example, Davy from his first name or Tom or Tommy from his middle name. When women marry, they may drop their maiden name and adopt their husband's last name, or they may keep both their maiden and husband's names. In this case, they may or may not hyphenate it, as in Elizabeth Parker-Jones or Elizabeth Parker Jones. Their children usually, but not always, take the husband's last name.

Family Roles and Organization
Head of Household and Gender Roles

Among Americans, it is acceptable for women to have a career and for men to assist with child care, household domestic chores, and cooking responsibilities. Both parents work in many families, necessitating placing children in child-care facilities. In some families, fathers are responsible for deciding when to seek health care for family members, but mothers may have significant influence on final decisions.

Prescriptive, Restrictive, and Taboo Behaviors for Children and Adolescents

For most Americans, a child's individual achievement is valued over the family's financial status. In many middle- and upper-class American families, children have their own room, television, and telephone, and even their own computer. At younger ages, rather than having group toys, each child has his or her own toys and is taught to share them with others. Americans encourage autonomy in children, and after completing homework assignments (with which parents are expected to help), children are expected to contribute to the family by doing chores, such as taking out the garbage, washing dishes, cleaning their own room, feeding and caring for pets, and helping with cooking. They are not expected to help with heavy labor except in rural farm communities.

Children are allowed and encouraged to make their own choices, including managing their own allowance money and deciding who their friends might be, although parents may gently suggest one friend as a better choice than another. American children and teenagers are permitted and encouraged to have friends of both the same and opposite genders. They are expected to be well behaved, especially in public. They are taught to stand in line—first come, first served—and to wait their turn. As they reach the teenage years, they are expected to refrain from premarital sex, smoking, using recreational drugs, and drinking alcohol until they leave the home. However, this does not always occur, and teenage pregnancy and use of recreational alcohol and drugs remain high. When children become teenagers, most are expected to get a job, such as babysitting, delivering newspapers, or doing yard work to make their own spending money, which they manage as a way of learning independence. The teenage years are also seen as a time of natural rebellion.

In American society, when young adults become 18 or complete their education, they usually move out of their parents' home (unless they are in college) and live independently or share living arrangements with nonfamily members. If the young adult chooses to remain in the parents' home, then she or he might be expected to pay room and board. However, young adults are generally allowed to return home when they are needed or for financial or other purposes. Individuals over the age of 18 are expected to be self-reliant and independent, which are virtues in the American culture.

Adolescents have their own subculture, with its own values, beliefs, and practices that may not be in harmony with those of their parents' wishes. Being in harmony with peers and conforming to the prevalent choice of music, clothing, hairstyles, and adornments may be especially important to adolescents. Thus, role conflicts can become considerable sources of family strain in many more traditional families who may not agree with the American values of individuality, independence, self-assertion, and egalitarian relationships. Many teens may experience a cultural dilemma with exposure outside the home and family.

Family Goals and Priorities

American family goals and priorities are centered on raising and educating children. During this stage in the American culture, young adults make a personal commitment to a spouse or significant other and seek satisfaction through productivity in career, family, and civic interests.

The median age at first marriage in the United States has gradually increased over the last 10 years from 26.8 years to 27.7 years for men; for women, the median age of first marriage has gradually increased from 25.1 years to 26 years (*Information Please Almanac*, 2009). In 1900, the divorce rate was 0.7 per year per 1000 marriages; this increased to 5.3 per year by 1981 and has gradually declined since then to 3.6 per year per 1000 (*Information Please Almanac*, 2009). As for births, currently 39.7 percent of all births are to unmarried women (Centers for Disease Control and Prevention, 2007).

The United States has seen an explosion in its older population during the 20th century, up from 3.1 million in 1900 to over 39.5 million in 2009 being over the age of 65 years (U.S. Census Bureau, 2009). The American culture, which emphasizes youth, beauty, thinness, independence, and productivity, contributes to some societal views of the aged as less important members and tends to minimize the problems of older people. A contrasting view among some emphasizes the importance of older people in society.

Americans also place a high value on egalitarianism, nonhierarchical relationships, and equal treatment regardless of their race, color, religion, ethnicity, educational or economic status, sexual orientation, or country of origin. However, these beliefs are theoretical and not always seen in practice. For example, women still have a lower status than men, especially when it comes to prestigious positions and salaries. Most top-level politicians and corporate executive officers are white men. Subtle classism does exist, as evidenced by comments referring to "working-class men and women." Despite the current inequities, Americans value equal opportunities for all, and most would agree that significant progress is being made.

Americans are known worldwide for their informality and for treating everyone the same. They call people by their first names very soon after meeting them, whether in the workplace, in social situations, in classrooms, in restaurants, or in places of business. Americans readily talk with waitstaff and store clerks and call them by their first names. Most Americans consider this respectful behavior. Formality can be communicated by using the person's last (family) name and title such as Mr., Mrs., Miss, Ms., or Dr. To this end, achieved status is more important than ascribed status. What one has accumulated in material possessions, where one went to school, and one's job position and title are more important than one's family background and lineage. However, in some families in the South and the Northeast, one's ascribed status has equal importance to achieved status. The United States does not have a caste or class system, and theoretically, one can move readily from one socioeconomic position to another. To many Americans, if formality is maintained, it may be seen as pompous or arrogant, and some even deride the person who is very formal. However, formality is a sign of respect and is valued by most older Americans.

Alternative Lifestyles

The American family is becoming a more varied community, including unmarried people, both women and men, living alone; single people of the same or different genders living together with or without children; single parents with children; and blended families consisting of two parents who have remarried, with children from their previous marriages and additional children from their current marriage.

The newest category of family, domestic partnerships, is sanctioned by many cities or counties in the United States and grants some of the rights of traditional married couples to unmarried heterosexual, homosexual, older people, and disabled couples who share the traditional bond of the family. Some states allow gay and lesbian couples to marry and to adopt children. The last 10 years have seen many hotly debated issues regarding same-sex marriages and civil unions. Among more rural subcultures, same-sex couples living together may not be as accepted or recognized in the community as they are in larger cities. As gay parents have become more visible, lesbian and gay parenting groups have started in many cities across the United States to offer information, support, and guidance, resulting in more lesbians and gay men considering parenthood through adoption and artificial insemination. Some national groups that have links to local and regional organizations are included on DavisPlus.

Workforce Issues

Culture in the Workplace

Americans are expected to be punctual on their jobs, with formal meetings, and with appointments. If one is more than a minute or two late, an apology is expected, and if one is late by more than 5 or 10 minutes, a more elaborate apology is expected. When people know they are going to be late for a meeting, the expectation is that they call or send a message indicating that they will be late. The convener of the meeting or teacher in a classroom is expected to start and stop on time out of respect for the other people in attendance. However, in social situations, a person can be 15 or more minutes late, depending on the importance of the gathering. In this instance, an apology is not really necessary or expected; however, most Americans will politely provide a reason for the tardiness.

The American workforce stresses efficiency (time is money), operational procedures on how to get things done, task accomplishment, and proactive problem solving. Intuitive abilities and common sense are not usually valued as much as technical abilities. The scientific method is valued, and everything has to be proven. Americans want to know *why*, not *what*, and will search for a single factor that is the cause of the problem and the reason why something is to be done in a specific way. Many are obsessed with collecting facts and figures before they make decisions. Pragmatism is valued. In the United States, everyone is expected to have a job description, meetings are to have a predetermined agenda (although items can be added at the beginning of the meeting), and the agenda is followed throughout the meeting. Americans prefer to vote on almost every item on an agenda, including approving the agenda itself. Everything is given a time frame, and deadlines are expected to be respected. In these situations, American values expect that the needs of individuals are subservient to the needs of the organization. However, with the postmodernist movement, where there are no absolute truths and most aspects of a person's worldview are based on perceptions and social contexts, greater credibility and recognition have been given to approaches other than the scientific method.

Issues Related to Autonomy

Most Americans place a high value on "fairness" and rely heavily on procedures and policies in the decision-making process. However, Americans' value for individualism, in which the individual is seen as the most important element in society, favors a person's decision to further her or his own career over the needs or wants of the employer. Therefore, individuals frequently demonstrate little loyalty to the organization and leave one position to take a position with another company for a better opportunity or higher salary. In organizations in which people generally conform because of the fear of failure, there is a hierarchical order for decision making, and the person who succeeds is the one with strong verbal skills who conforms to the hierarchy's expectations. This person is well liked and does not stand out too much from the crowd. Frequently, others view as a threat the person with a high level of competence and who stands out. Thus, to be successful in the highly technical American workforce, the individual must get the facts, control feelings, have precise and technical communication skills, be informal and direct, and clearly and explicitly state his or her conclusions.

During workforce shortages, American health-care facilities rely on emigrating nurses and physicians from the Philippines, Canada, England, Ireland, India, and other countries to supplement their numbers. Some foreign nurses, such as British and Australian, culturally assimilate into the workforce more easily than others but still have difficulty with *defensive* charting as is required in the United States. In their socialized health-care system, clients are not likely to initiate litigation (Purnell & Galloway, 1995). Others may have difficulty with the assertiveness expected from American nurses.

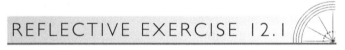

REFLECTIVE EXERCISE 12.1

Bonnie Jackson, a European American Roman Catholic age 42 years, was diagnosed with breast cancer 8 months ago and had bilateral mastectomies. She underwent chemotherapy and radiation therapy, but the cancer has metastasized to her lungs, ribs, and brain. She has decided to forgo additional allopathic medical treatments, but is open to herbal therapies. Because of intense pain, she has been admitted to a home hospice service. Bonnie has never been married and currently lives with her life partner of 22 years, Jeni Chambers, who has durable power of attorney for health-care decision making.

On the intake home hospice assessment, the nurse asked who was the next of kin and was told that it was Jeni. The nurses then asked what blood relative would make decisions about health care if she was unable to make decisions. Bonnie again gave Jeni's name and explained their relationship. The nurse stated she was unsure if this was acceptable and would ask her supervisor. Bonnie explained that both her parents were deceased and that she was estranged from her two older brothers and younger sister, at which point the nurse responded, "I can understand why!"

1. What is the incidence of breast cancer among women in the United States?
2. Is there a difference in breast cancer among different racial and ethnic groups?
3. Is there a difference between breast cancer rates in lesbians and heterosexual women?

Continued

4. What do you know about advance directives and durable power of attorney in health-care decision making? Can Jeni legally be the decision maker for Bonnie?
5. What family support systems does Bonnie have?
6. Would you ask Jeni if her family is supportive of their relationship?
7. What resources besides family might be available for Bonnie and Jeni?
8. What is your response to Bonnie deciding to forgo allopathic treatments but be willing to entertain herbal therapies?
9. How do you feel about same-sex intimate partnerships? What differences do you see between providing care to patients with same-sex partnerships and to patients from heterosexual partnerships?
10. If Bonnie and Jeni were to seek support from the Catholic Church, how do you think church members would respond? What is the Roman Catholic Church's view on same-sex intimate partner relationships?

Biocultural Ecology
Skin Color and Other Biological Variations
The majority of European Americans are generally fair-skinned, and thus prolonged exposure to the sun places them at an increased risk for skin cancer. Oxygenation determination can easily be determined from skin color as well as the nail beds.

Diseases and Health Conditions
In the United States, cardiovascular disease is the leading killer of both men and women. Factors that contribute to the development of cardiovascular disease include obesity, lack of physical activity, and smoking. For white male Americans, the leading sites for cancer include the prostate, lung, and colon. For white female Americans, the most common sites include the breast, lung, and colon. Although these same sites account for most cancers in other ethnic and racial groups, the order of occurrence differs. Almost 23.6 million Americans have been diagnosed with diabetes mellitus (DM), and the disease is undiagnosed in an additional 5.4 million people. The prevalence of DM among whites is 7.8 percent (Centers for Disease Control and Prevention, 2011).

The Centers for Disease Control and Prevention (CDC) estimate that more than 1 million people are living with HIV in the United States. One in five (21 percent) of those people living with HIV is unaware of the infection. Despite increases in the total number of people living with HIV in the United States in recent years, the annual number of new HIV infections has remained relatively stable. However, the level remains far too high, with an estimated 56,300 Americans becoming infected with HIV each year.

More than 18,000 people with AIDS still die each year in the United States. Gay, bisexual, and other men who have sex with men (MSM) are strongly affected and represent the majority of persons who have died. Through 2007, more than 576,000 people with AIDS in the United States have died since the epidemic began (Centers for Disease Control and Prevention, 2011).

Sexually transmitted infections (STIs) remain a major public health challenge in the United States. CDC's surveillance report as of 2007, the latest data available, includes data on the three STIs that physicians are required to report to the agency—chlamydia, gonorrhea, and syphilis—which represent only a fraction of the true burden of STIs. Some common STIs, such as human papillomavirus (HPV) and genital herpes, are not reported to CDC. In total, CDC estimates that there are approximately 19 million new STIs each year, which cost the U.S. health-care system $16.4 billion annually and cost individuals even more in terms of acute and long-term health consequences (Centers for Disease Control and Prevention, 2011).

Despite the continued high burden of STIs, the latest CDC data show some signs of progress:

1. The national gonorrhea rate is at the lowest level ever recorded.
2. Continuing increases in chlamydia diagnoses likely reflect expanded screening efforts and not necessarily a true increase in disease burden.
3. For the first time in 5 years, reported syphilis cases did not increase among women overall.
4. Likewise, cases of congenital syphilis (transmitted from mother to infant) did not increase for the first time in 4 years (Centers for Disease Control and Prevention, 2011).

Illnesses and diseases with an increased incidence in white ethnic groups in the United States include appendicitis, diverticular disease, cancer of the colon, hemorrhoids, varicose veins, cystic fibrosis, rosacea, osteoporosis and osteoarthritis, and phenylketonuria.

Since the late 1990s, every continent has had outbreaks of new or reemerging diseases. North America has had outbreaks of bubonic plague, campylobacteria, cyclospora, salmonella, *E. coli* in spinach, and Legionnaire's disease. See the Appendix for illnesses and diseases and their causes for specific ethnic and cultural groups common in the United States.

Variations in Drug Metabolism
Information regarding drug metabolism among racial and ethnic groups has important implications for health-care practitioners when prescribing medications. Besides the effects of smoking, which accelerates drug metabolism; malnutrition, which affects drug response; a high-fat diet, which increases absorption of antifungal medication, whereas a low-fat diet renders the drug less effective; cultural attitudes and beliefs

about taking medication; and stress, which affects catecholamine and cortisol levels on drug metabolism, studies have identified some specific alterations in drug metabolism among diverse racial and ethnic groups (Prows & Prows, 2004). The studies on drug metabolism across ethnicity and race have used white ethnic groups/race as the control. Thus, differences in drug metabolism variations among whites are not reported. Health-care providers need to investigate the literature for ethnic-specific studies regarding variations in drug metabolism, communicate these findings to other colleagues, and educate their clients regarding these side effects.

High-Risk Behaviors

The steady decline in smoking prevalence has been observed nationally; however, in certain segments of the population, incidence remains high, thus highlighting the need for expanded interventions that can better reach persons of low socioeconomic status and populations living in poverty. In 2009, the latest figures available, 20.6 percent of all adults (46.6 million people) continue to smoke. In the United States, tobacco use is responsible for about one in five deaths annually (i.e., about 443,000 deaths per year), and an estimated 49,000 of these tobacco-related deaths are the result of secondhand smoke exposure. On average, smokers die 13 to 14 years earlier than nonsmokers; the percentage varies by race and ethnicity, as evidenced by the following statistics:

- 23.2 percent of American Indian/Alaska Native adults
- 22.1 percent of white adults
- 21.3 percent of African American adults
- 14.5 percent of Hispanic adults
- 12 percent of Asian American adults (excluding Native Hawaiians and other Pacific Islanders) (Centers for Disease Control and Prevention, 2011)

Alcohol use is very common in the United States and has immediate effects that can increase the risk of many harmful health conditions. Excessive alcohol use, either in the form of *heavy drinking* (drinking more than two drinks per day on average for men or more than one drink per day on average for women) or *binge drinking* (drinking five or more drinks during a single occasion for men or four or more drinks during a single occasion for women), can lead to increased risk of health problems, such as liver disease or unintentional injuries.

According to the Behavioral Risk Factor Surveillance System (BRFSS) survey, more than half of the adult U.S. population drank alcohol in the past 30 days. Approximately 5 percent of the total population drank heavily, whereas 15 percent of the population binge drank. According to the Alcohol-Related Disease Impact (ARDI) tool, from 2001 to 2005, there were approximately 79,000 deaths annually attributable to excessive alcohol use. In fact, excessive alcohol use is the third leading lifestyle-related cause of death for people in the United States each year (Centers for Disease Control and Prevention, 2011). The conclusion of many studies suggests that alcohol-related violence is a learned behavior, not an inevitable result of alcohol consumption (Purnell & Foster, 2003a; 2003b).

Health-Care Practices

American society has become "obesogenic," characterized by environments that promote increased food intake, nonhealthful foods, and physical inactivity. Policy and environmental change initiatives that make healthy choices in nutrition and physical activity available, affordable, and easy will likely prove most effective in combating obesity. The Division of Nutrition, Physical Activity, and Obesity (DNPAO) is working to reduce obesity and obesity-related conditions through state programs, technical assistance and training, leadership, surveillance and research, intervention development and evaluation, translation of practice-based evidence and research findings, and partnership development. Although the obesity rate appears to be declining or (at least) leveling, obesity remains high among adults and children (Centers for Disease Control and Prevention, 2011). Obesity is a complex issue related to lifestyle, environment, and genes. Many underlying factors have been linked to the increase in obesity, such as increased portion sizes; eating out more often; increased consumption of sugar-sweetened drinks; increased television, computer, electronic gaming time; changing labor markets; and fear of crime, which prevents outdoor exercise. Health-care providers can assist overweight clients in reducing calorie consumption by identifying healthy choices among culturally preferred foods, altering preparation practices, and reducing portion size.

The practice of self-care using folk and magicoreligious practices before seeking professional care may also have a negative impact on the health status of some individuals. Overreliance on these practices may mean that the health problem is in a more advanced stage when a consultation is sought. Such delays make treatment more difficult and prolonged.

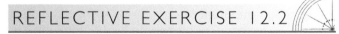

REFLECTIVE EXERCISE 12.2

Tammy Shorts, a 54-year-old patient care assistant, has worked on the same acute-care teenage pediatric unit for 12 years. She tells everyone that she loves her job and the teenagers. The unit got a new male nurse manager, Mr. Galway, 2 years ago. During that time, Mrs. Shorts has had six counseling sessions for coming to work more than 10 minutes late and leaving early. She insists that she still gets her work completed,
Continued

despite coming in late and leaving early. Besides, what is the big deal about 10 or 15 minutes? The nurse manager has informed her that if she is late or leaves early one more time, she will be suspended without pay. Mrs. Shorts believes she is being treated unfairly and, unknown to Mr. Galway, has gone to his supervisor and complained that he has touched her on the shoulder unnecessarily and that he is singling her out because she is female and he is male. In addition, he calls her "Tammy" instead of "Mrs. Shorts."

1. Is the expectation of punctuality on reporting on time consistent with the European American culture?
2. In the American workforce, when employees have a complaint or concern about their supervisor, who is the first person they should speak to about it?
3. What should Mrs. Shorts's first response be to being touched unnecessarily?
4. What should Mrs. Shorts's first response be if she is offended by Mr. Galway calling her by her first name? Is this common with the European American culture?
5. What is the first thing you would do to resolve this situation?
6. If your first action does not resolve the situation, what is your second action?

Nutrition

Meaning of Food

When Americans invite a guest to dinner for the first time, the guest frequently brings a gift, although this is not required, and one of the choices is often food. There are no specific rules as to what type of food to bring, but wine, cheese baskets, and candy are usually appropriate. Bread (unless it is a very special bread) and soft drinks are not usually appropriate unless specifically requested.

Common Foods and Food Rituals

American food and preparation practices reflect traditional food habits of early settlers who brought their unique cuisines with them. Accordingly, the "typical American diet" has been brought from elsewhere. Americans vary their mealtimes and food choices according to the region of the country, urban versus rural residence, and weekdays versus weekends. In addition, food choices vary by marital status, economic status, climate changes, religion, ancestry, availability, and personal preferences.

Many older people and people living alone do not eat balanced meals, stating they do not take the time to prepare a meal, even though most American homes have labor-saving devices such as stoves, microwave ovens, refrigerators, and dishwashers. For those who are unable to prepare their own meals because of disability or illness, most communities have a Meals on Wheels program through which community and church organizations deliver, usually once a day, a hot meal along with a cold meal for later and food for the following morning's breakfast. Other community and church agencies prepare meals for the homeless or collect food, which is delivered to those who have none. When people are ill, they generally prefer toast, tea, juice, and other easily digested foods.

Given the size of the United States and its varied terrain, food choices differ by region: beef in the Midwest, fish in coastal areas, and poultry in the South and along the Eastern Seaboard. Vegetables vary by season, climate, and altitude, although larger grocery stores have a wide variety of all types of American and international meats, fruits, and vegetables. Many television stations and major newspapers have large sections devoted to foods and preparation practices, a testament to the value that Americans place on food and diversity in food preparation.

Special occasions and holidays are frequently associated with specific foods and may vary according to the ethnicity of the family. For example, hot dogs are consumed at sports events, and turkey is served at Thanksgiving.

Dietary Practices for Health Promotion

Overall, the typical American diet is high in fats and cholesterol and low in fiber, according to the U.S. Department of Agriculture (USDA) (www.mypyramid. gov). The USDA recommends MyPyramid for Americans, which was originally adopted in 1950, revised in 1992, and revised again in 2005. This food pyramid is commonly taught in elementary and secondary education and is used as a guide for teaching healthy eating to the public. Daily recommendations include 6 to 11 servings of bread, cereal, rice, or pasta; 3 to 5 servings of vegetables; 2 to 4 servings of fruit; 2 to 3 servings of milk, yogurt, or cheese; 2 to 3 servings of meat, poultry, fish, dry beans, eggs, and nuts; and limited use of fats, oils, and sweets.

Nutritional Deficiencies and Food Limitations

Socioeconomic status may dictate food selections—for example, hamburger instead of steak; canned or frozen vegetables and fruit rather than fresh produce; and fish instead of shrimp or lobster. Most grocery stores have an adequate supply of frozen and canned fruits and vegetables, although they may be high in sodium and sugars. Given the size of the United States and proximity of farms to urban areas, there are few overall limitations for food choices for most Americans.

Pregnancy and Childbearing Practices

Fertility Practices and Views Toward Pregnancy

Commonly used methods of birth control among Americans include natural ovulation methods, birth

REFLECTIVE EXERCISE 12.3

Robert Northrop, a white 64-year-old manager in a large shoe store, presented at a neighborhood clinic with a chief complaint of difficulty urinating, especially in the morning. He has been divorced for over 20 years, lives alone, and has no children. He admits to weekend-only binge drinking when he is out with friends. During the week, he works 10-hour days and does not have time to go out with friends in the evening. His diet consists of frozen TV dinners, prepared fast foods, sandwiches made from deli meats and cheese, and snacks that include potato chips, pretzels, cheese twists, soft drinks, and energy drinks. Mr. Northrop's past medical history includes skin cancer, hemorrhoids, varicose vein surgery, and hypertension and hypercholesterolemia, for which he is on medication.

1. Name one occupation-related condition for which Mr. Northrop is at risk.
2. What lifestyle changes would you recommend to Mr. Northrop?
3. Do you think giving him the USDA MyPlate will help him change his dietary habits?
4. Can you suggest an alternative for Mr. Northrop for his weekend binge drinking?
5. Would you use low- or high-contexted communication with Mr. Northrop?
6. What health conditions does Mr. Northrop have that are consistent with European American Caucasians?

control pills, foams, Norplant, the morning-after pill, intrauterine devices, sterilization, vasectomy, prophylactics, and abortion. Although not all of these methods are acceptable to all people, many women use a combination of fertility control methods. The most extreme examples of fertility control are sterilization and abortion. Sterilization in the United States is strictly voluntary. Abortion remains a controversial issue in the United States, as it is in other countries. The "morning-after pill" also continues to be controversial to some. Anyone, male or female, over the age of 18 years can purchase the drug without a prescription. Those under the age of 18 years must have a prescription. Although some men have vasectomies, the literature is also scarce on the number of families who use vasectomy as a method of birth control.

Fertility practices and sexual activity, sensitive topics for many, are two areas where "outside" health-care providers may be more effective than health-care providers known to the client because of the concern about providing intimate information to someone they know.

Prescriptive, Restrictive, and Taboo Practices in the Childbearing Family

A prescriptive belief among Americans is that women are expected to seek preventive care, eat a well-balanced diet, and get adequate rest to have a healthy pregnancy and baby. The American health-care system encourages women to breastfeed, and many places of employment have made arrangements so women can breastfeed while at work.

A restrictive belief among Americans is that pregnant women should refrain from being around loud noises for prolonged periods of time. Taboo behaviors during pregnancy among Americans include smoking, drinking alcohol, drinking large amounts of caffeine, and taking recreational drugs—practices that are sure to cause harm to the mother or baby.

In the American culture, in which the father is often encouraged to take prenatal classes with the expectant mother and provide a supportive role in the delivery process, fathers with opposing beliefs may feel guilty if they do not comply. The woman's female relatives may provide assistance to the new mother until she is able to care for herself and the baby.

Additional cultural beliefs carried over from cultural migration and shared among other cultures as well as the European American culture include the following:

• A pregnant woman should not reach over her head because the baby may be born with the umbilical cord around its neck.
• If you wear an opal ring during pregnancy, it will harm the baby.
• Birthmarks are caused by eating strawberries or seeing a snake and being frightened.
• Congenital anomalies can occur if the mother sees or experiences a tragedy during her pregnancy.
• Nursing mothers should eat a bland diet to avoid upsetting the baby.
• The infant should wear a band around the abdomen to prevent the umbilicus from protruding and becoming herniated.
• A coin, key, or other metal object should be put on the umbilicus to flatten it.
• Cutting a baby's hair before baptism can cause blindness.
• Moving heavy items can cause your "insides" to fall out.
• If the baby is physically or mentally abnormal, God is punishing the parents.

In the past, the postpartum woman was prescribed a prolonged period of recuperation in the hospital or at home, something that is no longer as feasible the shortened length of confinement in the hospital after delivery.

The health-care provider must respect cultural beliefs associated with pregnancy and the birthing process when making decisions related to the health care of pregnant women, especially those practices that do not cause harm to the mother or the baby. Most cultural practices can be integrated into preventive teaching in a manner that promotes compliance.

REFLECTIVE EXERCISE 12.4

Margaret Schultz, age 15 years, is 3 months pregnant and making her first visit to the maternal child nurse practitioner. She is accompanied by her 17-year-old boyfriend, Billy, who is the father. Billy declines to give his last name but says he will take care of Margaret and the baby. Margaret and Billy currently live with Margaret's mother and three younger siblings. Margaret says she has no health problems and wants to keep the baby. She has made this appointment because she just wants to have a healthy baby. She is particularly concerned because her classmates tell her that she cannot lift heavy packages or carry her book bag because she might have a miscarriage. Her mother told her she could eat anything she wants, but Margaret is afraid that if she does, she will gain lots of weight like her mother, her boyfriend will leave her, and the baby might be born with a birthmark.

1. What is your overall first impression of this case?
2. Why might Billy not be willing to provide his last name?
3. What kind of support does Margaret have? Do you think this support will continue after the baby is born?
4. What is your response to Margaret's concern about lifting heavy objects?
5. What is your response to Margaret's concern about eating whatever she wants?
6. What is your response to Margaret's concern that the baby might be born with a birthmark?
7. What overall advice do you have for Margaret at this time? Do you think you should call Margaret's mother and discuss the pregnancy?

Death Rituals

Death Rituals and Expectations

For many American health-care providers educated in a culture of mastery over the environment, death is seen as one more disease to conquer, and when this does not happen, death becomes a personal failure. Thus, for many, death does not take a natural course because it is "managed" or "prolonged," making it difficult for some to die with dignity. Moreover, death and responses to death are not easy topics for many Americans to verbalize. Instead, many euphemisms are used rather than verbalizing that the person died: "passed away," "no longer with us," and "went to heaven."

The American cultural belief in self-determination and autonomy extends to people making their own decisions about end-of-life care. Mentally competent adults have the right to refuse or decide what medical treatment and interventions they wish to extend life, such as artificial life support and artificial feeding and hydration.

Most Americans believe that a dying person should not be left alone, and accommodations are usually made for a family member to be with the dying person at all times. Health-care providers are expected to care for the family as much as for the patient during this time.

Most people are buried or cremated within 3 days of the death, but extenuating circumstances may lengthen this period to accommodate family and friends who must travel a long distance to attend a funeral or memorial service. The family can decide whether to have an open or closed casket at the viewing (or wake). Significant variations in burial practices occur with other ethnocultural groups in the United States.

Responses to Death and Grief

American society has been launching major initiatives to help patients die as comfortably as possible without pain; one such initiative is Toolkit for Nurturing Excellence at End-of-Life Transition (TNEEL, 2003). As a result, more people are choosing to remain at home or to enter a hospice for end-of-life care where their comfort needs are better met.

One of the requirements for entering a hospice in the United States is that the patient must sign documents indicating that he or she does not want extensive life-saving measures performed. Bereavement support strategies include being physically present, encouraging a reality orientation, openly acknowledging the family's right to grieve, accepting varied behavioral responses to grief, acknowledging the patient's pain, assisting them to express their feelings, encouraging interpersonal relationships, promoting interest in a new life, and making referrals to other resources such as a priest, minister, rabbi, or pastoral care.

Spirituality

Dominant Religion and Use of Prayer

In the United States, major religious groups include Protestant (51.3 percent), Roman Catholic (23.9 percent), Mormon (1.7 percent), other Christian (1.6 percent), Jewish (1.7 percent), Muslim (0.6 percent), other or unspecified (2.5 percent), unaffiliated (12.1 percent), and none (4 percent) (*CIA World Factbook,* 2011). Many groups settled in America for religious freedom. Furthermore, specific religious groups are concentrated regionally in the United States, with Baptists in the South, Lutherans in the North and Midwest, and Catholics in the Northeast, East, and Southwest. Within this context, there is a separation of church and state, and the U.S. government cannot support a particular religion or prevent people from practicing their chosen religion. However, this does not include cults or extremist groups, which usually devote themselves to esoteric ideals and fads.

Even though there is a separation of church and state in the United States, many public events and ceremonies open with a prayer, and phrases such as "one nation under God" are often included. American money still has the phrase "in God we trust" printed on it. Most people see these religious symbols as harmless rituals. Instead of speaking to "religious values," politicians speak to "family values" as a way of getting around religious principles. However, these issues are subject to debate from time to time. Unlike many countries that support a specific church or religion and in which people discuss their religion frequently and openly, religion is not an everyday topic of conversation for most Americans.

The health-care provider who is aware of the client's religious practices and spiritual needs is in a better position to promote culturally competent health care. The practitioner must demonstrate an appreciation of and respect for the dignity and spiritual beliefs of clients by avoiding negative comments about religious beliefs and practices. Clients may find considerable comfort in speaking with religious leaders in times of crisis and serious illness.

Meaning of Life and Individual Sources of Strength

When Americans are asked what gives their lives meaning and where they find strength, a variety of answers are offered. Formal religion is one, but other common responses include family, work, self-improvement, friends, music, dance, hobbies, sports events, and meditation. For some, sources and meaning of life come from having a pet, such as a dog or cat.

Spiritual Beliefs and Health-Care Practices

Spiritual wellness brings fulfillment from a lifestyle of purposeful and pleasurable living that embraces free choices, meaning in life, satisfaction in life, and self-esteem. Practices that interfere with a person's spiritual life can hinder physical recovery and promote physical illness.

Health-care providers should inquire whether the person wants to see a member of the clergy even if she or he has not been active in church. Religious emblems should not be removed because they provide solace to the person and removing them may increase or cause anxiety. A thorough assessment of spiritual life is essential for the identification of solutions and resources that can support other treatments.

Health-Care Practices

Health-Seeking Beliefs and Behaviors

Currently, the United States is undergoing a paradigm shift from one that places high value on curative and restorative medical practices with sophisticated technological care to one of health promotion and wellness; illness, disease, and injury prevention; health maintenance and restoration; and increased personal responsibility. Most believe that the individual, the family, and the community have the ability to influence their health. For a few, good health may be seen as a divine gift from God, with individuals having little control over health and illness.

The primacy of patient autonomy is generally accepted as an enlightened perspective in American society. To this end, advance directives such as "durable power of attorney" or a "living will" are an important part of medical care. Accordingly, patients can specify their wishes concerning life and death decisions before entering an inpatient facility. The durable power of attorney for health care allows the patient to name a family member or significant other to speak for the patient and make decisions when or if the patient is unable to do so. The patient can also have a living will that outlines the person's wishes in terms of life-sustaining procedures in the event of a terminal illness. Each inpatient facility has these forms available and will ask the patient what his or her wishes are. Patients may sign these forms at the hospital or elect to bring their own forms, many of which are on the Internet.

Guidelines for immunizations were developed largely as a result of the influence of the World Health Organization (WHO). Specific immunization schedules and the ages at which they are prescribed vary widely among countries and can be obtained from the WHO Web site (http://www.who.int). Recently, controversy has arisen when some facilities have made the requirement that all employees must be immunized against the flu. Most employees comply, but a few see it as an infringement of their individual rights. In addition, some religious groups, such as Christian Scientists, do not believe in immunizations. Beliefs like this, which restrict optimal child health, have resulted in court battles with various outcomes.

Responsibility for Health Care

The United States is moving to a paradigm in which people take increased responsibility for their own health. In a society in which individualism is valued, people are expected to be self-reliant. In fact, people are expected to exercise some control over disease, including controlling the amount of stress in their lives. If someone does not maintain a healthy lifestyle and then gets sick, some believe it is the person's own fault. Unless someone is very ill, she or he should not neglect social and work obligations.

At the time of this writing, the Patient Protection and Affordable Care Act (PPACA) of 2010—aimed to provide health insurance for all Americans—is being instituted. The PPACA continues to be hotly debated, with some states declaring it unconstitutional. The next few years will determine the success of the PPACA. In the United States, everyone, regardless of socioeconomic or immigration status, can receive acute-care services. However, they will be charged a fee for the service, and they may not be able to get nonacute follow-up care unless they can prove they are able to pay for the service. Even if they are covered by health insurance, an insurance company representative may need to approve the visit and then have a list of procedures, medicines, and treatments for which it will pay.

Health-care providers should not assume that clients who do not have health insurance or practice health prevention do not care about their health. Many are included in the working poor where they make minimum wage, which is less than the cost of a family insurance policy.

Self-medicating behavior in itself may not be harmful, but when combined with or used to the exclusion of prescription medications, it may be detrimental to the person's health. A common practice with prescription medications is for people to take medicine until the symptoms disappear and then discontinue the medicine prematurely. This practice commonly occurs with antihypertensive medications and antibiotics. No culture is immune to self-medicating practices; almost everyone engages in it to some extent.

One cannot ignore the ample supply of over-the-counter medications in American pharmacies, the numerous television advertisements for self-medication, and media campaigns for new medications, encouraging viewers to ask their doctor or health-care provider about a particular medication for cholesterol, erectile dysfunction, and a host of other conditions.

Folk and Traditional Practices

Some Americans favor traditional, folk, or magico-religious health-care practices over biomedical practices and use some or all of them simultaneously. For many, what are considered alternative or complementary health-care practices may be mainstream medicine for another person. In the United States, interest has increased in alternative and complementary health practices. The U.S. government has an Office of Alternative Medicine at the National Institutes of Health that has awarded millions of dollars in grants to bridge the gap between traditional and nontraditional therapies.

As an adjunct to biomedical treatments, many people use acupuncture, acupressure, acumassage, herbal therapies, and other traditional treatments. Examples of folk medicines include covering a boil with axle grease, wearing copper bracelets for arthritis pain, mixing wild turnip root and honey for a sore throat, and drinking herbal teas. Most Americans practice folk medicine in some form; they may use family remedies passed down from previous generations.

An awareness of combined practices when treating or providing health education helps ensure that therapies do not contradict each other, intensify the treatment regimen, or cause an overdose. At other times, they may be harmful, conflict with, or potentiate the effects of prescription medications. Many times, these traditional, folk, and magico-religious practices are and should be incorporated into the plans of care for clients. Inquiring about the full range of therapies being used, such as food items, teas, herbal remedies, nonfood substances, over-the-counter medications, and medications prescribed or loaned by others, is essential so that conflicting treatment modalities are not used. If clients perceive that the health-care provider does not accept their beliefs, they may be less compliant with prescriptive treatment and less likely to reveal their use of these practices.

Barriers to Health Care

Barriers to health care for European Americans are essentially the same for any culture and include availability, accessibility, affordability, appropriateness, accountability, adaptability, acceptability, awareness, attitudes, approachability, alternative and complementary practices and providers, and health literacy (see Chapter 2). In order for people to receive adequate health care, a number of considerations need to be addressed. Several studies have identified that a lack of fluency in language is the primary barrier to receiving adequate health care in the United States (see Chapter 1).

Health-care providers can help reduce some of these barriers by calling an area ethnic agency or church for assistance, establishing an advocacy role, involving professionals and laypeople from the same ethnic group as the client, using cultural brokers, and organizationally providing culturally congruent and linguistically appropriate services. If all of these elements are in place and used appropriately, they have the potential of generating culturally responsive care.

Cultural Responses to Health and Illness

Significant research has been conducted on patients' responses to pain, which has been called the "fifth vital sign." Most Americans believe that patients should be made comfortable and not have to tolerate high levels of pain. Accrediting bodies, such as the Joint Commission, survey organizations to ensure that patients' pain levels are assessed and that appropriate interventions are instituted. Cultural backgrounds, worldviews, and the variant cultural characteristics profoundly influence the pain experience.

Additional resources for pain are the American Pain Foundation, the American Pain Society, the Boston Cancer Pain Education Center (in 11 languages), and the OUCHER Pain scale (OUCHER!, n.d,) for children, all of which are available on the Internet. The health-care provider may need to offer and encourage pain medication and explain that it will help the healing to progress. Research needs to be conducted in the areas of ethnic pain experiences and management of pain.

For some Americans, mental illness may be seen as being as important as physical illness. For some, mental illness and severe physical handicaps are considered a disgrace or cause a stigma. As a result, the family is likely to keep the mentally ill or handicapped person at home as long as they can. This practice may be reinforced by the belief that all individuals are expected to contribute to the household for the common good of the family, and when a person is unable to contribute, further disgrace occurs.

In previous decades, physically handicapped individuals in the United States were seen as less desirable than those who did not have a handicap. If the handicap was severe, the person was sometimes hidden from the public's view. In 1992, the Americans with Disabilities Act went into effect, protecting handicapped individuals from discrimination.

In the United States, rehabilitation and occupational health services focus on returning individuals with handicaps to productive lifestyles in society as soon as possible. The goal of the American health-care system is to rehabilitate everyone: convicted criminals, people with alcohol and drug problems, as well as those with physical conditions. Rehabilitation seems to now be well established in the United States.

Blood Transfusions and Organ Donation

Most Americans and most, but not all, religions favor organ donation and transplantation and transfusion of blood or blood products. Jehovah's Witnesses do not believe in blood transfusions. Health-care providers may need to assist clients in obtaining a religious leader to support them in making decisions regarding organ donation or transplantation.

Health-Care Providers
Traditional Versus Biomedical Providers

Most Americans combine the use of biomedical health-care practitioners with traditional practices, folk healers, and magico-religious healers. The health-care system abounds with individual and family folk practices for curing or treating specific illnesses. A significant percentage of all care is delivered outside the perimeter of the formal health-care arena. Many times folk and traditional therapies are handed down from family members and may have their roots in religious beliefs. Traditional and folk practices often contain elements of historically rooted beliefs.

The American practice is to assign staff to patients regardless of gender differences, although often an attempt is made to provide a same-gender health-care provider when intimate care is involved, especially when the patient and caregiver are of the same age. However, health-care providers should recognize and respect differences in gender relationships when providing culturally competent care because not all people accept care from someone of the opposite gender.

Status of Health-Care Providers

Individual perceptions concerning competence and acceptability of providers may be closely associated with previous contact and experiences with health-care providers. In general, health-care providers, especially physicians, are viewed with great respect, although recent studies show that this is declining among some groups. Although many nurses in the United States do not believe they have respect, public opinion polls usually place patients' respect of nurses higher than that of physicians. The advanced practice role of registered nurses is gaining respect as more of them have successful careers and the public sees them as equal or preferable to physicians in many cases. Evidence suggests that respect for professionals is correlated with their educational level, including baccalaureate-, master's-, and doctoral-level programs of study, and the impact of nursing interventions on health-care outcomes. In the United States, approximately 10 percent of nurses are men, with very active campaigns in some areas of the country to recruit men and other underrepresented groups into nursing (Purnell, 2007).

REFERENCES

Centers for Disease Control and Prevention. (2007). *Unmarried childbearing.* Retrieved from http://www.cdc.gov/nchs/fastats/unmarry.htm

Centers for Disease Control and Prevention. (2011). Retrieved from www.cdc.gov

CIA World Factbook. (2011). *United States.* Retrieved from https://www.cia.gov/library/publications/the-world-factbook/geos/us.html

Information Please Almanac. (2009). *United States.* Retrieved from http://www.gale.cengage.com/reference/peter/200901/info_almanac.htm

Munoz, C., & Hilgenberg, C. (2005). Ethnopharmacology. *American Journal of Nursing, 105*(8), 40–49.

OUCHER! (n.d.). Retrieved from http://www.oucher.org/

Prows, C.A., & Prows, D.R. (2004). Tailoring drug therapy with pharmacogenetics. *American Journal of Nursing, 104*(5), 60–71.

Purnell, L. (2007). Men in nursing: An international perspective. In C. O'Lynn & R. Tranbarger (Eds.), *Men in nursing* (pp. 219–235). New York: Springer Publishing.

Purnell, L., & Foster, J. (2003a). Cultural aspects of alcohol use: Part I. *The Drug and Alcohol Professional, 3*(3), 17–23.

Purnell, L., & Foster, J. (2003b). Cultural aspects of alcohol use: Part II. *The Drug and Alcohol Professional, 2*(3), 3–8.

Purnell, L., & Galloway, W. (1995). What to do if called upon to testify. *Accident and Emergency Nursing, 17*(4), 246–249.

Toolkit for Nurturing Excellence at End-of-Life Transition (TNEEL, 2003). Retrieved from http://www.tneel.uic.edu/tneel-ss/introduction.asp

U.S. Census Bureau. (2010). Retrieved from http://factfinder2.census.gov/faces/tableservices/jsf/pages/productview.xhtml?pid=ACS_10_5YR_S1701&prodType=table

DavisPlus For reflective exercises, review questions, and additional information, go to

http://davisplus.fadavis.com

Chapter 13

People of Filipino Heritage

Corazon C. Munoz

The author would like to thank Dula Pacquiao for her work on this chapter in previous editions.

Overview, Inhabited Localities, and Topography

Overview

The Philippines is located in Southeast Asia in the Western Pacific ocean. To its north lies Taiwan, and to its west is Vietnam. The tropical climate makes the Philippines prone to earthquakes and typhoons but has also endowed the country with natural resources and made it one of the richest areas of biodiversity in the world. The Philippines is an archipelago consisting of 7107 islands, with three main geographical divisions: Luzon, Visayas, and Mindanao (*CIA World Factbook,* 2011). With a landmass of 300,000 square kilometers (115,830 square miles), it is slightly larger than the state of Arizona. The terrain is mostly mountainous with narrow-to-extensive coastal lowlands. The tropical climate consists of dry and rainy seasons suitable for year-round agriculture and fishing, but it is affected by the seasonal northeastern and southwestern monsoons. With an estimated population of about 104 million, the population has decreased since 2005 (*CIA World Factbook,* 2012). Although the country is rich in natural resources and has a mixed economy of agriculture, light industry, and support services, almost 33 percent of the population lives below the poverty level (*CIA World Factbook,* 2011).

The Spaniards colonized the country for over 3 centuries from 1565 to 1898. Following the Spanish-American War, the islands were ceded to the United States and given the anglicized name "the Philippines." Filipinas (Pilipinas) and Philippines are used interchangeably today. Native speakers refer to the country as Filipinas or Pilipinas and use Philippines when speaking to outsiders or writing in English. In 1946, when the Philippines gained its independence from the United States, it adopted the Tagalog-based *Pilipino* as its national language. In 1959, Pilipino was officially declared the national language. In 1986, however, the national assembly declared the national language as *Filipino,* based on existing Philippine and other languages. Generally, *Filipino* is used interchangeably with *Filipino American.* The term *Pilipino* is generally used to distinguish indigenous identity and nationalistic empowerment.

Filipino Americans are a diverse group because of regional variations in the Philippines, which influence the dialect spoken, food preferences, religion, and traditions. Generational differences within families are associated with age and time of migration from the Philippines. Other factors influencing diversity include pre- and postmigration level of education, occupation, and intermarriage, as well as other variant cultural characteristics (see Chapter 1). This chapter discusses the major characteristics of mainstream Filipino culture, offering some insights into some differences among groups. The reader should avoid using this information as a universal template for every Filipino.

Heritage and Residence

The Filipino way of life is a tapestry of multicultural influences superimposed on indigenous tribal origins (Fig. 13-1). The people are predominantly of Malayan ancestry, with overlays of Chinese, Japanese, East Indian, Indonesian, Malaysian, and Islamic cultures (*CIA World Factbook,* 2012). The Philippine culture is distinct from its Asian neighbors largely because of the major influences from the Spanish and American colonization.

The Filipino sense of morality and justice evolved from tribal times. Close-knit, kin-based groups known as *barangays* emerged to protect communities from outside atrocities. Communal values of collective welfare and solidarity fostered security of its members in an unstable environment. Outsiders to the culture recognize these values in the Filipino traits of collective loyalty, generosity, hospitality, and humility. These basic values are strong components of childhood socialization in the family. Filipinos inculcate a strong

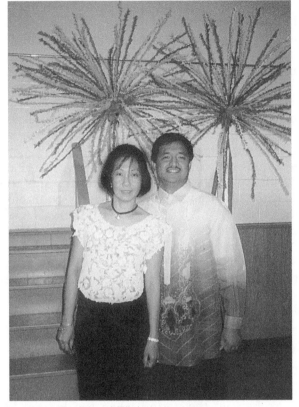

Figure 13-1 Traditional Filipino costumes.

along with social and cultural exchanges, have helped create transnational community networks and established multiple migration streams over time.

These early migrants were ineligible for citizenship and were denied privileges such as employment requiring citizenship, union membership, the right to own land, and the right to marry in states with antimiscegenation laws (laws prohibiting cohabitation, sexual relations, or marriage between people of different races). The Great Depression heightened racial animosity toward Filipino workers, and passage of the Tydings-McDuffie Act (Philippines Independence Act) in 1934 virtually ended immigration (Ceniza-Choy, 2003).

In 1946, immigration restrictions for Filipinos were eased and they were granted naturalization rights. Between 1946 and 1965, 33,000 immigrants entered the United States and contributed to a 44 percent increase in the Filipino population in America. The Immigration Act of 1965 initiated a period of renewed mass immigration by promoting family reunification and recruitment of occupational immigrants. Since the passage of the 1965 Act, the Philippines has become the largest source of immigrants from Asia. A search for better economic and educational opportunities and reunification with family members in the United States continue to be the primary motivating factors for emigration. Working adult children sponsor their older relatives to come to the United States to care for their young children. In turn, older people facilitate the subsequent immigration of other children.

Because the Philippine economy has been unable to provide jobs for college graduates, an estimated 6 million Filipino professionals work overseas, and as many as 300,000 Filipinos emigrated in 2006. Export of professional and skilled labor is one of the biggest industries in the Philippines. Remittances sent home by Filipinos overseas contribute as much as 10 percent to the country's gross domestic product, estimated at between 11 and 13 billion pesos (approximately US$278 million) in 2006 (IBON Foundation, 2007).

sense of family loyalty beyond the nuclear family. Family obligations extend to cousins, in-laws, and others who are intimately linked with the family by ceremonies such as serving as sponsors of marriage or baptisms (Bautista, 2002).

Most Filipinos in North America were born in the Philippines. The majority of Filipino Americans reside in the states of California, Hawaii, Illinois, New Jersey, New York, Washington, and Texas. Filipinos make up the second largest foreign-born population after Mexicans in the United States (Reeves & Bennett, 2004).

Reasons for Migration and Associated Economic Factors

Many Filipinos migrate to America and elsewhere primarily for economic prosperity. The economic challenges in the Philippines are exaggerated by its unemployment rate, foreign debt, population growth, and social inequities. These factors contribute to the migration of Filipinos to the United States, including physicians, nurses, engineers, information technology experts, and other laborers. American corporations, trade companies, and financial institutions partnering with Philippine companies have invested in promoting economic development and exchanges with the country. These larger political and economic influences,

Educational Status and Occupations

Around 1900, Americans introduced public education in the Philippines. Early training of schoolteachers was provided by the Thomasites, forerunners of the U.S. Peace Corps. The development of educational programs in the Philippines was highly influenced and patterned after those in the United States, as in the case of nursing and medicine. Early missionaries and philanthropic organizations such as the Daughters of the American Revolution, the Catholic Scholarship Fund, and the Rockefeller Foundation were instrumental in the Westernization of health-care education and practice in the Philippines. American nursing educators went to the Philippines, and Filipino nurses were sent to the United States for training. They subsequently returned to the Philippines and assumed leadership positions in nursing schools and hospitals. Since 1970, all nursing curricula have converted to a 4-year degree program leading toward a BSN (Pacquiao, 2004).

The Philippines has one of the highest literacy rates in Asia at 96 percent. Schools are either publicly or privately funded. Formal education starts at the age of 7 years, with 6 years of primary education. Nursery school and kindergarten are offered in most private schools. Students get 4 years of secondary education in either a vocational-technical or an academic school. A high school graduate is 2 years younger than those graduating from U.S. high schools because of the omission of middle school years.

Filipinos view educational achievement as a pathway to economic success, status, and prestige for both the individual and the family. A person's profession is always identified when introducing, addressing, or writing about the person (e.g., Doctor, *Magpantay*, or Engineer, *Paredes*). A family's status in the community is enhanced by the educational achievement of the child, and a child's education is considered an investment for the whole family. Both male and female children are expected to do well in school, and parents do their best to provide for their children's full-time education. Adolescents who closely identify with their families are found to be concerned with the potential effect of their scholastic achievement on their families' reputation (Salazar, Schuldermann, Schuldermann, & Hunyh, 2000). Family members and other relatives commonly contribute toward the education of their kin. Among lower- and middle-class families, siblings take turns going to college in order to maximize resources for one member to finish school, who can then contribute to the education of her or his siblings. One's choice of profession is generally a family decision and is based on potential economic return to the group. Hence, increased demand for nurses abroad attracts higher enrollment in nursing, as families view this occupation as a pathway to economic improvement.

Filipinos appear to be assimilated and successful and tend to blend into American society, which gives them a reputation as a "model minority." In reality, high educational attainment of American-born and immigrant Filipinos does not guarantee their entry into well-paying or high-status jobs. Significant discrimination confronts native-born and immigrant Filipinos in the American labor market linked with factors such as ethnicity, gender, region of residence, and level of education (Yamane, 2002). As is the experience of many foreign graduates, Filipinos' education and experience are rarely matched with a suitable job because of the restricted labor market, resulting in many individuals competing for low-level jobs for which many are overqualified. Only those who are educated in health-care fields tend to find jobs consistent with their education.

Whereas American nursing education stresses critical thinking, in the Philippines, mastery of facts and rote learning are emphasized. A defined hierarchy exists in schools, with the teacher as the expert authority. This hierarchy is congruent with the social organization in the broader society, in which age and position are markers of status and power. The younger generations are rewarded for accepting the ideas and counsel of older people and teachers. Challenging authority and asserting one's creative ideas are unnatural predispositions, especially for the young. Nursing faculty have identified the tendency of Filipino students to take things at face value, avoid conflict, communicate nonassertively, and learn by rote memorization. Students' traditional values at home were in conflict with values in school and teacher expectations (Pacquiao, 1996). Facilitating understanding of the dominant cultural values and norms in school, in addition to teaching the subject matter, is essential to facilitate these students' academic success.

Communication
Dominant Language and Dialects

Filipinos were influenced by American language and culture beyond the period when the United States recognized its independence in 1946. *Tagalog* is the primary language spoken in the Philippines. The two other official languages are English and Spanish. Within the Philippines there are approximately 75 ethnolinguistic groups who speak more than 100 dialects. For the sake of simplicity, the Philippine government has given all of these languages the collective name of Pilipino (Munoz & Luckmann, 2005).

English is the official language used for business and legal transactions, as well as taught in secondary schools and universities. This has an impact on how Filipinos adjust in the United States, making it easier and faster to navigate the systems in the United States as compared with other Asian immigrant groups. Business and social interactions commonly use a hybrid of both Tagalog and English (*Tag-Lish*) in the same sentence. Tag-Lish is often used in health education. Most Filipinos speak the national language, Filipino, which is based on Tagalog (Tatak Pilipino, 2003). This has created some regional tensions because the other dialects are not well represented in Tagalog as the national language, making it difficult for those in the Central and Southern regions of the country to learn and speak Tagalog.

Many Spanish words are found in the Filipino language such as *sopa* (soup), *calle* (street), *hija/hijo* (daughter/son), and *respeto* (respect). The influence of indigenous Filipino and Spanish languages produces distinct characteristics when Filipinos speak English. There is absence of certain sounds in the Filipino language such as short *i*, long *a*, and long *o*. Hence, *liver* may be enunciated as *lever*, *make* as *mik*, and *flow* as *flaw*. Many Filipinos are unable to differentiate *s* from *sh* (*physiology* as *fishiology*), *u* from short *o* or short *a* sounds (*cut* as *cot* or *cat*; *church* as *charts*). They have a tendency to place emphasis on the second syllable of a multisyllabic word (in ter´fe rence, pen ni´cill in, Ro bi´tus sin(™)).

Filipino social hierarchy is evident in the language. Specific nouns rather than pronouns are used to denote a person's age, gender, and position in the social hierarchy. For instance, *Manang* and *Manong* are used to refer to or address an older woman and man, respectively. These nouns are used to address the person or when speaking about her or him. There is absence of the "she/he" in the Filipino language. Rather, generic and gender-neutral pronouns *siya* (singular "she/he") and *sila* (plural "they/them") are used. Hence, many Filipinos may unconsciously use "she" and "he" interchangeably in reference to the same individual.

Although many Filipinos speak English, their ethnic language or dialect, knowledge and use of the English language, and age of migration to the United States often influence enunciation, pronunciation, and accentuation. Older Filipinos who originated from *non–Tagalog*-speaking regions may understand and speak better English than other Filipinos. In multigenerational Filipino American families, different languages may be used to communicate with family members and friends. Although many Filipinos speak and write fluently in English, they may have difficulty understanding American idiomatic expressions. For example, to a new immigrant, "How are you?" may be interpreted as a question about the person's well-being, requiring an elaboration of one's situation, rather than a mere greeting. Filipinos may have difficulty communicating their lack of understanding to others and may use ritualistic language and euphemistic behavior that appear to be the opposite of how they actually perceive the situation. Saving face, or concealment (Pasco, Morse, & Olson, 2004), is a characteristic pattern of behavior employed to protect the integrity of both parties, which is a consequence of the cultural value on maintaining smooth interpersonal relations. Desirous of group approval, the individual becomes sensitive to the feelings of others and, in turn, develops a high sense of sensitivity to personal insults.

Traditional Filipino communication is highly contextual. It is basically formal, addressing individuals by their academic titles such as Dr. or Mr. and Mrs. The communication pattern is also rooted in the past and is hierarchical, which is consistent with respect for older adults or those with known accomplishment and achievement (Munoz & Luckmann, 2005).

The individual is enculturated to attend to the context of the interaction and to adopt appropriate behaviors. Many Filipinos are keenly observant, displaying an intuitive feeling about the other person and the contextual environment during interactions. Contextual variables include the presence of *ibang tao* (outsiders) versus *hindi ibang tao* (insiders) and the age, social position, and gender of the other individual. In the company of insiders, such as one's family, each member develops an intuitive knowledge of the other so that words are unnecessary to convey a message and meanings are embedded in nonverbal communication. In the presence of outsiders, a child's emotional outburst may be met with adults' stern silence, indifference, or euphemistic grins. These behaviors imply to insiders that emotional outbursts are inappropriate in front of outsiders. One may not disagree, talk loudly, or look directly at a person who is older and who occupies a higher position in the social hierarchy. Honorific terms of address denoting an individual's status within the hierarchy exist in all dialects. In Tagalog, when communicating to an older person or a person of status, he or she is addressed using gender and age-specific honorific nouns such as *Lolo*/*Lola* (Grandpa/Grandma), and *ate*/*kuya* (older sister/older brother).

Filipino interpersonal and social life operates to maintain smooth interpersonal relationships; communication tends to be indirect and ambiguous to prevent the risk of offending others. Filipinos may sacrifice clear communication to avoid stressful interpersonal conflicts and confrontations. As saying no to a superior is considered disrespectful, it predisposes an individual to make an ambiguous positive response. Filipinos are often puzzled, and sometimes offended, by the precision and exactness of American communication. Newly recruited Filipino nurses are stunned by their American coworkers' abrasiveness and open expressions of anger toward one another and their subsequent behavior of sitting down at coffee "as if nothing happened."

To many traditional Filipinos, actions speak louder than words. They value respect and might find questions like "Do you understand?" or "Do you follow?" disrespectful. It is preferable for the speaker to say, "Please let me know if I understood you correctly." When speakers occupy different positions in the social hierarchy, an informal and familiar manner of speaking by the subordinate may be perceived as impolite and disrespectful. Allowing time for a Filipino to respond not only communicates respect but also gives time for translating the dialect into English. Speaking clearly and slowly facilitates appreciation of varying pronunciation and accentuation of the English language across cultures.

Cultural Communication Patterns

Relational orientation has been suggested as the essence of Asian social psychology. Enriquez (1994) posited that the Filipino core values of shame (*hiya*), yielding to the leader or majority (*pakikisama*), gratitude (*utang na loob*), and sensitivity to personal affront (*amor propio*) emphasize a strong sense of human relatedness. These values originate from the central concept of *kapwa*, which arises from the awareness of shared identity with others. *Kapwa* embraces the insider-outsider categories of human relations and prescribes different levels of interrelatedness or involvement with others. *Pakakikipagkapwa,* being one with others, implies accepting and dealing with the other individual as a fellow human being. *Kapwa* is grounded in the fundamental value of shared inner perception or feeling for another, from which all other attributes for human relations are made possible.

Eight levels of social interactions were identified by Enriquez within the core concept of *kapwa*. These levels demonstrate a hierarchy of human relatedness within the Filipino language and context of meanings. The contextual axis of interactions is conceptualized within a continuum of how the "other" is categorized—whether as an insider or outsider. The degree of sharing and involvement with outsiders may progress from levels 1 to 5, whereas interactions at levels 6 to 8 are observed with insiders. The eight levels are *pakikitungo* (civility, level 1), *pakikisalimuha* (interacting, level 2), *pakikihalok* (participating, level 3), *pakikibagay* (conforming, level 4), *pakikisama* (adjusting, level 5), *pakikipagpalagayang loob* (understanding and accepting, level 6), *pakikisangkot* (getting involved, level 7), and *pakikiisa* (being one with, level 8).

Developing working relationships with Filipinos requires an understanding of where one is situated within the insider-outsider continuum. Outsiders can move toward higher levels of interactions by observing cultural norms of communication, using trusted gatekeepers to mediate conflicts, seeking validation of perceptions of behaviors from more acculturated members of the group, and allowing face-saving opportunities to prevent embarrassment and personal denigration. When confronting a Filipino coworker, provide privacy, and point out positive attributes as well as the problem. Observing nonverbal behaviors and interpreting them within the Filipino cultural context help promote culturally congruent interactions. Accommodating differential sharing and involvement between insiders and with outsiders shows cultural understanding that enhances development of intercultural relationships. For example, a Filipino speaking Tagalog with another reinforces the value of being one with others. Learning and using some Filipino greetings and honorific terms of address facilitate movement of the relationship to higher levels of involvement. Defining work situations in which Filipino dialects may be spoken demonstrates cultural sensitivity and accommodation. The insider and outsider delineations may be less important to some Filipinos who are highly educated and take pride in their global outlook. Unlike other immigrants who settle in ethnic enclaves, more recent Filipino immigrants acculturate and relate well with people from various cultures.

Smiling and giggling are often observed, especially among young Filipino women. The meanings of these spontaneous and highly unconscious behaviors are embedded in the context of the situation and may range from glee, genuine interest, and agreement, to discomfort, politeness, or indifference. It is helpful to point out how the behavior can be misinterpreted by patients and others, if inappropriate to the situation. Behavior change can be expected if correction is done in a timely, respectful, and sincere manner.

Having a heightened sensitivity to personal insults, Filipinos have a remarkable ability to maintain a proper front to protect their self-esteem when threatened. Conflict-avoidance behaviors to conceal discomfort or distress are evident in euphemistic denial of anger, minimization of pain, and silence. However, pent-up emotions and accumulated resentment may result in explosive anger, depression, and somatization. Health-care providers should be sensitive to these behaviors and explore the underlying causes by establishing trust and maintaining respectful relationships. Offering pain medications and attending to nonverbal behaviors, rather than waiting for the patient to verbalize his or her needs, are culturally congruent approaches.

First-generation Filipinos in North America have high regard for health-care providers (Abe-Kim, Gong, & Takeuchi, 2004) and present themselves in therapy sessions as polite, cooperative, verbal, and engaging. However, agreement with health-care providers does not ensure that patients will follow through with the recommendations. Health-care providers should be comfortable with patients' deferential attitudes without resorting to authoritarian approaches, which may be perceived as oppressive and may encourage euphemistic complaint behaviors. Once trust is developed, expression of authentic feelings is possible. Filipinos who are accustomed to indirect communication may perceive focusing on action-oriented strategies and outcomes as intrusive and coercive.

Direct eye contact varies among Filipinos depending on the degree of acculturation, length of time in America, age, and education. Some individuals may avoid prolonged eye contact with authority figures and older people as a form of respect. Older men may refrain from maintaining eye contact with young women because it may be interpreted as flirtation or a sexual advance. Filipinos are comfortable with silence and may allow the other person to initiate verbal interaction as a sign of respect. During a teaching session, a Filipino patient's nod may have several meanings that can range from "Yes, I hear you," "Yes, we are interacting," "Yes, I can see the instructions," or some other message that may be difficult for the patient to disclose. Validating a patient's response in a sensitive and respectful manner, as well as observing her or his behaviors, can prevent miscommunication.

Touch is used freely, especially with insiders. Greater distance is observed when interacting with outsiders and people in positions of authority. Same-gender closeness and touching, which may be perceived as homosexual adult behavior in America, are considered normal. Young adults of the same gender may hold hands, put one arm over another's shoulder, or walk arm-in-arm. As they become more acculturated, many Filipinos become aware of the differences and adapt to the new culture.

The implicit rules of the social hierarchy are observed when conflicts arise. A subordinate does not confront his or her superiors. Rather, a mediator who is likely to be a trusted individual at the same level of hierarchy as the superior may be employed to mediate and approach the superior on behalf of the subordinate. This behavior may be interpreted as dishonest by those who value direct and assertive communication.

Temporal Relationships

Filipinos have a relaxed temporal outlook. They have a healthy respect for the past, an ability to enjoy the present, and hope for the future. Past orientation is evident in their respect for older people and dead ancestors (*galang*), and a sense of gratitude and obligation to kin (*utang na loob*). Future orientation is manifested in the family's commitment to provide for the education of the young, parental participation in the care of their children and grandchildren, and a strong work ethic. A strong present orientation is associated with the cultural emphasis on maintaining positive relationships with others. Permanent social bonds with kin and significant others outside of kin are nurtured. Filipinos enjoy their families, fiestas, and life. They spend generously to make family events memorable and enjoyable. Although most Filipinos have adapted to American punctuality in the business sphere, promptness for social events is situationally determined. "Filipino time" means arriving much later than the scheduled appointment, which can be from 1 to several hours. The focus is on the gathering rather than on the schedule. A Filipino host may invite American guests at least 1 hour later than the Filipino guests in the hope that both will arrive at the same time.

Format for Names

The Filipino family is bilineally extended to several generations. Kinship and family affinity can be legally and spiritually claimed equally from both sets of families, giving the child the identity of the extended family. This bilineal kinship is reflected in their names. Children carry the surnames of both parents. For example, Jose Romagos Lopez and Leticia Romagos Lopez are the children of Maria Romagos and Eduardo Lopez. The middle name or initial (R) is the mother's maiden name, Romagos. After marriage, Jose keeps the same name, whereas his sister's name becomes Leticia L. Lukban (her husband being Ernesto Lukban). Leticia's maiden name, Lopez, is abbreviated as her middle initial.

Many Filipino names are of Spanish origin. Symbolic of Filipinos' Catholic faith, saint names are often used with first names. Filipino females may have a Ma. (for Maria) before their given names—for example, Ma. Luisa stands for Maria Luisa. Although the name Maria is often given to girls, some males may use Maria as a first or second name—hence, Ma. Jose Romagos Lopez and Jose Ma. Paredes Castro. The saint name is an integral part of the first name, so an individual will use both first names: Maria Luisa or Jose Maria. Few Filipino American women keep their own surname after marriage, although this may increase among second- and third-generation Filipinos.

Adults use first names to address young children. Nicknames symbolizing affectionate regard for the person (*Nini*, Baby, *Bongbong*) are commonly used instead of the first name. These nicknames may indicate special meanings, positions, and/or outstanding characteristics of the child. First names are avoided when addressing older adults and those occupying higher positions in the hierarchy. In formal business transactions, prefixes such as Mr., Mrs., Miss, or Ms. or the person's professional degree are used before the person's last names (Dr. Abaya or Attorney Abaya).

REFLECTIVE EXERCISE 13.1

Marianita de la Fuente, a 95-year-old female, was admitted to a general medical unit for chest pain, generalized weakness, and dizziness. She has diabetes mellitus and hypertension for which she is on medication. With 8 children and 23 grandchildren, she proudly tells all the health-care providers that all her children finished college and her grandchildren are doing very well in school. The patient had several diagnostic tests in the first 2 days of her hospitalization.

On the third day of her hospitalization, her condition worsened. Because she is a devout Catholic, the family requested a Catholic priest to provide the sacrament for the sick. With a large and extended family, Mrs. de la Fuente's room is always crowded with visitors. The staff are complaining about the number of visitors and how there is not adequate room when providing care for the patient.

1. What cultural value regarding family does the staff need to consider in this situation?
2. What are some culturally sensitive strategies that nurses can do to provide care to this patient and address the number of visitors in the patient's room?
3. Describe the Filipino family kinship system and the roles of older parents and adult children.
4. How does Mrs. de la Fuente express her value of education?

Family Roles and Organization
Head of Household and Gender Roles

Since the pre-Spanish era, Filipino women have been held in high regard, having rights equal to those of men (Agoncillo & Guerrero, 1987). In contemporary Filipino families, although the father is the acknowledged head of the household, authority in the family is considered egalitarian. The mother plays an equal, and often major, role in decisions regarding health, children, and finances (Fig. 13-2).

Traditional female roles include caring for the sick and children, maintaining kinship ties, and managing the home. Parents and older siblings are involved in the care and discipline of younger children. In extended family households, older relatives and grandparents share much authority and responsibility for the care and discipline of younger members. Traditional Filipino families may not expect female children to engage in activities that are considered appropriate for men, such as driving, bicycling, and other functions requiring mechanical or technical skills. Blurring of roles between men and women occurs with increased education, urbanization, and emigration to a new culture, as in the United States and elsewhere.

In the United States, Filipino families predominantly consist of married couples with both spouses working. Filipino womanhood has evolved from the Spanish construct of modesty, demureness, and femininity to a contemporary image of a woman who is educated, working, and adept at balancing traditional roles and career demands. Traditional Filipino parents expect their male and female children to pursue college education and economically productive careers and also to have a family. Family members and Filipino friends or acquaintances are the preferred caregivers of young children when parents are working. Older adults, especially grandmothers, emigrate in time for the birth of their grandchildren and are

expected to take care of them on behalf of their working adult children (Pacquiao, 1993).

Prescriptive, Restrictive, and Taboo Behaviors for Children and Adolescents

Like other cultural groups, Filipinos highly value their children. They are seen as gifts from God and therefore are considered special blessings to the family. The strong in-group consciousness of Filipinos is rooted in the centrality of family and kin, to the exclusion of others, in the socialization of individuals. As the strongest unit of society, the family demands the deepest loyalties and significantly influences an individual's social interactions. Ascriptive and particularistic personal ties with kin are significant in the allocation of rank, authority, and power to individuals. Generational position conditions the status as well as the role performance of individuals. The family and one's familial role define and order authority, rights, obligations, and modes of interaction. Younger generations are taught to be respectful and heed the authority of older siblings and relatives, parents, and grandparents. Respect is manifested in both speech and actions by using honorific terms of address, avoiding confrontation and offensive language, keeping a low tone of voice, greeting older people by kissing their forehead or back of their hand, avoiding direct eye contact when being admonished, offering food, touching, and so forth. Husbands and wives address each other using the honorific terms that they wish to model for their children. In front of the children, a husband will address his wife as *Inay* (Mother) and the wife correspondingly refers to her husband as *Itay* (Father). Under no circumstance are children permitted to call their parents by their first names. Friends of Filipino children are expected to show respect to adult members of the family when they visit.

Reciprocal obligations among kin are embodied in the value of *utang na loob*, a personal sense of indebtedness and loyalty to kin, which carries an obligation to repay or perform services for one another. Filial respect and obligation for caring for one's parents is the ultimate confluence of generational respect and reciprocal obligation. Childhood socialization to the mechanism of shame (*hiya*) reinforces the value of *utang na loob* and generational respect. Failure to perform or recognize reciprocal obligations, as well as disrespect of older people or people of authority, results in the loss of one's self-esteem and status, as well as incurs shame to one's family.

Conditions such as mental illness, divorce, terminal illness, criminal offenses, unwanted pregnancy, homosexuality, and HIV/AIDS are not readily shared with outsiders until trust is established. The extent to which a Filipino patient may disclose personal information is contextualized. Family presence may act as a barrier to full disclosure of conditions that may be perceived as putting the family at risk for shame.

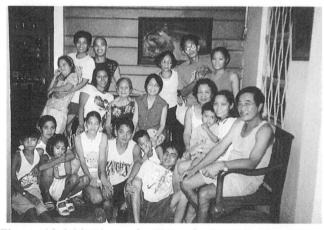

Figure 13-2 Members of a Filipino family that is bilaterally extended to three generations. *(Photograph by Rowena Legaspi.)*

Dating at an early age is discouraged for young daughters who are advised that a short courtship period may suggest that they are "easy to get." Young men with sincere intent must strive to get on the good side of the family and have patience with a long courtship. Open demonstrations of affection with sexual undertones are to be avoided by the young couple. Ideally, the groom's parents formally ask for the bride's parents' consent for the marriage of their children. Traditional families desire that their daughters remain chaste before marriage. Pregnancy out of wedlock brings shame to the whole family. Modernization and urbanization have changed the social mores in the Philippines; yet, many Filipino American families are still perceived by younger family members as having an overly protective attitude toward children in matters of "hanging out" with friends, dating, and courtship. Girls are subjected to greater limitations than boys, which contributes to higher reports of contemplating suicide by Filipino girls. Studies of second-generation Filipino students in high schools revealed greater parental control over daughters, with more latitude allowed for sons. For many Filipinas, high school achievement was met by parental control over their choice of colleges and pressure to remain close to home and family supervision (Wolf, 1997).

Family Goals and Priorities

In addition to blood relatives, fictive kinship is established through the *compadrazgo* system in which friends and associates are invited to become godparents or surrogate parents in religious ceremonies, such as baptism and marriage. Fictive kinship is a significant support system for Filipino Americans who left families or relatives in the home country. In times of illness, the extended family provides support and assistance. Sometimes, a family visit to the hospital takes on the semblance of a family reunion.

The family is the basic social and economic unit of Filipino kinship. Family relations strongly influence individual decisions and actions. Relatives and family constitute the reference group for individuals, determining their behavior as well as that of their relatives in any social exchange. Family loyalties and obligations supersede individual interests and residential migration. This is evident in migration patterns of adult children and aged parents, which are planned to maximize the economic welfare and support for group members.

Family emphasis on communal values and generational respect is highly institutionalized. Community activities generally center on the family. Fiestas, weddings, baptisms, illnesses, and funerals are occasions for reinvigorating relations with kin and rekindling local connections, in which the presence and, more importantly, the absence of relatives are viewed as highly significant. Early child-rearing practices are permissive, with emphasis on providing an emotionally secure environment for the child. Priority is placed on promoting the child's well-being and social acceptance. The child is introduced early into various mechanisms designed to impose compliance with family values. A family's prestige is measured by the upbringing of their children, judged by their adherence to traditional cultural values.

The family emphasis on faithfulness to religious obligations is tied with the cultural values of generational respect and reciprocal obligation. Child-rearing practices stress entire family participation in the religious education and adherence to rituals by young members. Older generations share the responsibility for reinforcing these values. Religious sacraments, such as marriage, are embedded in the age-grading activities of the extended family (Fig. 13-3).

As the basic economic unit of society, the family defines the economic obligations of kin to one another. Children are looked upon as economic assets and as sources of support for parents in old age. Thus, educating young members becomes a family priority. The socioeconomic status of the aged is closely linked with the family's wealth; if resources are limited, older people rely on children and relatives. Older parents and grandparents are integrated within the family, thus lessening the impact of advancing age. Traditional Filipinos consider institutionalization of aged parents tantamount to abandonment of filial obligation and respect for older people. Many older people aspire to return to the Philippines to spend their remaining years with loving kin.

The development of *pakiramdam* and *kapwa* is the defining goal of the family. Group cohesiveness, loyalty, and faithfulness to shared obligation are expectations that transcend distant migration, marriage, and adulthood. Students who feel obligated to maintain

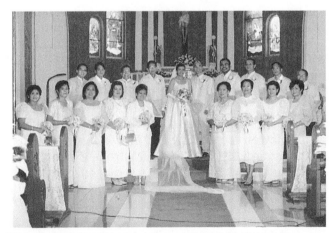

Figure 13-3 The Spanish influence in the Philippines is depicted in this Roman Catholic wedding featuring godparents as an important part of fictive kinship development for the couple and their families. *(Photograph by Rowena Legaspi.)*

their family's reputations believe that effort and interest, rather than ability, can result in school success (Salazar et al., 2000).

Filipino American older people have reported experiencing conflict between the maintenance of family obligations, such as babysitting for their grandchildren, and their desire to be more independent from their adult children. Family obligations may result in their inability to meet medical appointments, obtain needed medications, and make meaningful social connections because of lack of independent transportation. Depression has been associated with loneliness, feelings of isolation, and financial difficulty (McBride & Parreno, 1996). Older Filipino Americans identified integration in the family of their adult children, participation in community activities with family and close friends, and maintaining religious functions as highly important (Pacquiao, 1993).

Diversity exists in the degree to which Filipino Americans adhere to the traditional cultural values. Some middle-aged immigrant Filipino parents do not expect to live with their children in old age. Diversity in family member roles and priorities exists as a result of the financial resources of the family. Reciprocal obligations with kin are expressed differently based on the capacity of older people and adult children to meet them and include economic, physical, emotional, and social support dimensions.

Alternative Lifestyles

Traditional Filipino parents seldom provide sex education, and sex is not discussed openly at home. Homosexuality may be recognized and considered an aberrant behavior, but it is not openly practiced in order to save face and prevent shame for the family. In recent years, younger gay, lesbian, bisexual, and transgender Filipinos in the Philippines and in North America are taking a more active role in being recognized and expressing their rights.

Although the tenets of the Catholic Church have a direct bearing on sexual mores for older generations of Filipinos, they have less influence on younger generations, as is seen in the high incidence of HIV/AIDS among Filipinos compared with that of other Asian/Pacific Islanders (APIs). The family may not be the primary source of support for individuals, who may be isolated to prevent stigma to the family. The nuclear family may protect the affected member from outsiders and intentionally remove them from a network of friends and extended family. Providing an atmosphere that fosters the much-needed sense of belonging should be the goal of culturally congruent services.

Divorce can carry a stigma for older and more traditional Filipinos, especially those who are devout Catholics. The stigma may be worse for Filipinos in the Philippines for whom divorces are not allowed and are considered a religious taboo. Divorces among Filipino Americans generally result from failed marital duties, lack of mutual support between partners, and marital infidelity.

Workforce Issues
Culture in the Workforce

Experience with racism is a continuing theme voiced by Filipino nurses working with white American nurses (Spangler, 1992). Among Filipino American female nurses and nurse's aides, longer residence in the United States is associated with increased stress, evidenced by higher levels of serum norepinephrine, and higher diastolic pressure and lower dips in blood pressure readings during sleep (Brown & James, 2000). The requirement by the American Nurses Association for equal pay for the same job transformed foreign nurse recruitment into a competitive enterprise, in which employers and existing staff expected recruited nurses to be functionally competent on the job as soon as they received their American RN license because they will receive pay comparable with that of other RNs. In reality, providing transitional support for foreign nurses requires a significant commitment of time and financial investment and a prolonged acculturation process (Pacquiao, 2004).

Filipino nurses have been recruited in large numbers to staff mostly evening and night shifts in which acute shortages of American trained nurses exist. This has reinforced the cultural tendency toward collective solidarity by defining the context of interactions within the insider-outsider continuum. American nurses and administrators of health organizations with large contingents of Filipino nurses are becoming aware of the need for special knowledge and skills in understanding and managing a diverse workforce and in developing culturally specific staff development programs.

Cultural conflicts in the workplace stem from different communication patterns: the dominant norm of assertiveness versus the highly contextual Filipino communication. The cultural concept of shared identity with other Filipinos creates a propensity among Filipino nurses to speak in their own dialect with one another to the exclusion of non-Filipino coworkers and patients. A lack of fluency in speaking and in enunciating English words results in anxiety when interacting with outsiders. Assertive communication is difficult for Filipinos, who have been enculturated to avoid conflict. Filipino nurses may consider it impolite and disrespectful to confront or challenge the authority of a superior. When a problem with a manager occurs, a Filipino nurse may communicate through a mediator, usually another Filipino nurse, who is in the same level within the hierarchy as the manager. Communicating disagreement with a physician is difficult for many Filipino nurses. Conversely, Filipino registered nurses expect their subordinates to be deferential toward them.

Conflict can result from different cultural values about caring. Coming from a highly collective orientation, Filipinos define caring in terms of active caring for others. This perspective differs from the American value of self-care. Filipino nurses feel comfortable performing what they perceive as caring tasks for patients that American nurses expect patients to do for themselves. Initially, they may not be inclined to teach and demonstrate procedures to patients because of their traditional belief in doing the caring tasks for patients. Outsiders may misconstrue Filipino nurses' preoccupation with caring tasks as disorganization or lack of assertiveness.

Different views about a valued coworker may be another source of conflict. The Filipino values of shared perception and being one with others create a cooperative, rather than a competitive, outlook. A valued individual produces for the group and puts the group above her or his own personal gain. Humility, hard work, loyalty, and generosity are admired. The businesslike and competitive perspectives of Americans, in which behavior is internally motivated by individual gain, may be interpreted as selfish and uncaring. Self-proclamations of accomplishments are viewed as cocky and offensive. Instead, it is up to the group to recognize a member's achievement, which is assessed in terms of how the action benefited the group.

Health-care organizations are cultural entities defined by norms that reflect the dominant values of the host society. Professional schools mirror these dominant societal norms, which are congruent with those of health-care organizations. Among outsiders to the dominant American culture, the experience in nursing schools and health-care organizations is dissonant with previous life experiences, which require an understanding of both cultural and occupational role differences. Bicultural development of Filipino and non-Filipino staff should be the goal of occupational orientation and training. Biculturalism requires awareness of self and others and the ability to adapt behaviors that build positive relationships with others who may be different from oneself (Pacquiao, 2003). Understanding cultural differences and similarities allows for the development of intercultural understanding and skills that promote teamwork. Bicultural mentors who can teach cultural norms of the organization and work with diverse patients and staff will foster the individual's ability to adapt behaviors. Staff development requires training in frame switching—using different frameworks to understand behaviors of others and commitment to the belief that other perspectives are equally sound in explaining our experiences. Impression management is a bicultural skill that is grounded in the ability to interpret behaviors of others within their own cultural context and manifest behaviors that promote relationship and intercultural understanding (Pacquiao, 2001).

Issues Related to Autonomy

A core Filipino cultural concept is *bahala na*, which consists of the belief and predisposition to trust the divine providence and social hierarchy to resolve problems. Filipinos may avoid taking an active role in managing problems because of their fatalistic belief that a "greater power" will prevail. Outsiders may interpret this behavior as a lack of initiative or responsibility. Many Filipino nurses are hesitant to assume leadership roles and assert their points of view, especially with outsiders. After an initial effort, further attempts to resolve the problem are generally left to the leader or hierarchy. Providing support and acting as a role model help these nurses assert themselves and feel confident in problem solving and conflict resolution. Filipinos are proud people who place importance on maintaining self-esteem and dignity by saving face and avoiding shame. Their sensitivity and attention to other people's feelings are often exhibited as indecisiveness, which many Americans interpret as lack of assertiveness.

The Filipino hierarchy and emphasis on collectivity bring a consequent group-oriented sense of responsibility and accountability. The leader is respected, followed, and expected to make decisions on behalf of members. The leader is trusted to act in the best interests of the group. The concept of individual accountability and responsibility in a highly litigious society, such as the United States, may initially be difficult for Filipino nurses to understand. Supportive role modeling in assuming individual accountability is important for Filipino-educated nurses.

Biocultural Ecology
Skin Color and Other Biological Variations

Variations in anthropomorphic physical and biophysiological characteristics of Filipinos exist as a result of ethnic and racial intermingling. The people of one of the Filipino aboriginal tribes, the Aeta, are negroid and petite in stature. They are believed to have migrated from Africa through land bridges during the Ice Age. However, like other tribal groups in the Philippines, they are now a minority. The typical native-born or immigrant Filipino may be of Malay stock (brown complexion) with a multiracial genetic background.

The youthful features of Filipinos make it difficult for some to assess their age. Common Filipino physical features may include jet black to brunette or light brown hair, dark to light brown pupils with eyes set in almond-shaped eyelids, deep brown to very light tan skin tones, and mildly flared nostrils and slightly low to flat nose bridges. The eye structure may challenge health-care providers in assessments such as observing pupillary reactions for increased intracranial pressure, measuring ocular tension, and evaluating peripheral vision. The flat nose bridge may be overlooked by opticians when fitting and dispensing eyeglasses.

The high-melanin content of the skin and mucosa may pose problems when assessing signs of jaundice, cyanosis, and pallor. This feature also poses difficulty in diagnosing retinal, gum-related, and oral tissue abnormalities. When performing skin assessments, practitioners should consider the complexion and skin tone of the Filipino patient. The usual manifestations of anemia (pallor and jaundice) should be assessed in the conjunctiva. Newborns may have Mongolian spots— bluish-green discolorations on the buttocks—that are physiological and eventually disappear.

Filipinos range in height from under 5 feet to the height of average Americans. Body weight varies according to nativity and other factors such as nutrition, physical activity, and heredity. Filipinos commonly gain weight when they come to the United States. There are no definitive studies relating nutrition with standard height and weight measures for this population; therefore, it is essential to assess for weight changes on an individual basis.

Filipinos have a small thoracic capacity. Approximately 40 percent have blood type B and a low incidence of the Rh-negative factor (Anderson, 1983). As more interracial families emerge in Filipino communities, changes in their serologic profile will likely occur.

Diseases and Health Conditions

Filipino men and women have the highest prevalence of hypertension compared with whites (Ryan, Shaw, & Pilam, 2000) and compared with other Asians characterized by sodium sensitivity (Garde, Spangler, & Miranda, 1994). Despite the high prevalence of hypertension among Filipino Americans, the rate of controlled hypertension is lower than the rates for whites and other Asians.

Filipinos also had the highest rate and risk of type 2 diabetes at 32.1 percent, compared with 5.8 percent in whites and 12.1 percent in African American women. Filipino women were found to have higher visceral adipose tissues compared with non-Hispanic whites and African American women. Filipino Americans have a disproportionately high prevalence of diabetes in a nonobese population (Bateman, Abesamis-Mendoza, & Ho-Asjoe, 2009).

High incidence of hyperuricemia is attributed to a shift from a Filipino to an American diet (McBride, Mariola, & Yeo, 1995). Liver cancer tends to be diagnosed in the late stages of the disease and appears to be associated with the presence of the hepatitis B virus. Silent carriers of the virus are common among Asians, and its presence is detected only when other problems are being evaluated. Health-care providers should routinely screen for hepatitis B virus, especially among recent immigrants. A high incidence of glucose-6-phosphate dehydrogenase (G-6-PD), thalassemias, and lactose intolerance and malabsorption exist among the Filipino population (Anderson, 1983).

Compared with other APIs and white males, Filipinos are more likely to be diagnosed with advanced-stage colorectal and prostatic cancers. They have the worst survival rates from these cancers (Lim, Clarke, Prehn, Glaser, West, & O'Malley, 2002). Like other APIs, Filipinos underuse cancer screening tests (Kagawa-Singer & Pourat, 2000). Filipino Americans are at increased risk for type 2 diabetes and have higher visceral adipose tissue (VAT) than whites and African Americans (Araneta & Barrett-Connor, 2005). The three leading causes of mortality among Filipino Americans are cardiovascular disorders followed by stroke and cancer.

Lack of insurance, low income, and limited access to care were found to have a significant impact on APIs' use of health services (Coughlan & Uhler, 2000; Yu, Huang, & Singh, 2004). A Canadian study using the 2001 Community Health Survey revealed that minorities, including Filipinos, were less likely to be admitted in the hospital, tested for prostate-specific antigen (PSA), or given a mammogram or Pap test, despite the fact that they had more contact with a general practitioner than white Canadians (Quan et al., 2006). Among older Filipinas, length of residence in the United States and having had a checkup when no symptoms were present were associated with adherence to cancer screening (Maxwell, Bastani, & Warda, 2000).

Compared with white Americans, Filipinos have higher levels of depression. In contrast, strong ethnic identity characterized by sense of ethnic pride, involvement in ethnic practices, and cultural commitment to one's racial and ethnic identity were significant factors in mitigating depressive symptoms among Filipino Americans (Mossakowski, 2003). Strong bonds with members of the community and access to culturally congruent health services promoted commitment of older Filipinas to planned physical activity (Maxwell, Bastani, Vida, & Warda, 2002).

Variations in Drug Metabolism

Studying how ethnicity affects drug response is challenging, in part because of the tremendous variations that exists within each ethnic group. Many studies have used broad categories when classifying participants without differentiating among subgroups— for example, using the term *Asians* to refer to Filipinos, Korean, and Chinese, among others (Munoz & Hilgenberg 2006). Ethnographic research has uncovered significant differences in how people of color metabolize drugs differently. There are variations in both pharmacodynamics and pharmacokinetics mechanisms of action. Also, certain ethnic groups have more of these variations than others (Lin & Smith, 2000).

Compared with white Americans, Asians require lower doses of central nervous system depressants such as haloperidol, have a lower tolerance for alcohol, and are more sensitive to the adverse effects of alcohol (Levy, 1993). Owing to the sodium-sensitive nature of hypertension affecting Filipinos and the high-sodium content of their diet, use of diuretics should be considered. Culturally congruent stress management in addition to dietary modifications and physical activity should be included in the treatment plan to control high blood pressure.

Because of availability of over-the-counter antibiotics and lack of adequate medical monitoring of these drugs in the Philippines, Filipino immigrants may be insensitive to the effects of some anti-infectives. A positive reaction to tuberculin or the Mantoux test is observed because of the practice of giving bacille Calmette-Guérin (BCG) vaccinations in childhood. Chest x-rays and sputum cultures are recommended for screening and diagnosis of tuberculosis. More research is needed to determine pharmacodynamics among Filipinos, including gender differences. Health-care providers, as with all patients, need to assess Filipino patients individually when administering and monitoring medication effects.

High-Risk Behaviors

Gender differences are evident in the Filipino tolerance and acceptance of high-risk health behaviors related to alcohol, drugs, cigarettes, and safe sex. More Filipino men than women are heavy drinkers. Most Filipino Americans report drinking socially, with a small number reporting having three or more drinks per day (Garde et al., 1994). Because denial is closely associated with alcoholism, the frequency and amount of alcohol taken are generally underreported.

Cigarette smoking is more prevalent among Filipino men than women. Smoking rates have been positively correlated with lower educational levels and income and a tendency to think or speak in a Filipino language, and, for women, being born in the United States. Most Filipino youths reported living with an adult who smoked, and their first substance of choice was cigarettes, followed by alcohol and inhalants (Maxwell, Garcia, & Berman, 2007).

Filipinos constitute the largest number of reported HIV/AIDS cases among APIs in the United States (Reeves & Bennett, 2004). Low knowledge scores on information about HIV transmission and unprotected sex with multiple partners underscore the urgency of HIV and AIDS education and prevention.

Health-Care Practices

Cultural, social, and economic factors are implicated as reasons for Filipino Americans' underutilization of health services. Typical of the ethnically underserved, older people in the United States may be unaware of available services and are reluctant to access social and health services, particularly when culturally sensitive and bilingual providers are unavailable. Lack of transportation, fear of going to the area where services are located, and inappropriate program design are some of the other reasons for low utilization of services by this group. More recent Filipino immigrants differ significantly from their earlier counterparts in their access and utilization of health services. This group is highly educated and accesses many of the health-care services in the United States.

A study of the experiences of Filipino women with breast cancer screening services identified a pattern of avoidance. Factors contributing to this behavior included cultural beliefs, lack of health insurance, and lack of a familiar source of care (Wu & Bancroft, 2006). Some believe that undergoing the test and attempting to know one's condition could tempt faith, which can bring bad luck. Avoidance of an unpleasant diagnosis and concealment of serious illnesses are consequent behaviors of this belief. Many Filipinos seek a familiar and consistent health practitioner who has established a relationship with them. Gender-congruent health-care providers are preferred for conditions specific to women's or men's health. Preference for culturally congruent services and practitioners and the presence of supportive social connections increased participation and commitment among older Filipinas for health promotion (Maxwell et al., 2002).

Nutrition
Meaning of Food

Food to any group is symbolic and is associated with the affective state of the individual. It is a source of nourishment to the body, as well as a source of pleasure and satisfaction, depending on one's emotional and psychological state. To the Filipino, food is a fundamental form of socialization. Food and meal patterns are integral to the cultural emphasis on generosity, hospitality, and thoughtfulness that support group cohesiveness. No social gathering of Filipinos occurs without food. Food is offered as a token of gratitude and caring, to welcome others, to celebrate accomplishments and important events, to offer support in times of sickness or crisis, and to reinforce social bonds in everyday interactions. Sharing food with others, or at the very least inviting others to share one's food, is expected of Filipinos and considered a sign of good upbringing. The insider versus outsider context influences the choice of food offered (Enriquez, 1994).

In the Philippines, traditional Filipino meals are labor intensive, requiring the participation of several family members. Meats are costly, so small amounts are cut in pieces and expanded using vegetables and starches to feed an entire family. All family members, regardless of age, attend social gatherings at which a variety of dishes are prepared to accommodate individual choices. The hosting family serves large amounts of food to accommodate invited guests and those who happen to be around. Guests customarily linger for several meals because the focus is on the gathering. Latecomers are welcomed and expected to fully participate in the entire meal and the company of other guests. Dishes are served all at once from appetizers to desserts so guests are free to eat their courses without waiting for everyone to arrive. Guests are encouraged to return to the table to join arriving guests. More food means more portions for each one and vice versa.

Common Foods and Food Rituals

Indigenous Filipino cooking is characterized by boiling, steaming, roasting, broiling, marinating, or sour-stewing to preserve the fresh and natural taste of food. Spanish, Chinese, and American influences are integrated into contemporary Filipino cuisine. Foods may be sautéed, fried, or served with a sauce. Because of the tropical climate of the Philippines, many types of plants and animals flourish. Seafood (fish and shellfish) forms the bulk of the Filipino diet. Fresh, dried, and marinated fish are abundant in the diet.

In the Philippines, animal sources of protein are chicken and pork because cows and water buffalo are primarily used for farming. Because protein-rich foods are costly, meals generally consist of larger portions of carbohydrates, primarily rice. Plants are the second most important food source and include a variety of seaweeds, edible roots, delicate leaves, tendrils, tropical fruits, seeds, and some flowers. Fruits and vegetables are consumed in large quantities in a variety of ways. Rice is eaten at every meal—steamed, fried, or as a dessert. Less acculturated Filipinos tend to prepare and serve more traditional Filipino foods at home (de la Cruz, Padilla & Agustin, 2000). Filipino and Asian food stores are abundant in regions where many APIs reside.

Except for babies and young children, milk is almost absent in the Filipino diet. This may be partly due to lactose intolerance. However, milk in desserts such as egg custard (flan) and ice cream seems to be tolerated. In the Filipino food pyramid, milk and dairy products are incorporated in the major protein groups rather than as a separate category. Dietary calcium is derived from green leafy vegetables and seafood. Coconut milk is a common cooking additive among the Bicolanos of southern Luzon. Salty (soy sauce, fish sauce/*patis*, salted shrimp fry, or fermented fish/*bagoong*) and spicy sauces known as *sawsawan*

complement meals. These sauces are distinct from the salt added during cooking.

In the Philippines, breakfast consists of rice, meat or fish, and vegetable dishes or dinner leftovers. The breakfast beverage may be coffee, chocolate, or juice. In urban areas, Western-style meals are more common. For many Filipinos, breakfast, lunch, and dinner are not complete without steamed or fried rice served with fish, meat (especially pork), and vegetables. Snacks of bananas, yams, rice cakes, and rice-flour cakes are served as midday snacks, between meals, and before bedtime. The midday meal is the heaviest meal of the day, although this pattern is becoming more difficult among urban dwellers who cannot go home during lunchtime.

Dietary Practices for Health Promotion

Filipinos believe health is maintained by moderation. Although Filipinos enjoy food and love to eat, they adhere to the wisdom that too much of a good thing can be harmful. In some parts of the Philippines, it is considered polite to leave food on one's plate. For many Filipino Americans, moderation in food intake is a special challenge because of the abundance and great variety of quality products at reasonable costs. Significant increases in weight patterns among new immigrants are associated with changes in dietary habits.

The principle of hot and cold is observed by many traditional Filipinos to promote health. A warm beverage is served first at breakfast after a long evening fast, and hot soups are served as the first course to enhance digestion. Cold drinks may be avoided when one has a cold or fever to restore balance and promote harmony between the body and its environment. Eating rice is considered to be essential to a healthy life. *Arroz caldo,* chicken and rice soup, is generally offered to promote recovery after an illness. Chicken soup with *malunggay* leaves is believed to cleanse the blood.

Garlic and onions are believed to thin the blood and combat hypertension. Ginger root is boiled and served as a beverage to relieve sore throats and promote digestion. Guava shoots are eaten to treat diarrhea. Drinking coconut juice and water from boiled fresh corn silk promotes diuresis. Bitter melon is eaten as a vegetable to prevent diabetes. Greens such as *malunggay* and *ampalaya* leaves are used in stews to regain stamina for someone believed to be anemic or run-down.

Nutritional Deficiencies and Food Limitations

In the Philippines, nutrition is greatly affected by socioeconomic factors. Malnutrition persists in the country, especially among the poor and less educated, and is one of the leading causes of infant mortality. In the United States, Filipino immigrants may be at risk for nutritional deficiencies during their adjustment period, especially when they come with limited resources and without a support network of family and friends. Postmenopausal and pregnant women may be vulnerable to calcium deficiency owing to lactose intolerance and decreased intake of seafood and green leafy vegetables that were plentiful in the Philippines but limited in availability and variety in American food stores. Changing food patterns and lifestyle is associated with migration and acculturation. Filipino Americans experience similar problems such as obesity, hyperlipidemia, and diabetes seen in the general population. Knowledge of indigenous food sources and meal patterns, nutritional content of foods, changes in nutritional patterns, and accessibility of traditional ingredients is important for nutritional assessment and counseling.

Pregnancy and Childbearing Practices

Fertility Practices and Views Toward Pregnancy

The Roman Catholic Church and Filipino family values significantly influence childbearing and fertility practices. In marriage, the only acceptable method of contraception is the rhythm method. Abortion is considered a sin and is generally not acceptable. Whereas these beliefs remain strong among many Filipinos, education, global communication, and modernization are causing changes, particularly in metropolitan cities such as Manila. Recent Filipino immigrants who come from large urban areas are more educated and less committed to the Church's position on birth control and premarital sex.

Filipino culture is child-centered, and abortion evokes strong reactions, even among liberal Filipinos. Though some may support the right to abortion, they may have difficulty having one themselves and feel guilty for considering this option. Pregnancy is considered normal and is a time when a woman can demand attention and pampering from her husband and family members. Health-care providers who do not understand this special period for the pregnant Filipino woman may feel that the patient is "lazy and spoiled." Pregnancy and childbirth are times for the family to draw closer together. Everyone assists in anticipation of the new baby, especially the pregnant woman's mother, who has a strong influence during this period. For mother and daughter, this is a special event in which the bond between them becomes stronger.

In the Filipino American community, women openly give advice to pregnant women, share their own birthing experiences, and ask personal questions that may be considered rather intrusive by outsiders. Elaborate baby showers are hosted by family members and friends, and it is customary to invite male spouses, relatives, and friends as well as children. Male guests do not join in the activities and congregate separately from the women.

Prescriptive, Restrictive, and Taboo Practices in the Childbearing Family

Childbearing is widely celebrated by Filipino families. Children are perceived to be God's blessings and therefore to be accepted and be grateful. Filipino practices surrounding pregnancy are influenced by indigenous beliefs, Western practices, and socioeconomic factors. In the Philippines, most mothers receive prenatal care from a doctor, nurse, or midwife, although two-thirds of births are delivered at home. Traditional birth attendants (*hilots*) use massage and are consulted for physical, spiritual, and psychological advice and guidance (National Statistics Office, Philippines, 2005).

After childbirth, the new mother continues to be pampered. Relatives help with the new baby and in running the household. Eighty-eight percent of Filipino babies are breastfed for some time, with a median duration of 13 months. However, supplementation of breastfeeding with other liquids and foods occurs too early, with 19 percent of newborns less than 2 months of age receiving supplemental foods or liquids other than water (National Statistics Office, Philippines, 2005). Lactating mothers are encouraged to take plenty of hot soups (chicken with papaya) to promote milk production (Hawaii Community College, 2005).

Some Filipino American women refuse to take vitamins during pregnancy for fear that these could deform the fetus. Some believe that when pregnant women crave certain foods, especially during the first trimester, the craving should be satisfied to avoid harm to the baby. Some women believe that the baby takes on the appearance of the craved food. Thus, if the mother craves dark-skinned fruit or dark-colored food, the infant's skin will be dark. Pregnant women are protected from sudden fright or stress because of the belief that this may harm the developing fetus. Table 13-1 provides a summary of traditional beliefs and practices observed among some Filipinos in Hawaii. Becoming aware of the pregnant Filipino woman's network of family and community health advisers, whose opinions she respects, is important for building trust and rapport in the patient–health provider relationship.

Some women prefer to have their mothers rather than their husbands in the delivery room. Mothers of pregnant women serve as coaches and teachers and are often respected over health-care providers for their experience and knowledge. This may be puzzling to health-care providers who view pregnancy as an emancipating event. Conflicts are likely to occur if the coach and teacher believe in practices that are contrary to Western childbearing practices.

During postpartum, exposure to cold is avoided. Showers are prohibited because these may cause an imbalance and predispose illness. However, the

▐▌ Table 13-1   Traditional Filipino Beliefs and Practices Surrounding Pregnancy and Childbirth

Prenatal	Postpartum
Eating blackberries will make the baby have black spots.	Use warm water to drink and bathe for a month.
Eating black plums will give the baby dark skin.	Don't name the baby before it is born.
Eating twin bananas will result in twin births.	Don't name the baby after a dead person.
Eating apples will give the baby red lips.	Give money to charity or the needy when a baby comes to your house the first time.
When a woman's stomach is not round, the baby will be a boy.	Eating sour or ice-cold foods may cause abdominal cramps.
If a woman's face is blemished, the baby will be a boy.	Wrap the baby's abdomen with a cloth until the umbilical cord falls off.
Going outside during a lunar eclipse is harmful to the baby.	The mother and baby should not go out for a month except to visit a doctor.
Going out in the morning dew is bad for the baby because evil spirits are present.	Putting garlic, salt, or a rosary near the baby's crib will keep evil spirits away.
Funerals are avoided because the spirit of the dead person may affect the baby.	
Wearing necklaces may cause the umbilical cord to wrap around the baby's neck.	
Sitting by a doorway will make the delivery difficult.	
Sitting by a window when it is dark may let evil spirits come to the pregnant woman.	
Sweeping at night may sweep away the good spirits.	
Knitting might tangle the baby's intestines at birth.	

Source: Adapted from Hawaii Community College (2005).

mother is given a sponge bath with aromatic oils and herbs, or a *hilot* gives an aromatic herbal steam bath followed by full body massage, including the abdominal muscles, stimulating a physiological reaction that has both physical and psychological benefits.

Childbirth experiences of Filipino women immigrants in a hospital in Australia revealed language and communication problems as barriers to seeking antenatal care, perceived discrimination by the hospital staff, and conflicting expectations of delivery practices between the mothers and the health-care providers. The women preferred to be examined by female health-care providers and assume a squatting position for birthing. Contrary to their birthing practices, health-care providers expected the husbands to be with them during delivery. The women felt that they were not consulted about their care and preferred to deliver at home (Hoang, 2008).

Death Rituals

Death Rituals and Expectations

Death for Filipinos as a spiritual event is based on the Roman Catholic belief system and doctrine. Illness and death may be attributed to supernatural and magico-religious causes such as punishment from God, angry spirits, or sorcery. Religiosity and fatalism contribute to stoicism in the face of pain or distress as a way of accepting one's fate (Lipson & Dibble, 2005). Planning for one's death is taboo and may be considered tempting fate. Hence, many traditional Filipinos are averse to discussing advance directives or living wills (Pacquiao, 2001). When death is imminent, contacting a priest is important if the family is Catholic. Religious medallions, rosary beads, scapulars, and religious figures may be found on the patient or at the bedside. Family members generally wish to provide the most intimate care to the patient.

After death, a wake is planned. In the Philippines, the wake may last 3 days or longer to allow time for relatives to arrive from distant places. In the United States, the wake is much shorter because it is costly. Although a wake is generally held in the home in the rural regions, funeral parlors are used in urban areas and in the United States. Families and friends gather to give support and recall the special traits of the deceased. Food is provided to all guests throughout the wake and after the burial.

The burial rites are consistent with the religious traditions of the family, which may be Judeo-Christian, Muslim, Buddhist, or other religions. Among Catholics, 9 days of novenas are held in the home or in the church. These special prayers ask God's blessing for the deceased. Depending on the economic resources of the family, food and refreshments are served after each prayer day. Sometimes, the last day of the novena takes on the atmosphere of a *fiesta* or a celebration. Filipino families in the United States follow variations of this ritual according to their social and economic circumstances. Funerals in the Philippines can be simple or elaborate, with a band accompaniment, several priests officiating, and a large throng of mourners. Reciprocal obligation continues in death through the performance of rituals such as the wake, novenas, and establishing a burial site acceptable for the entire family.

On the 1-year anniversary of the death, family and friends are reunited in prayer to celebrate this memorable event. Most Filipino women wear black clothing for months or up to a year after the death of a spouse or close family member. The 1-year anniversary ends the ritual mourning. Before this period, family members postpone weddings and other celebrations in deference to the memory of the deceased. Memories and love for the deceased are shown on All Soul's Day, a Catholic feast day celebrated in November, when families visit and decorate the graves of their loved ones. Filipino American families may continue these traditions, particularly when strong kinship is present and the clan lives in close proximity. Many who die in the United States are buried in the Philippines, and the family in that country continues the tradition.

Beliefs related to cremation vary according to individual preference. Ordinarily, bodies are buried, but cremation is acceptable to avoid the spread of disease and limit the high costs of burial plots. Since the process of cremation has been accepted by the Roman Catholic Church in the Philippines, there has been an increase in this option. In America, some Filipinos who wish to return their deceased family members to the Philippines may choose cremation for practical and economic reasons.

Responses to Death and Grief

Most Filipinos believe in life after death. Caring for the spiritual needs of the dying is one way of ensuring peaceful rest of the soul or one's spirit. Family presence around the dying and immediate period after death to pray for the soul of the departed is considered a priority. If the patient is Catholic, the priest anoints the patient and gives Holy Communion if the patient is able to participate. Caring is shown by providing a peaceful environment, speaking in low tones, and praying with the ill person.

After death, grief reaction varies. Women generally show emotions openly by crying, fainting, or wailing. Men are expected to be more stoic and grieve silently. Young children are admonished for behaving inappropriately because this is considered disrespectful to the deceased. Family members gather together and provide physical and emotional support for each other. Praying for the deceased and following the implicit guidelines of behavior during mourning are ways of demonstrating grief appropriately. Wearing black or subdued colors (gray, white, navy blue, brown); avoiding parties and playing loud, distracting music; postponing weddings; or devoting time to one's studies to honor the dead are some of the acceptable ways of expressing grief. Honoring the memory of the deceased is a continuing obligation among close kin.

Spirituality

Dominant Religion and the Use of Prayer

The Philippines is the only predominantly Christian country in the Far East. In 2000, Roman Catholics accounted for 80.9 percent of the total population. Other religious groups include Muslims, other Christians, Evangelicals, Iglesia ni Kristo, Aglipay, and others (*CIA World Factbook*, 2012). The spread of the fundamentalist movement within Roman Catholicism is becoming more evident. Christianity in the Philippines is a blend of Spanish Catholicism, American Christianity, and surviving indigenous animistic traditions (Fig. 13-4).

Although Filipinos seek medical care, they believe that part of the efficacy of a cure is in God's hands or by some mystical power. Novenas and prayers are often said on behalf of the sick person. Families may bring religious items such as rosaries, medals, scapulars, and talismans for the sick person to wear. Talismans and amulets are believed to protect one from the forces of darkness, one's enemies, and sickness. Blessed holy water or oil is used to rub on the area in the body believed to be the source of distress. Performance of religious obligations and sacraments and daily prayers are some of the ways many Filipinos believe health and peaceful death are achieved. Providing for spiritual needs of Filipino patients requires accommodation to their various ways of practicing beliefs.

Meaning of Life and Individual Sources of Strength

Filipinos consider a meaningful existence to be a healthy and appropriate relationship with nature, God, and kin. Indigenous Filipino beliefs are embedded in the relationship between humans within the cosmology of the universe. This concept is demonstrated by the integration of supernatural, magicoreligious, and natural phenomena in the belief system and practices toward health and illness. Filipinos do not see themselves as victims but rather as part of the larger cosmos, subject to both the controllable and the uncontrollable forces of nature. To the traditional Filipino, strength comes from an intimate relationship

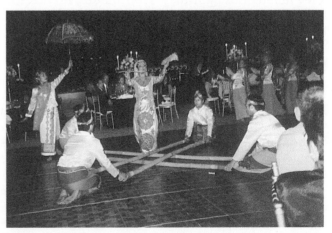

Figure 13-4 Filipino folk dance depicting indigenous Muslim and Malayan influences.

with God, family, friends, neighbors, and nature. The concept of self is formed from the relationship with a divine being and the social collective.

Many Filipinos find religion to be a source of strength in their daily lives. Some Filipinos are considered fatalistic in that they tend to accept fate easily, especially when they feel they cannot change a situation. Moreover, the acceptance of fate or destiny comes from their close relationship and healthy respect for nature. The acceptance of events they cannot change is tied to their religious faith. A common expression uttered by Filipinos is *bahala na*, originating from *bathala na* (it is up to God). *Bahala na* is often used when the person has used all resources to deal with a problem, and it is up to a higher power to take care of the rest (Enriquez, 1994). Nevertheless, an element of self-reliance exists among Filipinos, manifested by their confidence that the situation is within their sphere of influence through education and hard work.

Spiritual Beliefs and Health-Care Practices

Holism and integration characterize Filipino health-care beliefs and practices. Religious and spiritual dimensions are important components in health promotion. The importance of harmony between humans and nature and the role of natural and supernatural forces in health and illness are included in their beliefs about causes of illness and healing modalities. Prayers, religious offerings, appeasing natural spirits, and witchcraft may be practiced simultaneously along with biomedical interventions. Despite increasing notoriety and scandal associated with Filipino faith healers, this healing modality is widely sought in the Philippines. Many Filipinos seek biomedical and integrative ways of healing and do not subscribe to the competitive reductionism of the West. They believe in the synergistic relationship of differing modalities and have no problem subscribing to both ways of healing. Many Filipino American health-care providers participate in religious pilgrimages to Lourdes, France, and the shrine of Fatima in Portugal to pray for good health and healing.

Health-Care Practices

Health-Seeking Beliefs and Behaviors

Filipinos seek out family and close kin first for help when they are ill. When illness is more defined, mobilization of support occurs within the family. Decisions about when, where, and from whom to seek help are largely influenced by the intimate circle of family. Among Filipino older people in the United States, the choice of health-care providers is based on accessibility and availability to their working adult children (Pacquiao, 1993). Linguistically and ethnically congruent health-care providers are preferred. A dual

system of personal health care exists for many Filipinos, including those who are established in American communities. Filipinos may accept and adhere to medical recommendations and may use alternative sources of care suggested by trusted friends and family members. Often, they adhere to Western and indigenous medicine simultaneously, creating more choices to deal with their own or their family's health issues.

Many Filipinos consult an informal network of friends and family members, including physicians, nurses, pharmacists, or neighbors, who have had similar symptoms. Once the person finds the brand name of the "effective" medicine, the person can easily purchase the drug by asking family or friends to purchase medication in the Philippines. Hoarding prescription drugs and sharing medicine may be practiced by Filipinos in the United States. Those who do not believe in wastefulness or who believe that office visits are expensive may practice these behaviors.

When educating Filipino patients about medication, health-care providers should stress that medications need to be taken as prescribed; medications are ordered specifically for each ailment; unused drugs should be discarded; and the use of medications by individuals other than the intended patient may have serious consequences. Assessing these behaviors and delivering the message in a respectful, courteous, and unhurried manner may enhance the patient–health-care provider relationship, especially for traditional Filipino patients.

Health-care practices stress balance and moderation for the Filipino. Health is the result of balance, and illness is the consequence of imbalance. Imbalances that threaten health are brought about by personal irresponsibility or immorality. Care of the body through adequate sleep, rest, nutrition, and exercise is essential for health. A high value is also placed on personal cleanliness. Keeping oneself clean and free of unpleasant body odors is viewed as essential to health and social acceptance. To be slovenly and disorderly is to be shamelessly irresponsible. Aromatic baths are taken both for pleasure and to restore balance.

Responsibility for Health Care

Parents may seek all possible assistance that they can personally generate from family, friends, the church, the community, and the formal health-care system (often in that order) for a child with a serious illness such as cancer, eventually accepting the inevitability of death. From a Western perspective, the outcome may be slightly different than if formal services were accessed as early as possible. Adult children, especially those working in the United States, are responsible for the health care of their aged parents and extended kin. Responsibility may be in different forms, such as decision making, accepting financial responsibility, providing supportive presence, performing caretaking tasks, or negotiating with the health-care provider and the system.

In general, older adult women provide direct care for younger members. Older men participate in caring tasks such as driving the patient to the clinic. Decisions and financial support are relegated to family members who are deemed qualified and able. The family acts as a unit, and the individualistic paradigm commonly used by American caregivers is replaced by a social ethic of care. Before the decision is made to inform the patient about his or her terminal condition, a discussion among family members occurs, and they may request that the physician not divulge the truth to protect the patient. The ethical principles of beneficence and nonmaleficence take precedence over patient autonomy (Pacquiao, 2003).

Filipino family hierarchy may require consulting with family members before decisions are made. This may pose a problem to Western practitioners who believe in the adult patients' autonomy to make decisions about their own lives. The same perspective of Filipinos may result in their inability to question and assert ideas with physicians, who are regarded to be in a higher position of authority. Major decisions may be delegated to the physician rather than the patient or family taking an active collaborative role in decision making. Failure to develop a trusting relationship with the health-care provider can lead to noncompliance with prescribed regimens because of lack of participation in the decision-making process.

Folk and Traditional Practices

Supernatural and magico-religious beliefs about health and illness are integrated with scientific medicine. Mental illness may be attributed to an external cause such as witchcraft, soul loss, or spirit intrusion. Illness in infancy and childhood may be attributed to the evil eye. This belief system is consistent with the variety of Filipino folk healers. Healing rituals may involve religious rites (prayers and exorcism), sacrifices to appease the spirits, use of herbs, and massage.

Balance and moderation are embedded in the hot-and-cold theory of healing. The ideal environment is warm, moderate, and balanced. The underlying principle is that change should be introduced gradually. Sudden changes from hot to cold, from activity to inactivity, from fasting to overeating, and so forth introduce undue bodily stresses, which can cause illness. After strenuous physical activity, a rest should precede a shower; otherwise, the person could develop arthritis. Cold drinks or foods such as orange juice or fresh tomatoes are not served for breakfast to prevent stomach upset. Exposure to sudden cold drafts may induce colds, fever, rheumatism, pneumonia, or other respiratory ailments. Some Filipinos in the United States avoid hand washing with cold water after ironing or heavy labor. Exposure to cold such as showers is avoided during menstruation and the postpartum period.

The Department of Health in the Philippines (2005), through its Traditional Health Program, has endorsed 10 herbs that have been thoroughly tested and clinically proven to have medicinal value in the relief and treatment of various ailments (Table 13-2). The Philippine government has encouraged production of these herbal medicines to provide affordable medicines for the populations who have limited or no access to Western health care. Widespread acceptance of these herbal medicines is evident among educated and higher-income groups.

Barriers to Health Care

Studies of Filipinos in the United States show that, for many reasons, Filipinos generally do not seek care for illness until it is quite advanced. Some take minor ailments stoically and consider them natural imbalances that will run their normal course and disappear. Others claim to watch the progress of their illness so that the appropriate health-care provider can be consulted. Still others may not seek help because of economic reasons, lack of insurance, distrust of the health-care system, religious reasons, lack of knowledge, or an inability to articulate their needs (McBride et al., 1995).

Many Filipinos are reluctant to participate in health-promotion programs such as cancer screening

II▷ Table 13-2 | **Herbal Medicines Approved by the Department of Health in the Philippines**

Filipino Name/Generic Name	English Name	Uses
Akapulko (*Cassia alata*) "bayas-bayasan"	Ringworm bush	Ringworms and skin fungal infections
Ampalaya (*Momordica charantia*)	Bitter gourd or bitter melon	Non–insulin-dependent diabetes
Bawang (*Allium sativum*)	Garlic	Cholesterol reduction Blood pressure control
Bayabas (*Psidium guajava*)	Guava	Antiseptic to disinfect wounds Mouthwash to treat tooth decay and gum infection
Lagundi (*Vitex negundo*)	Five-leaf chaste tree	Relief of coughs and asthma
Niyog-niyogan (*Quisqualis indica*)	Chinese honeysuckle	Dried matured seeds to eliminate intestinal worms, particularly *Ascaris* and *Trichina*
Sambong (*Blumea balsamifera*)	Blumea camphora	Diuretic, helps in the excretion of urinary stones and treatment of edema
Tsaang gubat (*Ehretia microphylla lam*)		Taken as tea; used in treating intestinal motility and as a mouthwash because leaves have a high fluoride content
Ulasimang bato (*Pepperomia pellucida*) "pansit-pansitan"		Arthritis and gout; may be prepared as tea or eaten as a salad
Yerba buena (*Clinopodium douglasii*)	Peppermint	Analgesic to relieve body aches and pain; may be taken internally or applied locally

Source: Adapted from Department of Health (2005).

and health education. Aging Filipino veterans may be denied health services because of lack of insurance and consequently referred to various nonprofit community clinics. Older Filipino émigrés did not have adequate health benefits through their place of employment. Thus, they may have been used to postponing seeking care until the illness was quite advanced. Health-care providers should expect wide variations in health behaviors among Filipino American patients. A nonjudgmental history taking should be well documented. Turning on the "multicultural ear" and listening with care to the context of these actions can provide insight for a health-care provider, particularly when the health-care provider is under time pressure.

Cultural Responses to Health and Illness

Filipinos view pain as part of living an honorable life, as well as part of the process of spiritual purification while still on earth. Some view this as an opportunity to reach a fuller spiritual life or to atone for past transgressions. Thus, they may appear stoic and tolerate a high degree of pain. Health-care providers may need to offer and even encourage pain relief interventions for patients who do not complain of pain despite physiological indicators. Others may have a strong sensitivity to the "busyness" of health-care providers, quietly diminishing their own need for attention so that others can receive care, or they may simply have little knowledge of how pain management can be maximized.

Minimal expression of psychological and emotional discomfort may be observed. The discomfort in discussing negative emotions with outsiders may be manifested by somatic complaints or ritualistic behaviors, such as praying. Exploring the underlying meaning of somatization (loss of appetite, inability to sleep) and observing the patient's interactions with others can provide valuable information. Filipino patients may display visible evidence of their religion, such as religious medals, prayer cards, and rosary beads, to manage anxiety and pain. These artifacts should be incorporated into their treatment regimen. Using cultural mediators or brokers to probe innermost feelings of patients may be helpful if used appropriately. Pain assessment can include the role of prayer by the patient and members of the support network. Questions such as "Do you have someone praying for you?" or "Is there a special prayer to help you deal with pain?" may provide vital information for individualizing care.

Most Filipinos believe that mental illness carries a certain amount of stigma. The first choice is caring by family members, friends, and relatives rather than seeking health professionals (Gong, Gage, & Tacata, 2003) to minimize exposing the problem to outsiders.

Among rural residents and less-educated Filipinos in the Philippines, mental illness is generally attributed to external causes such as sorcery, soul loss, or spirit intrusion. Witch doctors, fortune-tellers, and faith healers are often sought. Filipinos in the United States seek professional interventions when symptoms are advanced. Psychiatric symptoms are precipitated by a loss in self-esteem, loss of status, and shame related to the stresses of immigration. Separation from family, inability to find suitable employment, uncertainty, lack of money, and other relocation stressors create serious psychological reactions among Filipinos. Among Filipino Americans, religiosity was correlated with seeking help from the religious clergy, whereas spirituality was associated with less help-seeking from professional mental health practitioners (Abe-Kim et al., 2004). Using sociocultural behaviors learned early in life, Filipinos have a remarkable ability to maintain a proper front to protect their self-esteem and self-image. Mental health-care providers should recognize that despite the possibility of a Filipino patient's refusing professional mental health services, involving a trusted family member or friends; initiating contact with a Filipino mental health worker, especially a Filipino physician; or using both practices may increase the odds of getting the person into a culturally compatible treatment program. Deference to authority may successfully bring the Filipino patient into treatment, with the patient's expectation that the authority figure will fix the problem.

Blood Transfusions and Organ Donation

The value of blood transfusion is recognized and accepted by Filipinos. However, organ donation may be less acceptable, except perhaps in cases in which a close family member is involved. Many Filipinos who follow Catholic traditions believe that keeping the body intact as much as possible until death is a reasonable preparation for the afterlife. Asian Americans, including Filipinos, hold more negative attitudes toward organ donation than European Americans. They are less likely to participate in large, urban organ donor program (Alden & Cheung, 2000).

Health-Care Providers

Traditional Versus Biomedical Providers

Western medicine is familiar and acceptable to most Filipinos. Many recent Filipino immigrants are educated in the health-care fields. Some Filipinos accept the efficacy of folk medicine and may consult both Western-trained and indigenous healers. Traditional healers are sought more in the rural areas of the Philippines. Folk healers are less common in the United States, with the exceptions of the West Coast and Hawaii. When available, they contribute by facilitating cultural rapport between health-care providers and the patient and by increasing utilization of needed health-care services. For example, the **hilot** is often willing to be included in the counseling session and provide support for the patient's adherence to the medical treatment. The *hilot* may provide a special prayer to be incorporated into the medically prescribed treatment plan to increase the patient's sense that all available resources are being used. In some areas on the West Coast, the *hilot* has a distinct role and function in the Filipino community. A few Filipino health professionals have learned the *hilot*'s art, skills, and spiritual approach, which they blend into their professional practice.

A health-care provider of the same gender and the same culture may encourage more Filipinos to take advantage of disease prevention services. The availability of Filipino primary-care providers and, whenever possible, a bilingual person are critical to improving health care for older Filipinos.

Status of Health-Care Providers

Filipinos generally consider the physician as the primary leader of the health-care team, and other providers are expected to defer to the physician. As Filipino families become more acculturated and aware of how health-care services are accessed in the United States, changes in attitude and behavior may be expected.

When ill, Filipinos may first consult a family member or a friend who is a physician or other professional before arranging a medical appointment. Some prefer physicians from their own region, when possible, whereas others indicate preference for physicians who are knowledgeable and competent and have good bedside manners regardless of culture or ethnic background. Factors considered in choosing health-care providers by middle-aged immigrant Filipino women

REFLECTIVE EXERCISE 13.3

Concepcion Miraflor had major depression for many years. Becoming progressively depressed for the past 6 months, she has expressed to her daughter that everyone would be better off if she were dead. Her daughter brought her to the mental health clinic for evaluation, where she was assessed to be a threat to herself and was admitted to the psychiatric unit and started on an antidepressant. She is 51 years old, has completed a sixth-grade education, is unemployed, and has no health insurance. Although she can speak limited English, she is unable to respond in English since she became depressed. She lives with her youngest daughter and her family and takes care of her two young grandchildren at home. Her son-in-law, who is from Pakistan, is a practicing Muslim. As a devout Catholic, Mrs. Miraflor was not happy with this inter-religious marriage. She is very concerned because her two grandchildren were not baptized in the Catholic Church.

1. How is the patient's level of spirituality influencing her relationship with her family and the possible area of conflict?
2. What issues can the nurse assist the patient in addressing while she is in the hospital?
3. Would you suggest a visit from a spiritual counselor?
4. Would you suggest involvement with a traditional healer?
5. What are some nursing implications related to ethnopharmacology that the nurse needs to consider while the patient is on antidepressant therapy?

were concern for privacy, feelings of modesty, approval from family members (especially the spouse), and, most important, the overall caring environment in the system.

Interactions of Filipinos with Canadian nurses in the hospital reflected their *kapwa*-oriented worldview, which categorized nursing approaches and interactions within the insider-outsider continuum. Patients based their preferences for which nurses to perform their personal and private tasks or receive information on the nurses' ability to provide spontaneous and unsolicited care and monitoring of their condition. Organizational policies and protocols, in addition to short hospital stays, were identified as barriers toward moving the patient–nurse relationship toward higher intimacy and trust (Pasco et al., 2004).

REFERENCES

Abe-Kim, J., Gong, F., & Takeuchi, D. (2004). Religiosity, spirituality, and help-seeking among Filipino Americans: Religious clergy or mental health professionals? *Journal of Community Psychology, 32,* 675–689.

Agoncillo, T., & Guerrero, M. (1987). *History of the Filipino people* (7th ed.). Manila, Philippines: Garcia Publishing.

Alden, D.L., & Cheung, A.H.S. (2000). Organ donation and culture: A comparison of Asian American and European American beliefs, attitudes, and behaviors. *Journal of Applied Social Psychology, 30*(2), 293–314.

Anderson, J.N. (1983). Health and illness in Pilipino immigrants. *Western Journal of Medicine, 139*(6), 811–819.

Araneta, M.R.G., & Barrett-Connor, E. (2005). Ethnic differences in visceral adipose tissue and type 2 diabetes: Filipino, African-American, and White women. *Obesity Research, 13,* 1458–1465.

Bateman, W., Abesamis-Mendoza, N., & Ho-Asjoe, H. (Eds.). (2009). *Praeger handbook of Asian American health: Taking notice and taking action.* Simi Valley: CA: ABC-CLIO.

Bautista, V. (2002). *The Filipino Americans (1763–present): Their history, culture, and tradition* (2nd ed.). Naperville, IL: Bookhaus.

Brown, D.E., & James, G.D. (2000). Physiological stress responses in Filipino-American immigrant nurses: The effects of residence time, life-style, and job strain. *Psychosomatic Medicine, 62,* 394–400.

Ceniza-Choy, C. (2003). Empire of care: Nursing migration in Filipino American history. Durham, NC: Duke University Press.

CIA World Factbook. (2012). *Philippines.* Retrieved from https://www.cia.gov/library/publications/the-world-factbook/geos/rp.html

Coughlan, S.S., & Uhler, R.J. (2000). Breast and cervical cancer screening practices among Asian and Pacific Islander women in the US, 1994–1997. *Cancer Epidemiology Biomarkers and Prevention, 9,* 597–603.

De la Cruz, F.A., Padilla, G.V., & Agustin, E.O. (2000). Adapting a measure of acculturation for cross-cultural research. *Journal of Transcultural Nursing, 11*(3), 191–198.

Department of Health. (2005). Ten herbal medicines approved by DOH. Retrieved from www.philippineherbalmedicine.org/doh_herbs.htm

Enriquez, V.G. (1994). From colonial to liberation psychology: The Philippine experience. Manila, Philippines: De La Salle University Press.

Espiritu, Y.L. (2003). Homebound: Filipino American lives across cultures, communities and countries. Ewing, NJ: University of California Press.

Garde, P., Spangler, Z., & Miranda, B. (1994). Filipino-Americans in New Jersey: A health study. Final Report of the Philippine Nurses' Association of America to the State of New Jersey Department of Health, Office of Minority Health.

Gong, F., Gage, S.-J.L., & Tacata, L.A., Jr. (2003). Help seeking behavior among Filipino Americans: A cultural analysis of face and language. *Journal of Community Psychology, 31*(5), 469–488.

Hawaii Community College. (2005). Traditional Filipino health beliefs. Retrieved from http://www.hawcc.hawaii.edu/nursing/tradfil2.htm

Hoang, Ha. (2008). Language and cultural barriers of Asian migrants in accessing maternal care in Australia. *International journal of Language Society and Culture 26*(6), 55-61. Retrieved from http://www.educ.utas.edu.au/users/tle/JOURNAL/issues/2008/26-6.pdf

IBON Foundation. (2007). Retrieved from http://www.ibon.org

Kagawa-Singer, M., & Pourat, N. (2000). Asian American and Pacific Islander breast and cervical carcinoma screening rates and *Healthy People 2000* objectives. *Cancer, 89*(3), 696–705.

Levy, R. (1993). Ethnic and racial differences in response to medicines: Preserving individualized therapy in managed pharmaceutical programmes. *Pharmaceutical Medicine, 7,* 139–165.

Lim, S., Clarke, C.A., Prehn, A.W., Glaser, S.L., West, D.W., & O'Malley, C.D. (2002). Survival differences among Asian subpopulations in the United States after prostate, colorectal, breast, and cervical carcinomas. *Cancer, 94*(4), 1175–1182.

Lin, K.M., & Smith, M.W. (2000). Psychopharmacology in the context of culture and ethnicity. In P. Ruiz (Ed.), *Ethnicity & psychopharmacology.* Washington, DC: American Psychiatric Press.

Lipson, J.G., & Dibble, S.L. (2005). *Culture and clinical care.* San Francisco: University of California San Francisco Nursing Press.

Maxwell, A.E., Bastani, R., Vida, P., & Warda, U.S. (2002). Physical activity among older Filipino-American women. *Women Health, 36*(1), 67–79.

Maxwell, A.E., Bastani, R., & Warda, U.S. (2000). Demographic predictors of cancer screening among Filipino and Korean immigrants in the United States. *American Journal of Preventive Medicine, 36*(1), 67–68.

Maxwell, A.E., Garcia, G.M., & Berman, B.A. (2007). Understanding tobacco use among Filipino American men. *Journal of Tobacco Research, 9*(7), 767–776.

McBride, M., Mariola, D., & Yeo, G. (1995). Aging and health: Asian Pacific Islander American elders. Stanford, CA: Stanford Geriatric Education Center.

McBride, M., & Parreno, H. (1996). Filipino American families and caregiving. In G. Yeo & D. Gallagher-Thompson (Eds.), *Ethnicity and the dementias.* Washington, DC: Taylor & Francis.

Mossakowski, K.N. (2003). Coping with perceived discrimination: Does ethnic identity protect mental health? *Journal of Health and Social Behavior, 44*(3), 318–331.

Munoz, C., & Hilgenberg, C. (2006). Ethnopharmacolgy: Understanding how ethnicity affects drug response. *Journal of Holistic Nursing Practice, 20*(5), 227–234.

Munoz, C., & Luckmann, J. (2005). Transcultural communication in nursing. Clifton Park: NY: Thomson Delmar Publishing Inc.

National Statistics Office, Philippines. (2010). Index of demographic and health. Retrieved from http://www.census.gov.ph/data/sectordata/datandhs.html

Pacquiao, D.F. (1993). Cultural influences in old age: An ethnographic comparison of Anglo and Filipino elders. Doctoral dissertation, Graduate School of Education, Rutgers University, New Brunswick, NJ. Ann Arbor, MI: University Microfilms, Inc. (number 9320788).

Pacquiao, D.F. (1996). Educating faculty in the concept of educational biculturalism: A comparative study of sociocultural influences in nursing students' experience in school. In V.M. Fitzsimons & M.L. Kelley (Eds.), *The culture of learning: Access, retention, understanding and mobility of minority students in nursing* (pp. 129–162). New York: National League for Nursing Press.

Pacquiao, D.F. (2001). Cultural incongruities of advance directives. *Bioethics Forum*, *17*(1), 27–31.

Pacquiao, D.F. (2003). Cultural competence in ethical decision-making. In M.M. Andrews & J.S. Boyle (Eds.), *Transcultural concepts in nursing care* (4th ed., pp. 503–532). Philadelphia: Lippincott.

Pacquiao, D.F. (2004). Recruitment of Philippine nurses to the US: Implications for policy development. *Nursing and Health Policy Review*, *3*(2), 167–180.

Pasco, A.C.Y., Morse, J.M., & Olson, J.K. (2004). Cross-cultural relationships between nurses and Filipino Canadian patients. *Journal of Nursing Scholarship*, *36*(3), 239–246.

Quan, H., Fong, A., De Coster, C., Wang, J., Musto, R., Noseworthy, T.W., et al. (2006). Variation in health services utilization among ethnic populations. *CMAJ: Canadian Medical Association Journal*, *174*(6), 787–791.

Reeves, T.J., & Bennett, C.E. (2004). We the people: Asians in the US. Census 2000 special reports. Washington, DC: U.S. Department of Commerce.

Ryan, C., Shaw, R., & Pilam, M. (2000). Coronary artery disease in Filipino and Filipino American Patients: Prevalence of risk factors and outcomes of treatment. *Journal of Invasive Cardiology 12*(3), 134–139.

Salazar, L.P., Schuldermann, S.M., Schuldermann, E.H., & Hunyh, C. (2000). The Filipino adolescents' parental socialization for academic achievement in the United States. *Journal of Adolescent Research*, *15*(5), 564–587.

Spangler, Z. (1992). Transcultural nursing care values and caregiving practices of Philippine-American nurses. *Journal of Transcultural Nursing*, *4*(2), 28–37.

Tatak Pilipino. (2007). Profile of the Philippines. Retrieved from http://www.filipinoheritage.com

U.S. Census Bureau. (2002). The Asian population: 2000. Retrieved from http://www.census.gov/prod/2002pubs/c2kbr01-16.pdf

Wolf, D.L. (1997). Family secrets: Transnational struggles among children of Filipino immigrants. *Sociological Perspectives*, *40*(3), 457–483.

Wu, T.-Y., & Bancroft, J. (2006). Filipino American women's perceptions and experiences with breast cancer screening. *Oncology Nursing Forum*, *33*(4), 1–11.

Yamane, L. (2002). Native-born Filipina/o Americans and labor market discrimination. *Feminist Economics*, *8*(2), 125–144.

Yu, S.M., Huang, Z.J., & Singh, G.K. (2004). Health status and health services utilization among US Chinese, Asian Indian, Filipino, and other Asian/Pacific Islander children. *Pediatrics*, *113*(1), 101–107.

DavisPlus *For reflective exercises, review questions, and additional information, go to*

http://davisplus.fadavis.com

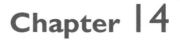

Chapter 14

People of German Heritage

Jessica A. Steckler

Overview, Inhabited Localities, and Topography

Overview

Germans are reserved, formal people who appreciate a sense of order in their lives. Their love of music and celebrations has permanently influenced many of the world's cultures. The Christmas tree (*Weihnachtsbaum*) with its brightly decorated ornaments, a universal symbol of the holiday season, is a German creation. Gingerbread houses (*Lebkuchen*), Christmas carols (*Weihnachtslieder*) and cards, the "Easter hare" (*Osterhase*), hot cross buns, valentines (*Freundschaftskarten*), Groundhog Day, chain letters (*Briefe zum Himmel*), the tooth fairy, and *Kaffeeklatsch* or "gossip sessions" all have their origins in German culture.

There are 51 million Germans in the United States (U.S. Census Bureau, 2008) and over 3.1 million in Canada (Statistics: Canada, 2006). Ethnic groups of European origin are usually categorized as "white" on applications, in surveys, and in research studies, so there is little culturally specific information available about them. This is unfortunate, because differences in worldviews, cultural beliefs, and health-care practices among white ethnic groups hold important implications for health-care providers.

The Federal Republic of Germany (*Bundesrepublik Deutschland*), comprising 16 states, boasts beautiful landscapes, high and low mountain ranges, sandy lowlands, rolling hills, lakelands, and ocean borders. Situated in the heart of Europe, Germany is a link between the East and the West and between Scandinavia and the Mediterranean. Germany has the largest economy in Europe, has the third largest economy in the world, and is the leading per-capita export nation in the world (*CIA World Factbook,* 2011). With a population of over 82 million, it is one of the most densely populated countries in Europe. Germany is a member of the United Nations and NATO and is a founding member of the European Union (*CIA World Factbook,* 2011). Most of Germany is located in the temperate zone, with temperatures ranging from 27°F in the mountains to 68°F in the valleys of the south. Temperatures are comparable with the climate in the northwest portion of the United States. The Upper Rhine has a mild climate; Upper Bavaria has warm Alpine winds from the south; and the Harz Mountains have cold winds, cool summers, and heavy winter snows.

Heritage and Residence

In the 18th century, the New World colonies from New England to the Deep South grew and flourished. Even though the colonial settlers shared an Old World heritage, they were a diverse people. German settlers, along with other immigrants from Britain, France, Scotland, and Ireland, shared a love of family and land—a love that would eventually bond them to one another to form a nation of Americans. The earliest German immigrants to the United States settled in the colonies along the eastern seaboard, including William Penn's colony in Pennsylvania. Religious tolerance and equitable land distribution contributed to the success of these Pennsylvania settlements. Mennonites, Dunkers, Amish, and Moravians from Germany made up the new Pennsylvania communities. The area in which they settled, known as *Pennsylvania Dutch Country*, was actually mislabeled by English neighbors who thought the word *deutsch*, meaning "German," stood for "Dutch." One hundred thousand strong, these Pennsylvania Germans were the main carriers of German culture to the mid-Atlantic area (Domer, 1994).

Other religious social idealists from Germany soon flowed into the colonies. Among them were the Harmonists, who broke from the German Lutheran Church under the leadership of George Rapp (Boorstin, 1987). The Harmonists built Harmony, Pennsylvania; Harmony, Indiana; and Economy (Ambridge), Pennsylvania. The Harmonists were followed by other German sects: the Zoars, who settled in Ohio, and the Inspirationists, who originally settled in western New York and later moved west to Iowa by "divine command."

The second wave of German immigrants arrived in the United States between 1840 and 1860. They were fleeing political persecution, starvation, and poverty in their homeland and settled on the western frontier (Weaver, 1979). This group of influential Germans was less interested in taking root in the United States than in establishing a German culture. These new immigrants kept the German language in their schools, published newspapers in German, joined their own singing societies and orchestras, and married only other Germans.

The 1930s and 1940s saw a third wave of German immigration. Artists, architects, social scientists, physicists, and mathematicians came to this country to escape the Nazi Holocaust. These new arrivals were highly educated and at the height of their careers. After witnessing the horrors of the Holocaust, they had no desire to transplant Old World institutions or to establish new European-style homelands (Boorstin, 1987). These third-wave immigrants became rapidly acculturated into American life and greatly enriched American culture in the fields of music, psychology, science, and mathematics. Among this prominent group were Albert Einstein and Hannah Arendt, an author and political scientist.

Historians have helped to further our understanding of the diffusion of German immigrants into the American heartland by tracing the existence of the "two-door house." These German-built houses, which architecturally copied their European counterparts, have two front doors. With their movement across the United States, two-door houses appeared in Pennsylvania, Maryland, West Virginia, the Blue Ridge Mountains, Ohio, Indiana, Illinois, Missouri, Iowa, Kansas, Nebraska, Michigan, and Texas (Domer, 1994).

Germans continue to embrace the United States as their own. The desire to become American has been nurtured by the presence of American troops in Germany, and many Germans have entered the United States as spouses of military personnel. For others, business ventures and the promise of career opportunities brought them to this country. Today, about one-fourth of all American citizens can trace their ancestry to German roots. Germans are the dominant ancestral group in St. Louis, Missouri; Milwaukee, Wisconsin; Chicago, Illinois; Cincinnati, Ohio; Buffalo and New York City in New York; and Baltimore, Maryland (U.S. Census Bureau, 2008).

Reasons for Migration and Associated Economic Factors

Germans have been very much a part of important events shaping U.S. socioeconomic history. They have been participants, observers, and victims in the Revolutionary War, the Civil War, the influenza epidemic, the Great Depression, World Wars I and II, the Vietnam War, the Persian Gulf War, and the current global recession. The reasons for their immigration to the United States vary according to historical antecedents and are, therefore, discussed under Heritage and Residence.

Educational Status and Occupations

Germans have a deep respect for education. In Germany, credibility, social status, and level of employment are based on educational achievement. In other words, Germans are very class conscious. Germans take pride in their school system, particularly in their craftsmanship and technology. Unlike in the United States, education is free at all levels, except kindergarten, which is optional, but entrance to university education is difficult and accomplished only by passing the *Abitur* examination. Literacy rates of Germany (99 percent) and the United States (98 percent) are comparable (*CIA World Factbook,* 2011).

In Germany, children can begin kindergarten at age 3 (Educational Aspects in the United States and Germany, n.d.). This is comparable with our preschool. At age 6, they enter grade school, which includes grades 1 to 4. At grade 5, they begin one of three tracks of education: *Hauptschule*, which is special education and the most basic educational path; *Realschule*, which is general education; or *Gymnasium*, which is like U.S. college preparatory courses. German students graduate at grade 10 and can then enter into vocational education, which prepares them for a trade or for working in business, or they can continue college preparation. Those students wishing to go to the universities must pass the *Abitur* test, which is both verbal and written.

Germans who immigrated to the United States in the 19th century influenced American preschool and higher-educational systems. The Johns Hopkins University in Baltimore, Maryland, was founded on the model of Humboldt University in Berlin, Germany (McKinnon, 1993). During this same period, many American historians and political scientists attended German universities, returning with their doctoral degrees, and were instrumental in developing prototypes for American graduate education. Many of the influences of the 19th-century German immigrants on the educational system remain visible today.

By the mid-19th century, *Turnvereins* were taking root in midwestern German American communities. These political and gymnastic organizations believed in a sound mind and body and provided opportunities to grow both physically and intellectually (Acton, 1994). In this same era, schools—many of which were parochial schools—were established in which only German was spoken. German Catholics also established parochial schools in this era, but unlike the Lutherans, their ethnic identity was not tied to the church (Coburn, 1992).

German immigrants were viewed as an internal threat in the United States during World War II and faced turbulent times. A growing anti-immigrant sentiment leading to calls for immigration restriction intensified the political climate. Some German immigrants' desire to maintain an identity apart from the American culture was expressed through the founding of the National German American Alliance. Many German Americans changed their names, made apologies, and displayed their loyalties in an effort to attenuate suspicions, embarrassments, and persecutions.

Today, German American families continue to value education. Most German Americans have a high school education at minimum. Twenty-four percent have attained post–high school education. However, in the age group 65 and older, 43 percent have less than a high school education (Rowland, 1992); no current information on educational levels of German Americans could be found. Vocational or university education is being sought more frequently by recent high school graduates attempting to prepare themselves for a highly competitive work environment and by adults who are pursuing second and third careers. By German standards, success means being employed, and education is seen as the way to achieve this success (McKinnon, 1993).

The earliest German immigrants were primarily farmers. Tobacco, wheat, rice, cotton, corn, and sugar were among the most widely grown crops. Plantations grew from Virginia to the colonies in the South as a result of these prosperous ventures. Planting and harvesting crops required many workers with strong backs, and because not all Germans could pay for their passage to the New World, many worked as indentured servants. They suffered many hardships and worked long hours at the mercy of their owners. Family members were commonly separated from one another, and often children were sold to pay the debt of their parents.

Between the Revolutionary War and the Civil War, many religious sects, including the Shakers, Harmonists, Zoars, and Inspirationists, founded hundreds of intentional communities (Boorstin, 1987). Known historically as the *Utopians*, they farmed the land; spun flax, cotton, and wool into beautiful textiles; and manufactured fine clocks and furniture. Unlike those who immigrated to the United States before the Revolutionary War, the Utopians formed caring and supportive communities instead of living in isolation from others. They worked happily for the settlement; built simple, strong dwellings; planted bountiful gardens; and established strong trade routes to the American West (Boorstin, 1987).

In the post–Civil War era, Germans who came to the United States often "chain-migrated" to the western frontier. Families and friends would leave one area to join family, friends, and neighbors in another place.

These groups became farmers, miners, millers, construction workers, shopkeepers, blacksmiths, and locksmiths. Many were artists and craft workers who created pottery, leather goods, soap, candles, and musical instruments (e.g., the dulcimer). These Germans established outstanding breweries, beer gardens (*biergarten*), and pubs (*kneipen*) everywhere they settled. They also brought many trades to the United States, including butchering, coppering, tailoring, and cabinetmaking. Whereas they dominated the trades, German immigrants were found less frequently in professional and management positions (Schied, 1993).

In the early decades of the 20th century, the Nazi Holocaust drove many German immigrants from their home country. Many who came in the 1930s and 1940s continued their gifted work in the United States. Germans continue to establish their homes in the United States. Newly arriving immigrants are highly educated and vocationally well trained. German workers are among the most skilled in the world. Germany and the United States have similar industries in manufacturing, construction, and service.

Communication

Dominant Language and Dialects

German, the official language of the Federal Republic of Germany, is spoken in Germany; Austria; and Liechtenstein; large parts of Switzerland and South Tirol; and small parts of Belgium, France, and Luxembourg. German is the native language of over 100 million people, and many literary works have been translated into German (Kappler & Grevel, 1993). Within Germany, there are many dialects along with high (more formal) and low (less formal and more conversational) German. Individuals' home regions can be easily identified through their speech, and citizens from neighboring regions may have difficulty understanding one another because of the differences in regional jargon and accents.

In addition to the German language, German children learn English at grade 5, and at grade 7, they learn a third language of their choice. At grade 9, Advanced English or, perhaps, a fourth language can be chosen (European Education Directory, 2006).

English is the dominant language of German Americans. Germans who originally emigrated from Germany learned American English at work, in school, and through socialization. Their children grew up speaking English in public schools and German at home.

Currently, U.S. schoolchildren are learning English, and some grade schools teach Spanish. In high school, Russian, French, and Advanced Spanish classes can be chosen. The opportunity to learn German became more available in 1997. German immersion programs were established and took the form of summer camps,

Saturday and after-school classes, independent, and private and public schools.

The purpose of the German immersion programs is to help students use a second language approximating that of a student who is native to that language. School-based immersion programs allow the student to use a second language for communicating in normal everyday situations as well as in subject content learning.

Some of the full-time German immersion programs are supported and accredited by the German government. The school must satisfy both the state and German school guidelines. When a student graduates from a German accredited school, they receive an American diploma and also earn the German International ABITUR. The first German immersion education programs were modeled after the French immersion programs developed in Canada. German immersion programs can currently be found in 20 states.

Some German American families turned to tutoring to help their children learn German when the German immersion programs were inconvenient or unavailable in their community. German tutors can be found online, as well as at the American Association of Teachers of German (AATG), which was established in 1926 (http://aatg.org/). The AATG is dedicated to the advancement of the language and culture of German-speaking countries.

Today, there is a growing awareness of endangered languages, and this is true about the dialects of German Americans. A language becomes endangered when there are so few speakers that it may no longer be used often enough and could be lost forever. For example, Texas German, a dialect found in the Texas hill country, is nearly extinct. This resulted from a change in school law mandating the use of English in all schools during World War I (Texas State Historical Association, n.d.). In German American homes where the German language is expected to be spoken and children are faced with speaking English in the schools, intergenerational conflicts may result. Parents do not speak English, but the children prefer to speak English.

Americans and Germans have some similar patterns of speech behavior. German is a low-contextual language, with a greater emphasis on verbal than nonverbal communication, showing a high degree of social approval to people whose verbal behavior in expressing ideas and feelings is precise, explicit, straightforward, and direct.

Forty-nine million people in the United States claim to have German ancestors, and 1.4 million of them can speak German (U.S. Census Bureau, 2005). Individuals in some German American communities mix English and German creatively when expressing humor. In Dubois County, a German American community in Indiana, linguistic competence is measured by a person's ability to switch between German and English to reflect bicultural roots and traditions (Salmons, 1988).

Cultural Communication Patterns

People of German ancestry enjoy discussing topics of interest after dinner. These conversations, sometimes debates, cover a range of issues from politics, religion, food, and work experiences to life in general. Jokes, funny stories, or anecdotes about family members are interspersed within the discussion.

Germans carry on their conversations at three levels. The first, *Gespräch*, is used for casual conversation and is more informal; the second, *Besprechung*, is conversation carried on in a work setting between employees and supervisors about performance; and the third, *Diskutieren*, is the common form of social discourse used in discussions about various issues and is the most formal use of the German language (S. Maubach, personal communication, 2007). Most Americans are often ill prepared to enter the debate on philosophical and political issues that are addressed at this level and are thus placed at a disadvantage. This cultural barrier can prevent Germans from developing deeper relationships with outside groups.

Feelings among Germans and German Americans are considered private and are often difficult to share. Sharing one's feelings with others often creates a sense of vulnerability or is looked on as evidence of weakness. The act of expressing fear, concern, happiness, or sorrow allows others a view of the personal and private self, creating a sense of discomfort and uneasiness. Therefore, philosophical discussions, hopes, and dreams are shared only with family members and close friends. Emotions are intensely experienced but are not always expressed among family or friends. "Being in control" includes harnessing one's emotions and not revealing them to others.

Newer-generation German Americans, influenced by the cultural values of the United States, are more overt in sharing their thoughts, ideas, and feelings with others. They have joined in the American belief that direct confrontation and open dialogue can be productive. In spite of this general pattern of acculturation, pockets of Germans in the United States continue to be reserved when sharing their private affairs, thoughts, and concerns, including their health concerns, with strangers. Their reluctance for socializing may make them appear unfriendly; yet, under their stern exterior, they want to be liked.

Good manners are very important to Germans. A display of politeness and courtesy is viewed as a sign of respect. Social distance, eye contact, touch, and facial expression define boundaries. Failure to adhere to these protocols is considered rude by Germans and may alienate people who are unaware of them. When some people think of the handshake in the context of the German culture, they conjure visions of comics imitating this German greeting—the quick stooping of the shoulders and the clicking of the heels (Friday, 1989). The handshake, still a structured phenomenon in Germany (without the clicking!), has been acculturated into a more casual form by German Americans and is a common method of greeting for both men and women, but the practice is to always shake hands with women first. When families and friends gather, handshaking is practiced along with pats on the arms or back.

Practices associated with personal touch and displays of affection, such as hugging and kissing, vary among German families. In families in which the father plays a dominant role, little touching occurs between the father and the children. This relationship, however, may become more demonstrative as parents and children age. Affection between a mother and her children is more evident. In other German families, there is outward expression of love from both fathers and mothers, grandparents, and extended family members; hugs and kisses are expected and often demanded as a "reaffirmation of love."

Whereas close friends are often extended warmth through handshakes, brief embraces, and sometimes kisses, strangers are kept at arm's length and greeted formally. As the author recalls from childhood, strangers, particularly those who were not German, were looked on with suspicion, even though some of these "strangers" were in-laws. Generally, Germans are careful not to touch people who are not family or close friends.

The distancing used by Germans to position themselves in relation to others is greater than the distancing used by some other cultural groups in the United States. More acculturated German Americans may control their space in a manner similar to that of other Americans. In health-care situations, providers frequently enter their patients' personal space. German Americans understand the need for this intrusion and voluntarily participate in such encounters, while preserving their dignity and privacy.

Germans place a high value on their privacy. Germans may live side by side in a neighborhood and never develop a close friendship. A German neighbor would not be expected to borrow a cup of sugar from another neighbor because doing so would be an admission that she or he failed to adequately stock the pantry. Germans would never consider dropping in on another German neighbor because this behavior is incongruent with their sense of order. Much preparation is completed to ready the house for guests. When invited into the home of a German, the guest may be surprised to find that the distance between pieces of furniture is not conducive to conversation; their philosophy is "German space is sacred" (Hall & Hall, 1990). In addition to spacing furniture, Germans use doors to protect their privacy. A closed door requires a knock and an invitation to enter regardless of whether the door is encountered in the home, business, or hospital. A closed door secures a sense of privacy and safety for Germans. Germans guard their privacy, which includes receiving phone calls at home. It is best to wait for an invitation or ask permission before contacting a new German acquaintance at home.

Germans maintain eye contact during conversation, but staring at strangers is considered rude. Even looking into a room from the outside is considered a visual intrusion; the interior of a room should not be entered without permission (Hall & Hall, 1990).

Smiling is reserved for friends and family. Because smiling does not occur during introductions, Germans are often considered unfriendly. Work is considered serious business; thus, Germans smile very little at work. Dealing with illness is also considered serious business, calling for "correct responses" (i.e., reserved, direct, and unsmiling).

Several unacceptable expressions of nonverbal behavior for Germans include chewing gum in public, cleaning one's fingernails in public, talking with one's hands in the pockets, placing one's feet and legs on furniture, pointing the index finger to one's own head (an insult), and public displays of affection. Younger, more nontraditional German American youths may not adhere to these perceptions. Americans cross their fingers for luck, whereas Germans squeeze the thumb between index and middle fingers. However, allowing the thumb to protrude more than its tip length is an offensive gesture (CultureGram, 1994).

Temporal Relationships

Germans use time to buy the future and pay for the past. Their focus on the present is to ensure the future. The past, however, is equally important, and Germans begin their discussion with background information, which always includes history. Americans generally do not understand the German people's need to lay a proper foundation for discussion. Conversely, Germans develop a deep understanding of their historical heritage through an intense analysis of past events. Friday (1989) explained this contradiction as the result of a difference in educational emphasis in German and American schools.

Germans pride themselves on their punctuality. Being on time is an obsession. People who expect to be late for appointments should call and explain. If this is not done, the German sense of order is disturbed. Work is completed by setting and meeting deadlines. "Keeping to the schedule" is extremely important. There is a sense of impatience and often intolerance in the German American who encounters a situation in which someone else is not performing on schedule. This impatience can be stirred to anger in the work setting, in the supermarket, on the highway, in the hospital, or in the health-care provider's office. In the mind of a German, who is always on time, there are rarely good excuses for tardiness, delays, or incompetence that disturb the "schedule" of events. Within this cultural continuum model, Western Europeans and North Americans attend to details in a linear, orderly manner, measuring days, hours, and seconds. Time has value for both groups, often equated with money.

Format for Names

Traditionally, Germans keep social relations on a formal basis. Even neighbors of long-standing acquaintance are addressed as *Herr* (Mr.), *Frau* (Mrs.), or *Fräulein* (Miss) and their last name. Those in authority, older people, or subordinates are always formally addressed. Only family members and close friends address one another by their first names. Many German Americans born in the 1930s and 1940s continue to be formal in their social and business interactions. If this consideration is not returned, or if someone presumptuously calls them by their first name, it may be considered a sign of disrespect or poor upbringing. Hall and Hall (1990) explain, "The taboo against first-naming should not be dismissed as an empty convention." In their book they describe an old custom, *Brüderschaft-trinken*, in which "two friends formalize their shift to the more intimate form of address. They hook arms and each sips from a glass. Then they shake hands and announce their first names" (p. 49).

Germans combine a person's professional title with *Herr, Frau, Fräulein,* or other titles and their last name. For example, a director of a business is addressed as *Frau* or *Fräulein Direktorin*. The title is often used without the name. A physician may be addressed simply as *Doktor*. Younger generations or more acculturated Germans may be less formal in their interactions. Because of cultural blending, health-care providers will find that German Americans vary widely in their observance of these rules of etiquette. Therefore, these health-care providers should ask their patients how they would like to be addressed. This approach lessens the possibility of the provider unintentionally offending the patient.

Family Roles and Organization
Head of Household and Gender Roles

Traditional German families view the father as the head of the household. In the United States, the husband and wife are more likely to make decisions mutually and share household duties. Stay-at-home dads are uncommon in Germany (S. Maubach, personal communication, 2006). Often, when illness, dependence, and disability interfere and prevent family members from carrying out their roles, others assume decision-making responsibilities either temporarily or permanently.

In Germany, where emphasis is on **Ordnung** (order), and **Gemeinschaft** (community), older people are not expected to be self-reliant. Health and social programs for older people are considered part of the institutional approach of European programs. Because of the comprehensiveness of these benefits, there is less financial reliance on the family. One home may remain in the same family for generations. Often, more than one generation live under the same roof. Older family members who live with their children are included in family celebrations as well as in the daily routine of the families. As they become unable to perform their roles and duties, other family members assume their responsibilities.

Older people within German American families are sought for their advice and counsel, although the advice may not always be followed. They are admired for maintaining their level of independence and their continued contributions to society. Many live alone or with aging spouses. Helping older parents or grandparents to remain in their own home is important to German American families. By providing a helping hand with home maintenance, shopping, and finances, the family is able to safeguard and prolong a state of independence, even when living hundreds of miles away. For those who grow dependent, moving in with children or residing in a nursing home is a viable choice for German American families.

The differences in the family role for older people in Germany and in the United States may be due to the far-reaching mobility of the American population that does not exist in Germany, where families generally live in close proximity. When Americans moved to the western frontier, they were required to adopt attitudes that included a degree of individualism, self-reliance, and initiative not demanded in a more geographically stable and settled society in which families had support because they were geographically close. The emphasis on these traits, as well as the concept of "America, land of unlimited opportunity," has made life in the United States difficult.

The Older Americans Act, Medicare, and Medicaid legislation, which are considered residual approaches for meeting one's social needs, support the context of the German belief in self-reliance and the supportive role of the family. Such residual approaches are offered when the normal channels such as family, marketplace, and church are not sufficient for meeting needs. Strong advocacy groups such as the American Association of Retired Persons and the National Council of Senior Citizens, which have mobilized older Americans as a self-interest group, also support this idea of self-reliance (Gelfand, 1988).

In the United States, 24 percent of older people live alone (Lamanna & Riedman, 2008), whereas in Germany, 16 percent live alone. The significant proportion of older women living alone in both countries can be attributed to the heavy loss of life among German men in World War II. Although families may live close to one another, a significant portion of the older population (24 percent) report feeling lonely (Rowland, 1992). With both spouses working to maintain economic security, many people have less time available to interact socially with older family members living on their own. An interesting fact is that the Germans love their dogs, and in Germany, it is acceptable to take the family dog everywhere—restaurants, visiting, and the hospital. In the United States, however, animals, except for seeing-eye dogs, are restricted from most public places. Other pets in German households may be cats, rabbits, birds, hedgehogs, and, of course, horses (S. Maubach, personal communication, 2006).

Prescriptive, Restrictive, and Taboo Behaviors for Children and Adolescents

Prescriptive behaviors for children include using good table manners, being polite, doing what they are told, respecting their elders, sharing, paying attention in school, and doing their chores. Additional behaviors include keeping one's nose clean, eating all food that is placed on their plates, looking at a person who is talking, and sitting up straight. Prescriptive behaviors for adolescents include staying away from bad influences, obeying the rules of the home, sitting "like a lady," and wearing a robe over pajamas. Restrictive and taboo behaviors for children include talking back to adults, talking to strangers, touching another person's possessions, and getting into trouble. Restrictive and taboo behaviors for adolescents include smoking, using drugs, chewing gum in public, having guests when parents are not at home, going without a slip (girls), and having run-ins with the law.

Germany has regulations about noise levels in public areas such as athletic fields where people gather to watch soccer games, tennis, and riding events. These regulations are enforced for both children and adults. On occasion, schools in highly populated areas apply similar restrictions for playground activities (German Noise Law, 2010).

Family Goals and Priorities

In Germany, history, family, and lifelong friendships are highly valued. Concern for one's reputation is a strong value. One's family reputation is considered part of a person's identity and serves to preserve one's social position (good and bad). The author recalls her mother admonishing her about the proper behavior for a young woman. She always pointed out, "You never know whom you will run into." This admonition meant that you might meet someone, at any time and without your being aware, who could draw conclusions from your behavior that might tarnish the family's reputation.

Alternative Lifestyles

Pregnancy outside marriage results in disapproval, which can be overt or subtle. Because German families are concerned about their reputations in the community, the presence of an unwed mother taints their reputation and may result in the family being ostracized. If marriage follows the pregnancy, less sanctioning occurs, but just the fact that the pregnancy occurred before the marriage creates a stigma for the woman—and sometimes the child—that may last for the rest of their lives. The family members rarely forget this embarrassment, although it may never be discussed openly.

Today, acculturation and realignment of the moral rules of society, in which one out of four children is born out of wedlock, have lessened the seriousness of teenage pregnancy. These changes, together with the availability of more options for pregnant teenagers and greater social acceptance for unwed mothers than existed in the 1970s, have not lessened the shock for parents.

When couples delay having children, families may pressure the couple about producing children. Understanding a couple's decision not to have children is often difficult for German American families, and it may never be accepted.

Many middle-aged gay and lesbian German Americans may fear exposure because of the extreme discrimination homosexuals experienced in Nazi Germany. In addition, religious education plays an important role in anchoring family conceptions and leads to denial of homosexual feelings. When healthcare providers encounter gays and lesbians who need religious support, a referral to one of the gay and lesbian religious groups may be helpful (see Chapter 2).

Workforce Issues
Culture in the Workplace

Germans are among the most skilled and educated workers in the world. Much of Germany's success is due to advanced technologies, and it is a leading nation in Nobel Prizes for physiology and medicine. Some of its most important contributions are in rocketry, material science, and chemical products (Solar Navigator, 2006). German workers are educated to meet the needs of a highly industrialized country. The atmosphere of German business is very formal.

Several considerations must be remembered when working with Germans and some German Americans. First, it is important to be on time for work and business appointments and to complete work assignments on time. Second, business communication should remain formal: shaking hands daily, using the person's title with the last name, keeping niceties to a minimum, and avoiding the adjustment of office furniture during meetings. Employees are not addressed by their first names. Third, one should respect privacy by not entering rooms with a closed door before knocking and being invited inside. Fourth, dress, opinions, and activities should be conservative. Finally, learning to speak German is important if an employee is living in Germany and working for a German company (Hall & Hall, 1990).

The current trend toward a global economy has encouraged many American companies to establish sites in Germany and many German corporations to have subsidiaries in the United States as well as other places throughout the world. Many German managers are transferred to the United States by their companies and easily enter and adapt to the American business climate. Others trained in the health professions, the physical sciences and education, and technologies join the ranks of practicing professionals in the United States.

In the workplace, American values and beliefs often oppose German traditions. Friday (1989), in exploring the problems of transcultural adaptation for American and West German managers, noted that "the management style of German and American managers within the same multinational corporation is more likely to be influenced by their nationality than by the corporation culture" (p. 436). Although Friday's work was done outside the health-care industry, some of his findings have implications for relationships across a broad range of work settings, including health-care services. For one, German and American managers hold different perceptions of their relationship with their employer. Germans see themselves as part of the corporate family, whereas many Americans do not identify with their corporation. Germans anticipate lifelong employment with the same company, whereas Americans may move to other companies should a good opportunity arise. Another difference is that American managers expend much energy to be liked, whereas Germans prefer being credible in their positions to being liked. To satisfy their need to be liked, American managers encourage informality in the workplace, such as by addressing peers, subordinates, or superiors by their first names; by asking personal questions; and by believing in equality and making themselves at home in one another's offices. For the German manager, credentials and education confirm their credibility and lead to power.

Issues Related to Autonomy

Germans and German Americans expect to receive respect for their work and for their ability to make decisions about their work. They find a hovering supervisor annoying and demeaning. Balancing control and freedom in the workplace is necessary to foster productivity in German and German American workers (Hall & Hall, 1990). American and German managers use different styles of assertiveness. Whereas Americans model their approach within the idea of equality or "fair play," Germans, who have no translation for "fair play," are assertive by putting other people in their

place. As in all languages, nuances and jargon can frustrate the individual whose second language comes only from the textbook and who does not understand idioms and colloquial expressions. The Germans' use of two distinctive manners of communication—*gesprach*, casual talking, and *besprechung*, the workplace discussion about performance—continues into the workplace.

Biocultural Ecology

Skin Color and Other Biological Variations

Germans range from tall, blond, and blue-eyed to short, stocky, dark-haired, and brown-eyed. Because many Germans have fair complexions, skin color changes, and disease manifestations can be easily observed. For those with fair skin, prolonged exposure to the sun increases the risk for skin cancer.

Diseases and Health Conditions

Because Germany is highly industrialized, Germans suffer from many of the same life-threatening diseases that afflict groups from other highly industrialized countries. Leading causes of death for German Americans follow the patterns of the dominant American society and include heart disease, cancer, cerebrovascular disease, and accidents. Because of the poor management of industrial contaminants, people in the Eastern regions often suffer from pollution-related illnesses (*Health Industry Today*, 2011). When assessing recent German immigrants, it is helpful for health-care providers to know where in Germany the patient resided before entering the United States.

HIV/AIDS rates in Germany are low (0.1% in 2007) (*CIA World Factbook*, 2011). Germany offers guidance and care to those who are infected, as well as a comprehensive prevention program for its citizens. Because prostitution has been legal in Germany since 1987, frequent health checks are required for those in this profession (*WordIQ Dictionary*, 2010).

In 1998, research localized the genetic cause for a syndrome of symptoms for a new form of myotonic muscular dystrophy. A second study conducted in Minnesota, Texas, and Germany identified the same causative mutation (Mackle, 2001). This new form of the disease, called *DM2*, appears to be most common in Americans of German descent (Mackle, 2001).

Another genetic disease, hereditary hemochromatosis, is also found in German Americans. Hemochromatosis, a toxic level of iron accumulation, can cause diabetes, chronic fatigue, liver disease, impotence, and even heart attacks. The disorder is due to a mutation in the *HFE* gene located on chromosome 6. German Americans can avoid, prevent, and treat these maladies with genetic testing and early diagnosis. Hemochromatosis is treatable through the removal of iron through phlebotomy (withdrawal of blood or bloodletting). The person can expect a normal life expectancy with aggressive treatment. Diagnosis can be established through a blood test known as an *iron profile*.

Sarcoidosis, a disorder found mostly in women between the ages of 20 and 40, occurs in all races, but people of German descent are at a higher risk (Gottfried, 2001). Sarcoidosis causes persistent cough or no symptoms. The cause is unknown, but doctors speculate that it involves an adverse reaction of the immune system; the diagnosis is often missed.

Dupuytren's disease, a slowly progressive disorder, is a deformity of the hand in which the fingers are contracted toward the palm. This often results in a functional disability. Dupuytren's disease is frequently found in people of German descent. Affecting mostly older males, the disease causes the synthesis of excessive amounts of collagen. The excess collagen is deposited in a ropelike fashion from the palm into the fingers, permanently fixing the fingers in a state of flexion. Although the cause is uncertain, Peyronie's disease is often found in people with Dupuytren's disease (NIH, n.d). A benign plaque forms within the erectile tissue of the penis, which causes it to bend, resulting in reduced flexibility and causing pain during erection. This can prohibit sexual intercourse. The disease occurs mostly in middle-age men and often in men who are related, suggesting that genetic factors may increase the likelihood of developing this disease. Some researchers have theorized that Peyronie's disease may be an autoimmune disorder. A surgical approach to treatment has had some success. Candidates for surgery are men with curvature so severe that it prevents sexual intercourse.

Lowenfels and Velema (1992) examined the incidence of cholelithiasis in people from Denmark, Germany, India, Italy, Norway, and England. Although the study revealed prevalence rates from each of these countries, Norway ranked first and Germany ranked second for the overall incidence of gallbladder disease. Although the study addresses populations in Germany, the results may be applicable to Germans in other parts of the world.

A cohort study of white men of Norwegian, Swedish, and German ancestry conducted between 1966 and 1986 revealed an increased risk of stomach cancer among foreign-born and first-generation German Americans living in the north-central states (Kneller et al., 1991). This study suggests an interrelationship among ethnic, geographic, and dietary factors as the cause. High concentrations of immigrants from northern Europe, which includes the high-cancer-risk countries of Germany and Scandinavia, settled in the north-central region of the United States. Low educational attainment; employment in laboring and semiskilled occupations; and ingestion of salted fish (at least once a month), bacon, milk, cooked cereal, and apples increased the risk factors for the foreign-born and first-generation individuals. These findings support the theory of ethnic risk. Subjects who smoked 30 or more cigarettes per day exhibited a five-fold risk for the development of stomach cancer. In addition, those who smoked a pipe and chewed smokeless tobacco had an increased risk for stomach cancer (Kneller et al., 1991).

According to Zielenski and colleagues (1993), an increased incidence of cystic fibrosis (CF) is found among Hutterite German–speaking communal farmers living on the Great Plains of North America. Mutations in the Hutterite population, a genetic isolate with an average inbreeding coefficient of about 0.05, exhibit an increased prevalence of CF carriers. Maternal-child health professionals providing care to this ethnic group can assist patients by encouraging genetic counseling to ensure early diagnosis of CF in their infants.

Hemophilia, a genetic bleeding disease found in Germany and the United States, can be traced from Queen Victoria of England, who, through a gene mutation, passed hemophilia to her son and through her daughters (Kilcoyne, 2004). The disease was then spread into Europe through the royal families, including the House of Hohenzollern, which consisted of kings and emperors of Prussia, Germany, and Romania. World War I led to the German Revolution, and the House of Hohenzollern abdicated, ending the monarchy. Historians believe that the source of hemophilia in the United States is a woman in Plymouth, New Hampshire, most likely English. There are currently over 20,000 people in the United States with hemophilia, accounting for over 75 percent of all cases of hemophilia (CDC, 2011). As in the United States around 1993, those with hemophilia in Germany were contaminated with the AIDS virus through the administration of blood products and anticlotting factors. Health-care providers may want to be mindful of the German history of hemophilia and the AIDS issues while diagnosing bleeding issues in newly arrived German immigrants.

S. Maubach (personal communication, 2006) described the back pain experienced by schoolchildren who must carry their books everywhere during school sessions. No lockers are provided in the school building, so all supplies, including heavy books, are carried all day long. Only public transportation is available to transport children to school, and children must carry their books and personal belongings with them. Again, during medical examinations of newly arrived immigrant children complaining of back pain, the health-care provider should question whether this situation existed in their former school.

Variations in Drug Metabolism

Few research studies have been completed on variations in drug metabolism and interactions specific to people of German ancestry. Aggregate data on white populations report that there are no slow metabolizers of alcohol in this population (Levy, 1993). One study reported that 5 percent of Germans are poor metabolizers of debrisoquine (Levy, 1993), and therefore this group may need lower dosages of propranolol to control blood pressure.

High-Risk Health Behaviors

Germans are known for their breweries and their *Gasthäuser*, or "restaurant that serves spirits." Beer is also served at the pubs (*kneipen*). In Germany, drinking beer is a way of life. German youth can legally drink beer at age 16 and drive at age 18. Beer is served with meals, whereas water is rarely consumed. Sparkling mineral water (*mineralwasser*) is commonly served if water is requested by a patron. Even lactating mothers are encouraged to drink malt beverages to increase breast milk production. This long-standing tradition of beer consumption is not without its abuses.

Health-Care Practices

Germans, whether born in Germany or in the United States, share a love of nature. They enjoy the great outdoors. Fresh air and exercise are highly valued. Hiking, walking, swimming, skiing, cycling, soccer, horseback riding, and playing tennis are just a few of the activities enjoyed by people of German ancestry. Walking is a way of life. Sports are played for exercise and the pleasure of participating in group activities. Water sports are very popular and are encouraged among older people, disabled people, mothers, and small children. Because many German Americans are joiners, health club memberships appeal to German Americans.

Ruhezeit, or quiet time, is nearly sacred in Germany. This time-honored tradition occurs between 1 p.m. and 3 p.m. Monday through Saturday and all day Sunday. During this time, older Germans take naps, and older retired German Americans may follow this ritual as well. Stores in Germany close during this time period. Neighbors and friends are expected not to create noise, telephone, or interrupt in any other manner. This quiet time is often followed by *Kaffe and Kuchen*, coffee and cake time, around 4 p.m. (The German Connection, 2006).

Nutrition
Meaning of Food

Food is a symbol of celebration for Germans and is often equated with love. Food and food rituals are powerful identification symbols for ethnic groups. The diet of immigrants is modified by the availability of foods and their financial status. The desire to maintain ethnic food habits has prompted children and grandchildren of immigrants to retain their ethnic heritage.

Common Foods and Food Rituals

Traditional methods of food preparation with high-fat ingredients add to nutritional risks for many German Americans. Real cream and butter are used in German cooking. Gravies and sauces that are high in fat content, as well as fried foods, rich pastries, sausages, and boiled eggs, are only a few of the culinary favorites. Germans have traditional ways to prepare their favorite foods. Meats, turkey, chicken, pork, and fish are stewed, roasted, or marinated and are often served with gravies. Vegetables (fresh is preferred) are often served in a butter sauce. Foods are also fried in butter, bacon fat, lard, or margarine. *Bratwurst* (*currywurst*) served with curry ketchup and *pommes frites* (french-fried potatoes) with mayonnaise are found at the top of the list in Germany.

One-pot meals such as string beans and potatoes, *snipply* cabbage and potatoes, chicken pot pie, pork and sauerkraut, stews, and soups are served as family meals. Casseroles are also popular. Foods prepared with vinegar and sugar as flavorings are also favorites. Potato salad, cucumber salad, coleslaw, chow, pickled eggs, pickled cucumbers, cauliflower, tongue, and herring are common examples of favored foods prepared with these flavorings. Sour cream, mayonnaise, and mustards are used frequently in food preparation.

The nutritional habits of some Germans may be a significant health risk factor. Food is an integral part of a German's life. Food is served at celebrations and during visits and is taken on trips. The German infatuation with food can lead to overeating, which results in obesity. Children are rewarded for good behavior with food. Those who are ill receive Jell-O, egg custards, ginger ale, or tomato soup (not creamed) to settle their stomachs. Sending food with loved ones who will be away from the family for a time is quite common: Homemade cakes, cookies, and jams are a few of the offerings.

Nothing pleases German cooks more than witnessing people with hearty appetites at the table. Generous amounts of food are prepared, and second helpings are encouraged. Burping, with an apology, to honor the good food is acceptable at the German table (S. Maubach, personal communication, 2006). In choosing foods for German Americans, the health-care provider should consider cutting portion size, overcoming harmful food rituals, and reducing fat intake.

Some German American food practices reflect acculturation. For example, the rice pudding enjoyed by many German Americans is originally a European American dish. However, unlike European Americans who serve rice pudding as a common dessert dish, German Americans reserve it for special occasions such as weddings. Celebration versions of rice pudding often contain dried fruit, such as raisins or currants, rum for flavoring, or a meringue topping.

Corn, frequently served as a vegetable in North America, is not eaten in Germany, where it is considered food for farm animals. Visitors from Germany are often startled when corn is served to them, but once they taste it, they are easily converted. Many early German immigrants turned to farming to conquer starvation, raising grains (including corn), fruits, and vegetables that were popular in North America. Foods associated with special events such as weddings, holidays, and religious occasions are the last to yield to acculturation. German cooks produce their best culinary efforts for holidays. Weeks of baking and preparation often precede the actual holidays. Selection of foods for the meal, proper preservation, and artistic presentation of tasty dishes are attended with care.

Table 14-1 lists common foods in the German American diet, based on the author's experience,

Table 14-1 Common Foods in the German American Diet

Beverages	Rice pudding	Salami
Coffee (with sugar and cream)	*Springerle* (cookies)	Saage (veal)
Herbal teas	*Stollen*	Tongue
Kümmel (caraway seed)	Strudel	Veal
Light and dark beers	**Fish**	Venison
Schnapps	Anchovy paste	*Vonname* (smoked pork chop)
Steinhager (juniper beverage)	Carp (*karpfen*)	*Weissbratwurster*
White wine	Dover sole	Wild boar
Breads, Noodles, and	Pickled herring	**Preserves**
Dumplings	Roe	Apple butter
Rolls	Rollmops	Crabapple jelly
Dumplings	Smoked cisco	**Vegetables**
Knöpfle	**Fruits**	Beets
Potato dumplings	*Apfel* (apple)	Cabbage
Pretzels	Dried apples	Carrots
Pumpernickel	Dried pears	Celery root
Ribbles	*Madelkerr* (fruits)	Mushrooms
Spätzle	*Nüsse* (nuts)	Onions
Cheese	Prunes	Potatoes
Camembert	**Meats and Fowl**	Sauerkraut
Limburger	Bacon	White asparagus
Desserts	Beef	White radishes
Baumkuchen (tree trunk cake)	Bratwurst	**Miscellaneous**
Kranz (almond and hazelnut cake)	Chicken	Caraway seeds
Lebkuchen (honey cakes)	Duck	Castor sugar (pearl sugar)
Lübecker marzipan	Frankfurter	Cilantro
Pfannkuchen	Game bird	Honey
Pfefferkuchen (gingerbread)	*Gänseleberwurst* (goose liver)	Juniper berries
	Goose	Molasses
	Knockwurst	Paprika
	Liver dumplings	Vanilla beans
	Mettwurst	
	Mutton	
	Pork	

REFLECTIVE EXERCISE 14.2

Marian Graybill is a 27-year-old single mother. She has a 6-year-old daughter. Marian has been diagnosed with hypertension and is on Lasix 20 mg daily, which she takes only when she has swelling in her feet. Her doctor has asked her to be mindful of her sodium consumption. Marian's family lives in Germany and delights in sending packages of German food favorites. Often these are envelopes of dried seasonings that can be added to fish and meat. The sodium content of the seasonings is very high. Marion loves these dishes and prepares them for her daughter and herself. It is important to Marian that her daughter be familiar with food from Germany.

1. Marian is only 27 years old and is hypertensive. Understanding Marian's need to enculturate her daughter in light of German cooking, how would she be impressed with the importance of following the doctor's request to lower her sodium intake?
2. What could be done to help ensure that she will take her Lasix on a daily basis?

personal interviews, the literature, and a marketing analysis conducted at a meeting of a local DANK (*Deutsch Amerikanischer National Kongress* [German American National Congress]) for a new food chain planning an international market concept. DANK has been in existence in the United States since 1959 (DANK, 2010).

Dietary Practices for Health Promotion

Because of apartment living in Germany, many Germans love to garden, and they bring this love to the United States. Gardening provides the fresh vegetables that Germans enjoy. What is not eaten is canned, pickled, dried, or frozen for future use.

Having a full larder is very important to Germans and German Americans.

A few foods are used to prevent or treat illnesses. Prune juice is given to relieve constipation. A special soup from fresh tomato juice is used to treat a migraine headache. Ginger ale or lemon-lime soda relieves indigestion and settles an upset stomach. After gastrointestinal illnesses, a recuperative diet is administered to the sick family member, beginning with sips of ginger ale over ice. If this is retained, hot tea and toast are offered. The last step is coddled eggs, a variation of scrambled eggs prepared with margarine and a little milk. If these foods are tolerated, the sick person returns to the normal diet. Garlic and onions are eaten daily to prevent heart disease.

Nutritional Deficiencies and Food Limitations

The literature does not report any enzyme deficiencies or food intolerances specifically related to Germans. However, those of lower socioeconomic status may lack the financial ability to purchase foods essential for a nutritious diet.

Pregnancy and Childbearing Practices

Fertility Practices and Views Toward Pregnancy

In her book, *Life at Four Corners*, Coburn (1992) captured a bit of the history of maternal-child health in Block Corners, Kansas, a German Lutheran settlement of the mid-19th century. She provided a glimpse into the daily life of a woman in the Midwest: "A woman's role within the family centered on supporting the farm economy, childbearing, child rearing, and providing continuous services to feed, clothe, and nurture all family members" (p. 88).

Coburn's research showed that large families were common in Block Corners. Farms needed a labor force, and a large family often addressed that need. First-generation Block Corners women had at least seven or eight children. Babies were born every 2 years, and miscarriages and stillbirths were common. Accidents and disease claimed the lives of many children. Second-generation women had an average of 6.5 children, and third-generation women had an average of 2.5 children. This drop in birth rate of the third generation is attributed to assimilation.

Bearing large numbers of children, coupled with the hard life of supporting a farm economy and continuously providing food, clothes, and nurturing, caused physical strain on women, which often limited their longevity. In spite of these hardships, birth control was not sanctioned by the church until the 1930s and was not openly discussed. Educational information was passed verbally from one woman to another. Although it was known that breastfeeding decreased the likelihood of pregnancy, little else about pregnancy prevention was known.

Large families are rare in Germany. Most couples have only two children. This may be a result of limited living space; most Germans rent apartments rather than own homes. The German government recognizes the importance of family and provides child-rearing allowances and work leaves. The state pays a monthly allotment for each child up to 18 months of age and allows a child-rearing leave of 3 years for each child. Employers cannot sever parents from their employment, and leave time counts toward their pension. These benefits also apply to the care of sick family members (Helmert, Beck, Marstedt, Muller, Muller, & Hebel, 1997; Kappler & Grevel, 1993). Family leave legislation in the United States is more restrictive. Although maternity or paternity leave may be available after childbirth or adoption, it is often provided without pay and for a shorter duration.

A variety of birth control practices and interventions for improving fertility among Germans are readily available. On the one hand, the German respect for authority and love for scientific facts and data encourage the use of methods to control, as well as to enhance, fertility practices. On the other hand, the use of medication or devices might be viewed as interrupting the natural progression of things. Cathy Seibold (Personal communication, 1995) explains, "These approaches may be contradictory to the German love and appreciation of the world of nature."

For German Catholics, the influence of religious beliefs on birth control matters should not be overlooked. Heterologous artificial insemination, use of contraceptive pills, and unnatural contraception are forbidden. In addition, therapeutic or direct abortion is forbidden as the unjust taking of innocent life. Teachings of Protestant sects on fertility control vary from no official position to forbidding the behavior (see the discussion under Spirituality).

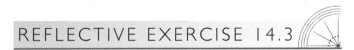

REFLECTIVE EXERCISE 14.3

Fourteen-year-old Lydia Shultz is 2 months pregnant. She is being seen in the health-care provider's office and is accompanied by her mother and grandmother. Both her mother and grandmother occasionally weep as they wait in the office with Lydia. They tell of their disbelief that Lydia is pregnant at 14 and how embarrassed they are. They ask for names of homes for unwed mothers.

1. Discuss the impact of teenage pregnancy on this German American family.
2. Understanding the German American family culture, how can this family be helped through this life crisis?

Prescriptive, Restrictive, and Taboo Practices in the Childbearing Family

Germans share some of the prescriptive, restrictive, and taboo practices of other cultures concerning pregnancy. Some examples of prescriptive practices include getting plenty of exercise and increasing the quantity of food to provide for the fetus. Some restrictive practices include not stretching and not raising the arms above the head to minimize the risk of the cord wrapping around the baby's neck.

Predicting the sex of the child was, and may still be, an important practice. For example, if the child is carried low, it is a girl; if the child is carried high, it is a boy. If the mother is "all out in the front," it is a girl, and if the mother is broad in the back, it is a boy.

A review of the literature and personal interviews did not reveal any prescriptive, restrictive, or taboo practices related to the birthing process. Birthing rooms that allow fathers and other family members to be present are popular among German Americans. In Germany, midwives commonly deliver babies ("Birth and Midwifery in Germany," 2011). The author's grandmother, who assisted with many home deliveries in the 1930s and 1940s, related one belief concerning the delivery of an infant. A child born with the membrane (the amniotic sac, also known as a *veil*) over its head is believed to be a special child, a belief shared by many cultures.

Prescriptive practices for the postpartum period include getting plenty of exercise and getting fresh air for the baby; if the mother is breastfeeding, she should eat foods that enhance the production of breast milk. Many believe that a new baby will soon arrive in the household that is visited first by a newborn. The author's mother often said, "Come visit us, but go somewhere else first."

Death Rituals

Death Rituals and Expectations

Germans and German Americans traditionally observe a 3-day period of mourning activities after the death of a family member. The body of the deceased is prepared and "laid out" in the home, where support from family and friends is readily available. Neighbors come to do the chores and to sit with the family of the deceased until the burial. A short service is held in the home before the body is taken to the church, where family and friends can attend a funeral service. After the church services, the body is taken to the cemetery for burial. After a short graveside service, the minister invites everyone in attendance to the home of the deceased for food.

As embalming practices emerged at the turn of the 20th century and funeral homes became more popular, particularly in the urban areas, this tradition changed. Today, German Americans usually have a family funeral director. The family may go to the funeral home together to select a coffin. Following the directions of loved ones about what should be done after their death is very important. Careful selection of the clothes to be worn by the deceased and the flowers that represent the immediate family is equally important. These selections are based on their knowledge of the deceased's way of life and on preserving the family's reputation and good name. Even in death rituals, Germans are quick to judge the quality of attention given to these details. The author can recall her family's suspicion about the possibility that a certain family in the community took shortcuts to decrease the cost spent on the funeral process. The insinuation was that the family pocketed the money instead of honoring the family member.

Responses to Death and Grief

The viewing provides an opportunity for family, friends, and acquaintances to view the body; offer their condolences; and extend their offers of assistance should the family need help in the future. Crying in public is permissible in the author's family, but in some German American families, the display of grief is done privately. A tradition of wearing black or dark clothing when attending a viewing or a funeral may be expected of both family and friends. Another expectation is that the bereaved family limits socialization activities for the following several months.

The traditions that surround the provision of food for the mourners have changed over the years. From the 1940s through the early 1960s, women in the neighborhood prepared the food and served it as people arrived at the home following the burial. More recently, families have become the primary providers of food and may hire caterers to prepare food or use a restaurant, as is done in Germany, where homes are too small to accommodate large groups of people.

For Germans and German Americans, death is seen as part of the life cycle, a natural conclusion to life. Individuals who embrace a set of religious beliefs may look forward to a life after death, often a better life. Death is a transition to life with God. Because illness is sometimes perceived as a punishment, the length and intensity of the dying process may be seen as a result of the quality of the life led by the person.

Spirituality

Dominant Religion and Use of Prayer

Martin Luther launched the Reformation in the early 16th century. Ninety percent of the population has some religious affiliation. Protestants and Catholics share equal portions of the population (33 percent). Other religions of German Americans include Judaism (the third largest population of Jews in Western Europe), Islam, and Buddhism (Solar Navigator, 2006). Similar to the United States, Germany has no state church; church and state remain separate. Religion is seen as a personal matter for German Americans, but those with an active interest in religion often discuss their beliefs with others (CultureGram, 1994).

A provision made by the Basic Law of Germany guarantees that "freedom of faith and conscience as well as freedom of creed, religious, or other beliefs, shall be inviolable. The undisturbed practice of religion shall be guaranteed" (Kappler & Grevel, 1993). Although there is no state church in Germany, churches, as independent public corporations, have a partnership relationship with the state. They can claim state grants, which in turn support schools and kindergartens. Churches can levy taxes on their membership, but the taxes are collected by the state. German churches also serve a charitable and social purpose by running nursing homes, retirement centers, hospitals, schools, training centers, and consultation and caring services.

Table 14-2 reflects the formal positions or the relationships between spiritual beliefs and health practices of several Protestant religions and the Roman Catholic Church. The Jewish, Muslim, and Greek Orthodox faiths are addressed in other chapters. Health-care providers must recognize that individuals' decisions may vary from the formal position of their religious groups. Therefore, the table serves only as a guide, not as an exclusive basis for decision making in health care.

Most German religious philosophies do not divorce physical health from the actions of God. Many hold the view that God works through health-care providers as well as through the resources of medicine. Prayer is used to ask for healing, for effectiveness of treatments, for strength to deal with the symptoms of the illness, and for acceptance of the outcome of the illness. Prayers are often recited at the sickbed, with all who are present joining hands, bowing their heads, and receiving the blessing from the clergy.

Reading the Bible is also an important spiritual activity. Most German and German Americans have a family Bible, which is passed down through the generations. It serves as spiritual comfort and as a reservoir of family historical data such as the dates of births, marriages, and deaths.

Meaning of Life and Individual Sources of Strength

Individual sources of strength for most Germans and German Americans are their beliefs in God and in nature. Although they may not attend church on a regular basis, a German's faith is deep. Family and other loved ones are also sources of support in difficult times. Home, family, friends, work, church, and education provide meaning in life for individuals of German heritage. Family loyalty, duty, and honor to the family are strong values.

Spiritual Beliefs and Health-Care Practices

Teachings of the churches joined by German people provide direction and counsel on many health-care issues. Many of these churches have taken a formal position on abortion, artificial insemination, and prolongation of life. The church prescribes when individual choice is important in deciding on accepting or refusing treatments and provides advice when seeking spiritual counseling.

Health-Care Practices

Health-Seeking Beliefs and Behaviors

Germans receive regular medical and dental checkups, immunizations, and routine screening because most of the population is covered by statutory health insurance. Germany has one of the slowest-growing economies in Europe. Supporting the East German modernization, high unemployment, and a growing aging population since the mid-1990s have stressed the economy. In addition, Germany has faced health-care reform, embracing an approach that mirrors the United States' HMOs with protest from German physicians, similar to the reactions of physicians in the United States. The health-care systems are sharing more similarities than in the past. Germans are facing challenges of access experienced in the United States.

Responsibility for Health Care

Although health care in Germany is considered "the individual's own responsibility, it is also a concern of the society as a whole" (Kappler & Grevel, 1993, p. 353). The average life expectancy in Germany is 76.41 years for men and 82.57 years for women versus 75.78 years for men and 80.81 years for women in the United States. Germany's infant mortality rate of 3.95 per 1000 infants is comparable with the United States' infant mortality rate of 6.41 per 1000 (*CIA World Factbook*, 2011).

Women in the family often administer remedies and treatments. In traditional families, the mother usually sees that children receive checkups, immunizations, and vitamins. German Americans use a variety of over-the-counter drugs. C. M. Weicksel (personal communication, 1995) summed up the practice as "people tend to self-medicate with over-the-counter drugs until these medications are ineffective; then they go to the doctor." The use of over-the-counter drugs may stem from the belief that individuals are responsible for their own health and from the beliefs and traditions about the treatment of sickness learned within the family system. In Germany, however, over-the-counter drugs can be purchased only from a pharmacy, which increases the cost to the consumer. Therefore, over-the-counter drugs are not as accessible to Germans as they are to German Americans. Today, prescription drugs are more complex, and numerous

Table 14-2 Positions of Roman Catholic and Selected Protestant Religions Regarding Various Health-Care Practices

Health-Care Practice	Baptist	Roman Catholic	Brethren	American Lutheran	Missouri Methodist	Presbyterian	Synod Lutheran	Wisconsin Lutheran	Church of Christ	Salvation Army
Administration of drugs, blood, and vaccine	Acceptable	Justifiable as long as for the good of the whole	Acceptable	Acceptable	Acceptable	Acceptable	Acceptable	Acceptable	No position	Acceptable
Biopsies	Acceptable	Acceptable	Acceptable	Encouraged	Acceptable	Acceptable	Acceptable	Acceptable	No position	Acceptable
Loss of limb	Acceptable	Acceptable (principle of totality)	Acceptable	Acceptable	Acceptable	Acceptable	Has no position	Acceptable if done to save a life	No position	Acceptable
Transplants	Acceptable	Permissible	Acceptable	Encouraged	Acceptable	No position	Acceptable	Acceptable	No position	Acceptable
Prolongation of life	Discouraged in clearly terminal cases	Advocates taking into consideration benefit and burden to patient	Allowed to preserve individual's freedom and dignity	Extraordinary and heroic efforts sometimes deemed justifiable	When death inevitable, allows freedom to direct or encourage a physician to remove artificial support systems	Quality of life viewed as more important than length of life	Permitted only in extraordinary cases after careful deliberation	Disapproves of prolongation of the agony of death	No position	Acceptable if prolongation of life is desired by individual; comfort and appropriate measures should be provided
Euthanasia	Left to individual choice for no extraordinary measures	Not permissible	Decision left to doctor and family	Advocates death with dignity	Discouraged	Favors right to die	Opposed	Advocates use of drugs to relieve pain	Favors death by natural means and processes	Unacceptable
Donation of body parts	Encouraged	Deemed justifiable	Acceptable	Encouraged	Encouraged	No official position	No position	Acceptable	No position	Acceptable
Autopsy	Encouraged	Permissible	Acceptable	Strongly approved	Encouraged	No position	Left to individual choice	Relatives encouraged to give permission	No position	No restriction
Disposal of body	Burial or cremation permitted	Burial favored; cremation permitted if unusual circumstances exist (e.g., infection)	Left to individual or family	Burial favored, but cremation acceptable	Burial and cremation permitted, and customary procedures for disposal of body after use for research	Burial favored, but cremation acceptable	Allowed if done with honor	Burial favored, but cremation permitted under epidemic conditions	No position	Left to individual and family

Eugenics, genetics	No position	Opposed	Advised for assessment of serious illness	Acceptable; marriage and procreation discouraged if offspring likely to inherit hereditary defects	Research and parental counseling encouraged	No position	No position	Viewed as great blessing	No position
Birth control	Left to individual choice	Only natural means permitted	Acceptable	Disapproved	Family planning favored	Acceptable	No position	Unacceptable, except if hereditary defects likely to occur	No position
Artificial insemination	No restrictions for mates	Viewed as illicit	Left to individual choice	Acceptable	Theological barriers	No position	No position	Left to husband and wife; adoption acceptable	No position
Sterility tests	Acceptable	Permissible	Left to individual choice	Approved if necessary to ensure health of mother	Acceptable, but counsel with physician and pastor encouraged	No position	Left to individual choice	Acceptable	No position
Therapeutic abortion	Left to individual choice	Permitted only indirectly (e.g., removal of uterine cancer)	Left to individual choice	Approved if necessary to ensure health of mother	Acceptable, but counsel with physician and pastor encouraged	Justifiable by circumstances (e.g., rape or incest)	Permitted to save life of mother	Justifiable to save mother's life or in case of rape or incest	Decision of physician accepted
Abortion on demand	Left to individual choice	Prohibited	Opposed	Opposed	Same as above	Deemed justifiable by circumstances (e.g., rape or incest)	No position	Opposed	Opposed

over-the-counter medications have become more accessible to German Americans. The two used in combination may lead to dangerous drug interactions for those who practice self-medication. Thus, health-care providers need to ascertain if over-the-counter and folk remedies are being used to determine whether there are contraindications with prescription medications.

Folk and Traditional Practices

Among the early German immigrants, women practiced folk medicine, which often included singing and the laying on of hands. Families passed this knowledge on from mother to daughter. Common natural folk medicines included roots, herbs, soups, poultices, and medicinal agents such as camphor, peppermint, and spirits of ammonia. The author's mother and grandmother had an arsenal of remedies that were a combination of folk and over-the-counter preparations to treat a variety of ills. A list of these remedies and their uses can be found in Table 14-3.

Magico-religious folk medicine includes "powwowing," *brauche*, use of special words, and the wearing of charms. Some stories told by the author's mother referred to the powwow sessions she attended as a child to cure her frequent ear infections and her inability to gain weight. She attempted to cure a plantar's wart by rubbing it with a sliced onion and burying the onion where water flowed. The expectation was that as the onion deteriorated, so would the wart. When this failed, an appointment with the podiatrist soon followed. Another belief is that carrying a nut from the buckeye tree guarantees health. Some individuals have a strong belief that being hexed brings bad luck, which can manifest itself as illness. The extent to which today's German American population continues to follow these practices is unknown.

Barriers to Health Care

Germany blends a private health-care delivery system with universal coverage and social solidarity. The financing is inexpensive and equitable with portable coverage. People are never uninsured in Germany, so families are not burdened with hefty health-care bills (Underwood, 2009). In the United States, access to care is limited for those who live in rural areas. Although efforts are being made to reduce these barriers, economic and geographic barriers to health care continue to exist for a large number of German Americans.

Cultural Responses to Health and Illness

When asked to describe a German's response to pain, the word most often used is "stoic." Even when Germans are experiencing pain, they may continue to carry out their family and work roles. Research reveals that older German Americans are less likely to complain, more accurate in their description of pain, and more likely to follow the physician's advice (Wright, Saleebey, Watts, & Lecca, 1983). Although results of studies that examine ethnicity and pain remain problematic, one significant finding does exist: Regardless of the degree of acculturation, individual expressions of pain may follow those of the more traditional members of the culture. Thus, health-care providers may not be able to identify verbal or nonverbal cues among Germans. Careful interviewing and astute observation must be used to accurately assess the level of pain experienced by Germans.

Although both Germany and the United States provide care for the mentally ill, mental illness may continue to be viewed as a flaw and is perhaps not as acceptable to German Americans as it is for some other cultures. If this is accurate, members of this group may be slow to seek help because of the lack of acceptance as well as the stigma attached to needing help. German people's discomfort with expressing personal feelings to strangers may impede the counseling process and influence the counseling methods used. The German need to discuss the past without expressing

Table 14-3 German Folk Remedies for Various Afflictions

Affliction	Remedy
Abrasions, burns	Vaseline
Boils	Black salve
Bumps and burns	Butter
Cleaning cuts and abrasions	Hydrogen peroxide
Colds	Vicks VapoRub as chest rub or placed in a vaporizer
Colds	Camphorated oil (chest rub; soft cloth covered with oil is placed over chest and neck area)
Colic in infants	Catnip and fennel (diluted in water and flavored with a little sugar)
Constipation	Castor oil
Cuts	Mercurochrome
Diaper rash	Cornstarch
Diarrhea	Paregoric in water
Earache	Warm oil
Headaches	Warm oil
Menstrual cramps	Hot tea
Muscle aches	Alcohol with wintergreen
Muscle stiffness	Hot or cold compresses
Nervousness	Spirits of ammonia in water
Sunburn	Noxzema
Teething in infants	Whiskey in water (rubbed on infant's gums)
To enhance health	Cod liver oil
Toothache	Oil of cloves
Upset stomach	Hot tea with peppermint oil

personal feelings should be recognized within the counseling process.

Even though the people with mental illness have been assimilated into American culture, many may remain stigmatized in the German American culture. Since the passage of the Americans with Disabilities Act, more people are aware of the needs of the physically disabled, including acculturated German Americans. Physical disabilities caused by injury are more acceptable to German Americans than those caused by genetic problems. The latter bring feelings of guilt and a sense of responsibility.

Returning people to the highest level of health possible appeals to the German nature. The European American culture believes in helping people, including older people, to recover their health. Rehabilitation has become an integral part of patient care in both Germany and the United States, and rehabilitation facilities abound in both countries. In Germany, rehabilitation is also a vital component of care in psychiatric facilities (Wuerth, 1993). For Germans, the rapid return to their roles in society is paramount, and rehabilitation represents the transition to these roles.

Once others become aware of illness, sick individuals are excused from their responsibilities. Even through German Americans are allowed to assume the sick role, some individuals may have difficulty doing so. The stoicism of some may delay their seeking medical care and allow the problem to become more severe or chronic. This may result in the need for more complex treatments for relief of symptoms. As individuals recover, they are expected to relinquish the sick role and resume their normal responsibilities. It is important to note that it is the physician in Germany who determines whether a person can attend work. The physician determines the length of absence from work, and the employer must provide employees with their salaries.

Blood Transfusions and Organ Donation

German Americans identify blood transfusions, organ donation, and organ transplants as acceptable medical interventions. Many religions followed by German Americans provide guidance on each of these issues. See Table 14-2 for a more complete description of these beliefs and practices.

Health-Care Providers
Traditional Versus Biomedical Providers

In Germany, folk medicine and midwifery are highly revered. Midwifery is a "family-based tradition" (Coburn, 1992, p. 93), with skills passed from mother or close female relatives to daughters. Through interviews with the residents of Block Corners, Kansas, Coburn was able to describe the work of a local midwife, Grandma Block. In addition to her midwifery, she passed along folk remedies for a variety of illnesses. The local physicians respected Grandma Block. She knew when their skills and knowledge were needed, and if she called them, they knew to come immediately (Coburn, 1992). Adolescent girls were pressed into service when illness and childbirth occurred. Older or widowed women also provided help in preparing food, cleaning house, and nursing the sick in families of both relatives and nonrelatives. Currently, in Germany, medical-care regulations deem that a physician must have a midwife (*Hebamme*) present during a birth. However, a physician does not have to be present if the midwife is doing the delivery ("Birth and Midwifery in Germany," 2011). This is the opposite of the practice in the United States, where a physician must be present if the birth is complicated. In Germany, alternative medicine such as acupuncture and homeopathy is used also during childbirth to control pain.

The use of certified nurse-midwives is currently growing in the United States. Choosing a nurse-midwife over an obstetrician is a personal, not a cultural, decision for German Americans. German Americans accept the care of health-care providers of the opposite gender. However, this is probably due to cultural indoctrination rather than an ethnic mandate.

Status of Health-Care Providers

Health-care providers hold a relatively high status among Germans. This admiration stems from the German love of education and respect for authority. German Americans appreciate the status symbols of money, power, and institutional affiliations held by these professionals. German families are proud to have a health-care provider in their midst, and it is common for family members to seek counsel from them. Because Germans may find asking for help difficult, they may feel more comfortable confiding in a family member.

Health-care providers' strange language, unusual practices, and "secret" body of knowledge often create barriers to forming relationships with patients. Because of their indoctrination into the culture of the health professions, health-care providers can become shortsighted and fail to meet the personal needs of German patients. To deliver culturally conscious health care, providers must understand their own ethnic and professional culture as well as the ethnic cultures of their patients. Today, the entry of more women into nontraditional work roles in health care has forced changes in the health-care environment in the United States.

REFERENCES

Acton, R. (1994). A remarkable immigrant: The story of Hans Reimen Claussen. *The Palimpsest, 75*(2), 87–100.

Birth and midwifery in Germany. (2011). *Midwifery Today*. Retrieved from http://www.midwiferytoday.com/international/Germany.asp

Boorstin, D.J. (1987). *Hidden history*. New York: Harper & Row.

Centers for Disease Control and Prevention (CDC). (2010). *Hemophilia*. Retrieved from http://www.cdc.gov/ncbddd/hemophilia/facts.html

CIA World Factbook. (2011) Germany. Retrieved from https://www.cia.gov/library/publications/the-world-factbook/

Coburn, C.K. (1992). *Life at four corners*. Overland Park, KS: University of Kansas Press.

CultureGram. (1994). *Germany '95*. Provo, UT: David M. Kennedy Center for International Studies.

DANK. (2010). Retrieved from http://www.dank.org/

Domer, D. (1994). Genesis theories of the German-American two-door house. *Material Culture, 26*(1), 1–35.

Educational Aspects in the United States and Germany. (n.d.). Retrieved from http://sitemaker.umich.edu/schubert.356/kindergarten

European Education Directory. (2006). Retrieved from http://www.euroeducation.net/prof/germanco.htm

Friday, R. (1989). Contrasts in discussion behaviors of German and American managers. *International Journal of Intercultural Relations, 13*(42), 429–446.

Gelfand, D. (1988). Directions and trends in aging services: A German-American comparison. *International Journal of Aging and Human Development, 27*(1), 57–68.

The German Connection. (2006). *Autrata family's home page—Behavioral norms in German: Siestas and Sundays*. Retrieved from www.seoprofiler.com/analyze/autrata.com

Gottfried, M. (2001). *Duff's a true model patient*. Life and Breath Foundation. Retrieved from www.lifeandbreath.org/

German Noise Law. Retrieved from http://www.guardian.co.uk/world/2010/aug/16/germany-children-noise-law

Hall, E.T., & Hall, M.R. (1990). *Understanding cultural differences*. Yarmouth, ME: Intercultural Press.

Health Industry Today. (2011). Retrieved from http://health.einnews.com/news/germany-diseases

Helmert, U., Beck, B., Marstedt, R., Muller, G., Muller, H., & Hebel, D. (1997). Effects of decreasing sick leave benefits: Results of a survey of social health care insurance members. Retrieved from http://www.ncbi.nlm.nih.gov/entrez/query.fcgi?cmd=Retrieve&db=PubMed&list_uids=9440911&dopt=Abstract

Kappler, A., & Grevel, A. (1993). *Facts about Germany*. Frankfurt, Germany: Westermann, Braunschweig.

Kilcoyne, R. F. (2004). Hemophilia, musculoskeletal complications. Medscape, 10. Retrieved from http://emedicine.com/radio/topic909.htm

Kneller, R.W., McLaughlin, J.K., Bjelke, E., Schuman, L.M., Blot, W.J., Wachouslder, S., Gridley, G., Cochien, H.T., & Fraumeni, J.F. (1991). A cohort study of stomach cancer in a high-risk American population. *Cancer, 68,* 672–678.

Lamanna, M., & Riedmann, A. (2008). Marriages and families: Making choices in a diverse society. UK: Cengage.

Levy, R. (1993). Ethnic and racial differences in response to medicines: Preserving individualized therapy in managed pharmaceutical programmes. *Pharmaceutical Medicine, 7,* 139–165.

Lowenfels, A.B., & Velema, J.P. (1992). Estimating gallstone incidence from prevalence data. *Scandinavian Journal of Gastroenterology, 27*(11), 984–986.

Mackle, B. (2001). *New gene found for myotonia muscular dystrophy: Unusual mutation involved*. MDA News. Retrieved from http://www.mdaa.org/news/010803dm_mutation.html

McKinnon, M. (1993). In the American grain: The popularity of living history farm. *Journal of American Culture, 3,* 168–170.

National Institutes of Health (NIH). (n.d.). *Kidney and urological disease*. Retrieved from http://kidney.niddk.nih.gov/kudiseases/a-z.asp

Rowland, D. (1992). A fine nation. *Health Affairs, 11*(3), 205–215.

Salmons, J. (1988). In the social function of some southern Indiana German-American dialect stories. *Humor, 1 & 2,* 159–175.

Schied, F.M. (1993). *Learning in a social context*. DeKalb, IL: LEPS Press.

Solar Navigator. (2006). Retrieved from www.solarnavigator.net

Statistics, Canada. (2006). Retrieved from http://www12.statcan.ca/census-recensement/index-eng.cfm.

Texas State Historical Association. (n.d.). Retrieved from http://www.tshaonline.org/handbook/online/articles/ryh02

Underwood, A. (2009). *Health care abroad: Germany*. Retrieved from http://prescriptions.blogs.nytimes.com/2009/09/29/health-care-abroad-germany/

U.S. Census Bureau. (2005). *American community survey*. Retrieved from http://www.census.gov/acs/www/

U.S. Census Bureau. (2008). *American community survey*. Retrieved from http://factfinder.census.gov/servlet/IPTable

Weaver, W. (1979). Food acculturation and the first Pennsylvania-German cookbook. *Journal of American Culture, 2*(3), 420–429.

WordIQ Dictionary. (2010). Prostitution in Germany. Retrieved from http://www.wordiq.com/definition/Prostitution_in_Germany

Wright, R., Saleebey, D., Watts, R., & Lecca, P. (1983). Attitudes toward disabilities in a multicultural society. *Social Science and Medicine, 36,* 616–620.

Wuerth, U. (1993). An open psychiatric unit in the U.S. and Germany. *Journal of Psychosocial Nursing, 31*(3), 29–33.

Zielenski, J., Fujwara, T.M., Markiewicz, D., Paradis, A.J., Anacleto, A.I., Richards, B., Schwartz, R. H., Klinger, K., Tsui, L., & Morgan, K. (1993). Identification of the M1101K mutation in the cystic fibrosis transmembrane conductance regulator (CFTR) gene and complete detection of cystic fibroses mutations in the Hutterite population. *American Journal of Human Genetics, 52,* 609–615.

DavisPlus *For case studies, review questions, and additional information, go to*
http://davisplus.fadavis.com

Chapter 15

People of Haitian Heritage

Jessie M. Colin and Ghislaine Paperwalla

The authors would like to thank Ingrid Parenteau and Sheran Kegerise, graduate students at Barry University, for their assistance in the literature review and preparation of the manuscript.

Overview, Inhabited Localities, and Topography

Overview

Haiti, located on the island of Hispaniola between Cuba and Puerto Rico in the Caribbean, shares the island with the Dominican Republic. With a population of 9.7 million inhabitants, Haiti covers an area of 27,750 square kilometers (10,714 square miles), about the size of the state of Maryland (*CIA World Factbook,* 2011).

In 1492, Christopher Columbus landed on the island and named it *Hispaniola,* which means "Little Spain." Haiti, or *Ayti,* meaning "land of mountain," was given its name by the first inhabitants, the Arawak and the Caribe Indians. Before 1492, there were five well-organized kingdoms: the Magua, the Marien, the Xaragua, the Managua, and the Higuey (Dorestant, 1998). Two-thirds of Haiti contains mountains, great valleys, and extensive plateaus; small plains mark the rest of the country.

The capital and largest city, Port-au-Prince, has a population of over 800,000. Widespread unemployment and underemployment exist; more than two-thirds of the labor force do not have formal jobs owing to the marked decrease in assembly sector jobs. In addition, Haiti's economy suffered a severe setback when a magnitude 7.1 earthquake devastated its capital city, Port-au-Prince, in January 2010. About 80 percent of the population had already lived under the poverty line, with 57.4 percent living in abject poverty (*CIA World Factbook,* 2011). After the earthquake, the GDP per capita was $1200 (*CIA World Factbook,* 2011). Prior to the earthquake, two-thirds of Haitians depended on the agricultural sector, mainly small-scale subsistence farming, and are still vulnerable to damage from frequent natural disasters, exacerbated by the country's widespread deforestation. U.S. economic engagement under the Haitian Hemispheric Opportunity through Partnership Encouragement (HOPE) Act, passed in 2006, has boosted apparel exports investment by providing tariff-free access to the United States (*CIA World Factbook,* 2011).

The infant mortality rate is high, with 54.02 deaths per 1000 live births; the average life expectancy is 62.17 years (*CIA World Factbook,* 2011); and in 2008, only 70 percent of the urban population (50 percent in rural areas) had access to improved drinking water sources (WHO, 2010). The World Health Organization (WHO) estimated that prior to the disaster in 2010, diarrheal diseases accounted for 16 percent of deaths among children less than 3 years of age. In October 2010, an outbreak of cholera added to the devastation of the earthquake, killing an additional 3000 people and infecting approximately 130,000 more (*BBC News,* 2011).

The Haitian population in the United States is not well documented; this may be because of the U.S. Census Bureau's inability to track the large numbers of undocumented immigrants. According to the 2010 census, over 830,000 Haitians, or 0.3 percent of the population, live in the United States (U.S. Census Bureau, 2009). Most of them live in Florida, New York, Massachusetts, New Jersey, and Connecticut. However, some Haitian leaders and activists believe that close to 1.5 million Haitians live in the United States. An additional 122,000 live in Canada, of which 90 percent live in Quebec (Statistics Canada, 2006). Haitians, like other ethnic groups, are very diverse. They come from urban and rural Haiti and represent all socioeconomic classes. Factors affecting Haitians' acculturation and assimilation include variant cultural characteristics (see Chapter 1).

Heritage and Residence

Before the time of Columbus, the various indigenous tribal groups intermarried. With the arrival of Europeans, and then Africans, the people of Haiti became more diverse. Today, Haitians range from light- to dark-skinned, and social identity is shaped by sharp class stratification and color consciousness.

In 1697, Haiti came under French rule. By the end of the 18th century, the slave population numbered 500,000. In 1791, a slave insurrection broke the chain of slavery, and on January 1, 1804, Haiti gained its independence from France. The French plantation owners were removed and replaced by the generals of the indigenous Haitian Army, which ruled mercilessly (Louis-Juste, 1995). Agricultural workers and peasants were trapped in a semifeudal system: They were exploited by landowners, terrorized by the section chiefs of police, and forced to obey laws explicitly. The coffee fields of the peasants served as the primary source of revenue for the government coffers, thereby guaranteeing all government debt payments between 1826 and 1932 (Louis-Juste, 1995). These harsh conditions did not prevent the peasants from rising up against injustice and exploitation, as evidenced by the Goman uprising in 1820, the Acaau in 1880, and the peasant movement of Jean Rabel (Louis-Juste, 1995).

Haitian immigrants have a sense of national pride, including a high level of self-esteem regarding their blackness, although in both public and private discourse, they may focus on color and class division—two painful wedges within Haitian society.

Haiti's independence from France in 1804 did not resolve the division among the descendants of French colonists, the African slaves, and the core of the population, who were largely of African descent and culture. Many members of the upper class used the markers of **mulatto** (color), the French culture, and the French language to differentiate themselves from the lower class, who were mostly black and **Creole** and spoke a predominantly African language.

Ti Manno, a Haitian singer who migrated to New York, used satire and irony to expose and deride the type of thinking that divides Haitians in Haiti and abroad. The following lyrics depict the turmoil and struggle that promote the division within the Haitian society (Jean-Baptiste, 1985):

The Black Man
Neg Kwens dil pa Kanmarad neg Brooklyn.
Neg Potopwens dil pa anafe ak neg pwovens.
Mon Che se-m nan fe yon ti pitit.
M'rayi ti pitit la
A fos li led.
Li nwa tankou bombon siwo.
Nen-l pa pwenti.
Ti neg mwe ala nou pa gen chans o.
La vi nou toujou red o.
Nou deyo, pi red.
Se neg nwe cont milat o.
Nou deyo nap soufri.
Nou lakay se pi red.

Translation:
Haitians in Queens feel superior to those who live in Brooklyn.
Haitians in Port-au-Prince despise those who live in the provinces.
My dear, my sister had a little baby.
I hate this little kid.
This baby is ugly.
He is as dark as sugarcane syrup cake.
His nose is not pointy.
We Haitians, we are so unlucky.
Life is always hard for us.
Away from home we suffer more.
It's black against mulatto.
Abroad we suffer.
At home it is even worse.

Despite independence, colonial prejudices about skin color have persisted. Internal social rivalries and the scale of Haitian mobility are tied to a European color, race, and class model. This model relates to skin pigmentation, hair texture, the shape of the nose, and the thickness of the lips. Whereas the structure of Haitian society continues to be built on a neocolonial model, relationships based on color are extremely complex. For example, dark skin color tends to be associated with underprivileged status. Although more black-skinned people have entered the circle of the privileged, most blacks are poor, underprivileged, and unemployed.

Haiti defines itself as a black nation. Therefore, all Haitians are members of the black race. In Haiti, the concept of color differs from the concept of race. The Haitian system has been described as one in which there are no tight racial categories but in which skin color and other phenotypic demarcations are significant variables.

In the 1940s, a black middle class emerged in Haiti and claimed to represent the majority. The development of this class and its rhetoric served as a springboard for Francois Duvalier, a rural physician who was elected president for a 4-year term in 1957. In 1964, he became president-for-life, using the issue of black empowerment and a promise to eliminate the color and class privileges of the mulattos. By the late 1970s, a group of dark-skinned, primarily American-educated and English-speaking technocrats had attained positions of prominence and influence in the government. However, the mulatto retained social prominence, and color continued to play a major role in the perception of class in Haiti.

Reasons for Migration and Associated Economic Factors

Haitian immigration and travel to the United States have continued for many years. Most, but not all, of those who emigrated were members of the upper class.

Before 1920, Haitians traveled to North America and Europe only for educational purposes. In 1920, the United States occupied Haiti, and the first wave of Haitian migration to North America soon followed. Over the next decade, more than 40,000 Haitian peasants were forced to go to Cuba and the Dominican Republic to cut sugarcane in the *bateys* (plantations). Haitian land was taken and used for apple and banana plantations, and many acres of land throughout Haiti were controlled by the United States (*Haiti: Early History to Independence*, 2007).

The late 1950s showed signs of weakness in Haitian agriculture. The peasants started leaving the provinces in search of work and a better life. Migrating to the capital, Port-au-Prince, they established Lasalin, the first slum of Port-au-Prince (Aristide, 1995). Today, over 2 million people live in and around the capital, many in large slums (*CIA World Factbook,* 2011). A significant turning point in Haitian migration occurred in 1964 when Duvalier declared himself president-for-life. As a result of his government, many Haitians began fleeing the island. These immigrants were primarily relatives of politicians who opposed the political philosophy of Duvalier. When Duvalier died in 1971, his son, Jean Claude (a.k.a. "Bébé Doc"), age 19, was appointed president-for-life. In addition, during this era, Haiti was suffering from economic deprivation, which motivated a major exodus of urbanites and peasants. Because many Haitians were unable to pay for their transportation, passports, and visas, some covertly emigrated to the United States in small sailboats.

From 1980 until recently, Haitian immigrants have been divided into two groups: those who have arrived in the United States legally and those who have entered through the underground. An explosion of immigration took place in 1980, in part because of a short-lived (April to October) change in U.S. immigration policy during the period of the Mariel boat lift from Cuba. The influx of Cuban refugees required that a special status be created by the State Department called "Cuban-Haitian entrant: status pending." According to Health and Rehabilitation Services, Haitian refugees were included in this status to prevent the policy from being discriminatory. This group of immigrants were referred to as **boat people**, a term associated with extreme poverty. Today, this term does not evoke as much negativism, although it continues as a reminder of a painful emigration period in Haitian history.

From the 1990s to 2010, political unrest, coups, and protests occurred. The tides of history were changing, and Jean-Bertrand Aristide was elected in the first democratically held election in many years. The democratic process did not last; in that same year, a coup d'état on Aristide and a hemisphere-wide embargo was imposed on Haiti. In 2001, Aristide was reelected in a flawed election. In February 2004, an armed rebellion led to the departure of President Jean-Betrand Aristide; an interim government took office to organize new elections under the auspices of the United Nations Stabilization Mission in Haiti (MINUSTAH). Continued violence and technical delays prompted repeated postponements, but Haiti finally did inaugurate a democratically elected president, Réné Preval, and parliament in May of 2006. Haitian migration took on a new face when the earthquake of January 2010 occurred. Today, more than 1 million people still remain displaced—380,000 being children (Simon, Kleschnitzki, & Shusterman, 2011). Although thousands of Haitians remain in an immigration holding pattern since before the earthquake, 55,000 Haitians have gained family visas but continue on waiting lists because of immigrations quotas (Zissis, 2010). The Dominican Republic has accepted as many as 50,000 people since the earthquake (Paravisini, 2010). Since the earthquake, 2500 Haitians have been granted temporary resident visas or permits allowing them to go to Canada. In addition 3700 students and temporary workers from Haiti have been permitted to stay in that country (Power, 2010). France is home to approximately 80,000 Haitians and allowed for a temporary residence by undocumented Haitians soon after the disaster in Haiti (McKenzie, 2010).

Prior to the earthquake, more than two-thirds of the population was living on less than US$2 daily (PAHO, 2011). Approximately 250,000 people lost their lives in this catastrophic event, marked as one of the worst in world history. Roughly 2.8 million people were affected, and nearly 1.5 million became homeless. After one year, many countries and organizations, including the Pan American Health Organization (PAHO) and the World Health Organization (WHO) launched initiatives to assist Haiti in restructuring and rebuilding their infrastructure. A Post Disaster Needs Assessment (PNDA) was initiated on February 18, 2010, by the United Nations, the World Bank (2010), the European Commission, and the inter-American Development Bank, at the request of the prime minister of Haiti. This group led other groups in assessing restructuring needs (PAHO, 2011). Disease, structural instability, hunger, and an inability to reach all those outside of the city have been some of the many obstacles after the earthquake (Simon, Kleschnitzki, & Shusterman, 2011).

A special focus was placed on the 1.5 million people in IDP (internally displaced person) camps (PAHO, 2011). In late October 2010, there was an outbreak of cholera that required specific reporting and handling (PAHO, 2011). Many hospitals were totally destroyed, and many others were seriously damaged. The disposal of medical waste continues to pose an environmental risk to everyone in Haiti. Haiti has suffered a catastrophic tragedy that will take continued support from many to rebuild.

Educational Status and Occupations

Following Haiti's independence in 1804, the new rulers of Haiti began advocating French cultural patterns and replicating the French value system. A French model of education was informally adopted and codified in 1860, in accord with the Roman Catholic Church. This resulted in two major changes: The Catholic Church became the official church of Haiti, and Catholic missionaries became responsible for education. The accepted language for communication was now French. During this era, Creole, the language of the uneducated, was perceived as inferior. Social mobility was possible only for French-speaking Haitians. While the educated elite became acculturated into the European value system, the illiterate masses tended to perpetuate the traditional values and customs of their African heritage.

Even though Haitians value education, few are privileged enough to attain a formal education. The Haitian school system is based on the French model and offers free primary and secondary education. Public schools include those operated and controlled by religious orders as well as those under the direct jurisdiction of the Minister of Education. Children from families with financial means attend private schools. The educational model emphasizes liberal arts and humanities rather than technical and vocational studies.

The Haitian educational system continues to emphasize 19th-century values, which promote good manners, the classics, literature, philosophy, Latin, and Greek. It deemphasizes the physical and social sciences. The Haitian educational system is based on a two-level curriculum. In the first level, the student receives a certificate of primary education. To receive this certificate, the student must sit for a rigorous test, which includes spelling, reading comprehension, composition, Haitian history and geography, general knowledge, arithmetic, and biology. At this level, the student can speak, read, and write French at the basic level.

The next level consists of two parts: The first is reached after 6 years of secondary education. To receive this diploma, the student must pass examinations in French, English, and Spanish; Haitian literature and history; mathematics; and sciences such as physics, chemistry, biology, and botany. Students in the classical track also take Latin and Greek examinations. A student who has received the first-level certificate should be able to enter the first year of college in American schools. The second-level baccalaureate is likened to the first year of college in North America; the emphasis is on the liberal arts. Again, the student must pass an examination in all the areas covered in the first level, plus philosophy. The results of these national examinations are announced on the radio over a 2-day period or posted on a board in front of the school.

Although Haiti has several universities, they are mainly located in Port-au-Prince. Most of them are state universities. With proper credentials, anyone can enter the university system. However, since the early 1980s, only those in positions of influence have been able to benefit from the state universities. Haitian professionals mirror those of American society; they are lawyers, physicians, nurses, engineers, educators, electricians, plumbers, and construction workers.

The literacy rate, which means that those age 15 and over can read and write, is 52.9 percent (*CIA World Factbook,* 2011). The level of illiteracy continues to be a major concern in Haiti. Since 1940, the government has conducted several literacy programs. In 1948, Haiti had its first experience with community education. This public educational system was based on the growth model of development, a UNESCO education project, which duplicated experiences in Latin America (Jean-Bernard, 1983).

Among Haitian immigrants, women work in hotels, hospitals, and other service industries in domestic and nursing assistant roles. Men work as laborers and factory helpers. Many more Haitians are in the workforce today than there were in the early 1980s, although data for the years 1974 and 1994 from the U.S. Immigration and Naturalization Service (2006) revealed that a disproportionate number of legal Haitians were not employed. In addition, when comparing data by specific groups, a dramatic increase in the number of Haitians in all work environments is found. Data about the work structure of undocumented people are not available because these people technically are "underground" and do not exist.

In Haiti, most major industries are owned and operated by the government. Unemployment is 66 percent (*CIA World Factbook,* 2011). Those who are employed often work under such poor conditions that they have become unmotivated and take little pride in their work, which results in low productivity. In general, Haitians are entrepreneurial, operating their own shops, marketplaces, or schools. Among these entrepreneurs, the motivation, spirit, and pride in their work are readily apparent.

Communication

Dominant Language and Dialects

The two official languages in Haiti are French and Creole. Creole, a rich, expressive language, is spoken by 100 percent of the population, whereas French is spoken by 15 percent of the population. Since 1957, Creole has been the unofficially accepted language in the internal affairs of the Haitian government, but in

1987, during the Aristide presidency, it was designated in the Haitian Constitution as one of the official languages. Because Creole is the official language, it is used for internal communication within the island.

In contemporary society, the Haitian dilemma can best be understood through this dual-language system. Language is one of the vehicles used to depersonalize those of the lower classes. French is the dominant language of the educated and the elite, whereas Creole is the language of those who are suppressed, the lower classes. The emphasis on French served as a barrier to the early social dynamism that permitted Creole to develop and serve as a unifying force among the African slaves, who came from many different tribes and spoke different languages. In spite of its suppression in formal education, Creole has inspired a very rich and interesting oral literature comprising songs, proverbs, and tales. This oral literature is the most significant aspect of Haitian folklore.

Understanding the language dilemma and the literacy issues assists health-care providers in developing creative tools for educating Haitians. Some of these tools may include video programs, audiocassettes, and radio programs in Creole. Because of the masses of people who are unable to read, printed literature in Creole is not a helpful educational tool.

Cultural Communication Patterns

Haiti has an oral culture with a long tradition of proverbs, jokes, and stories reflecting philosophical systems. These are used to pass on knowledge, convey messages, and communicate emotions. For example, the Creole phrase *Pale franse pa di lespri pou sa* translates to "To speak French does not mean you are smart." *Crayon Bon Die pa gin gum* ("God's pencil has no eraser") conveys the concept of fatalism. Another proverb frequently used is *Sonje lapli ki leve mayi ou* ("Remember the rain that made your corn grow"), which means that one must show gratitude to those who have helped them or done good for them.

Haitians are very expressive with their emotions. By observing them, one can tell whether they are happy, sad, or angry. Haitians' communication patterns include loud, animated speech and touching in the form of handshakes and taps on the shoulder to define or reconfirm social and emotional relationships. Pain and sorrow are very obvious in facial expressions. Most Haitians are very affectionate, polite, and shy. Uneducated Haitians generally hide their lack of knowledge to non-Haitians by keeping to themselves, avoiding conflict, and, sometimes, projecting a timid air or attitude. They smile frequently and often respond in this manner when interacting with Americans or when they do not understand what is being said. Many may pretend to understand by nodding; this sign of approval is given to hide their limitations. Therefore, health-care providers must use simple and clear instructions. Because Haitians are very private, especially in health matters, it is inappropriate to share information through friends. Many may prefer to use professional interpreters who will give an accurate interpretation of their concerns. Most importantly, the interpreter should be someone with whom they have no relationship and will likely never see again.

Voice intonations convey emotions. Haitians speak loudly even in casual conversation among friends and family; the pitch is moderated in formal encounters. When the conversation is really animated, the conversants speak in close proximity and ignore territorial space, especially when emphasizing a point or an issue. Sometimes, the conversation is at such a high pitch and speed that, to an outsider, the conversation may appear disorganized or angry. Haitians love political discussions. In these instances, the conversation may appear stressful and hostile; however, to the participants, the conversation is enjoyable, motivating, and meaningful.

Traditional Haitians generally do not maintain eye contact when speaking with those in a position of authority. In the past, maintaining direct eye contact was considered rude and insolent, especially when speaking with superiors (e.g., children speaking with parents, students with teachers, or employees with supervisors). However, the influence of American education seems to be changing this trend. Most adults maintain eye contact, which means "We are on equal terms, no matter who you are. I respect you and you respect me as an equal human being." For children, however, the custom of not maintaining eye contact with superiors remains deferential. Thus, health-care providers may need to assist children in dealing with conflicting messages.

Haitians touch frequently when speaking with friends. They may touch you to make you aware that they are speaking to you. Whereas Haitian women occasionally walk hand-in-hand as an expression of their friendship, this trend is disappearing both in Haiti and in Haitian communities in North America. This behavior may be changing because of the concept of homosexuality, which is taboo within the Haitian culture.

Haitians greet one another by kissing and embracing in informal situations. In formal encounters, they shake hands and appear composed and stern. Men usually do not kiss women unless they are old friends or relatives. Children greet everyone by kissing them on the cheek. Children refer to adult friends as Uncle or Auntie out of respect, not necessarily because they are related by blood.

Temporal Relationships

The temporal orientation of Haitians is a balance among the past, the present, and the future. The past is important because it lays the historical foundation from which one must learn. The present is cherished and savored. The future is predetermined, and God is the only Supreme Being who can redirect it. One often hears *Bondye bon* ("God is good"), meaning if you conduct yourself conservatively and the right way, God will be there for you. The future is left up to God, who is trusted to do the right thing. In a study by Prudent, Johnson, Carroll, and Culpepper (2005), several of the informants voiced their belief in God's will when talking about whether or not they would survive being HIV positive and/or having AIDS.

Haitians have a fatalistic but serene view of life. Some believe that destiny or spiritual forces are in control of life events such as health and death, so they say, *Si Bondye vle* ("If God wants"). Given the belief in a predetermined path of life, one can understand this view. Haitians believe that they are the passive recipients of God's decisions. Health-care providers must be clear, honest, and open when assessing Haitian individuals' perceptions and how they perceive the forces that have an influence over life, health, and illness. Acceptance of these beliefs is an important factor in building trust and ensuring adherence.

Most Haitians do not respect clock time; flexibility with time is the norm, and punctuality is not valued. They hold to a relativistic view of time, and although they try, some find it difficult to respond to predetermined appointments. Arriving late for appointments, even medical appointments, is not considered impolite. In North America, Haitians may be more readily compliant with business appointments, but socially, the margin around expected time is very wide—anything or anyone can wait. It is not unusual to see an invitation to a social function listed with an invitation time an hour earlier than the actual time of the function. For example, a wedding invitation may say 6:00 p.m. when the ceremony is actually scheduled for 7:00 p.m. to ensure that all invitees are there on time. Health-care providers should be mindful of this time orientation by making reminder calls for appointments and encouraging the patient in a respectful and caring manner about the importance of timeliness. A thorough assessment of time and temporal view helps health-care providers to plan appointments so that clinic or office backlogs and disruptions are minimized.

Format for Names

Haitians generally have a first, middle, and last name—for example, Marie Maude Guinard. Sometimes the first two names are hyphenated as in Marie-Maude. The family name, or *nom de famille,* is very important in middle- and upper-class society; it helps to promote and communicate tradition and prestige. However, friends call individuals by their first names. Families usually have an affectionate name or nickname for individuals. The father, mother, grandparent, or any close family member gives this affectionate name at birth.

When a woman marries, she takes on her husband's full name. For example, if Marie-Carmel Guillaume marries Charles Guy Lespinasse, she is always called Mrs. Lespinasse. In an informal setting, she might even be called Mrs. Charles. She loses her name except on paper. Her name and identity are subsumed by her husband's name. This is a reflection of Haitian society in which women are considered subservient to men. Haitian names are primarily of French origin, although many Arabic names are now heard since the migration of Arabs and Jews to Haiti in the 1920s. Haitians are formal and respectful and, as such, should be addressed by their title: Mr., Mrs., Miss, Ms., or Dr.

Family Roles and Organization
Head of Household and Gender Roles

Traditionally, the head of the household was the man, but in reality, most families today are matriarchal. Haitian men prefer and choose to believe that they make the decisions, but most major decisions are made by the wife and/or mother, with the man remaining a distant figure with a great deal of authority. Today, joint decisions are common. The man is generally considered the primary income provider for the family, and governance, rules, and daily decision making are considered his province. Sociopolitical and economic life centers around men. Men are expected to be sexual initiators, and the concept of **machismo** prevails in Haitian life. Women are expected to be faithful, honest, and respectable. Men are usually permitted freedom of social interaction, a freedom not afforded to women. The opportunities offered in North America for women to become income providers, together with their observations of different male-female interactional styles, have encouraged many Haitian women to reject their native, subservient role. This change in the marital interaction has created much stress on marital relationships and an increase in domestic violence, although domestic violence remains one of those closeted issues that are not publicly discussed.

Prescriptive, Restrictive, and Taboo Practices for Children and Adolescents

Children are valued among Haitians because they are key to the family's progeny, cultural beliefs, and values. Children are expected to be high achievers because *Sa ki lan men ou se li ki pa ou* ("What's in your hand is what you have"). In other words, education can never be taken away from you. Children are expected to be obedient and respectful to parents and elders, which is their key to a successful future. They are not allowed to express anger to elders. **Madichon** is a term used when children are disrespectful; it means that their future will be marred by misfortune. Another proverb used to scare and compel children to behave is *Ti moun fwonte grandi devan baron* ("An impudent or insolent child will grow under the Baron's eye [Baron Samedi is the guardian of the cemetery in the voodoo religion] and therefore won't have a long life").

Physical punishment, which is often used as a way of disciplining children, is sometimes considered child abuse by American standards. Fear of having their children taken away from them because of their methods of discipline can cause parents to withdraw or not follow through on health-care appointments if such abuse is evident (e.g., bruises or belt marks). Haitians need to be educated about American methods of discipline and laws so that they can learn new ways of disciplining their children without compromising their beliefs or violating American laws.

Many parents feel confused about how to raise their children in the United States. Their authoritarian behavior is challenged in American society, which they perceive as being too permissive. They feel powerless in understanding how to raise their children in America while still retaining Haitian traditions. The liberal American approach to child rearing poses a great dilemma for Haitian children. They find themselves living in two worlds: the American world, which allows and supports self-actualization and oneness, and the Haitian world, which promotes silence, respect, and obedience.

In the summer, Haitian parents engage their children in certain health-promotion activities such as giving them *lok* (a laxative), a mixture of bitter tea leaves, juice, sugarcane syrup, and oil. In addition, children are also given *lavman* (enemas) to ensure cleanliness. This is supposed to rid the bowel of impurities and refresh it, prevent acne, and rejuvenate the body.

Because Haitian life is centered on males, particularly firstborns, the education of boys is different from that of girls. The family is more indulgent of the behavioral deviations of boys. Boys are given more freedom and are even expected to receive outside initiation in social and sexual life. However, girls are educated toward marriage and respectability. Their relationships are closely watched. Even when they are 16 or 17 years of age, they cannot go out alone because any mishap can be a threat to the future of the girl and bring shame to her family. These beliefs increase Haitians' frustrations and challenges of rearing their children, especially girls, in America.

Health-care providers need to be aware of these various challenges and be prepared to assist children and family members to work through these cultural differences, while still conveying respect for family and cultural beliefs. Health-care providers can play a significant role by helping children and their parents to better understand American practices.

Approximately 300,000 **restavec** children are in Haiti. *Restavec* is translated to mean "to live with." It was started as an economically motivated action to relieve some parents of the hardship of feeding, clothing, and paying for the education of their children by loaning them out to relatives (Saint-Domingue, 2011). Unfortunately, this has not proven to be true and has not met its original intent. *Restavec* children work long hours and rarely go to school. They are regularly abused. They usually eat scraps of food and sleep on the floor (Schaaf, 2009). Although they are not chained or locked up, they stay to avoid severe abuse and beatings (Schaaf, 2009). Sixty-five percent of the population of children are girls between 6 and 14 years old. After the earthquake, the incidence of *restavec* rose dramatically because many lost their parents or were abandoned (Schaaf, 2009). Organizations like International Organization for Migration (IOM) have started an initiative to end the *restavec* system (Saint-Domingue, 2011). Because of the homelessness and desperation after the quake, there has been a surge in the practice. In 2009, CNN aired a program describing the practice and posted it into a blog so people around the world would become aware of the situation (Schaaf, 2009). IOM is working to stop it, along with an organization headed by a man who was a *restavec* as a child: the Jean Robert Cadet Foundation (Saint-Domingue, 2011).

Family Goals and Priorities

The family is a strong component of the Haitian culture. The expression "Blood is thicker than water" reflects family connectedness. An important unit for decision making is the *conseil de famille,* the family council. This council is generally composed of influential members of the family, including grandparents. The family structure is authoritarian and includes linear roles and responsibilities. Any action taken by one family member has repercussions for the entire family; consequently, all members share prestige and shame.

The family system among Haitians is the center of life and includes the nuclear, consanguine, and affinal relatives, some or all of whom may live under the same roof. Families deal with all aspects of their members' lives, including counseling, education, crises, and marriage. Each family has its own traditions, which form the basis for a family's reputation and are generalized to all members of the family. The prestige of a family is very important and is based on attributes such as honesty, pride, trust, social class, and history. Even families who experience economic difficulties are well respected if they are from a *grande famille*. Wealthy families who have no historical background or tradition are referred to as *nouveaux riche* and find it difficult to marry into the more well-established *grandes familles*, even though they have money.

The family is an all-encompassing concept in the Haitian culture. By including family members in the care of loved ones, health-care providers can achieve more trusting relationships, which foster greater adherence to treatment regimens. Haitians believe that when family members are ill, there is an obligation to be there for them. If a family member is in the hospital, all family members try to visit. Many visitors may cause concern to health-care providers who are not accustomed to accommodating large numbers of visitors. Health-care providers need to be patient with them and facilitate their visits.

When grandparents are no longer able to function independently, they move in with their children. The house is always open to relatives. Elders are highly respected and are often addressed by an affectionate title such as "Aunt," "Uncle," "Grandma," or "Grandpa," even if they are not related. Their children are expected to care for and provide for them when self-care becomes a concern. The elderly are family advisers, babysitters, historians, and consultants. Migration to America poses a tremendous challenge in caring for elderly Haitians. The nursing home concept does not exist in the Haitian culture; therefore, Haitians are generally very reluctant to place their elderly family members in nursing homes.

Alternative Lifestyles

Homosexuality is taboo in the Haitian culture, so gay and lesbian individuals usually remain closeted. If a family member discloses that he or she is gay, everyone keeps it quiet; there is total denial. Gay and lesbian relationships are not talked about; they remain buried. There are no gay bars in Haiti, and overt homosexual conduct is not publicly displayed, although this trend seems to be changing.

Although divorce is common among Haitians, before it becomes final, family members, friends, the church, and elders try to counsel the couple. Health-care providers must approach this issue carefully and establish a trusting relationship before discussing divorce.

Single parenting, widespread in Haiti, is well accepted and closely tied to the issue of concubinage. In Haitian society, a well-accepted practice is for men to have both a wife and a mistress, with the latter relationship referred to as *placage*. Both women bear children. The mistress raises her children alone and with minimal support from the father. These children are often known by the man's family but are not known to the wife. Haitian women in general know that their husbands are involved in extramarital relationships but pretend not to know. Health education, birth control, and safe sex are issues that should be approached with sensitivity and acceptance within cultural boundaries.

Workforce Issues

Culture in the Workplace

Haitians living in America have demonstrated a very strong motivation for work and a continued commitment to the entrepreneurial spirit. They can be found in every sector of the American workforce. They are hard workers, and many work two jobs to provide for their American family while sending money to Haiti for those left behind. In the first year of migration, they are generally forced to take lower-status and low-paying jobs. These jobs are used as stepping-stones to better jobs until they are able to communicate in English and legalize their immigrant status. According to the U.S. Census Bureau (2010), in 2009, 71 percent of Haitians over the age of 16 years were in the civilian workforce, compared with 65 percent of the total workforce. At the same time, median earnings for Haitian males were $33,000 for men and $29,000 for Haitian women, compared with $45,000 for men and $36,000 for women in the total workforce. In addition, 20 percent of Haitians were living below the poverty line compared with the total population of 14 percent. Work is a necessity, and they conform to the rules and regulations of the workplace. Haitian immigrants have taken menial, low-paying jobs that many Americans would not accept even when unemployed. Haitians appreciate comfort, and they work to be able to afford the necessities of life. The economic survival of Haiti is closely tied to the financial support provided to family members in Haiti by Haitians who have migrated to the United States and Canada.

Issues Related to Autonomy

In America, educated Haitians seek job opportunities in their fields. Those who have a trade try to find employment in that area. Uneducated, undocumented, and illiterate individuals experience much more difficulty in entering the job market, where employment opportunities are restricted to working in places in which there is overcrowding, poor ventilation, and high pollution, all of which place them at high risk for occupational diseases.

Immigrants from various Haitian villages and cities tend to settle in clusters with their relatives or neighbors from their areas of origin. This pattern of settlement by area of origin helps immigrants adapt to the demands of their new environment and ensure that they have someone living nearby whom they can call on in times of illness or other crises. However, when people live and work primarily in an ethnic enclave, the native culture becomes a barrier to assimilation and acculturation into the dominant society.

The educational level of health-care providers in Haiti is different from that in America. For example, medical education is not research-based, and nursing programs for the most part are at the diploma level with an apprenticeship. The only nursing baccalaureate program is the *Faculté des Sciences Infirmières de L' Université Episcopale D'Haiti* (Faculty of Nursing Science of the Episcopal University of Haiti), in

Leogane on the southern coast of the island. Establishing this school and adopting this name were major accomplishments. Nursing is finally accepted on par with the medical community, as well as with the other professional schools. All other professional schools start with the words "*Faculté des Sciences*" and end with whatever the science is (e.g., medicine, law, engineering).

Haitian health-care providers who migrate to the United States have experienced a great deal of difficulty in obtaining licensure to practice. Those who learned their profession in Haiti were taught in French and the test-taking approach is different; multiple-choice examinations are a new and difficult concept for Haitians.

Haitian nurses are very skilled clinically; however, sometimes they may experience difficulty in applying theoretical knowledge to practice. This may be due in part to language barriers, socialization, and their diploma education, which focuses on tasks and skills development. Haitian professionals struggle with professional cohesiveness and collegiality. Many groups have established professional societies whose goals are to support one another, to promote professional development, and to promote collegial relationships. Some examples of these professional groups are the Haitian Nurses Association, the Haitian-American Medical Association, the Haitian Educator Association, the Haitian-American Engineers, and the Haitian-American Lawyers.

Sometimes Haitians in the workplace greet one another in their native tongue because it is easier to articulate ideas and feelings and to express support in their native language. This may be irritating to non-Haitians, who consider it rude.

Biocultural Ecology

Skin Color and Other Biological Variations

Different assessment techniques are required when assessing dark-skinned people for anemia and jaundice. One must examine the sclera, oral mucosa, conjunctiva, lips, nailbeds, palms of the hands, and soles of the feet when assessing for cyanosis and low blood hemoglobin levels. To assess for jaundice, one must examine the conjunctiva and oral mucosa for patches of bilirubin pigment because dark skin has natural underlying tones of red and yellow.

Diseases and Health Conditions

Because Haiti is a tropical island, prevalent diseases include cholera, parasitosis, and malaria. Haiti has no mosquito control, so newer immigrants should be assessed for signs of malaria such as chills, fever, fatigue, and an enlarged spleen. Other diseases of increased incidence among Haitian immigrants are hepatitis, tuberculosis, HIV/AIDS, venereal diseases, and parasitosis

from inadequate potable water sources in their homeland. Actual tuberculosis rates for Haitians are misleading because, until a few years ago, Haitians living in Haiti were routinely vaccinated with *Bacille bilié de Calmette-Guérin*, thus making all subsequent skin tests positive, even though they may not actually have had the disease. Unfortunately, upon immigration, many Haitians continue to live in overcrowded areas, are malnourished, and live in very poor sanitary conditions, factors that increase their risk for infectious diseases.

Haitians are prone to diabetes and hypertension—a reflection of genetics and their diet, which is high in fat, cholesterol, and salt. Data on the prevalence of diabetes and hypertension among Haitian Americans are difficult to assess because they are categorized as black. In addition to type 1 and type 2 diabetes, there is a type 3 malnutrition-related diabetes, also known as *tropical diabetes*. The prevalence ranges from 2 to 8 percent, accounting for different parts of the island (Pan American Health Organization, 2001). In addition, Haitians experience a high incidence of heart disease. Cerebrovascular diseases are the third leading cause of death; other cardiopathies are in 5th place, and arterial hypertension is in 11th place. More deaths are registered among females than males. In addition to cardiovascular diseases, there is a high incidence of cancer. The National Cancer Institute statistics showed that the most frequent type of cancer treated was cervical cancer, representing 40 percent of cases. Breast cancer ranked second with 30 percent. Nasopharyngeal cancer ranked in third position with 10 to 15 percent of the cases (Pan American Health Organization, 2001). Both cancer and heart disease are related to a high-fat diet. Today, Haitians in Haiti and in the United States are very conscious of the need to limit the fat content in their diets; as a result, the Haitian diet is not as fatty as it once was.

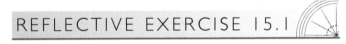

REFLECTIVE EXERCISE 15.1

Marie-Sandra is a 36-year-old Haitian woman. She was para 2 gravida 2, is 18 months postpartum, and has been breastfeeding her child. She noticed a change in the color of the breast milk from the right breast. She previously had a lesion in her right breast that was initially diagnosed as an abscess and appeared to have been there for 3 months. She returned to her physician after seeing the change in the color of her breast milk. The examination revealed a mass measuring 8 × 10 cm in the superior aspect of the breast.

A biopsy confirmed carcinoma infiltrate of the right breast. Marie had a sister who died of breast cancer at age 31. Her mother died at age 51 from "some interabdominal cancer." The oncologist believed that it was suggestive of breast and ovarian syndrome of a mutation gene.

Continued

Marie-Sandra had chemotherapy in Haiti that made her very ill, so she went to Cuba for continuation to complete four cycles of chemotherapy. Because definitive care was not available in Haiti, a university medical center in the United States enrolled her in a pro bono program. She came for the first time to the United States alone and that afternoon saw the surgeon, had a mammogram, and had preoperative diagnostic studies. A French translator was used.

The next day, Marie-Sandra had bilateral mastectomies. The left mastectomy was prophylactic because of her family history and no ability for mammography monitoring in Haiti. She remained in the United States without any family for 1 year while undergoing treatment and additional surgery. She received a 1-year course of chemotherapy, radiation therapy to the chest wall, genetic testing, Herceptin therapy, and prophylactic bilateral oophorectomies. Genetic BRCA 1 and BRCA 2 results were negative.

Marie-Sandra did well, and after 1 year, she returned to Haiti and started working again.

1. Given what you know about Marie-Sandra's history, how could she be helped to understand to change this major health event?
2. What suggestions might be provided for Marie-Sandra regarding her nutrition?
3. How might the health-care team assist with Marie-Sandra's acculturation in the United States?
4. How do traditional Haitians deal with family separation?
5. How might she be helped with being separated from her family?

Attention-deficit/hyperactivity disorder (ADHD) is a commonly diagnosed chronic mental condition in Haitian children (Prudent, Johnson, Carroll, & Culpepper, 2005). This disease has a large genetic component (McCann, Scheele, Ward, & Roy-Byrne, 2006). In the Haitian culture, there is no conceptual term for ADHD, nor is there a Creole term to describe it. Unfortunately, in the Haitian culture, the behavior displayed with this diagnosis may be interpreted as an ill-behaved or a "poorly raised" child or a psychically victimized child suffering from an "unnatural" condition. Parents may believe that this behavior can be controlled by parental discipline, or they may seek an alternative health consult such a *Hougan* or voodoo priest. Although medications are the preferred treatment for ADHD, which may be combined with psychological intervention, Haitians are fearful of psychoactive drugs because they see them as the cause of substance abuse and even possibly mental illness (Prudent et al., 2005). Therefore, assessing the parents' perceptions of the cause of the ADHD behavior and assisting them in holistic treatment are important.

Variations in Drug Metabolism

The literature reveals no studies on drug metabolism specific to Haitians or Haitian Americans. When Haitians are included in drug studies, it is assumed that they are included under the category of African American. Therefore, health-care providers may need to start with the literature for this broad category of ethnicity to posit and test theories of ethnic drug metabolism among Haitian Americans.

High-Risk Behaviors

Haitian refugees are one of the most at-risk populations living in the United States. Therefore, it is important for health-care providers to consider a number of factors in providing health-care services. An in-depth assessment of the person's environmental, occupational, socioeconomic, demographic, educational, and linguistic status enables the development of strategies that are culturally appropriate, adequate, and effective. As a new group of immigrants, Haitians bring to the health-care system a different set of beliefs and values about health and illness. These differences challenge health-care providers who must try to explain treatments while acknowledging, but not changing, their patients' cultural convictions. Attempts to change firmly held beliefs are counterproductive to establishing trusting health-care provider–patient relationships.

Behaviors that may be considered high risk in American society are generally viewed as recreational or unimportant among Haitians. Alcohol, for example, plays an important part in Haitian society. Drinking alcohol is culturally approved for men and is used socially when friends gather, especially on weekends. Women drink socially and in moderation. Cigarette smoking is another high-risk behavior practiced by Haitian men, whereas Haitian women have a very low rate of tobacco use. The trend toward decreasing cigarette use in America has not influenced Haitian society. Drug abuse among Haitians used to be low, but drug abuse in the adolescent population is increasing. In 1982, Haiti became the first developing country to be incorrectly blamed for the beginning of the AIDS epidemic. As a result, Haitians have had to endure the stigma associated with the belief that Haitians are "AIDS carriers." Unfortunately, HIV/AIDS has continued to spread in the Haitian community both in Haiti and the United States. Heterosexual transmission is the primary mode of HIV transmission in the Haitian community and is rapidly becoming an infection of women and children (Santana & Dancy, 2000). Health-care providers need to recognize the impact the stigma has had on male–female relationships, as well as familial relationships, in the Haitian community. Health providers must broaden their scope and approaches to HIV prevention by incorporating societal, contextual, and economic factors designed to modify traditional gender roles germane to influencing beginning negotiations of safer sex practices.

High-risk behavior in the Haitian culture includes the nonuse of seat belts and helmets when driving or riding a motorcycle or bicycle. Most cars in Haiti do not have seat belts, and there are no laws regarding the use of seat belts and helmets. Haitian cities are extremely overpopulated and traffic laws are very loose, resulting in hazardous driving conditions. Everyone tries to gain the upper hand. Haitian Americans must be educated about traffic laws, seat belt use, car seats for youngsters, and the need for helmets. Health-care providers may have to use graphic videos or skits when instructing patients about these safety practices. Health-care providers may also use Haitian radio stations for educational programs when they are available. Other strategies that may be used to help promote behavioral changes are through church and community group activities. Through these avenues, health-care providers can have a significant impact on health promotion and health risk prevention among Haitian Americans.

Health-Care Practices

To Haitians, good health is seen as the ability to achieve internal equilibrium between *cho* (hot) and *fret* (cold) (see also Nutrition and Health-Care Practices). To become balanced, one must eat well, give attention to personal hygiene, pray, and have good spiritual habits. To promote good health, one must be strong, have good color, be plump, and be free of pain. To maintain this state, one must eat right, sleep right, keep warm, exercise, and keep clean.

Haitians who believe in voodoo (see Dominant Religion and Use of Prayer) and other forms of folk medicine may use several types of folk healers. These healers include a voodoo practitioner, a *docte fey* (leaf doctor), a *fam saj* (lay midwife), a *docte zo* (bonesetter), and a *pikirist* (injectionist). Depending on whether the individual believes that the illness is natural or unnatural, she or he may seek help other than Western medicine from one of these healers.

Nutrition

Meaning of Food

For many Haitians in lower socioeconomic groups, food means survival. However, food is relished as a cultural treasure, and Haitians generally retain their food habits and practices after emigrating. Food practices vary little from generation to generation. Most Haitians are not culinary explorers. They prefer eating at home, take pride in promoting their food for their children, and discourage fast food. When hospitalized, many would rather fast than eat non-Haitian food. Haitians do not eat yogurt, cottage cheese, or "runny" egg yolk. Haitians drink a lot of water, homemade fruit juices, and cold, fruity sodas.

Common Foods and Food Rituals

The typical Haitian breakfast consists of bread, butter, bananas, and coffee. Children are allowed to drink coffee, which is not as strong as that consumed by adults. Generally, the largest meal for Haitians is eaten at lunch. At lunchtime, a basic Haitian meal might include rice and beans, boiled plantains, a salad made of watercress and tomatoes, and stewed vegetables and beef or cornmeal cooked as polenta. Table 15-1 lists popular foods in the Haitian community.

Dietary Practices for Health Promotion

Hot and cold, acid and nonacid, and heavy and light are the major categories of contrast when discussing food. Illness is caused when the body is exposed to an imbalance of cold (*fret*) and hot (*cho*) factors. For example, *soursop*, a large, green prickly fruit with a white pulp that is used in juice and ice cream, is considered a cold food and is avoided when a woman is menstruating. Eating white beans after childbirth is believed to induce hemorrhage. Foods that are considered heavy, such as plantain, cornmeal mush, rice, and

Table 15-1	**Popular Foods in the Haitian Community**
Bouillon	Soup made with beef broth mixed with various green vegetables (e.g., spinach, cabbage, watercress, string beans, carrots), meat or poultry, plantain, sweet potato, and Malaga, a sweet aromatic wine
Chiquetaille	Codfish or smoked herring, unsalted, shredded finely, mixed with onions, shallots, finely chopped hot pepper, vinegar, and lime
Fritters	*Marinade:* flour, water, eggs, parsley, onions, garlic, salt and pepper, chicken, hot pepper, and a pinch of baking soda, mixed together to pancake consistency and deep-fried
	Acra: chopped parsley, eggs, garlic, and onion mixed with Malaga; finely shredded codfish or smoked herring and hot pepper may be added
	Beignet: sweet ripe banana, sugar, and eggs, mixed with cinnamon, milk, margarine, flour, nutmeg, and vanilla extract
Green plantain	Boiled or fried, usually eaten with *griot*
Griot	Marinated pork cut up in small pieces and fried
Lambi	Conch meat softened and prepared in a sauce
Legume	Vegetables such as chayote and eggplant cooked with meat
Patee	Pastry dough filled with choice meat, chicken, or smoked herring
Pumpkin squash soup	Meat or poultry mixed with vegetables and pureed cooked squash and spices
Tomtom	Similar to dumplings, cooked and made into round balls and eaten with beef stew and okra

meat, are to be eaten during the day because they provide energy. Light foods, such as hot chocolate milk, bread, and soup, are eaten for dinner because they are more easily digested. Table 15-2 presents a classification of hot and cold foods.

To treat a person by the hot-and-cold system, a potent drink or herbal medicine of the class opposite to the disease is administered. Cough medicines, for example, are considered to be in the hot category, whereas laxatives are in the cold category. Certain food prohibitions are related to particular diseases and stages of the life cycle. Teenagers, for example, are advised to avoid drinking citrus fruit juices such as lemonade to prevent the development of acne. After performing strenuous activities or any activity that causes the body to become hot, one should not eat cold food because that will create an imbalance, causing a condition called *chofret*. A woman who has just straightened her hair by using a hot comb and then opens a refrigerator may become a victim of *chofret*. This means she may catch a cold and/or possibly develop pneumonia.

When they are sick, Haitians like to eat pumpkin soup, bouillon, and a special soup made with green vegetables, meat, plantains, dumplings, and yams. The Haitian diet is high in carbohydrates and fat. Eating "right" entails eating sufficient food to feel full and maintain a constant body weight, which is often higher than weight standards medically recommended in the United States. Men like to see "plump" women. Furthermore, weight loss is seen as one of the most important signs of illness. Additional components of what Haitians consider a healthy diet are tonics to stimulate the appetite and the use of high-calorie supplements such as *Akasan*, which is either prepared plain or made as a special drink with cream of cornmeal, evaporated milk, cinnamon, vanilla extract, sugar, and a pinch of salt.

A thorough nutritional assessment is very important to effectively promote nutritional health. Understanding food rituals assists health-care providers in designing individualized dietary plans, which can be incorporated into the diet to facilitate compliance with dietary regimens that promote a healthier lifestyle.

Nutritional Deficiencies and Food Limitations

Many Haitian women and children who come from rural areas have significant protein deficiencies owing to Haiti's economic deprivation. A cultural factor contributing to this problem is the uneven distribution of protein among family members. However, the problem is not one of net protein deficiency in the community but, rather, the unwise distribution of the available protein among family members. Whenever meat is served, the major portion goes to the men, under the assumption that they must be well fed to provide for the household. This same pattern exists today among Haitian immigrants. Being aware of this cultural factor enables health-care providers to prepare nutritional plans that meet patients' dietary needs.

Another major concern in this area is that of food insecurity and short intervals between births, chronic malnutrition, and anemia, which are widespread among Haitian women of childbearing age. These health inequalities result in a high prevalence of low birth weight, estimated at 15 percent; anemia, ranging from 35 to 50 percent; a body mass index under 18.5 kg/m², estimated at 18 percent; and a high maternal mortality rate, estimated at 456 per 100,000 live births (Pan American Health Organization, 2001).

Pregnancy and Childbearing Practices

Fertility Practices and Views Toward Pregnancy

Pregnancy and fertility practices are not readily discussed among Haitians. Most Haitians are Catholic and are unwilling to overtly engage in conversation about birth control or abortion. This does not mean that these two practices do not occur, but rather that they are just not openly discussed. Abortion is viewed as a woman's issue and is left to her and her significant other to decide. Accurate assessments and teaching related to these sensitive areas require tact and understanding. Initially, health-care providers should be cautious in assessing and gathering information related to fertility control. Pregnancy is not considered a health problem but rather a time of joy for the entire family. Pregnancy does not relieve a woman from her work. Because pregnancy is not a disease, many Haitian

ID Table 15-2	Haitian Hot and Cold Food Classification				
Very Cold (−3)	Quite Cold (−2)	Cool (−1)	Neutral (0)	Warm (+)	Very Hot (+2)
Avocado	Banana	Tomato	Cabbage	Eggs	Rum
Cashew nuts	Grapefruit	Cane syrup	Conch	Pigeon	Nutmeg
Mango	Lime	Orange	Carrot	Soup	Garlic
Coconut	Okra	Cantaloupe	Watercress	Bouillon	Tea
Cassava	Watermelon	Chayote	Brown rice	Pork	Cornmeal mush

Source: Adapted from M.S. Laguerre (1981, pp. 194–196).

women do not seek prenatal care. Pregnant women are restricted from eating spices that may irritate the fetus. However, they are permitted to eat vegetables and red fruits because these are believed to improve the fetus's blood. They are encouraged to eat large quantities of food because they are eating for two. Pregnant women who experience increased salivation may rid themselves of the excess at places that may seem inappropriate. They may even carry a "spit" cup in order to rid themselves of the excess saliva. They are not embarrassed by this behavior because they feel it is perfectly normal.

Fifty percent of women living in Port-au-Prince give birth in a hospital, compared with 31 percent of births in other urban areas, and only 9 percent of births in rural areas. The leading causes of maternal deaths are obstructed labor (8.3 percent), toxemia (16.7 percent), and hemorrhage (8.3 percent). The high maternal mortality rate is mainly the result of inadequate prenatal care (Pan American Health Organization, 2001).

The most popular methods of contraception are the birth control pill, female sterilization, injections, and condoms (3 percent each). Among sexually active women, 13 percent use a modern method of contraception and 4 percent rely on traditional methods. Among sexually active men, 17 percent use a modern method (6 percent use condoms) and 16 percent rely on traditional methods (Pan American Health Organization, 2001).

Prescriptive, Restrictive, and Taboo Practices in the Childbearing Family

During labor, the woman may walk, squat, pace, sit, or rub her belly. Generally, Haitian women practice natural childbirth and do not ask for analgesia. Some may scream or cry and become hysterical, whereas others are stoic, only moaning and grunting. What they need is support and reassurance; for example, applying a cold compress on the woman's forehead demonstrates caring and sensitivity on the part of the health-care provider. Since migrating, some Haitian women have adopted American childbearing practices and request analgesics. Cesarean birth is feared because it is abdominal surgery. Women in higher social strata are more amenable to having cesarean deliveries. Fathers do not generally participate in the labor and delivery, believing that this is a private event best handled by women. The woman is not coached; female members of the family give assistance as needed.

The crucial period for the childbearing woman is postpartum, a time for prescription and proscription. The woman takes an active role in her own care. She dresses warmly after birth as a way to become healthy and clean. Haitians believe that the bones are "open" after birth and that a woman should stay in bed during the first 2 to 3 days postpartum to allow the bones to close. Wearing an abdominal binder is another way to facilitate closing the bones.

The postpartum woman also engages in a practice called *the three baths*. For the first 3 days, the mother bathes in hot water boiled with special leaves that are either bought or picked from the field. She also drinks tea boiled from these leaves. For the next 3 days, the mother bathes in water prepared with leaves that are warmed by the sun. At this point, the mother takes only water or tea warmed by the sun. Another important practice is for the mother to take a vapor bath with boiled orange leaves, a practice believed to enhance cleanliness and tighten the internal muscles. At the end of the 3rd to 4th week, the new mother takes the third bath, which is cold. A cathartic may be administered to cleanse her intestinal tract. When the process is completed, she may drink cold water again and resume her normal activities.

In the postpartum period, Haitian women avoid white foods such as lima beans, as well as other foods, including okra, mushrooms, and tomatoes. These foods are restricted because they are believed to increase vaginal discharge. Other foods are eaten to give the new mother strength and vitality. Foods associated with this prescriptive practice are porridge, rice and red beans, plantains boiled or grated with the skins and prepared as porridge (the skin is high in iron, which is good for building the blood), carrot juice, and carrot juice mixed with red beet juice.

Breastfeeding is encouraged for up to 9 months postpartum. Breast milk can become detrimental to both mother and child if it becomes too thick or too thin. If it is too thin, it is believed that the milk has "turned," and it may cause diarrhea and headaches in the child and, possibly, postpartum depression in the mother. If milk is too "thick," it is believed to cause impetigo (*bouton*). Breastfeeding and bottle-feeding are accepted practices. If the child develops diarrhea, breastfeeding is immediately discontinued. Practices that do not put the mother or the child at risk should be supported and encouraged. Respecting the patients' cultural beliefs and practices helps to establish trust between the patient and the health-care provider and demonstrates caring. By being familiar with these health practices and beliefs, health-care providers can assist women in making culturally safe decisions related to pregnancy and plans for delivery.

Another prescriptive postpartum practice among Haitian women is to feed their infant a *lok* similar to the one administered to the older children in the summer. The laxative is administered with the initial feeding and is intended to hasten the expulsion of meconium. Because Haitians are fearful of diarrhea in children, health-care providers should stress the risks associated with *lok* and any other type of bowel-cleansing cocktails in infants and children. It is important to stress the impact of laxative use on the body system and educate the woman about the need to prevent dehydration.

Death Rituals
Death Rituals and Expectations

Generally, Haitians prefer to die at home rather than in the hospital. Since migrating to America, many have accepted death in a health-care facility to alleviate the heavy burden on the family during the last stage of the loved one's life. When death is imminent, the family may pray and cry uncontrollably, sometimes even hysterically. They try to meet the person's spiritual needs by bringing religious medallions, pictures of saints, or fetishes. When the person dies, all family members try, if possible, to be at the bedside and have a prayer service. If possible, and if it is not too disturbing to other patients, health-care providers should encourage this practice and involve a family member in the postmortem care.

Responses to Death and Grief

Death in the Haitian community mobilizes the entire family, including the matrilineal and patrilineal extensions and affines. Death arrangements in America are similar to those in Haiti. Generally, a male relative of the deceased makes the arrangements. This person may also be more fluent in English and more accustomed to dealing with the bureaucracy. This person is also responsible for notifying all family members wherever they might be in the world, an important activity because family members' travel plans influence funeral arrangements. In addition, he is responsible for ordering the coffin, making arrangements for prayer services before the funeral, and coordinating plans for the funeral service.

The preburial activity is called *veye*, a gathering of family and friends who come to the house of the deceased to cry, tell stories about the deceased's life, and laugh. Food, tea, coffee, and rum are in abundant supply. The intent is to show support and to join the family in sharing this painful loss. Another religious ritual is called the *dernie priye*, a special prayer service consisting of 7 consecutive days of prayer. Its purpose is to facilitate the passage of the soul from this world to the next. It usually takes place in the home. On the 7th day, a mass called *prise de deuil* officially begins the mourning process. After each of these prayers, a reception/celebration in memory of the deceased is held.

Haitians have a very strong belief in resurrection and paradise; thus, cremation is not an acceptable option (Fr. Darbouze Gerard, personal communication, 2001). Haitians are very cautious about autopsies. If foul play is suspected, they may request an autopsy to ensure that the patient is really dead. This alleviates their fear that their loved one is being *zombified*. According to this belief, this can occur when the person appears to have died of natural causes but is still alive. About 18 hours after the burial, the person is stolen from his or her coffin; the lack of oxygen causes some of the brain cells to die, so the mental facilities cease to exist while the body remains alive. The zombie then responds to commands, having no free will, and is domesticated as a slave.

Spirituality
Dominant Religion and Use of Prayer

Patients' cultural beliefs and religion can have a great impact on their acceptance of and adherence to health care and, therefore, on the outcomes of treatment.

REFLEXIVE EXERCISE 15.2

Manou is a 59-year-old Haitian American woman who lives in the Midwest United States. About 6 years ago, Manou lost her only son, age 20, who died tragically after dropping out of college and joining the military. Two years after her son's death, Manou fell ill and was diagnosed with cancer of the gallbladder. Her husband, a Lutheran pastor, had moved to Florida to build a church and to serve the Haitian American population living in the area. Manou stayed in the Midwest to care for her youngest daughter, who was then finishing high school. Manou was able to function for a number of years without ever mentioning her illness to her husband or daughter. She isolated herself from her family, including her parents.

Recently, Manou fell gravely ill while she was alone in the house. Her husband, who was still in Florida at the time, had to call a family member to check on her condition. She was taken to the nearest hospital emergency room and then transferred to a nursing home. She suffered with pain on her left abdominal quadrant and had difficulty eating. Her family members rushed to care for her, although they were unaware of her condition. They made leaf teas (parsley, garlic) in the hope of alleviating her pain and epigastric discomfort.

Manou was transferred from the nursing home to another hospital for further testing. There, it was revealed to her family that she was terminally ill and needed to be admitted to a hospice care facility. The family refused and wanted to take her home to care for her.

You happen to be a nurse and a member of the family. Manou's family was in disbelief; her husband and daughter looked to you for answers and to assist them in coping with this news. They need to be prepared for her imminent death.

1. What do you need to know about the health practices that Manou had engaged in at home? Why would this be important?
2. How can you help the family come to terms with this major event that Manou kept from them?
3. Do you think Manou kept her illness a secret because of lack of trust, or was she trying to protect her family? Is this behavior typical in the Haitian community, or is this out of the ordinary?
4. How can you assist this family in their grief?
5. What can you do to assist Manou in coming to terms spirituality/religiously with her imminent death?

REFLECTIVE EXERCISE 15.3

Lélé, a young Haitian man, survived the earthquake in Haiti on January 12, 2010. Prior to the earthquake, he was active, full of life, and pursing his studies. He lived in one of the small towns in Haiti and was going to school at the same time. Soon after the earthquake, Lélé developed some signs and symptoms that baffled many of the health-care providers who were giving assistance to the earthquake survivors. Lélé started losing weight, his skin color changed, and he became discolored. As his condition became worse, he had difficulty swallowing. Suspecting scleroderma, Lélé was brought along with his mother to the United States for treatment.

After 6 weeks, Lélé's mother returned home because there was nothing that Western/conventional medicine could do for him. She stated that she did not want to witness Lélé's death and would rather remember him alive. After 3 months of a languishing illness, Lélé died alone and far away from his young wife, his mother, and the rest of his family. Lélé's wish was to be buried in his homeland. Given the high cost of sending the body home for burial, his wife contemplated cremation and sending his ashes home. However, Lélé had converted to the Mormon faith, which prohibits cremation. When Lélé's wife was informed of this, she sought out a spiritual leader from the Mormon faith to assist her in making such an important decision.

1. Should Lélé's mother be brought into the decision-making process regarding cremation?
2. How important is family in the Haitian culture?
3. What resources might be made available to have Lélé's body returned to Haiti?
4. If the decision was made for cremation, which is contrary to Haitian culture, how might a nurse assist his wife with the grieving process?

Catholicism is the primary religion of Haiti. Since the early 1970s, however, Protestantism has gained in popularity throughout the island and has seriously challenged the Catholic Church, especially among the lower socioeconomic classes. Even though Haitians are deeply religious, their religious beliefs are combined with **voudou** (voodooism), a complex religion with its roots in Africa (Fig. 15-1). Voudou, in the most simplistic sense, involves communication by trance between the believer and ancestors, saints, or animistic deities. Voudou is not considered paganism among those who practice it, even though many of the rituals resemble paganism. Participants gather to worship the *loa* or *mystere*, deities or spirits who are believed to have received their powers from God and are capable of expressing themselves through possession of a chosen believer. With their great powers, the *loa* or *mystere* can provide favors such as protection, wealth, and health to those who worship and believe in them.

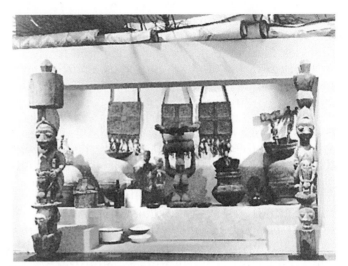

Figure 15-1 Santeria evolved from two main cultural antecedents: the worship of orisha among the Yoruba tribe of Nigeria and the cult of saints from the Roman Catholicism of Spain.

Meaning of Life and Individual Sources of Strength

The family system among Haitians is the center of life and includes the nuclear, consanguine, and affinal relatives. They may all live under the same roof. The family deals with all aspects of a person's life, including counseling, education, crises, marriage, and death.

The best way to understand and assess the spiritual beliefs and needs of Haitian American patients is to understand their culture. This is especially important because Haitian patients may express their concerns in ways that are unique to their cultural and religious beliefs. To ensure accurate assessments of these patients, it is essential to ask questions carefully and to completely understand the answers in order to gain an understanding of patients' perceptions of health and illness as dictated by their culture and religious beliefs. By recognizing and accepting patients' beliefs, health-care providers may alleviate barriers, and patients may feel more at ease to discuss their beliefs and needs.

Spiritual Beliefs and Health-Care Practices

Voudou believers may often attribute their ailments or medical problems to the doings of evil spirits. In such cases, they prefer to confirm their suspicions through the *loa* before accepting natural causes as the problem, which would lead to seeking Western medical care. For Haitian patients, the belief in the power of the supernatural can have a great influence on the psychological and medical concerns of the patients.

Health-Care Practices

Health-Seeking Beliefs and Behaviors

For Haitians, illness is perceived as punishment, considered an assault on the body, and may have two different etiologies: natural illnesses, known as *maladi Bondye* ("disease of the Lord"), and supernatural illnesses. Natural illnesses may occur frequently, are of short duration, and are caused by environmental factors such as food, air, cold, heat, and gas. Other causes of natural illness are movement of blood within the body, disequilibrium between hot and cold, and bone displacement. Supernatural illnesses are believed to be caused by angry spirits. To placate these spirits, patients must offer feasts called *manger morts*. If individuals do not partake in these rituals, misfortunes are likely to befall them. Illnesses of supernatural origin are fundamentally a breach in rapport between the individual and her or his protector. The breach in rapport is a response from the spirit and a way of showing disapproval of the protégé's behavior. In this instance, health can be recovered if the patient takes the first step in determining the nature of the illness. This can be accomplished by eliciting the help of a *voudou* priest and following the advice given by the spirit itself. To accurately prescribe treatment options, health-care providers must be able to differentiate between these belief systems.

Physical illnesses are thought to be on a continuum beginning with "*Kom pa bon*" ("I do not feel well"). In this phase, the affected person is not confined to bed; illness is transitory, and the person should be able to return to his or her normal activities. The next phase is *Moin malad* ("I am sick"), in which the individuals stay at home and avoid activity. The third phase is *Moin malad anpil* ("I am very sick"). This means that the person is very ill and may be confined to bed. The final phase is *Moin pap refe* ("I am dying").

Haitians believe that gas (*gaz*) may provoke pain and anemia. Gas can occur in the head, where it enters through the ears; in the stomach, where it enters through the mouth; and in the shoulders, back, legs, or appendix, where it travels from the stomach. When gas is in the stomach, the patient is said to suffer *kolik*, meaning stomach pain. Gas in the head is called *van nan tet* or *van nan zorey*, which translates to "gas in one's ears," and is believed to be a cause of headaches. Gas moving from one part of the body to another produces pain. Thus, the movement of gas from the stomach to the legs produces rheumatism, to the back causes back pain, and to the shoulder causes shoulder pain. Foods that help dispel gas include tea made from garlic, cloves, and mint; plantains; and corn. To deter the entry of gas into the body, one must be careful about eating "leftovers," especially beans. Since migrating to the United States, Haitians have begun eating leftovers, which is believed to cause many of their ailments. After childbirth, women are particularly susceptible to gas, and to prevent entry of gas into the body, they tighten their waist with a belt or a piece of linen.

Responsibility for Health Care

Haitians engage in self-treatment and see these activities as a way of preventing disease or promoting health. Haitians try home remedies as a first resort for treating illness. They are self-diagnosticians and may use home remedies for a particular ailment, or if they know someone who had a particular illness, they may take the prescribed medicine from that person. They keep numerous topical and oral medicines on hand, which they use to treat various symptoms. For example, an individual who suspects a venereal disease may buy penicillin injections and have someone administer them without consulting a physician. In Haiti, many medications can be purchased without a prescription, a potentially dangerous practice. However, health-care providers must be very discrete in assessing, teaching, and guiding the patient toward safer health practices. Admonishing patients may cause them to withdraw and not adhere to instructions. Haitians may also lead health-care providers to believe that they are interested, when in fact they have already discredited the health-care provider. When taking the patient's history, the health-care provider should inquire if the patient has been taking medication that was prescribed for someone else. Moreover, when prescribing a potentially dangerous drug, the health-care provider should be sure to caution the patient not to give the medication to ailing friends or relatives. Even though the health-care provider may not be completely successful at stopping the practice of exchanging medications, with continued reminders, she or he may be successful later.

Folk and Traditional Practices

Haitians may use others' experiences with a particular illness as a barometer against which to measure their symptoms and institute treatment. If necessary, a person living in the United States may ask friends or relatives to send medications from Haiti. Such medications may consist of roots, leaves, and European-manufactured products that are more familiar to them. Therefore, it is very important to ascertain what the patient is taking at home to avoid serious complications.

Constipation, referred to as *konstipasyon*, is treated with laxatives or herbal teas. Sometimes, Haitians use enemas (*lavman*). Diarrhea is not a major concern in adults; however, it is considered very dangerous in children and sometimes interpreted as a hex on the child. Parents may try herbal medicine, may seek help from a *voudou* priest or *hougan*, or if all else fails, may consult a physician. It is very important to assess the child carefully because he or she may have been ill for quite some time.

A primary respiratory ailment is *oppression*, a term used to describe asthma. However, the term really describes a state of anxiety and hyperventilation rather than the condition. *Oppression* is considered a cold state, as are many respiratory conditions. A home remedy for *oppression* is to take a dry coconut and cut it open, fill it with half sugarcane syrup and half honey, grate one full nutmeg and add it to the syrup mix, reseal the coconut, and then bury it in the ground for a month. The coconut is reopened, the contents are stirred and mixed together, and 1 tablespoon is administered twice a day until all of the contents have been consumed. By the end of this treatment, the child is supposed to be cured of the respiratory problem.

Barriers to Health Care

Because orthodox medicine is often bypassed or perceived as a second choice among Haitians, the potential delay of medical care can pose an increased risk to patients. The view that physicians of conventional medicine do not understand *voudou* and, therefore, cannot cure magical illness or that an illness worsens if the bewitched person seeks a physician is enough to persuade these individuals to seek unconventional modes of therapy with which they are more comfortable. The health-care team should understand some of the basic principles and practices of folk medicine, particularly root medicine, because this can play a significant role in determining the progress of the client's health status.

Many Haitians are in low-paying jobs that do not provide health insurance, and they cannot afford to purchase it themselves. Thus, economics acts as a barrier to health promotion. In addition, for those who do not speak English well, it is difficult for them to access the health-care system, fully explain their needs, or understand prescriptions and treatments.

Cultural Responses to Health and Illness

The *root-work system* is a folk medicine that provides a framework for identifying and curing folk illnesses. When illness occurs, or when a person is not feeling well or is "disturbed," root medicine distinguishes whether the symptoms and illness are of natural or unnatural origin. An imbalance in harmony between the physical and the spiritual worlds, such as dietary or lifestyle excesses, can cause a natural illness. For example, diabetes is considered a natural illness, but most Haitians do not seek immediate medical assistance when they detect the symptoms of polyuria, excessive thirst, and weight loss. Instead, they attempt symptom management by making dietary changes on their own by drinking potions or herbal remedies. When the person finally seeks medical attention, she or he may be very sick. At this point, the health-care provider should be cautious in explaining the condition and use a culturally specific approach when explaining the medical regimen, diet, and medications.

Pain is commonly referred to as **doule**. Many Haitians have a very low pain threshold. Their demeanor changes, they are verbal about the cause of their pain, and they sometimes moan. They are vague about the location of the pain because they believe that it is not important; they believe that the whole body is affected because disease travels. This belief makes it very difficult to accurately assess pain. Injections are the preferred method for medication administration, followed by elixirs, tablets, and capsules.

Chest pain is referred to as *doule nan ke mwen*, abdominal pain is *doule nan vent*, and stomach pain is *doule nan ke mwen* or *doule nan lestomak mwen*. Oxygen should be offered only when absolutely necessary because the use of oxygen is perceived as an indicator of the seriousness of the illness.

Nausea is expressed as *lestomak/mwen ap roule*, *M santi m anwi vomi, lestomak/mwen chaje*, or *ke mwen tounin*. Those who are more educated may express their discomfort as nausea. Because of modesty, they may discard vomitus immediately so as not to upset others. Specific instructions should be given regarding keeping the specimen until the practitioner has had a chance to see it.

Fatigue, physical weakness known as *febles*, is interpreted as a sign of anemia or insufficient blood. Symptoms are generally attributed to poor diet. Patients may suggest to the health-care provider that they need special care—that is, to eat well, take vitamin injections, and rest. To counteract the *febles*, the diet includes liver, pigeon meat, watercress, bouillon made of green leafy vegetables, cow's feet, and red meat.

REFLECTIVE EXERCISE 15.4

Marie was raised by her grandmother since typhoid took the lives of her parents. Marie said that when her brother, Jean-Claude, contracted the disease, her grandmother used a paste-like mixture of sour oranges, the leaves of a sour orange tree, and papaya leaves and placed it on his forehead to reduce the fever. This was used for 3 days, at which time her grandmother realized that the treatment was ineffective. At that point, Marie and her grandmother took Jean-Claude via a donkey-pulled cart to the nearest clinic. The trip took 8 hours. Even though the staff immediately started intravenous fluids and medication, Jean-Claude died the next day.

1. What were some of the major obstacles to treating Jean-Claude?
2. What are some of the variant cultural characteristics from the Purnell Model in this vignette?
3. What other traditional remedies do Haitians use?
4. What are traditional Haitian burial practices?

Another condition is fright or *sezisman*. Various external and internal environmental factors are believed to cause *sezisman*, thereby disrupting the normal blood flow. *Sezisman* may occur when someone receives bad news, is involved in a frightful situation, or suffers from indignation after being treated unjustly. When this condition occurs, blood is said to move to the head, causing partial loss of vision, headache, increased blood pressure, or a stroke. To counteract this problem, the patient may sit quietly, put a cold compress on the forehead, drink bitter herbal tea, take sips of water, or drink rum mixed with black, unsweetened coffee.

Haitian Americans may strongly resist acculturation, taking pride in preserving traditional spiritual, religious, and family values. This strong hold on cultural views sometimes creates stress leading to depression. The stigma attached to mental illness is strong, and most Haitians do not readily admit to being depressed. A major factor to remember is the strong prevalence of *voudou*, which attributes depression to possession by malevolent spirits or punishment for not honoring good, protective spirits. In addition, depression can be viewed as a hex placed by a jealous or envious individual. Factors that may trigger depression are memories of family in the homeland, thoughts about spirits in Haiti, dreams about dead family members, or guilt and regrets about abandoning one's family in Haiti for the abundance in America. Health-care providers need to be sensitive to the underlying causes of problems and ascertain the need for comfort within specific religious beliefs.

In the case of an unnatural illness, the person's poor health is attributed to magical causes such as a hex, a curse, or a spell that has been cast by someone as a result of family or interpersonal disagreement. The curse takes place when the intended victim eats food containing ingredients such as snake, frog, or spider egg powder, which cause symptoms of burning skin, rashes, pruritus, nausea, vomiting, and headaches (Fishman, Bobo, Kosub, & Womeodu, 1993). These symptoms often coincide with psychological problems manifested by violent attacks, hallucinations, delusions, or "magical possession." Because, under Western medical standards, an evil spirit would be classified as a true psychiatric problem with "culturally diverse manifestations" and not as an actual case of possession, the health-care provider is challenged in assessing and making the appropriate intervention (Fishman et al., 1993). If the health-care provider is aware of witchcraft, *voudou* practices, and the symptoms associated with them, it may prevent (1) incorrectly diagnosing an individual as mentally ill, (2) giving advice that frightens or confuses the patient into thinking an illness is unnatural in origin, or (3) initiating symptomatic treatment that does not reach the underlying stress. The role of the health-care provider is to be sensitive and understanding toward the patient who holds a belief in these traditional practices. Health-care providers should realize that hesitating to offer a specific diagnosis might be more detrimental to the patient than a negative diagnosis.

Blood Transfusions and Organ Donation

Most Haitians are extremely afraid of diseases associated with blood irregularities. They believe that blood is the central dynamic of body functions and pathological processes; therefore, any condition that places the body in a "blood-need" state is believed to be extremely dangerous. Patients and their families become emotional about blood transfusions. Thus, these are received with much apprehension. In addition, as in all societies, blood transfusions are feared because of the potential for HIV transmission. Health-care providers should explain the need for a blood transfusion factually and carefully clarify the procedure along with the involved risks. Health-care providers should involve patients and their families in the care as much as possible. Precautionary measures that have been taken to prevent blood contamination should also be explained.

Because Haitians hold strong religious beliefs about life after death, the body must remain intact for burial. Thus, organ donation and transplantation are not generally discussed. Since migrating to the United States, some Haitians have, with considerable distress, participated in organ transplantation. A prime concern is transference, believing that through the organ donor, the donor's personality will "shift" to the recipient and change his or her being. Health-care providers should assess Haitian patients' beliefs about organ donation and involve a religious leader to provide support and help facilitate a decision regarding organ donation or transplantation. Because some Haitians' knowledge and understanding in this area is limited, the health-care provider should be proactive by promoting health education.

Health-Care Providers
Traditional Versus Biomedical Providers

In general, most Haitians resort to symptom management with self-care first and then spiritual care. They commonly use traditional and Western health-care providers simultaneously (see Spirituality and Folk Practices).

Status of Health-Care Providers

Haitians are very respectful of physicians and nurses. Physicians are men and nurses are women. Nurses are referred to as "Miss." By incorporating culturally specific strategies in their program, health-care providers inspire confidence and trust. Haitian patients who have had limited contact with American health-care systems may have limited understanding of biomedical concepts. Health-care providers need to take the time to explain and reexplain relevant points to compensate for patients' deficient knowledge or language limitations. Health-care providers who show compassion and sensitivity toward Haitian patients achieve greater success in educating patients, families, and the community.

REFERENCES

Aristide, M.V. (1995). Economics of liberation. *Roots, 1*(2), 20–24.

BBC News. (2011, January 7). Retrieved from BBC: http://www.bbc.co.uk

CIA World Factbook. (2012). Retrieved from https://www.cia.gov/library/publications/the-world-factbook/geos/ha.html

Dorestant, N. (1998). *A look at Haitian history from a Haitian perspective.* Retrieved from http://www.geocite.com

Fishman, B.M., Bobo, L., Kosub, K., & Womeodu, R.J. (1993). Cultural issues in serving minority populations: Emphasis on Mexican Americans and African Americans. *American Journal of Medical Science, 306,* 160–166.

Jean-Baptiste, A.R. (1985). *The black man: Ti Manno in public.* New York: St. Aude Records.

Jean-Bernard, L. (1983). *Impossible alphabetization.* Port-au-Prince, Haiti: Des Antilles SA.

Haiti: Early history to independence. (2007). Retrieved from http://www.infoplease.com/ce6/world/A0858544.html

Laguerre M.S. (1981). Haitian Americans. In L. Sana (Ed.), *Handbook of immigrant health* (pp. 194–196). New York, NY: Springer Publishing Co.

Louis-Juste, A. (1995). Popular education and democracy. *Roots, 2*(1), 14–19.

McCann, B.S., Scheele, L., Ward, N., & Roy-Byrne, P. (2006). Childhood inattention and hyperactivity symptoms self-reported by adults with Asperger syndrome. *International Journal of Descriptive and Experimental Psychopathology, Phenomenology and Psychiatric Diagnosis, 39,* 45–54.

McKenzie, A.D. (2010, January 17). *France: Time to pay back Haiti.* Retrieved from IPS Interpress Service: http://ipsnews.net

Pan American Health Organization (PAHO). (2001). *Regional core health data.* Retrieved from http://www.paho.org/English/SHA/glossary.htm

Pan American Health Organization (PAHO). (2011, February 10). *Disaster in Haiti—One year later.* Retrieved from http://www.paho.org/disasters

Paravisini, L. (2010, February 7). *Dominican Republic fears increased migration from Haiti.* Retrieved from http://repeatingislands.com

Power, C. (2010, July 13). *Citizenship and Immigration Canada secures fast family reunification or Haitians affected by earthquake.* Retrieved from http://www.cic.gc.ca

Prudent, N., Johnson, P., Carroll, J., & Culpepper, L. (2005). Attention deficit disorder: Presentation and management in the Haitian American child. *Primary Care Companion Journal Clinical Psychiatry, 7*(4), 190–197.

Saint-Domingue. (2011, January 24). *Stamping down on Haiti's restavek shame.* Retrieved from http://citizenhaiti.com

Santana, M.A., & Dancy, B.L. (2000). The stigma of being named "AIDS carriers" on Haitian-American women. *Health Care for Women International, 21,* 161–171.

Schaaf, B. (2009, July 16). *Child slavery in Haiti: CNN covers Jean Robert Cadet Foundation.* Retrieved from http://haitiinnovation.org/fr/about/about_haiti_innovation

Simon, J.J., Kleschnitzki, S., & Shusterman, J. (2011, January). *Children in Haiti: One year after—The long road from relief to recovery.* Retrieved from http://unicef.org

Statistics Canada. (2006). Retrieved from http://www40.statcan.gc.ca/z01/cs0001-eng.htm

U.S. Census Bureau. (2009). *The population with Haitian ancestry in the United States: 2009.* Retrieved from http://www.census.gov/prod/2010pubs/acsbr09-18.pdf

U.S. Immigration and Naturalization Service. (2006). *Statistical yearbook of the Immigration and Naturalization Service 2005.* Washington, DC: U.S. Government Printing Office.

World Bank. (2010). *The World Bank annual report 2010.* Retrieved from http://www.worldbank.org

World Health Organization (WHO). (2010, September 3). *WHO weekly epidemiology record.* Retrieved from http://www.who.int/wer

Zissis, C. (2010, January 27). *The Haitian migration debate.* Retrieved from http://www.as-coa.org

DavisPlus *For case studies, review questions, and additional information,*

go to http://davisplus.fadavis.com

Chapter 16

People of Hindu Heritage

Jaya Jambunathan

Overview, Inhabited Localities, and Topography

Overview

India, located in southern Asia, has a landmass approximately one-third that of the United States. With over 1.18 billion people, India is currently the world's second largest country. Of the population, more than 80 percent are Hindus; 13.4 percent are Muslim; 2.3 percent are Christian; 1.9 percent are Sikh; 1.8 percent are other; and 0.1 percent are unspecified (*CIA World Factbook,* 2011). These divisions have historically caused tensions between different religious groups. Although different religious sectors share many common cultural beliefs and practices, they differ according to the variant cultural characteristics (see Chapter 1). Hindi and English are India's official languages, but there are also 17 regional languages that are considered official. India has several cities that have undergone place name changes, such as Bombay being renamed Mumbai. These changes were mainly done in an effort to return the city names to local dialects instead of British translations.

Seventy-two percent of the population of India is Indo-Aryan, 25 percent Dravidian, and 25 percent and 3 percent Mongoloid and other, respectively. Table 16-1 provides the demographic trends related to population, fertility, mortality, and migration.

The Indus Valley civilization, one of the oldest in the world, dates back at least 5000 years. Aryan tribes from the northwest infiltrated onto the Indian subcontinent about 1500 B.C.; their merger with the earlier Dravidian inhabitants created the classical Indian culture. Arab incursions starting in the 8th century and Turkish in the 12th were followed by those of European traders, beginning in the late 15th century. By the 19th century, Britain had assumed political control of virtually all Indian lands. Indian armed forces in the British army played a vital role in both world wars. Nonviolent resistance to British colonialism led by Mohandas Ghandi and Jawaharlal Nehru brought independence in 1947. The subcontinent was divided into the secular state of India and the smaller Muslim state of Pakistan. A third war between the two countries in 1971 resulted in East Pakistan becoming the separate nation of Bangladesh (*CIA World Factbook,* 2011). Despite problems related to overpopulation, environmental degradation, extensive poverty, and ethnic and religious strife, India is rising on the world stage due to rapid economic development. In January 2011, India assumed a nonpermanent seat in the UN Security Council for the 2011–2012 term (*CIA World Factbook,* 2011).

Physical characteristics influencing the history and civilization of India are the size of the country and the comparative isolation provided by the Himalayas. The country suffers from droughts; flash floods and widespread and destructive flooding from monsoonal rains; severe thunderstorms; earthquakes; deforestation; soil erosion; overgrazing; desertification; air pollution from industrial effluents and vehicle emissions; and water pollution from raw sewage and runoff of agricultural pesticides. Tap water is not potable throughout the country.

India's long-term challenges include widespread poverty, inadequate physical and social infrastructure, limited nonagricultural employment opportunities, insufficient access to quality basic and higher education, and accommodating rural-to-urban migration. Despite these challenges, India has capitalized on its large educated English-speaking population to become a major exporter of information technology services and software workers (*CIA World Factbook,* 2011).

Heritage and Residence

Immigrants from India come predominantly from urban areas and include all major Indian states. Earlier immigrants represented a small and transitory community of students, Indian government officials, and businesspeople, and came from a diverse linguistic, religious, regional, and caste population (*caste* is a hereditary social class, discussed later under Spirituality). Asian Indian immigrants to America came in

II Table 16-1   **Demographic Trends in India**

Demographic Indicators for India	2011	1995	2005	2015	2025
Population					
Midyear population (in thousands)	1,189,173	920,585	1,090,973	1,251,696	1,396,046
Growth rate (percent)	1.3	1.9	1.5	1.2	1
Fertility					
Total fertility rate (births per woman)	2.6	3.4	2.8	2.5	2.3
Crude birth rate (per 1000 population)	21	28	23	20	17
Births (in thousands)	24.9	26	25.5	25	23.7
Mortality					
Life expectancy at birth (years)	67	60	65	68	71
Infant mortality rate (per 1000 births)	48	75	58	42	30
Under 5 mortality rate (per 1000 births)	65	109	81	56	39
Crude death rate (per 1000 population)	7	10	8	7	7
Deaths (in thousands)	8.9	8.8	8.7	9.2	10.2
Migration					
Net migration rate (per 1000 population)	–0	–0	–0	–0	–0
Net number of migrants (in thousands)	–59	–74	–55	–50	–56

From U.S. Census Bureau, International Data Base (2010).

two waves (Fenton, 1988). The first wave began in the early 20th century and continued to the mid-1920s. Conditions such as racial discrimination and lack of access to economic advancement made it difficult for the first wave of Asian Indians to sustain themselves or their culture. More than three-quarters of the 7000 Asian Indian immigrants in this wave came from the northwest of India, primarily from Punjab, and 90 percent of the Punjabis were Sikhs. Most Punjabis worked as manual laborers, first in Canada and later on the West Coast of the United States. Other Asian Indian immigrants, who were professionals and businesspeople, were mostly Hindus and Muslims who settled in San Francisco, Los Angeles, New York City, and the Midwest. The second wave of immigration began after 1965 and still continues. Most individuals from this wave are highly educated, skilled professionals and were predominantly from the urban middle class. The colonial authority of the British Raj engrained in the Indian mentality that foreign education is better than indigenous training.

Asian Indians in the United States as reported by the American Community Survey and reported in *Little India*, currently number over 2.4 million, with the largest Indian American populations in California, New York, New Jersey, Texas, and Illinois, in that order ("Asian Indian Population in 2005," 2005). There are also large Indian American populations in Florida, Georgia, Maryland, Michigan, Pennsylvania, Ohio, and Virginia. The New York metropolitan area, consisting of New York City and adjacent areas in the state of New York, as well as nearby areas in New Jersey, Connecticut, and Pennsylvania, are home to approximately 600,000 Indian Americans ("Asian Indian Population in 2005," 2005).

In relation to cultural value systems of the first-generation and second-generation Asian Indian immigrants, first-generation Asian Indians are acutely aware of readily apparent cultural differences. Their modern and traditional ideas are in conflict, with Indian culture clashing with American culture, and theory clashing with practice, inside and outside the home. The basis for interactions outside the home is the dominant culture, whereas inside the home, first-generation Asian Indians attempt to preserve their cultural and religious heritage and abide by Indian cultural values. For second-generation Asian Indians, the conflict of being the "in-betweens" become accentuated. Like their parents, the second-generation Indians also compartmentalize their life inside and outside the home. Conflicts typically arise from the cultural clash of how second-generation Asian Indians perceive American Individualism versus Indian communitarianism, in which career decisions are based on their impact on the family's financial well-being, not the individual's.

Reasons for Migration and Associated Economic Factors

Asian Indians leave their country for a variety of reasons, the most important of which is to attain a higher standard of living. The reasons for an overwhelming majority were financial factors. Although Asian Indians did migrate for financial reasons, they also left for professional, educational, and social opportunities. For many Asian Indians, emigration was thought prestigious. The prospect of greater material prosperity, combined with better working conditions, enhances the appeal of a wider range of job opportunities in the United States. Secondary reasons included opportunities for additional education as well as Indian perceptions of America as a land of opportunity and freedom. Immigrants include parents (who come for the sake of their children) and those who come on student visas and later change to permanent resident status.

India is a source, destination, and transit country for men, women, and children trafficked for the purposes of forced or bonded labor and commercial sexual exploitation. The large population of men, women, and children—numbering in the millions—in debt bondage face involuntary servitude in brick kilns, rice mills, and embroidery factories, whereas some children endure involuntary servitude as domestic servants. Internal trafficking of women and young girls for the purposes of commercial sexual exploitation and forced marriage also occurs; the government estimates that 90 percent of India's sex trafficking is internal. Young boys from Afghanistan, Pakistan, and Bangladesh are trafficked through India to the Gulf States for involuntary servitude as child camel jockeys. Indian men and women migrate willingly to the Persian Gulf region for work as domestic servants and low-skilled laborers, but some later find themselves in situations of involuntary servitude, including extended working hours, nonpayment of wages, restrictions on their movement by withholding their passports or confinement to the home, and physical or sexual abuse. Despite the reported extent of the trafficking crisis in India, efforts are in progress to prosecute traffickers and protect trafficking victims and to rescue victims of commercial sexual exploitation, forced child labor, and child armed combatants. The critical challenge overall is the lack of punishment for traffickers, effectively resulting in impunity for acts of human trafficking (*CIA World Factbook,* 2011).

Educational Status and Occupations

Most Asian Indians speak English, and many also speak another language. Because the immigration laws of 1965 granted immigrant visas only to people with certain professional and educational backgrounds, most Hindus in the United States possess high educational qualifications. However, those granted visas on the basis of marriage or relationships, such as parents, do not necessarily have the same educational backgrounds.

Communication
Dominant Language and Dialects

Although English enjoys associate status in India, it is the most important language for national, political, and commercial communication. **Hindi**, with 1652 dialectical variations, is the national language and primary tongue of 41 percent of the people. Other official languages are Bengali, Telugu, Marathi, Tamil, Urdu, Gujarati, Malayalam, Kannada, Oriya, Punjabi, Assamese, Kashmiri, Sindhi, and Sanskrit. Hindustani is a popular variant of Hindi/Urdu spoken widely throughout northern India, but it is not an official language (*CIA World Factbook,* 2011).

Because of regional dialects in the main language, health-care providers must be simple and direct in their communication and clear in their enunciation. Communication difficulties may not be apparent in well-educated Hindus. However, with the arrival of parents and grandparents who may not speak English, it is of utmost importance for health-care providers to have an interpreter available to provide quality health care. Hindus, especially women, often speak in a soft voice, making it difficult to understand or decipher what they say. The speech is coupled with an accent, further compromising communication with individuals of other cultures.

Cultural Communication Patterns

Hindus have close-knit family ties. Men especially may become intense and loud when they converse with other family members. To an onlooker, it might seem disruptive, but in general, this form of communication can be construed as meaningful when it is conducted with close friends.

Women are expected to strictly follow deference customs—that is, direct eye contact is avoided with men, although men can have direct eye contact with one another. Direct eye contact with older people and authority figures may be considered a sign of disrespect. More often, men and women use head movements and hand gestures to emphasize the spoken word. Strangers are greeted with folded hands and a head bow that respects their personal territory. Touching and embracing are not acceptable for displaying affection. Even between spouses, a public display of affection such as hugging or kissing is frowned upon, being considered strictly a private matter. Despite these societal constraints regarding the outward display of affection, Hindus are extremely family oriented and nurture one another in sickness, whether at home or in the hospital setting.

Temporal Relationships

According to the Hindu theory of creation, time (in Sanskrit *kal*) is a manifestation of God. The past, the present, and the future coexist in God simultaneously. Hence, the Hindu concept of time is past, present, and future oriented, depending on generation, socioeconomic status, and educational level. The Hindu value on educational attainment denotes a futuristic temporality.

Because of the Indian worldview of the cyclic nature of the universe and belief in reincarnation, Indians have a relaxed attitude toward time (Jain, 1992). Due to the Hindu broad concept of time, adherence to the North American parameters of time may not be rigid. Punctuality in keeping scheduled appointments may not be considered important. Health-care providers must understand the value placed on time by Hindus and not misconstrue being late for appointments as a sign of irresponsibility or not valuing their health.

Format for Names

Women adhere to a specified linguistic style when talking with their husbands. The hierarchical structure of interrelationship is built into the structure of language. The woman refers to the man in the plural *Avar* and *Aap*, meaning "you" (with respect), whereas the man can use a singular "you" like *Ne, Aval*, or *Thum. Aap* means "thou" and is used for elderly family members and for strangers. Older family members are usually not addressed by name but as elder brother, sister, aunt, or uncle. A woman never addresses a man by name because the woman is not considered an equal or a superior. However, exceptions to this practice occur when the woman is older than the man.

The system of "naming" customs in India is complex and relative to the social and cultural structures. The naming customs are closely related to Hindusim, chaturvarna system of castes (see section on Spirituality), clan, and lineage (Jayaraman, 2005).

Family Roles And Organization
Head of Household and Gender Roles

No institution in India is more important than the family. The family was originally patriarchal and the joint family evolved from it, the transition arising from the death of the common ancestor or the patriarch of the family. The hierarchical structure of authority in the patriarchal joint family, based on the principle of superiority of men over women, is the most important instrument of social control. The rights and duties of individuals are prescribed by the hierarchical order of power and authority. The male head of the family is legitimized and considered sacred by caste and religion that delineate relationships.

The central criteria of the Hindu joint family include (1) family property jointly owned by men and inheritable only by the male lineage (although by law it is to be shared equally among both male and female offspring); (2) the hierarchical structure of authority according to gender and age; and (3) the dependence of women and children. Central relationships in this system are based on continuation and expansion of the male lineage through inheritance and ancestor worship, related to the father–son and brother–brother relationships.

Family plays a significant role in the Indian culture. For generations, India has had a prevailing tradition of the joint family system. It is a system under which extended members of a family—parents, children, the children's spouses and their offspring, and so on—live together. Usually, the eldest male member is the head in the joint Indian family system. He makes all important decisions and rules, and other family members abide by them.

Within the joint family system, the patrilineal system created a sense of worthlessness, servitude, and dependence for women characterized by a lack of freedom, as well as constraints and limitations that suppressed individual development. A submissive and acquiescent role is expected of women in the first few years of married life, with little or no participation in decision making. Strict norms govern contact and communication with the men of the family, including a woman's husband. However, in recent times, many families, especially in urban areas, have stopped abiding by the extended family system and have started living as a nuclear family.

Although a patrilineal system is not characteristic of the nuclear family, the distinctions between men and women persist. This is also true of the matrilineal system that exists in a few areas in the southwestern and northeastern regions of the country. In a matrilineal system, the lineage is counted through the woman, but power rests with the men in the woman's family. Hence, even in a matrilineal system, constraints abound for women because of power distribution that promotes male dominance.

In the Indian household, lines of hierarchy and authority are clearly drawn, shaping structurally and psychologically complex family relationships. Ideals of conduct are aimed at creating and maintaining family harmony. All family members are socialized to accept the authority of those ranked above them in the hierarchy. In general, elders rank above juniors, and among people of similar age, males outrank females. Among adults in a joint family, a newly arrived daughter-in-law has the least authority. Males learn to command others within the household but expect to accept the direction of senior males. Ideally, even a mature adult man living in his father's household acknowledges his father's authority on both minor and major matters. Women are especially strongly socialized to accept a position subservient to males, to control their sexual impulses, and to subordinate their personal preferences to the needs of the family and kin group. Reciprocally, those in authority accept responsibility for meeting the needs of others in the family group.

Much has changed in the status and roles of women; however, most Hindu women remain subservient to their closest male relatives, a situation that is gradually changing. Hindu society is trying to redefine the role of women in the institution of family and society. Politically Hindu women today enjoy an equal status with men and wider opportunities than their counterparts in many Western countries. Although there is ongoing discussion to provide them with new privileges and rights, including inheritance rights, much still needs to be done on the social and economic front. Women in Hindu society still suffer from gender bias and a number of other problems such as dowry, inheritance, domestic abuse, sexual exploitation, rape, and harassment.

Changing role status is further illustrated by Varghese and Jenkins (2009), who studied the variables that might be related to high cultural conflict among first- and second-generation Asian Indian immigrant women and the psychological consequences of cultural value conflict. Self-report data from 73 community-dwelling women were used to examine women's recollections of parental overprotection, their reports of cultural value conflict, and their ratings of self-esteem and depression symptoms. Varghese and Jenkins found that the results supported the hypotheses that unmarried and second-generation women would report greater maternal control and cultural value conflict than married and first-generation women. Second-generational status, high maternal control, and high cultural value conflict correlated with higher depressive symptoms, while being married, low maternal control, and low cultural conflict were related to high self-esteem.

Prescriptive, Restrictive, and Taboo Behaviors for Children and Adolescents

Hindu parents in general want their children to be successful and strongly encourage and emphasize scholastic achievement in fields that promise good employment and a high social status. Hindu parents in America want their children to be successful and maintain ties with their families and the Indian community. Thus, parents face a dilemma between aspiring for the American dream of success for their children and holding on to their desire to maintain Indian values. Status indicators such as education, income, and community and occupational leadership tend to replace ascribed social status.

The birth of a male child is considered important, and the desire for a male child rather than a female child is often prevalent. Furthermore, widowhood, especially for women, is considered a negation of marriage (Duvvurry, 1991). In America, Hindu parents may have reservations about eventual marriage partners for their children and concerns about the issues of dating, premarital sex, and freedom. Although many Hindu parents expect and accept the Westernization of their children, the question of marriage is still a concern for Hindu parents who have opinions about how their children should be married, whether "arranged" or partly arranged. Hindu parents or Indians from all religious traditions want their children to marry other Indians. Health-care providers should understand the various types of families (joint, extended, or nuclear) and should determine which individual has control within the hierarchy.

Arranged marriages at a young age are considered most desirable for women. This practice is related to the importance of virginity and restrictions placed on marriage within the same clan. For centuries, arranged marriages have been the tradition in Indian society. Even today, the vast majority of Indians have their marriages planned by their parents and other respected family members, with the consent of the bride and groom. They also demand a dowry, which has been outlawed by the Indian government, but Indian society and culture still promote and maintain it. They avoid detection by not letting authorities know about any money arrangements. Arranged matches are made after taking into account factors such as age, height, personal values and tastes, the backgrounds of their families (wealth, social standing), their castes, and the astrological compatibility of the couple's horoscopes.

In India, since marriage is thought to be for life, the divorce rate is extremely low, and arranged marriages generally have an even lower divorce rate. Divorce rates have risen significantly in recent years. There is conflict of opinion over what the phenomenon means—whether, for traditionalists, the rising number of divorces portends the breakdown of society or, for modernists, creates a healthy new empowerment for women.

Although arranged marriages are still a preferred choice among the younger generation, education and liberalization of ideas in urban areas have led to changes in selecting a marriage partner. The practice of an arranged marriage continues in the United States to minimize the stress associated with differences in caste, lifestyles, and expectations between the male and the female hierarchy.

The two major types of transfer of material wealth accompanying marriage are bride price and a dowry. The bride price is customarily prevalent among patrilineal tribes and the middle and lower castes of nontribal populations. Bride price is payment in cash and other materials to the bride's father in exchange for authority over the woman, which passes from her kin group to the bridegroom's kin group. In communities that follow this custom, a daughter is not regarded as a burden, and parents do not dread the thought of marriage. A daughter brings wealth to the family as a result of marriage.

Regional variations exist in understanding the dowry system. Dowry may be seen as the gift given to the bride and often settled prior to marriage, which may not be regarded as her property; as a gift given to the bridegroom before and at the time of marriage; or as a present to the groom's relatives. The practice of dowry in the Hindu community has a number of cultural and social sanctions. Dowry is regarded as essential to obtain a suitable match for a young woman, ensuring a high standard of life.

The increase in social and economic inequality is one of the most important inducements for a dowry and operates at all levels of society. Wealth ranges from a few hundred to thousands of rupees (Indian currency), and behind this transaction is a direct desire to improve the daughter's social status, which indirectly assists the social status of the bridegroom's family. The desire to obtain security and good status for the daughter places the bride's parents in a vulnerable position, in which they are faced with demands bearing no relation to their economic capacity. This may reduce them to a state of indebtedness.

Family Goals and Priorities

In the joint family structure, Hindu women are considered "outsiders" and are socialized and incorporated in such a way that the "jointness" and residence are not broken up. This means that a close relationship between the husband and the wife is disapproved because it induces favoring the nuclear family and dissolving the joint family.

The Hindu family's goals and priorities include the most important Hindu sacrament, the Vivaha (marriage), which is a religious and social institution. The marital union is a matter for the husband and wife, society, guardians, and supernatural powers that symbolize spirituality. Therefore, a marriage is regarded as indissoluble. The sacrament of marriage impresses on a person that earthly life is not to be despised; rather, it should be consciously accepted and elevated to the level of a spiritual experience.

In patrilineal societies, marriage signifies a transfer of a woman from her natal group to that of her husband. Marriage is not considered primarily an affair of the man and woman who are getting married but an event that involves the kin of both spouses. Hence, the institution of marriage is a means by which alliances are created or strengthened between two or more groups.

Family elders are held in reverence and cared for by their children when they are no longer able to care for themselves. Families believe that knowledge is transmitted through an oral tradition derived from experience, and the elderly are repositories of such knowledge.

Alternative Lifestyles

Religion has played a role in shaping Indian customs and traditions. While homosexuality has not been

REFLECTIVE EXERCISE 16.1

Revathy Srinivasan, a Hindu woman aged 25 years, has lived in the United States for 9 years, and her parents have just arrived. She wishes to marry Velayudham Mani (Vel), a man she met in graduate school, who is also a Hindu. However, her parents will not allow her to marry Vel because he is of a lower caste than she is. Besides, her parents want her to marry their friends' son Ajay, who is well established. Revathy's parents feel that both their and their friends' family backgrounds (wealth and social standing) are congruent, in addition to the astrological compatibility of both children's horoscopes. If Revathy insists on marrying Vel, they will not give Vel's family any dowry.

1. How common are arranged marriages among Hindus in India? In the United States?
2. What is a dowry?
3. What is the significance of a dowry?
4. Describe the caste system of Asian Indians.
5. Should Revathy seek counseling to help her solve her dilemma? If so, from what type of counselor should she seek help?

explicitly mentioned in the religious texts central to Hinduism, it has taken various positions, ranging from positive to neutral or antagonistic. Historical literary evidence indicates that homosexuality has been prevalent across the Indian subcontinent throughout history and that homosexuals were not necessarily considered inferior in any way. Whereas homosexuality probably occurs as frequently as in any group, this lifestyle may cause a social stigma, and there is a high degree of stigma associated with homosexuality in India. However, attitudes toward homosexuality have shifted slightly in recent years. In particular, there have been more depictions and discussions of homosexuality in the Indian news media. In mid-2009, the New Delhi High Court decriminalized homosexual intercourse between consenting adults, throughout India, making HIV education and surveillance very difficult. Outreach workers are often harassed and even arrested for "promoting homosexuality." It is estimated that 42 percent of all men who have sex with men are also married, fueling the increasing HIV infection rate among women of India (Cichocki, 2007).

Gay people in India may not be completely liberated, but they are more willing than ever before to challenge curiosity, even rejection, without allowing it to damage their conscience. In the past two years, many 18- to 24-year-olds have come out. They are honest with their parents. This is different from the times when parents would force a heterosexual marriage on them to "normalize" things. But in modern India the acceptance is different for male gays and lesbians because of lack of resources or educational opportunities. The Sahayatrika group of Kerala, which recently did a study on lesbian suicides, has catalyzed a reconsideration of same-sexuality. There has been an increase in support groups with separate help lines catering to Hindi-speaking, English-speaking, and transgender groups. In West Bengal, the "coming out" phenomenon is seen even in smaller districts, with networks like Manas Bangla, headquartered in Kolkata (Vasudev, Radhakrishnan, Ravindran, & Dangor, 2004).

A paucity of information exists regarding Hindu gay or lesbian couples in the professional literature. Healthcare providers can refer lesbian, gay, or bisexual Hindu Americans to the Gay and Lesbian Vaishnava Association Inc. (2005), a resource for Hindus and other Southeast Asian groups. Single-parent, blended, or communal families are not well accepted by Hindus. In addition, two magazines, *Trikone*, the first quarterly magazine for gay South Asian men and women, and *India Currents*, a monthly arts and entertainment magazine, are targeted to Indo-Americans living in California.

Workforce Issues

Culture in the Workplace

With comparative ease, most Hindus have become part of the skilled workforce in America. Hard work, interest in saving and investment, and business acumen enable many to become financially successful. Because of their educational and professional background, it is not difficult for most to find suitable employment and improve their economic status.

Many Hindus have a singular devotion to their career, profession, or business, which results in a personal cost evidenced in family relationships or in health status. Demonstrating hospitality is important to Hindus. A new friendship is not formally acknowledged among Hindus without the reciprocity of home visits. Thus, Americans who refer to their Indian acquaintances and colleagues as "friends" without having extended hospitality to them in their homes might confuse the Hindu immigrant's notions of friendship.

At work, Hindus adopt American practices and cultural habits, but at home and at Indian gatherings, they retain many of their own cultural practices. Active participation in Indian organizations is a growing phenomenon, especially in the absence of the cultural milieu available in India. Hindu Americans believe that such participation is the only way their children can become aware of their Indian heritage. Currently in America, numerous regional Indian organizations are available throughout the country, resulting in a vast network of communication. Religious revivalism and social conviviality are the hallmarks of Hindu adaptation.

Issues Related to Autonomy

An early realization of immigrants in a new country is that they must build new relationships and find new reference groups. Hierarchies of age, gender, and caste prescribe transactions among Hindus. At work, relationships are a reproduction of the authority-dependence characteristic of family and social relationships. In seeking to establish a personal and benevolent relationship, Hindus may be seen as too eager to please, ingratiating, or docile, all antithetical to the task of assertion and independence.

Hindus speak English as well as their regional languages at home. Therefore, they rarely have any difficulty with communication in the American workforce. However, because most Hindus have learned and speak British English, those unfamiliar with British English and idioms may have difficulty understanding them and should ask for clarification.

Biocultural Ecology

Skin Color and Other Biological Variations

Asian Indian Hindus evidence a diversity of physical types. Asian Indians can be divided into three general groups according to the color of their skin: white in the north and the northwest, yellow in the east, and black in the south. Whites, Indids, have a light brown skin color, wavy black hair, dark or light brown eyes; are tall or of medium height; and are either dolichocephalic (i.e., long-headed) or brachycephalic (i.e., short-headed). The physical type of the Indids varies according to regions, ranging from a light to a brown skin color. The yellow races are found in the periphery of India in the areas bordering Tibet and Assam.

Black-skinned people, Melanids, are often referred to as the *Dravidians*, the population of southern India. The Melanids have dark skin (ranging from light brown to black), elongated heads, broad noses, thick lips, and black, wavy hair; they are usually less than 5 feet 6 inches tall. The most characteristic Melanids are the Tamils, a major linguistic and cultural group in South India.

Because skin color varies regionally, health-care providers must be careful when arriving at a diagnosis that may be applicable only to white-skinned people. Pallor in brown-skinned patients may present as a yellowish-brown tinge to the skin. Pallor in dark-skinned individuals is characterized by the absence of the underlying red tones in the skin. Furthermore, jaundice may be observed in the sclera and should not be confused with the normal yellow pigmentation of the dark-skinned black patient. In addition, the oral mucosa of dark-skinned individuals may have a normal freckling or pigmentation. Cyanosis can often be difficult to determine in dark-skinned individuals. A close inspection of the nailbeds, lips, palpebral conjunctivae, and palms of the hands and soles of the feet shows evidence of cyanosis.

Diseases and Health Conditions

The rainy season in the tropics is associated with an increase in malaria. Asian Indians migrating to the

United States from the tropical regions may be susceptible to malaria, which intensifies during the monsoon season. Filariasis is prevalent in some parts of India. Respiratory infections such as tuberculosis and pneumonia are also widely prevalent in the midlatitudes and, in the rainy season, in monsoon areas. Respiratory infections occur in the most densely populated river valleys and coastal lowlands and in dark, intensely crowded urban areas. Major infectious diseases include food- or water-borne diseases like bacterial diarrhea, hepatitis A and E, and typhoid fever; vector-borne diseases like chikungunya, dengue fever, Japanese encephalitis, and malaria; animal contact diseases like rabies; and water contact diseases like leptospirosis. Highly pathogenic H5N1 avian influenza has also been identified (*CIA World Factbook,* 2011).

When performing health assessments, health screenings, and physical examinations, health-care providers must be alert to possible signs and symptoms of the risk factors associated with different diseases linked to migration from different regions of India.

The four leading chronic diseases in India, as measured by their prevalence, are, in descending order, cardiovascular diseases (CVDs), *diabetes mellitus* (diabetes), chronic obstructive pulmonary disease (COPD), and cancer. All four of these diseases are projected to continue to increase in prevalence in the near future given the demographic trends and lifestyle changes underway in India (Shetty, 2002). Heart disease tends to develop at a very early age in Asian Indians. The major causes of cardiovascular disease are tobacco use, physical inactivity, and an unhealthy diet. India suffers disproportionately from cardiovascular disease. A 2008 article in *The Lancet* (Crosta, 2008) reported that "India will bear 60 percent of the world's heart disease burden in the next two years [2008–2010]. In addition, researchers have determined that compared to people in other developed countries, the average age of patients with heart disease is lower among Indian people, and Indians are more likely to have types of heart disease that lead to worse outcomes."

Diabetes mellitus, insulin resistance, and central obesity are also prevalent among this population, as are high serum levels of lipoprotein (Blesch, Davis, & Kamath, 1999). Diabetes is second only to CVD as a health burden in India, and, of course, the two are highly correlated and interdependent. The International Diabetes Federation (IDF) reports a projected prevalence of 70 million patients in India by the year 2025 (Sicree, Shaw, & Zimmet, 2006; Taylor, 2010), and the World Health Organization (WHO) estimates that India will have 80 million cases of diabetes by 2030 (Wild, Roglic, Green, Sicree, & King, 2004).

Hindu immigrants have a higher mortality rate than that of the local population. Rheumatic heart disease, together with high blood pressure, is a major cardiac problem. Dental caries and periodontal disease affect 90 percent of the adult population. Sickle cell disease is highly prevalent; the gene is detected in 16.48 percent of selected populations.

Breast cancer is one of the leading causes of morbidity and premature death among women in India (Sadler, Dhanjal, Shah, Ko, Anghel, & Harshburger, 2001). Based on studies in India, Choudhry, Srivastava, and Fitch (1998) implied that immigrant women from India share the same risk as their Western counterparts.

In India, the most prevalent forms of cancer among men are tobacco-related cancers, including lung, oral, larynx, esophagus, and pharynx. Almost 50 percent more Indian men smoke than men in the United States. Among Indian women, in addition to tobacco-related cancers, cervix, breast, and ovarian cancers are also prevalent. India currently has the highest prevalence of oral cancer cases in the world as a result of the popularity of chewing tobacco in its rural regions.

Sexually transmitted infections (STIs) in children are not uncommon in India, though systematic epidemiological studies to determine the exact prevalence are not available. STIs in children can be acquired via sexual routes or, uncommonly, via nonsexual routes such as accidental inoculation by a diseased individual. Neonatal infections are almost always acquired intrauterine or during delivery.

Sexual abuse and sex trafficking remain important problems in India. Surveys indicate that nearly half of the children are sexually abused. Most at-risk children are street-based, homeless, or those living in or near brothels. The last two decades have shown an increase in the prevalence of STIs in children, though most of the data are from the northern part of the country and from major hospitals. However, due to better availability of antenatal care to the majority of women, cases of congenital syphilis have declined consistently over the past 2 to 3 decades. Other bacterial STIs are also on the decline. On the other hand, viral STIs such as genital herpes and anogenital warts are increasing. This reflects trends of STIs in the adult population. Concomitant HIV infection is uncommon in children. Comprehensive sex education, stringent laws to prevent sex trafficking and child sexual abuse, and antenatal screening of all women can reduce the prevalence of STIs in children (Dhawan, Gupta, & Kumar, 2010).

Variations in Drug Metabolism

Asians are known to require lower doses and to have side effects at lower doses than whites for a variety of different psychotropic drugs, including lithium, antidepressants, and neuroleptics (Levy, 1993). Asians are also more sensitive to the adverse effects of alcohol, resulting in marked facial flushing, palpitations, and tachycardia.

Dietary variations may significantly alter the metabolic rate or plasma levels of medicines in Asian Indians (Levy, 1993). The metabolism of antipyrine in Asian Indians living in rural villages in India has been compared with that of Indian immigrants in England. The results indicate that drug metabolism among Indian immigrants becomes more rapid when they adopt the British lifestyle and dietary habits (Levy, 1993). Hence, because of ethnic differences in the rates of drug metabolism, more consideration should be given to individualizing treatment regimens in special population groups, such as Hindus. Health-care providers should question therapeutic regimens that do not consider racial or ethnic differences.

High-Risk Behaviors

Alcoholism and cigarette smoking among Hindu Americans, especially among men, may cause significant health problems. Adolescents face tremendous pressure to keep up the image of "wiz kids" and to meet the expectations of their parents, which may override individual aptitudes and choices. This may create anxiety and frustration, thereby leading to failure and anger toward parents, which may predispose them to using drugs as a coping strategy. However, adequate literature or studies to substantiate these behaviors are not available.

Other high-risk behaviors include those that lead to contracting HIV. According to Cichocki (2007), the following populations are at the highest risk:

• *Sex workers*—Because of widespread poverty throughout India, women often resort to prostitution as a means of making money for their families. Others are forced into sex work due to an underground of violence and disrespect toward women. Finally, women involved in marital breakups will often begin prostituting themselves as a means of surviving financially after being left with children to feed and a household to support. In some areas of India, it is estimated that one in every two sex workers are HIV infected, many of whom are unaware of it.
• *IV drug use (IVDU)*—The recreational use of drugs often overlaps with the sex trade. While IVDU seems to be worse in the northeastern parts of India, it is common throughout the country. Many attribute the widespread problems of IVDU and HIV to government policies that do not support HIV prevention and risk reduction among IV drug users. Because IVDU is a crime and is consistently enforced and prosecuted, getting prevention messages to users is very difficult. There have been instances of prevention workers themselves being arrested while trying to help and educate IV drug users. Official estimates actually report the HIV prevalence among IV drug users to have gone

down from 13 percent in 2003 to 10 percent in 2005.
• *Truck drivers*—India's economy depends a great deal on its very large trucking network across the country. While truckers help move goods and services throughout India, they also contribute a great deal to the huge HIV population and the spread of HIV from one area of India to another. Truckers will pick up sex workers along their route, engage in unprotected sex activity, and then drop off the sex worker at the trucker's next stop along the route. This has contributed to the spread of HIV from urban areas into the rural towns and villages. The most damaging fact about truckers and their use of sex workers is that they usually do not know they are infected.
• *Migrant workers*—As is the case in the United States, migrant workers in India are very transient and mobile, moving from town to town wherever the work takes them. Unfortunately, they take their risky behavior along with them, fueling the spread of HIV throughout India. While there are attempts at HIV education, the variety of languages, dialects, and cultures makes HIV education very difficult.

High-risk behaviors contribute to the spread of HIV, which has progressed from a disease found in only the highest-risk populations to one found in all segments of the Indian population, including men and women, rich and poor, urban and rural. Populations thought at one time to be low risk are now being infected, as are high-risk groups. Some groups are being infected at a higher rate than others. For instance, women are being infected by way of heterosexual transmission at an alarming rate. Women now make

REFLECTIVE EXERCISE 16.2

Dabeet Singh, a practicing Hindu man aged 22 years, has been a student majoring in computer technology for 2 years at a nearby university. His roommate convinced him to see the nurse at the school health clinic because he has been demonstrating high-risk behaviors such as smoking two packs of cigarettes a day and drinking four 12-oz cans of beer every day. In addition, over the last 2 weeks, he has not been attending his classes but sitting in his room, acting anxious and frustrated with his friends and teachers. In a low voice, he tells the nurse that he wants to quit school and return home where people are more polite and can understand him better.

1. Give two plausible reasons for Dabeet's high-risk behaviors from a cultural context.
2. What evidence is there to show that Dabeet might be depressed?
3. What type of spiritual counseling might the nurse suggest?

up about 39 percent of those living with HIV. Most are being infected by husbands or boyfriends who have multiple sexual partners, many of whom are infected with HIV and do not know it.

Health-Care Practices

Patterns of health-seeking behaviors among Hindus are strongly influenced by their sociocultural networks. Customs and beliefs often affect medical-care decisions and choice of health-care services. The actions of supernatural forces and certain human excesses are considered important in causing illness, even among highly educated Hindus. Furthermore, regional variations in the intensity and strength of the belief system are significant. For example, some individuals believe that excessive consumption of sweets may cause roundworms and that too much sexual activity and worry are associated with tuberculosis. In addition, some believe that diarrhea and cholera are caused by a variety of improper eating habits. Therefore, health-care providers cannot take for granted that all Hindu immigrants have the same belief systems with the same degree of intensity. Deep-rooted beliefs about illnesses will inhibit the acceptance of scientific causes for diseases. This may result in difficulty with treatment.

Nutrition

Meaning of Food

Many cultures have influenced Indian food practices. Dietary habits within the Indian subcontinent are complex, regionally varied, and strongly influenced by religion. Hindus believe that food was created by the Supreme Being for the benefit of humanity; thus, growing, harvesting, preparing, and consuming food are steeped in rituals. Sacred Hindu texts contain aspects related to food, dietary habits, and recommendations.

The influence of religion is pervasive in food selection, customs, and preparation methods. Noble and Dutt (1982) stated that the classification of the regional food habits can be twofold, based on the types of cereals and fresh foods consumed. In the first category are rice and bread eaters; in the second category are vegetarians and nonvegetarians. Whereas Buddhism and Jainism turned people to vegetarianism, the influence of the Vedic religion and later the influx of outsiders made Indians nonvegetarians. In modern India, vegetarianism is firmly rooted in culture and the term *nonvegetarian* is used to describe anyone who eats meat, eggs, poultry, fish, and, sometimes, cheese. Many Brahmins in northern India consider eating meat to be religiously sanctioned. In some parts of India, Brahmins' eating fish is acceptable, whereas in other parts, eating meat of any source is sacrilegious (Kilara & Iya, 1992). Many Indians are vegetarians

because of agricultural traditions and adverse economic conditions.

Common Foods and Food Rituals

Although India is essentially an agricultural country, food production is insufficient to adequately feed the entire population. Geographic influences favor the production of grains, rice, wheat, jowar, *bajra*, jute, oilseeds, peanuts, and mustard. The principal food crop consists of rice in the better-watered regions and wheat in the Punjab. Sesame millet, maize, and peas grow throughout the country. Sugarcane and jute are cultivated extensively. The coconut palm is a valuable resource in the southern coastal areas. Cereals supply a large percentage of the total calorie requirements. Rice, wheat, millet, barley, maize, and *ragi* make up the bulk of the diet.

A variety of "pulses" (legumes such as lentils), cooked vegetables, meat, fish, eggs, and dairy products are also consumed. Heavily spiced (curry) dishes with vegetables, meat, fish, or eggs are favored, and hot pickles and condiments are common. Spice choices include garlic, ginger, turmeric, tamarind, cumin, coriander, and mustard seed. Vegetable choices include onions, tomatoes, potatoes, green leaves, okra, green beans, and root vegetables. Milk is used in coffee and tea and in preparing yogurt and buttermilk. Water is the beverage of choice with meals and as a thirst quencher.

One of the most common food items in southern India is boiled rice containing spices and vegetables; it is usually served with a lentil-based sauce, *sambar*. Other common foods in the south are *rasam* (a dilute liquid made from tomatoes, tamarind, and boiled rice served with spices) and *thayir* (yogurt with boiled rice). The traditional southern Indian vegetarian preparations of rice and lentil flour dishes are called *idli*, *dosai*, or *vadai*. Snacks are also consumed either as breakfast items or substituted in place of regular meals. Food is usually served in a *thali*, a round plate. Coffee is popular in southern India, whereas tea is the beverage of choice in the rest of the country. In the north, *chapati*, a bread made from wheat flour, is common, as is *puris*, which is similar to *chapati* except that it is deep-fried, whereas the former is baked on a round iron plate. Seasonal products such as groundnuts (peanuts), mangoes, and bananas are consumed between meals. Savory items such as deep-fried preparations of grains, vegetables, and spices are also consumed as snacks between meals. In northern India, wheat is the staple food. Other cereals are *jowar*, *bajra*, and *ragi*, which are consumed in porridges, gruels, and *rotis* (baked pancakes).

Customs and prejudices often remove certain food items from the diet, although the prohibitions vary from place to place. Thus, *bajra*, a staple food in Maratha families, is not looked on favorably in

Uttar Pradesh. People from Punjab do not favor fish, whereas people from the south generally dislike the idea of meat of any kind. In Saurashtra in the south, fish, fowl, meat, and eggs are taboo practically everywhere.

Women generally serve the food and may eat separately from men. Food preparation has strict rules. Women are not allowed to cook or have contact with other members of the family during their menstrual periods. Brahmins are the preferred cooks because the cook must be as pure as the eater (Kilara & Iya, 1992). Health-care providers must assess for food rituals practiced by Hindus in relation to mealtimes and food selections before attempting to teach them about medication regimens.

Dietary Practices for Health Promotion

Foremost among the perceptions of Hindus is the belief that certain foods are "hot" and others "cold," and, therefore, should be eaten only during certain seasons and not in combination. The geographic differences in the hot and cold perceptions are dramatic; many foods considered hot in the north are considered cold in the south. Such perceptions and distinctions are based on how specific foods are believed to affect body functions. The belief is that failure to observe rules related to the hot-and-cold theory of disease results in illness. When the three basic principles or humors— *vata, pitta,* and *kapha*—are in the state of equilibrium, digestion and metabolism are in order, the foundations of the tissues and excretion of waste products are normal, and an individual is physically and mentally happy.

Nutritional Deficiencies and Food Limitations

Nutritional deficiencies are regionally patterned, indicating preferences for a certain variety of cereals. For example, beriberi is found in rice-growing areas, pellagra in maize-millet areas, and lathyrism in Central India. Thiamine deficiency is common among people who are mostly dependent on rice. Thoroughly milling rice, washing rice before cooking, and allowing the cooked rice to remain overnight before consumption the following day result in the loss of thiamine.

Commitment to the concept of the "sacred cow" has a significant impact in India's economic life and ecology, most notably by encouraging dairy farming and milk use. However, lactose intolerance affects up to 1 percent of infants and more than 10 percent of adults, resulting in an inability to produce the enzyme needed to digest lactose, or milk sugar. The ability or inability to digest lactose may be due to genetic differences among Asian Indians.

The consumption of a single cereal, such as rice, as the bulk of a diet results in a poor intake of lysine and other essential amino acids. Pellagra, a nutritional deficiency causing skin and mental disorders and diarrhea,

occurs largely where people consume mostly maize and sorghum (*jowar*). Both cereals have high leucine content and provide strong evidence for the pathogenesis of pellagra. Lathyrism is a crippling disease causing paralysis of leg muscles that is seen mostly in adults who consume large quantities of seeds of the pulse *khesari* (*Lathyrus sativus*) over a long period of time. Thus, protein malnutrition is serious and widespread in India.

Goiters are common along the sub-Himalayan tracts, resulting from an iodine deficiency in food and water. Fluorosis occurs in parts of Punjab, Haryana, Andhra Pradesh, and Karnataka, resulting from drinking water with high fluoride content. Osteomalacia is prevalent in northwestern India, where diets are deficient in calcium and vitamin D. Endemic dropsy is prevalent in western Bengal as a result of the use of mustard oil for cooking (Noble & Dutt, 1982).

The high incidence of stomach cancer in the south may be due to the excessive intake of fried fatty foods and chilies and rapid food consumption. By contrast, cancer of the stomach is infrequent in people in the north who consume milk and dairy products. In several north Indian states, many people chew betel (paan), which is offered as a sign of hospitality. Paan contains arecanut, cardamom, fennel, lime (calcium hydroxide), tobacco, and other ingredients, and among users cancers of the mouth and lip are common, especially since tobacco can induce oral cancer. Beta carotene from Spirulina or other sources such as carrots can prevent such cancer (Garewal, 1995). Strachan, Powell, Thaker, Millard, and Maxwell (1995) found a vegetarian diet to be an independent risk factor for tuberculosis among immigrant Asians in south London. Using a case-control method, Asian immigrants from India diagnosed with tuberculosis during the previous 10 years were compared with two Asian control groups. The results confirmed earlier findings that Hindu Asians had an increased risk for tuberculosis compared with Muslims. Religion had no independent influence after adjustment for vegetarianism. The authors concluded that decreased immunocompetence associated with a vegetarian diet might result in increased mycobacterial reactivation among Hindu Asians.

Food practices of the Hindus may remain unchanged with increasing numbers of immigrants to America. In a study of the dietary habits of 73 Asian Indians in relation to the length of residence in the United States, Raj, Ganganna, and Bowering (1999) found that, in contrast to recent immigrants (less than 10 years), long-time immigrants reported eating mostly Indian foods for dinner and weekend meals. The authors also found that regardless of the length of residence in the United States, consumption of white bread, roots, tubers, vegetable oils, legumes, and tea changed little. Self-reported data indicated that high serum cholesterol levels, increased weight, hypertension, arthritis, and diabetes were diagnosed in respondents older than age 30 years. The authors concluded that despite the small sample size, although Asian Indians in the study included many American foods in their diets, they continued to eat many traditional foods, perhaps in an effort to retain cultural identity.

All major food groups of the Hindus are generally available through Indian grocery and spice stores located in major metropolitan areas throughout the United States. The flavor, spices, and diversity of ethnic foods are making many Indian restaurants popular. Given the diversity of Hindus in America, health-care providers must individually assess dietary practices and nutritional deficiencies of their patients according to their ethnic origins and area of residence.

For the majority of Hindu Americans who are vegetarians, their protein comes from pulses, lentils, legumes, and dairy products. Because the production of pulses has not kept pace with increasing poulation, the protein-calorie imbalance is widened. The scarcity of commodity such as pulses predisposes to infectious diseases and nutritional deficient disorders, especially in young children (Kumar, 2004). Other forms of malnutrition are caused by deficiency of micronutrients like iron, vitamin A, and iodine. Deficiency of vitamin A results in nutritional blindness in children. Iodine deficiency disorders are associated with impairment of mental and intellectual functions in children and adults, and in severe case with deafness and mutism, neuromuscular disorders, and perinatal and infant mortality (Kumar, 2004).

In remote and inaccessible areas where there is a lack of qualified physicians and modern health facilities, medicinal plants have traditionally been used. Certain foods and/or food additives such as *Spirulina* microalgae enhance the immune system and have antiaging properties and, in combination with turmeric and oil from the *neem* tree (an evergreen tree found in India), can ward off many infectious and noninfectious diseases, incuding cancer, gastrointestinal disorders, diabetes, skin troubles, dental problems, and cardiovascular disorders (Kumar, 2004). Also, beta carotene as an important antioxidant has been reported to inhibit oral carcinogenesis (Sankaranarayanan et al., 1997).

Pregnancy and Childbearing Practices

Fertility Practices and Views Toward Pregnancy

Methods of birth control among Hindus include intrauterine devices (IUDs), condoms, and the rhythm and withdrawal methods. Because of their cultural orientation, Hindu women may desire education in family planning from a same-sex health-care provider, as well as assistance with delivery from female physicians, midwives, or nurse practitioners. Fisher, Bowman, and Thomas (2003) enumerate the issues surrounding sexuality and childbirth in Asian Indian women. For many Indian women, intercourse experiences are painful because of lack of sex education. In general, women are not educated about contraceptive options until after the first child. For this reason, most couples have their first child within the first year of marriage. The birth of a healthy first child reassures both families about the couple's health and that they are a "good match." Couples are commonly sent to fertility specialists if a child is not born after the first or second year of marriage. Husbands do not accompany pregnant women to physician visits, but mothers do. Only the nurse and the obstetrician (who is a female) attend to the patient at the time of delivery, although the woman's mother and other female relatives are usually nearby for assistance with her personal needs. Husbands usually come to the hospital or birth center, but they are not permitted to watch the delivery. If the husband is visiting during postpartum rounds, he will leave the room for the wife's examination.

Fisher, Bowman, and Thomas (2003) also state that pregnancy can be a frightening time for a young wife, especially if there are no female relatives available to educate her. Indian men might prefer to wait outside the room or stay away from the hospital during this time in contrast to American hospitals and birthing centers, where it is the norm for the new father to be present at the birth of his child. Most often in the United States, the woman and her physician discuss birth control options. In the case of the Asian Indian woman, it is important for the physician to ask if contraception should be discussed first between the physician and her husband. The physician might want to ask the husband for his permission to discuss birth control with his wife.

It is important to understand Indian cultural mores and values surrounding sexual education, sexual behavior, and the childbirth experience, as otherwise these might serve as barriers for Indian immigrants in need of health care. The lack of formal sexual education, importance of the birth of the first child, premarital contraceptive education, dominance of the husband in contraceptive decisions, and predominant role of women and lack of role for men (including the husband) in the childbirth process are all factors that can enhance the understanding of the health-care provider in providing effective care with a positive outcome.

Prescriptive, Restrictive, and Taboo Practices in the Childbearing Family

In the traditional East Indian culture, a family member's advice is highly valued and implemented. Grandmothers, mothers, and mothers-in-law are considered to have expert knowledge in the use of home remedies during pregnancy and the postpartum period. Many older women frequently travel to the United States to assist new mothers in antenatal and postnatal care consistent with traditional customs. For example, in India, it is believed that colostrum is unsuited for infants. Most women think that the milk does not "descend to the breast" until their ritual bath on the third day; as a result, newborns are fed sugar water or milk expressed from a lactating woman.

Many East Indian women seek medical advice only when all available resources fail, so they may not seek medical advice or go to a health-care provider for regular prenatal checkups. In addition, health-care providers may experience difficulty assessing the pregnant mother's sexual history because of the personal and private nature of the information and the discomfort associated with responding to a stranger about their personal lives.

Physical examinations and procedures, particularly pelvic examinations, are especially traumatic to Hindu American women who may not have experienced or heard about these examinations in the past. It is important to explain the procedures, provide privacy, and assign a female health-care provider to decrease the stress and perceived discomfort associated with a pelvic examination. Most Hindu women are not accustomed to being cared for by male health-care providers.

Childbirth is a social and religious event in the Hindu culture. Pregnancy rituals to protect the pregnant mother and the unborn child from evil spirits are performed during specific months of pregnancy. Pregnancy rites are performed in the woman's house during the 5th month of pregnancy. Another ritual is performed in the husband's house during the 8th month of pregnancy. A *bangle*, meaning to surround, must be worn by all auspicious women (barring widows, who are not considered auspicious) especially during pregnancy, when women are considered susceptible to the influence of evil spirits. Bangles act as a sort of "ring-pass-nots" and are believed to create barriers that prevent evil spirits from approaching pregnant women (Duvvurry, 1991).

Dietary restrictions also exist during pregnancy. There are a diversity of practices related to foods that can be consumed or avoided during pregnancy, and the perceptions of foods as "hot" and "cold." The general belief is that hot foods are harmful and cold foods are beneficial during a pregnancy. Since pregnancy is thought to produce a state of "hotness," it is desirable to to balance it out by eating cold foods (Nag, 1994). During early pregnancy, cold foods are recommended to avoid miscarriage, while hot foods are recommended during the last stages of pregnancy to aid in the delivery (Choudry, 1997).

Based on the hot-and-cold theory of disease, certain hot foods like eggs, jaggery (traditional, unrefined, whole-cane sugar), coconut, groundnut, maize, mango, papaya, fruit, and meat are avoided during pregnancy because of a fear of abortion caused by heating the body or inducing uterine hemorrhage.

Pregnancy is a time of increased body heat, so cold foods such as milk, yogurt, and fruits are considered good. However, certain cold foods, such as buttermilk and green leafy vegetables, are avoided because of the belief that these foods cause joint pain, body aches, and flatulence (Raman, 1988). Whereas increased heat is deemed natural during pregnancy, overheating is considered dangerous. Minor swelling of the hands and feet is seen as increased heat and is not of much concern. However, a burning sensation during urination, scanty urine, and a white vaginal discharge are considered serious signs of significant overheating. Muhkopadhyay and Sarkar (2009) surveyed 199 women in Sikkim in northeast India about pregancy-related food beliefs. The authors found that women of social, literacy, or economic standing were more likely to eat special foods. Women with fewer children were more likely to follow dietary practices, in contrast with mothers who had several children. Pregnant women tended to increase their intake of foods such as milk and green vegetables, while decreasing their fruit intake.

Beliefs surrounding what facilitates a good pregnancy and associated outcome, as well as negative sanctions, are often held by immigrating women from India. Most Indian women have fatalistic views about life, including pregnancy. The practice of eating less or "eating down" during pregnancy is common, as it is believed that excessive eating results in large newborns and difficult deliveries (Choudry, 1997). Also, the consumption of high-protein foods, including milk, are avoided because they result in an exaggerated growth of the baby that may lead to a difficult delivery.

In addition to concern about the size of the baby, other factors that influence dietary practices of pregnant women include bodily movement, constitution, and morning sickness. These factors influence both the quality and the quantity of foods consumed. Morning sickness is caused by an increase in *pitta* or bodily heat. *Pitta*—an ayurvedic (*ayur*, longevity; *veda*, science; **Ayurveda** is the traditional system of medicine in India)—means "bile" and is a symptom complex associated with dizziness, nausea, yellow body excretions, a bitter taste in the mouth, and overheating of the body.

Anemia caused by iron deficiency is one of the nutritional disorders affecting women of childbearing age. This condition may be aggravated because of the practice of reducing the consumption of leafy vegetables to avoid producing a dark-skinned baby.

Other beliefs during pregnancy, such as physical activity like fetching water and carrying heavy loads until labor begins, continue in working-class class and farm women, in contrast to wealthy women who are coddled by their families. Although some beliefs can be rationalized, others may seem to have a lack of explanation. Profuse bleeding prior to delivery is seen as a good sign because it will purify the uterus and produce a clean child; bleeding during the 5th month is a sign that the baby is a male (Choudry, 1997).

There is no taboo against the father being in the delivery room, but men are usually not present during birthing. The men do not stay in the delivery rooms and hold their wives' hands during delivery. Instead, they tend to wait outside the delivery room and allow female relatives to support the pregnant mother during labor and delivery. Hence, in relation to the role of men during childbirth, the role of the husband is minimal. Traditional families are reluctant to accept the changes such as shared responsibility and joint decisions. However, these changes are embraced by affluent, educated, and urban families. An awareness of these cultural practices will enable nurses to better understand husbands' reluctance to be present in the delivery room. Miller and Goodin (1995) stated that for Hindu American women, one important factor to achieve a balance in health and wellness is self-control of strong feelings. These women often manifest this belief by suppressing their feelings and emotions during labor and delivery. Nurses can assist in meeting new mothers' needs by closely observing their nonverbal communication such as a change in body posture, restlessness, and facial expressions.

In the Hindu culture, the birth of a son is considered a blessing, not only because the son can carry the family name but also because he can take care of the parents in their old age. Furthermore, a son is also required for the performance of many sacred rituals. In contrast, the birth of a daughter is cause for worry and concern because of the traditions associated with dowry, a ritual that can impoverish the lives of those who are less affluent.

Since the male child is expected to support his parents in their old age, a male child is regarded to be superior to a female child, who is considered a liability because of dowry expectations at the time of marriage (Ranadive, 1994). Raman (1988) noted that women fast and consume herbal medicines in the hope of delivering a son, the birth of which is usually celebrated, while that of a daughter is more restrained and quiet. The preference for a male child exists even among immigrating women from India.

After the birth of a child, both the mother and the baby undergo purification rites on the 11th day postpartum. The postpartum mother is considered to be impure and is confined to a room. The pollution is said to last for 10 days (Duvvurry, 1991). This period of necessitated and mandatory confinement assists in bonding between the mother and the newborn, with the mother given adequate rest and time to tend to the baby's needs. After the 10th day, a ritual bath and religious ceremony are performed by the priest to purify the mother and to end the mandated confinement (Mahat, 1998). The baby is officially named on the 11th day during the "cradle ceremony," and several rituals are performed to protect the baby from evil spirits and to ensure longevity. A sponge bath for the newborn is recommended until the umbilical cord falls off. Soft massage to the extremities is recommended prior to bathing the infant. Washing the infant's hair daily is believed to improve the quality of the hair.

During the postpartum period, hot foods such as chicken drumsticks, dried fish, and greens are considered good for lactation, whereas cold foods are believed to produce diarrhea and indigestion in the infant. Cold foods such as buttermilk and curds, gourds, squashes, tomatoes, and potatoes are restricted because they produce gas. Such abstentions are practiced primarily for the baby's health because harmful influences might be transmitted through the mother's breast milk. Sources of protein such as eggs, curds, and meat are avoided because they might adversely affect the baby. A soft massage for the mother improves the quality and quantity of breast milk.

Breast milk is commonly supplemented with cow's milk and diluted with sugar water. A child's stomach is considered weak as a result of diarrhea; therefore, the child is given diluted milk. The mother's diet the first few days is restricted to liquids, rice, gruel, and bread. Boiled rice, eggplant, curry, and tamarind juice are added to the diet between 6 months and a year after the birth of the baby (Edmundson, Sukhatme, & Edmundson, 1992). Thus, for teaching to be effective, health-care providers must obtain dietary preferences and practices from the family before planning nutritional counseling.

During the postpartum period, the mother remains in a warm room and often keeps the windows closed to protect herself against cold drafts. Exposure to air conditioners and fans, even in warm weather, may be considered dangerous. Nurses can help the new mothers wear warm clothing and provide additional blankets to keep them warm. In summary, in order to provide culturally congruent care, the health-care provider must determine the belief systems regarding prescriptive, restrictive, and taboo practices in the Hindu American childbearing family.

In the United States and Canada, childbirth is viewed within the context of the nuclear family (Choudry, 1997). The role and extent of involvement of grandparents and other immediate family members are decided by the new parents. This is in contrast with the role of the family in the Indian culture, which extends beyond immediate family relatives because it is considered a part of social order providing emotional and social support during a time of need.

The postpartum period has its own taboos in that the mother's movements are constrained within the house. This confinement period is usually 40 days, during which the mother is assisted in her personal care, fed a special nourishing diet, and receives body massages. It is believed that pregnancy produces a state of hotness, with delivery disturbing the balance achieved during pregnancy, and weakens the woman. In order to regain the balance, milk, ghee (clarified, unsalted butter without any solid milk particles), nuts, and jaggery are included in the diet of the new mother. Dried ginger is also eaten, since it is believed to help control postpartum bleeding and acts as a uterine cleansing agent (Choudry, 1997). The newborn is cared for by the local "dai" or midwife, who visits every day to provide massages for both mother and baby. Cold baths or showers are generally avoided. Various purification ceremonies are performed on odd days after delivery.

There are variations in the practices of breastfeeding depending on the education and socioeconomic status of the women. For example, breastfeeding was found to be taboo for the first two days among slum dwellers, while 58 percent of educated mothers in an airforce community initiated breastfeeding within 4 to 12 hours (Mukopadhya & Achar, 1992). In a cross-sectional study of 57 lactating mothers in a rural community, Ray, Biswas, Choudhury, thereference is correct and Biswas (1993) found that mothers breast-fed their newborns within 24 hours. Delaying breast-feeding might be related to beliefs surrounding the colostrum because it is seen as indigestible or puslike and is therefore not good for the newborn. To facilitate weaning, the bottle is introduced early. Powdered formula and cow's milk are common subsitutes for breast milk. Solid food is introduced when the infant begins to reach out for food from the mother's plate. Ray and colleagues (1993) stated that the most common first food is soft rice and mashed vegetables. The introduction of solid food is celebrated with rituals and religious ceremonies and is called *annaprasan* (introduction of cereal).

Iyengar, Iyengar, Martines, Dashora, and Deora (2008) conducted a study on family, community, and provider practices during labor and childbirth—factors likely to influence newborn health outcomes. Data were collected through qualitative methods of interviews, observations, and focus group discussions. The authors found that there were still strongly held beliefs in favor of home-based childbirth, although it appeared that help was available if the mother needed to be taken to a health-care facility pending any problems. Health facility deliveries were preferred for first births, especially among adolescents. During home childbirth, a team of birth attendants or an older female relative made decisions and performed key functions. Also, to hasten home delivery, providers were commonly invited to administer oxytocin injections, whereas health staff did the same during facility deliveries. The practice of applying forceful fundal pressure was universal in both situations. Also, monitoring of labor was restricted to repeated unhygienic vaginal examinations, with little attention to monitoring fetal or maternal well-being. Babies born at home lay on the wet floor until the placenta was delivered. The cord was tied using twine or a ceremonial thread and cut using a new blade. In facility settings, drying and wrapping of the baby after birth were delayed, and there was minimal preparedness for resuscitation. Breastfeeding was postponed until 3 days after birth, when they believed breast milk became available. Mothers and newborns were discharged from the facility without efforts to initiate breastfeeding. The authors recommended communication interventions and improvements in the health system after a clear understanding of people's beliefs about childbirth and their rationale for restrictions in the use of health facilities for delivery.

Implications for nursing care abound in how nurses approach and care for the childbearing women immigrating from India. Nurses should avoid sterotyping Asian Indian women because there are regional and cultural variations, and a lack of understanding of the variations might lead to misinterpretation of behaviors. Choudry (1997) retiterated appreciating cultural meanings, since it sensitizes nurses and helps them provide appropriate care. Nurses can provide culture-specific perinatal education and care by understanding beliefs and practices related to pregnancy, since many immigrant families may want to preserve their tradition and values.

Death Rituals
Death Rituals and Expectations

Death is seen as a family and communal affair. Family members perform all the rites and rituals, with males dealing with the male body and females with the female body, from washing, anointing, and dressing, to the construction of the bier on which the corpse is laid and secured with choir ropes (Laungani, 1996). The deceased is cremated in less than 24 hours following death for hygienic, pollution and purification, and spiritual reasons. Also, Hindus traditionally cremate their dead for swifter, more complete release of the soul.

Hindus prefer to die at home. The eldest son is responsible for the funeral rites. In accordance with Hindu scriptures, it is the sacred duty of the eldest son to perform the funeral rites of his father. The following day, the ashes and charred bones are gathered by the crematorium attendants for later collection by relatives and performance of the final ceremony on the banks of the holy Ganges River. The ashes are immersed in the river to ensure the spiritual salvation of the deceased (Laungani, 1996). Hindus in America may save their family's ashes to later scatter them in holy rivers when they return to their homeland.

The death rite is called *antyesti*, or last rites. The basic purpose is to purify the deceased and console the bereaved. A tenet of Hinduism is that the soul survives the death. Therefore, performing a ritual bath, sprinkling holy river water over the body, covering the body with new clothes, daubing parts of the body with ghee, and chanting Vedic utterances purify and strengthen the deceased for the postmortem journey (Lipner, 1994). The priest pours water into the mouth of the deceased and blesses the body by tying a thread around the neck or wrist. The priest may anoint with water from the holy Ganges River or put the sacred leaf from the *Tulsi* plant in the mouth. At the yearly death anniversary (according to the lunar calendar), *Shradda* ceremonies (usually associated with funeral and postfuneral activities) are held in the home with the offering of *pinda* or balls of cooked rice (pindadana) to one's ancestors. Although individual Hindu community rites vary and can be simple or exceedingly complex, the basic rationale is the same.

Responses to Death and Grief

Hindu families share sacred moments and celebrate important events as a unit, and deaths are considered family events. The eldest son completes prayers for ancestral souls, but all male descendants perform the *Shradda* rites (Wolpert, 1991). Death is considered rebirth. Women may respond to the death of a loved one with loud wailing, moaning, and beating their chests in front of the corpse, attesting to their inability to bear the thought of being left behind to handle situations by themselves. This is significant for women because widowhood is considered inauspicious.

Mourning is a family as well as a social and communal affair. During the 12 days of mourning, female mourners visit female members of the bereaved family at a fixed hour every afternoon. With progression of days, wailing becomes less intense. The functional value of these practices may indicate the provision of intense security and comfort for bereaved people. At a psychological level, it provides catharsis for the entire family and may assist with speeding up the process of recovery from the loss of a loved one and making positive adjustments. Hence, health-care providers need to offer support and understanding of the Hindu culture with respect for death and grief beliefs.

Spirituality

Dominant Religion And Use Of Prayer

The cultural heritage of India is found primarily in philosophy and religion. Sources of philosophical ideas and religious beliefs lie in the *Vedas* and *Upanishads*, repositories of Hindu culture. They explain the two great objects of human life: duty and liberation. The relationship between religion and social structure is intricate. Religion provides the legitimacy and ideology for social and economic practices, whereas social structures produce particular religious beliefs. Two concepts are primary in the Hindu belief system: *karma* (all human actions lead to consequences (as you sow, so shall you reap) and *dharma* (righteousness action). Dharma forms the basis of karma, and the principles of dharma come from the karma theory (Rao, 2010). The doctrine of karma, dharma, reincarnation, the concept of the four ends or stages of life, and the caste system are conducive to maintaining these beliefs.

In Hindu philosophy, the external world is seen as being illusory, called *maya*. Since the world of the senses, the empirical world, is constantly changing, it is seen as an inconstant, illusory world. The ultimate purpose of human existence is to attain *moksha* (Laungani, 2006).

Hinduism represents a set of beliefs and a definite social organization. Hinduism connotes the belief in the authority of Vedas and other sacred writings of the ancient sages, the immortality of the soul and belief in a future life, the existence of a Supreme God, the theory of karma and rebirth, the worship of ancestors, a social organization represented by the four castes, the theory of the four stages of life, and the theory of the four *Purusarthas*, or ends of human endeavor.

The social structure of Hinduism revolves around two fundamental institutions: The caste and the joint family (explained earlier in this chapter) relate to everything connected with the Hindu people outside their religion. The Orthodox Hindu view is that society has been divinely ordained on the basis of the four castes: Brahmanas, Kshatriyas, Vaisyas, and Sudras. The fourfold caste system— *Chaturvarna*—is a theoretical division of society in which tribes, clans, and family groups are affiliated. Yet, the theory of society based on caste still governs Hindu life (see earlier in this chapter). All of the innumerable subcastes claim to belong to one of the four castes. The essential principles of *Chaturvarna* are unchangeable inequality based on birth, the gradation of professions and their inequality, and restrictions on marriage outside one's own group. Although religion does not bestow the caste system with a religious sanction, the great Hindu legal codes are based on the caste system.

In America, individual worship may take different forms within the Hindu religious tradition. Popular Hindu forms of worship require no special arrangements and can be carried out in private. A household shrine is an aid rather than a requirement for worship. Shrines may be set up in the living room or the dining room but are most often located in a back room or a closet. The shrine typically contains representations or symbols of one or more deities.

Almost all family and group religious observances take place on the weekend to fit the American work schedule, even though the lunar liturgical calendar could fall within the normal workweek. Indian worship includes praying, singing hymns, reciting scripture, and repeating the names of deities. For some Hindus, worship is the identification with, or merging of, the inner self with the ultimate reality, Brahma. Temples serve as important support institutions for the practice of the Hindu religion. The installation of a Hindu temple and the invocation of God into its central image make God present in that place, and the land becomes holy. The first Hindu temple constructed in America was in Pittsburgh, Pennsylvania, in 1976; it was modeled after the most popular Hindu temple in India: the Sri Venkateswara temple at Tirupathi.

Meaning of Life and Individual Sources of Strength

One of the main concepts that form the basis of the Hindu attitude toward life and daily conduct is the *Purusartha*, the four ends of humanity. The first of these is characterized by righteousness, duty, and virtue. Other activities through which a person seeks to gain something for self or pursue pleasures are material gain and love or pleasure. Finally, the renunciation of all these activities is to devote oneself to religious or spiritual activities for liberation from a worldly life.

Karma stresses the individual's responsibility for one's actions and is interpreted in terms of past life. One's present condition is seen as a result of one's actions in a past life or lives. Hence, the doctrine of karma by itself enunciates only the principle of an individual's moral responsibility for his or her own deeds. Actions lead to certain consequences, and an individual needs to be aware of this when taking an action. The doctrine of karma has persisted in India from the Vedic times of about 1000 B.C. and is a vital concept that permeates the lives and thoughts of the rich and poor.

To Hindus, religion and family are considered primary sources of strength. Dharma places a high priority on the family. Family is considered to be a critical stage in the path of action, which leads to ultimate spiritual liberation (Fenton et al., 1993). A number of rituals and spiritual practices are connnected with the family because it is through the families that Hindus fulfill many religious obligations. Common life-cyle rituals of Hindus in the United States include prenatal rituals, birth and childhood naming ceremonies, marriage, and cremation within 24 hours after death. All these involve the extended family whenever possible.

Hinduism is concerned with questions regarding ultimate reality and the individual's relationship with it. Spiritual support gives hope to life, ensures courage to face the consequences of illness, and directs the thinking of the person in a positive direction. Because of the strength of the kinship organization and a sense of kinship obligation, the individual seeks solace and strength in such an organization.

Spiritual Beliefs and Health-Care Practices

Hindus believe that all illnesses attack an individual through the mind, body, and soul. The body is the objective manifestation of a subjective mind and consciousness. Spiritual beliefs act mainly as diversional therapies during illness. Suffering of any kind produces hope, which is essential to life. Spiritual support gives hope and helps control emotions and behavior. The Ayurvedic view of health emphasizes social, environmental, and spiritual contexts. The key concept is harmony within the organism and within the system of which the organism is a part. In the Ayurvedic philosophy, people, health, and the universe are said to be related, and when these relationships are in imbalance, health problems can result. Herbs, metals such as copper or zinc, massages, and other techniques are used to clean the body and restore balance. A goal of Ayurvedic practice is to cleanse the body of substances that can cause disease and establish harmony and balance (Fugh-Berman, 1996).

Misra, Balagopal, Klatt, and Geraghty (2010) conducted a cross-sectional survey on the use of complementary and alternative medicine (CAM) by gender and its association with acculturation, health behaviors, and access to health care. Subjects consisted of 1824 Asian Indian adults in six states. The majority of the respondents were male, immigrants, college graduates, and had access to care. Sixty-three percent of Asian Indians used at least one type of CAM; most common was a vegetarian diet, followed by use of dietary and herbal supplements and alternative medical systems. Females reported a significantly higher use of CAM, a vegetarian diet, and use of dietary and herbal supplements than males. Older Asian Indians used Ayurvedic and homeopathic treatments, which are still widely practiced in India and growing in popularity in the West. Higher income had an impact on dietary and herbal supplement use, indicating that cost is a possible factor associated with its utilization.

The concept of palliative care in India is in a relatively early stage of development. Rajagopal and Venkateswaran (2003) noted that without government involvement, the development of the palliative-care specialty will be hampered at the national level. The authors examined practices related to the availability of strong opioids for pain relief in cancer patients. Stringent narcotic regulations often prevent the availability of morphine to patients who need this drug. Hence, patients are administered less potent but more expensive alternatives. In addition, educating the family and having open communication among the patient, family, and health providers can prevent emotional distress and isolation and enhance information and awareness. The author recommends developing a system of quality assurance and doing assessments in the areas of drug availability, education, and policy, and then developing plans of action based on need.

In India, people who live in the rural areas live below the poverty line; with approximately 2.5 million people suffering from cancer at any given time, provision of palliative care, although indicated, becomes expensive. Almost 80 percent of these patients reach hospitals in an advanced stage of the illness. McGrath, Holewa, Koilparampil, Koshy, and George (2009) compared aspects of palliative care in India and Australia. The author found that in both countries terminally ill patients preferred to die at home. Despite the succesful growth of palliative care in a decade, most people prefer to spend the last days of their lives at home surrounded by their family, although patients were encouraged to spend their last days in the hospital. This is in contrast to Australia, where the movement was toward allowing terminally ill patients to go home and rely on community-based services.

Limited studies have been published on how Asian Indian immigrants view hospice services as they may face or are currently facing end-of-life care decisions. Doorenbos (2003) examined whether absence of information about hospice, lack of financial resources, and cultural differences explain the lack of hospice service use in Asian Indian immigrant populations. Results indicated that in a sample of 43 first-generation Asian Indian immigrants, only 12 percent knew what a hospice program was, 22 percent had a little knowledge of hospice, and 22 percent had no knowledge of hospice. The results also indicated that some hospice staff misunderstood Asian Indian death and dying rituals. There was no indication from the participants that financial resources were a barrier to hospice use. Most of the respondents (86 percent) indicated their preference to die at home. However, only 11 percent were aware that the individual's home is the primary site for hospice care. The results demonstrate that although hospice would be the appropriate end-of-life care for this population, the main barrier was knowledge related to the site of hospice care. The majority also rated death and dying beliefs and rituals as important to them.

Gupta (2011) explored Asian Indian American Hindu (AIAH) cultural views related to death and dying through three focus group (senior citizens, middle-aged adults, and young adults) interviews, using both open-ended and semistructured questions. Focus group discussions were related to meaning attributed to death and pre- and postdeath practices. Results indicated that while all three generations believed in the afterlife and karmic philosophy, they exhibited differences in the degree to which Hindu traditions surrounding death and bereavement were influenced by living in the United States.

Health-care providers should assess the extent to which religion, beliefs and values, or socioeconomic status is a part of the individual's life, as these are related to the individual's perception of health and illness and daily practices. Also, assessing spiritual life is essential for identifying resources and solutions for therapy. In the Doorenbos (2003) study, completion of a cultural assessment at the time of admission into hospice care would assist hospice staff in identifying the beliefs that Asian Indian immigrants considered important.

Health-Care Practices
Health-Seeking Beliefs and Behaviors
In Indian culture, rituals are closely connected with religious beliefs about the relationships of human beings with supernatural forces. To maintain harmony between the self and the supernatural world, the belief that one can do little to restore health by oneself provides a basis for ceremonies and rituals. Worshipping goddesses, pilgrimages to holy places, and pouring water at the roots of sacred trees are believed to have medicinal effects for healing the sick person.

Asian Indians experience mental distress biomedically and assign it to ill-defined medical conditions, a phenomenon called somatization. Instead of admitting that they feel sad or depressed, Asian Indian women may say that they are experiencing weakness. Since most individuals who present with somatic complaints report some psychological distress on closer scrutiny, the health-care provider should probe about mental distress when presented with ill-defined somatic complaints.

Responsibility for Health Care
In general, Hindus are responsible for their own health care, but they mobilize personal, social, and religious resources in the face of a crisis. The resolution ranges from a denial of discomfort to acceptance of limitations of somatic or other psychological symptoms. Medical beliefs are a blend of modern and traditional theories and practices. In *Ayurveda*, the primary emphasis is on the prevention of illnesses. Individuals have to be aware of their own health needs. One of the principles of *Ayurveda* includes the art of living and proper health care, advocating that one's health is a personal responsibility. In *Ayurvedic* theory, the key to health is an orderly daily life in which personal hygiene, diet, work, and sleep and rest patterns are regulated. Depending on an individual's constitution, a daily routine has to be established and changed according to the season. Individuals must have information and awareness about living well. Hence, it is important to include prevention, health education, and health-care services.

A common health-care problem among Hindus is self-medication. Pharmacies in India generally allow the purchase of medications such as antibiotics without a prescription. Thus, Hindus migrating to America are accustomed to self-medicating and may bring medications with them or obtain them through relatives and friends. Self-treatment is also more likely if the symptoms are stigmatizing, such as psychiatric or STI symptoms. Use of CAM is widely prevalent among Hindus.

Many feel that modern medicine may be good only for acute conditions, while the traditional systems of medicine are better and more effctive for chronic conditions (Gupta, 2010). The use of CAM depends on the severity of the illness. Individuals will use CAM for minor illnesses before taking allopathic medications, while they use allopathic medications for severe conditions as the first choice. Often patients do not tell physicians they are using CAM for fear of offending the physician (Gupta, 2010).

Folk and Traditional Practices

Numerous practices taken from the hot-and-cold theory of disease causation and folk practices are related to illnesses. Traditional healers, *nattuvaidhyars*, use *Ayurvedic*, *Siddha*, and *Unani* medical systems. These systems are all based on the Tridosha theory. The *Ayurvedic* system uses herbs and roots; the *Siddha* system, practiced mainly in the southern part of India, uses medicines; and the *Unani* system, similar to the *Siddha*, is practiced by Muslims.

According to the *Tridosha* theory, the body is made up of modifications of the five elements: air, space, fire, water, and earth. These modifications are formed from food and must be maintained within proper proportions for health. A balance among three elements or humors—phlegm or mucus, bile or gall, and wind—corresponds to three different types of food required by the body. The following are some types of foods and the allopathic equivalents of diseases associated with them:

1. **Heat-producing foods:** *Brinjals* (Indian eggplant), dried fish, green chilies, raw rice, and eggs.
   Pittham foods include cluster beans, groundnuts, almonds, millet, oil, and runner beans. Allopathic equivalents of heat-producing diseases include diarrhea, dysentery, abdominal pain, and scabies. Allopathic equivalents of *pittham* diseases include vomiting, jaundice, and anemia.
2. **Cooling foods:** Tomatoes, pumpkin, gourds, greens, oranges, sweet limes, carrots, radishes, barley, and buttermilk. Cold, headache, chill, fever, malaria, and typhoid are allopathic equivalents of cool diseases.
3. **Gas-producing foods:** Root vegetables like potato, sweet potato, and elephant yam; plantain; and chicken drumsticks. Joint pains, paralysis, stroke, and polio are disorders related to gas-producing foods.

Heating and cooling effects are produced in the body and thus are not related to the temperature or spiciness of foods. An imbalance leads to disease. If too much heat is in the body from consuming heat-producing foods, then cold foods need to be eaten to restore balance.

Blood is considered one of the seven *dhatus* (body tissues) in the *Tridosha* theory of *Ayurveda*. The strength or weakness of the *dhatus* depends on the "richness or poverty of the blood." Blood is equated with life and is preserved with great care. Special foods like beet root (red foods) are required for good blood, whereas "no blood" is the concept nearest to that of malnutrition.

Thus, in terms of health practices, cultural patterns in India are regionally specific. Health-care providers must be extremely careful in their assessments and not stereotype health-care practices. In addition, providers must also be aware of practices related to the hot-and-cold theory of disease causation and treatment.

Barriers to Health Care

Dependency and reliance on family and friends may be considered a barrier among Hindus. In addition, the practice of self-medicating behaviors may mask disease symptoms until the health condition is at a more advanced stage, making treatment regimens more complex.

In relation to mental health, the stigma associated with mental illness can serve as a barrier to seeking professional treatment. Families may attempt to deny the illness because they may not want outsiders to know about the family member's mental illness (Kumar & Nevid, 2010).

Barriers to seeking preventive services for terminal illnesses like cancer are low awareness of cancer risk and methods of early detection (Surani, Baezconde-Garbanati, Bastani, & Montano, 2003). A barrier to mammography and other screening procedures to detect reproductive organ cancer is fear of taking off clothes or modesty. Hindu women also do not like to discuss genitourinary symptoms or undress in front of others, nor do they want to see a physician during their menstrual periods because it is considered "dirty." However, this might be changing as Hindu women are increasingly more educated and are joining the workforce (Gupta, 2010).

Cultural Responses to Health and Illness

Hindus have a fatalistic attitude about illness causation. Because of their religious beliefs of *karma*, they attempt to be stoic and may not exhibit symptoms of pain. Furthermore, pain is attributed to God's will, the wrath of God, or a punishment from God and is to be borne with courage. As a result, health-care providers may need to rely more on the nonverbal aspects of pain when assessing Hindu patients.

Kodiath and Kodiath (1992; 1995) studied the different attitudes of pain sufferers in India and in the United States. They found that while Americans tended to focus on finding a cure for their pain, Indians tried to find meaning in their pain. Also, while Americans favored analgesics, Asian Indians preferred herbal remedies.

Many Hindus are steadfast in their fatalistic spiritual belief. An individual's *dharma* and *karma* mold one's destiny and worldview. This may be a reason for Hindus' underutilization of psychological or counseling services as options for coping. Health-care providers must assess individual attitudes and comfort levels when counseling Asian Indian patients.

Because of the stigma attached to seeking professional psychiatric help, many Hindus do not access the health-care system for mental health problems. Instead, family and friends seem to be the best help, and there is a general belief that time is the best healer. Physical and mental illnesses are considered God's will, past *karma*, and are associated with a fatalistic attitude. The sick role is assumed without any feeling of guilt or ineptness in doing one's tasks. Because of strong family and kinship ties, the sick role is well accepted. The individual is cared for and relieved of responsibilities for that time. Because of strong family ties and joint and extended families, Hindus are not likely to use long-term-care facilities.

Psychological distress may be demonstrated through somatization, which is common, especially in women. The symptoms may be expressed as headaches, a burning sensation in the soles of the feet or the forehead, and a tingling pain in the lower extremities. Also, the belief in *Ayurveda* in the interrelatedness of mind, body, and spirit may make those with mental health symptoms delay treatment, since they seek spiritual, mind, and body treatments before seeking professional mental health services. Because family is important and family members may accompany the patient to the health-care provider's office, it may pose a problem for the American health-care system's emphasis on autonomy and privacy.

Kermode, Bowen, Arole, Pathare, and Jorm (2009) conducted a cross-sectional mental health literacy survey in Maharashtra, India. The authors administered a questionnaire to 240 systematically sampled community members and 60 purposively sampled Village Health Workers (VHW). Participants were presented with two vignettes describing people experiencing symptoms of mental disorders (depression and psychosis) and were asked about attitudes toward and desired social distance from the people in the vignettes (the latter being a proxy measure for stigma). Results indicated that although the community was relatively accepting of people with mental disorders, false beliefs and negative attitudes were still evident. Desired social distance was consistently greater for the person depicted in the psychosis vignette compared to the depression vignette. Furthermore, while a vast majority verbalized positive answers to all of the questions, they were not willing to have afflicted people marry into their family. Participants did not agree that the problems experienced in the vignettes were "a real medical illness," indicating that attitudes toward people with mental illness were not positive.

Pillai, Patel, Cardozo, Goodman, Weiss, and Andrew (2008) conducted a study on nontraditional lifestyles and prevalence of mental disorders in adolescents in Goa, India. The authors found that the current prevalence of mental disorders in adolescents was very low compared with studies in other countries. Strong family support was a critical factor associated with low prevalence of mental disorders, while factors indicative of adoption of a nontraditional lifestyle (going to the disco) and having an intimate friend of the opposite gender were associated with an increased prevalence. Nontraditional lifestyles may lead to an increased conflict with traditional values and create stressful environments that may predispose adolescents to mental disorders. Health-care providers must understand the role of the family in promoting mental health of the adolescents, as this study demonstrated the independent protective effect of family support.

Families tend to be protective of an ill member. They may not want to disclose the gravity of an illness to the patient or discuss impending disability or death for fear of the patient's vulnerability and loss of hope, resulting in death. The conflict between medical ethics and patients' values may pose a problem for health-care providers, who need to be cognizant of the importance of the family members' wishes and values regarding the care of their loved ones.

Blood Transfusions and Organ Donation

Very little literature is available related to blood transfusion, organ donation, or transplantation practices among Hindus. Seth and colleagues (2009) studied the prevalence of brainstem death and causes of nondonation. Families of those with brainstem death were approached for organ donation by the transplant coordinator. Results indicated that of 33 families counseled, 16 (48 percent) consented to organ donation. In 14 families (42 percent), organs and tissues retrieved and transplanted included 13 livers, 23 kidneys, 25 corneas, and 5 cardiac valves. Consent was more likely in females (10 out of 14 compared with 6 out of 19 males; $p = 0.037$). Consent did not correlate with age of donor or medical-legal issues ($p = 0.227$ and 0.579, respectively). Trained staff with requisite systems in place produced significant organ donation rates. Religious issues and medical-legal concerns were not a major hurdle for organ donation. Female patients with brainstem death were more likely to become organ donors. Thus, no Hindu policy exists that prevents receiving blood or blood products. Donating and receiving organs are both acceptable.

Health-Care Providers

Traditional Versus Biomedical Providers

Although Hindus in general have a favorable attitude toward American physicians and the quality of medical care received in the United States, relatives and friends are consulted first rather than a health-care provider. Kinship and friendship ties remain strong, even in medical matters.

Because any open display of affection is taboo, Hindu women are especially modest. Women generally seek female health-care providers for gynecologic examinations. Health-care providers need to respect their modesty by providing adequate privacy and assigning same-gender caregivers whenever possible.

In the area of mental health, traditional healers, such as *Vaids*, practice an empirical system of indigenous medicine; *mantarwadis* cure through astrology and charms, and *patris* act as mediums for spirits and demons. Health-care providers must specifically ask if their Hindu patients are using these folk practitioners and what treatments have been prescribed.

Status of Health-Care Providers

The Indian patient's view of the physician consists of omnipotence in that God grants cures through the physician. Indian patients tend to be subservient and may not openly question physicians' behaviors or treatments. If they are not pleased with the treatment, they just change physicians. However, they tend to be appreciative of the information that physicians provide about their illness. The physician is also viewed as an older person who is protective, authoritative, and in a teacher–disciple relationship. Through these, the patient expects the physician to teach her or him about the disease and how to get cured in a friend-to-friend relationship.

The physician is seen as the leader of the health-care team, and other medical personnel take on a lower status. However, some patients and their family members may want to be involved in their treatment and may request information. The acceptance of traditional and folk practitioners is highly variable among Western health-care providers and may depend on their previous experiences with CAM providers.

REFERENCES

Blesch, K.S., Davis, F., & Kamath, S. (1999). A comparison of breast and colon cancer incidence rates among native Asian Indians, U.S. immigrant Asian Indians, and whites. *Journal of the American Dietetic Association, 99*(10), 1275–1277.

Choudry, U.K. (1997). Traditional practices of women from India: Pregnancy, childbirth, and newborn care. *JOGNN, 26*(5), 533–539.

Choudhry, U.K., Srivastava, R., & Fitch, M. (1998). Breast cancer detection practices of south Asian women: Knowledge, attitudes, and beliefs. *Oncology Nursing Forum, 25*(10), 1693–1701.

CIA World Factbook. (2011). *India.* Retrieved from https://www.cia.gov/library/publications/the-world-factbook/geos/in.html

Cichocki, M. (2007). HIV around the world—India. Retrieved from http://aids.about.com/od/clinicaltrials/a/india.htm

Crosta, P.M. (2008). India to carry majority of world's health disease burden by 2010. *Medical News Today.* Retrieved from http://www.medicalnewstoday.com/articles/105302.php

Dhawan, J., Gupta, S., & Kumar, B. (2010). Sexually transmitted diseases in children in India. *Indian Journal of Dermatology, Venereology, and Leprology, 76,* 489–493.

Doorenbos, A. (2003). Hospice access for Asian Indian immigrants. *Journal of Hospice and Palliative Nursing, 5*(1), 27–33.Duvvurry, V.K. (1991). *Play, symbolism, and ritual.* New York: Peter Lang.

Edmundson, W.C., Sukhatme, P.V., & Edmundson, S.A. (1992). *Diet, disease, and development.* New Delhi, India: MacMillan India Ltd.

Fenton, J.Y. (1988). *Transplanting religious traditions: Asian Indians in America.* New York, NY: Praeger.

Fisher, J.A., Bowman, M., & Thomas, T. (2003). Issues for South Asian Indian patients surrounding sexuality, fertility, and childbirth in the U.S. health-care system. *Journal of American Board of Family Practice, 16*(2), 180–181.

Fugh-Berman, A. (1996). *Alternative medicine: What works.* Tucson, AZ: Odonian Press.

Garewal, H. (1995). Antioxidants in oral cancer prevention. *American Journal of Clinical Nutrition, 62,* 1410S–1416S

Gay and Lesbian Vaishnava Association Inc. (2005). Retrieved from http://www.galva108.org/faq.html

Gupta, R. (2011). Death beliefs and practices from an Asian Indian American Hindu perspective. *Death Studies, 35*(3), 244–266.

Gupta, V.B. (2010). Impact of culture on healthcare seeking behavior of Asian Indians. (2010). *Journal of Cultural Diversity, 17*(1), 13–19.

Iyengar, S.D., Iyengar, K., Martines, J.C., Dashora, K., & Deora, K.K. (2008).

Childbirth practices in rural Rajasthan, India: Implications for neonatal health and survival. *Journal of Perinatology, 28,* S23–S30.

REFLECTIVE EXERCISE 16.3

Harini Chaturvedi, a Hindu woman aged 60 years, recently moved to the United States from India to assist her son, his wife, and their four children (two sons, ages 13 and 11 years, and two daughters, ages 6 and 2 years) with child rearing while the parents work. One day, Ms. Chaturvedi complains of lower abdominal pain. Her son takes her to the emergency room. The male nurse who is on duty explains that he needs to assess her in order to obtain data about her pain. Ms. Chaturvedi does not maintain eye contact with the male nurse, and she is reluctant to let him examine her. She states she would prefer to talk with a female nurse. She also states that she does not want any pain medications.

1. Why would Mrs. Chaturvedi not maintain eye contact with the male nurse?
2. Why is Mrs. Chaturvedi reluctant to let a male nurse examine her?
3. Identify from a cultural and religious standpoint reasons for not wanting pain medications.

Jain, N.C. (1992, February). Teaching about culture and communicative life in India. Paper presented at the Annual Convention of the Western States Communication Association, Boise, ID.

Jayaraman, R. (2005). Personal identity in a globalized world: Cultural roots of Hindu personal names and surnames. *The Journal of Popular Culture, 38*(3), 467–490.

Kermode, M., Bowen, K., Arole, S., Pathare, S., & Jorm, A.F. (2009). Attitudes to people with mental disorders: A mental health literacy survey in a rural area of Maharashtra, India. *Social Psychiatry & Psychiatric Epidemiology, 44*, 1087–1096.

Kilara, A., & Iya, K.K. (1992). Food and dietary habits of the Hindu. *Food Technology, 46*, 94.

Kodiath, M.F., & Kodiath, A. (1992). A comparative study of patients with chronic pain in India and in the United States. *Clinical Nursing Research, 1*, 278–291.

Kodiath, M.F., & Kodiath, A. (1995). A comparative study of patients who experience chronic malignant pain in the United States. *Cancer Nursing, 18*(3), 189–196.

Kumar, H.D. (2004). Management of nutritional and health needs of malnourished and vegetarian people in India. In E.L. Cooper & N. Yamaguchi (Eds.), *Complementary and alternative approaches to biomedicine* (pp. 311–321). Kluwer Academic/Plenum Publishers.

Kumar A., & Nevid, J.S. (2010). Acculturation, enculturation, and perception of mental disorders in Asian Indian immigrants. *Cultural Diversity and Ethnic Minority Psychology, 16*(2), 274–283.

Laungani, P. (1996). Death and breavement in India and England: A comparative analysis. *Mortality, 1*(2), 191–212.

Levy, R.A. (1993). Ethnic and racial differences in response to medicines: Preserving individualized therapy in managed pharmaceutical programmes. *Pharmaceutical Medicine, 7*, 139–165.

Lipner, J. (1994). *Hindus: Their religious beliefs and practices.* New York, NY: Routledge.

Asian Indian population in 2005. (2005). *Little India.* Retrieved from http://www.littleindia.com/news/132/ARTICLE/1389/2006-11-12.html

Mahat, G. (1998). Eastern Indians' childbearing practices and nursing implications. *Journal of Community Health Nursing, 15*(3), 155–161.

McGrath, P., Holewa, H., Koilparampil, T., Koshy, C., & George, S. (2009). Learning from each other: Cross-cutural insights on palliative care in Indian and Australian regions. *International Journal of Palliative Nursing, 15*(10), 499–509.

Miller, S.W., & Goodin, J.N. (1995). East Indian Hindu Americans. In J.N. Geiger & R.E. Davidhizar (Eds.), *Transcultural nursing: Assessment and intervention* (pp. 475–499). St. Louis: Mosby.

Misra, R., Balagopal, P., Klatt, M., & Geraghty, M. (2010). Complementary and alternative medicine use among immigrant Asian Indians in the United States: A national study. *Journal of Alternative and Complimentary Medicine, 16*(8), 843–852.

Mukhopadhya, J., & Achar, D.P. (1992). Infant feeding practices among educated mothers in an airforce community. *Health and Population: Perspectives and Issues, 15*(3 and 4), 89–93.

Mukhopadhyay, S., & Sarkar, A. (2009). Pregnancy related food habits among women of rural Sikkim, India. *Public Health Nutrition, 12*, 2317–2322.

Nag, M. (1994). Beliefs and practices about food during pregnancy: Implications for maternal nutrition. *Economic and Political Weekly, 29*(37), 2427–2428.

Noble, A.G., & Dutt, A.K. (1982). *India: Cultural patterns and processes.* Boulder, CO: Westview Press.

Pillai, A., Patel, V., Cardozo, P., Goodman, R., Weiss, H.A., & Andrew, G. (2008). Nontraditional lifestyles and prevalence of mental disorders in adolescents in Goa, India. *The British Journal of Psychiatry, 192*, 45–51.

Raj, S., Ganganna, P., & Bowering, J. (1999). Dietary habits of Asian Indians in relation to length of residence in the United States. *Journal of the American Dietetic Association, 99*(9), 1106–1108.

Rajagopal, M.R., & Venkateswaran, C. (2003). Pallaitive care in India: Success and limitations. *Journal of Pain & Palliative Care Pharmacotherapy, 17*(3–4), 121–128.

Raman, A.V. (1988). Traditional practices and nutritional taboos: Effect on mothers and perinatal outcome. *Nursing Journal of India, 79*(6), 166.

Ranadive., J.R. (1994). Gender implications of adjustment policy programme in India. *Economic and policial Weekly, 29*(8), WS12–WS18.

Rao, R.N. (2010). Talking to the dying: Hindu views, Hindu ways. *International Journal of Sociology of the Family, 36*(1), 65–76.

Ray, B., Biswas, R., Choudhury, G., & Biswas, A.B. (1993). Infant feeding practices in a rural community of West Bengal. *Indian Journal of Public Health, 37*(1), 26–28.

Sadler, G.R., Dhanjal, S.K., Shah, R.B., Ko, C., Anghel, M., & Harshburger, R. (2001). Asian Indian women: Knowledge, attitudes and behaviors toward breast cancer early detection. *Public Health Nursing, 18*(5), 357–363.

Sankaranarayanan, R., Mathew, B., Varghese, S.P.R., Menon, V., Jaydeep, A., Nair, M.K., Mathews, C., Mahalingam, T.R., Balaram, P., & Nair, P.P. (1997). Chemoprevention of oral leukoplakia with vitamin A and betacartoene: An assessment. *Oral Oncology, 33*, 231–236.

Seth, A.K., Nambiar, P., Joshi, A., Ramprasad, R., Choubey, R., Puri, P., Murthy, M., Naidu, S., Saha, A., & Bhatoe, H. (2009). First prospective study on brain stem death and attitudes toward organ donation in India. *Liver Transplantation, 15*(11), 1443–1447.

Shetty, P.S. (2002), Nutrition transition in India, *Public Health Nutrition, 5*(1) 175–182.

Sicree, R., Shaw, J., & Zimmet, P. (2006). Diabetes and impaired glucose tolerance. In D. Gan (Ed.), *Diabetes atlas. International Diabetes Federation* (3rd ed., pp. 15–103). Belgium: International Diabetes Federation.

Strachan, D.P., Powell, K.J., Thaker, A., Millard, F.J.C., & Maxwell, J.D. (1995). Vegetarian diet as a risk factor fortuberculosis in immigrant south London Asians. *Thorax, 50*, 175–180.

Surani, Z., Baezconde-Garbanati, L., Bastani, R., & Montano, B. (2003). Improving community capacity to develop cancer awareness programs. *American Journal of Health Studies, 18*, 203–210.

Taylor, W.D. (2010). The burden of non-communicable diseases in India. Hamilton, ON: The Cameron Institute.

U.S. Census Bureau. (2010). *International data base.* Retrieved from http://www.census.gov/ipc/www/idb/worldpopinfo.php

Varghese, A., & Jenkins, S.R. (2009). Parental overprotection, cultural value conflict, and psychological adaptation among Asian Indian women in America. *Sex Roles, 61*, 235–251.

Vasudev, S., Radhakrishnan, G.L., Ravindran, N., & Dangor, K. (July, 2004). The gay spirit. *India Today, 46*, 235–251.

Wild, S., Roglic, G., Green, A., Sicree, R., & King, H. (2004). Global prevalence of diabetes: Estimates for the year 2000 and projections for 2030. *Diabetes Care, 2*, 1047–1053.

Wolpert, S. (1991). *India.* Berkeley: University of California Press.

DavisPlus *For reflective exercises, review questions, and additional information, go to*

http://davisplus.fadavis.com

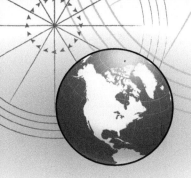

Chapter 17

People of Hmong Heritage

Larry Purnell

The author thanks the contribution of Sharon Johnson, PhD, RN, FNP, who contributed a chapter on the Hmong in Guide to Culturally Competent Health Care, 2nd ed. Philadelphia: F.A. Davis Co.

Overview, Inhabited Localities, and Heritage

Overview

The Hmong (pronounced Mong; the H is silent) are thought to originate in the Yellow River Valley of China and primarily lived in the mountainous areas shared by China, Burma, Vietnam, Thailand, and Laos. The Hmong in the United States mostly come from Laos and were an agrarian society that practiced "slash and burn" agriculture. Mountainous areas were cleared of underbrush, burned, and then used for crops. When the soil became depleted, they moved on, often moving their village as well. Twenty-one percent of the Hmong population in the United States are civilian veterans (U.S. Census Bureau, 2009).

Paj ntaub (*pan dow*) is a form of embroidery that Hmong women do to decorate their clothing and make historical story cloths. Story cloths were the way the family history was passed from generation to generation, since literacy was uncommon. Even today, remarkable story cloths are made that show the Hmong fighting the communists in the jungles, Hmong being killed, yellow rain falling on villages, and people fleeing through jungles and floating across the Mekong River to the refugee camps of Thailand. Story cloths also show the remarkable animals and vegetation of the areas where the Hmong lived. These are now made commercially by Thai Hmong and are sold at craft fairs (Duffy, Harmon, Ranard, Thao, & Yang, 2004).

Heritage and Residence

Over 186,000 Hmong currently live in the United States, of whom 44 percent were born in the United States. Thirty-seven percent live below the poverty line, and they have a very young median age of 16 years (U.S. Census Bureau, 2009). The overall figure of 204,000 for Hmong in the United States has been disputed because many Hmong in census data self-identify as Laotian, Thai, or Vietnamese; thus, actual numbers may be much

higher (Carroll & Uldova, 2005). Smaller numbers of Hmong have also settled in France, Canada, Australia, and Asian countries (Yau, 2005).

Although no Hmong initially settled in the Central Valley of California, many now live there, with California having the largest numbers of Hmong residents, followed by Minnesota and Wisconsin. Small groups migrate where they perceive that economic opportunities exist and are found in North Carolina, Georgia, Florida, Washington State, Oregon, Michigan, and Colorado (U.S. Census Bureau, 2009).

Reasons for Migration and Associated Economic Factors

Hmong began to immigrate to the United States and other countries in 1975 after the Vietnam War. These refugees came from the mountainous regions of Laos, where they had fought on the side of the CIA during the war. They were targeted for genocide because they had fought against the communist Pathet Lao, so they had to flee their county. Many Hmong died because of the war, from genocide, or in their attempts to leave Laos. Many Hmong immigrants in the United States bear the scars of war, bullet and shrapnel wounds, and the lasting effects of exposure to biological warfare, which they call "yellow rain" (Lindsay, 2010). The last large wave of Hmong to the United States occurred in 2004 when the U.S. State Department officially announced the acceptance of roughly 15,000 Hmong refugees from camp Wat Tham Krabok in Thailand (Grigoleit, 2006). Many lingered for years in these camps, and some are still in Thailand, although not all in refugee camps (Doctors Without Borders, 2008; Duffy et al., 2004).

Educational Status and Occupations

Hmong in Laos generally had no education; they were primarily illiterate, lived in very primitive circumstances, and had no access to the modern world or modern medicine. When immigrating to the United States, many Hmong experience shock in a world that is completely foreign to them. The Hmong have embraced the necessity of education in the United States and other places. More recent immigrants have had some education and exposure to the modern world, with 24 percent having completed high school and 13 percent holding baccalaureate degrees or higher (U.S. Census Bureau, 2009). Hmong have achieved higher education and degrees as registered nurses, physicians, psychologists, and social workers.

Communication

Dominant Language and Dialects

Hmong did not have a written language until the 1950s, when Christian missionaries began to develop a written form of their language. That is why Hmong written language today uses the Roman alphabet rather than the characters or scripts that are used in most other regional Southeast Asian languages (Encarta® Online Encyclopedia, 2003). Because of the lack of written Hmong language, many Hmong, especially older adults, are not literate in their own language.

Hmong is a dialectic, monosyllabic, tonal language. Pronunciation seems highly nonintuitive for English and Hmong speakers alike. The letter "P" is pronounced as "B"; "PH" as "P"; "X" as "S"; "S" as "SH"; "T" as "D"; and "R" as something like "DR." Tones are indicated by one of the consonants *j, g, b, v, s,* or *d* at the end of each word, or no consonant for the midrange level tone (Lindsay, 2011).

Hmong in the United States speak either White or Green Hmong, sometimes called Blue. These languages may not be understandable to those who speak the other Hmong dialects, where the same word can have totally different meaning. Therefore, it is advisable to obtain a professional interpreter. Do not provide Hmong-language written instructions unless someone in the household can read them. Instructions written in English may be a better choice because school-age children may know English.

Cultural Communication Patterns

Many Hmong believe that Americans are rude because they look directly in the eyes when speaking, and they are too direct with their questions. Proper communication when speaking to a Hmong person is to use fleeting glances without staring. Making light conversation prior to asking questions about health is proper and important (Caregiver Minnesota, 2006).

Hmong also use the word "yes" to indicate that they can hear you, but that does not mean that they understand what you are asking or that they will do what you are asking them to do (Caregiver Minnesota, 2006). Health-care providers should not rush to questions;

small talk first is considered more polite (Johnson, 2009). To determine if treatments are understood, the patient should be asked to provide a demonstration.

Hmong in general have a strong desire to be seen positively by people in authority. For this reason the social desirability factor may result in them telling the health-care provider what they believe the health-care provider wants to hear, not what is actually happening; this is considered being respectful (Caregiver Minnesota, 2006). When questioning Hmong about their compliance with treatment recommendations, it is best to ask them to demonstrate what they are doing—for example, how they do the blood sugar testing. To determine if they are taking medication correctly, the number of pills in the bottle and the date the prescription was filled should be checked.

Obtaining informed consent is a legal requirement for health-care providers in the United States, but it is directly oppositional to Hmong traditional decision making. In the Hmong culture, the male head of the family or clan makes decisions for family members; individuals do not have the right to make decisions for themselves. Because the Hmong lack experience with Western medicine and surgical procedures, they often have a great deal of fear of medical situations (Samovar, Porter, & McDaniel, 2009). They do not understand what is happening, and they sometimes distrust medical personal, especially if the person is a student. Rumors persist among the Hmong that they are used for practice by students, so if a treatment is called experimental, this confirms their beliefs, and they will most likely refuse treatment. Needing to obtain consent from the head of a family may result in delays for treatment as well, as the head of the clan may live in another state (Samovar, Porter, & McDaniel, 2009).

To be successful in obtaining consent, it is always important to respect the wishes of the individual, to wait until family members have arrived, to meet with the family members to explain the situation, and to accept their decision. If the patient's wishes are different from the head of the family, that must be followed, but most patients will go along with the decisions that are made for them (Johnson, 2009).

Hmong believe that it is inappropriate to say negative things in front of sick people. In illiterate societies, words have great power, and Hmong believe that if you speak negatively in front of an ill person, the words themselves can make bad things happen. Family members usually gather around the bed of a dying loved one, telling that person they are going to get better. Thus, telling a person what complications may occur as part of obtaining informed consent can create great concern to the family (Samovar, Porter, & McDaniel, 2009).

In Western culture, the achievement of education and position engenders respect and authority. In the Hmong culture, however, patients may not feel the same way about Hmong health-care providers and will treat them according to their position in the Hmong family/community hierarchy. This creates additional stressors for health-care providers and interpreters who may be expected to defer to the wishes of Hmong patients who have higher status in their community. Be aware that Hmong health-care providers and interpreters may be related to the patient, and they could be placed in an untenable situation because of a clan hierarchy that Western individuals may not understand (Samovar, Porter, & McDaniel, 2009).

Do not touch the head of a Hmong adult or child. It is considered the most sacred part of the body. Do not point with your feet, step over someone else's feet, show the bottoms of your shoes, or step in front of a Hmong person. These behaviors are considered offensive (Caregiver Minnesota, 2006).

Do not signal using an upturned finger, especially the index finger, since some may use this type of gesture to call animals. Do not point at a Hmong because it is considered aggressive and threatening. Do not touch a Hmong patient's back or shoulder. For many adults, male–female touching, including shaking hands, is considered inappropriate (Caregiver Minnesota, 2006).

Temporal Relationships

Hmong born in Laos may not have their true age on their documents. In Laos, the Hmong had no calendars or clocks, so these concepts were foreign to them. Many of them did not know their age, so an age was assigned to them by immigrant officials when they entered the United States; thus, Hmong may appear older or younger than the age on official documents. Appointment times are a difficult concept, and Hmong may sometimes arrive early in the morning when they had an afternoon appointment (Johnson, 2009). Therefore, the health-care provider must be flexible with appointments. When they first arrive, most Hmong tend to be present oriented. However, once they become more familiar with U.S. culture, they become more futuristic, as evidenced by taking advantage of educational opportunities.

Format for Names

The Hmong naming system is undergoing change. Today, a clan name often serves as a last name. In the West, a Hmong man usually has two names, a first and a last name, but he may have three names: his first name, an honorific name, and his clan name. A man uses his original name after marriage until he is given an honorific name, usually after he becomes a father for the first time. The name of a Hmong man is very important, as his wife and children will be identified with it (Stratis Health, 2004). Hmong do not call each other by their first name. They address one another by their title, such as aunt,

uncle, brother, etc. Demonstrate respect by asking Hmong patients how they would like to be addressed (Stratis Health, 2004).

A married Hmong woman might retain her clan name as her last name, but this practice is not common among Hmong Americans. More commonly, a Hmong woman adopts her husband's clan name as her last name or joins her own clan name and her husband's clan name to form a new hyphenated last name. For example, Kazoua Kong-Thao is from the Kong clan but is married to a member of the Thao clan. A Hmong American may have a first name made up of two or more words. Ka Ying Yang, Maykao Y. Hang, and Yue Pheng Xiong are all examples of well-known young Hmong Americans who have adopted this practice (Stratis Health, 2004).

Many Hmong American parents have begun to give their children English first names, using the clan name or the grandfather's name as the last name. Hmong parents tend to name their children according to gender and birth order. Many parents name their oldest son Toua ("the first"), their second son Lue ("the second"), and the third son Xang ("the third"). Tou ("boy" or "master") is a very common name for a Hmong boy, and many parents use this nickname for their sons, even though the actual name is different. May ("girl" or "miss") is a common name for a Hmong girl, and many families use this nickname for their daughters (Stratis Health, 2004).

The most common names for boys are Long, Pao, Teng, Thai, Tou, Toua, and Xang. Parents tend to name their daughters Bao or Bo, Kia, May, May Ia, Mee, Pa, Xi, and Yi. There are many Hmong names that can be

REFLECTIVE EXERCISE 17.1

Mr. Kong, a Hmong man age 66 years, has been living in Wisconsin for 25 years. He is a Vietnam War veteran but speaks very little English. Mr. Kong has been complaining of shortness of breath and swollen legs for several weeks but has delayed coming to an allopathic health-care provider because he prefers the herbs he has been taking, although they do not seem to be helping him. Because he had severe shortness of breath this morning, he agreed to come to the local Veterans Administration Hospital and is accompanied by his daughter and two sons.

1. How can a Hmong who does not speak English be a veteran?
2. Would his daughter or sons be used as interpreters? Why? Why not?
3. When Mr. Kong is discharged, how would it be decided what language to use for the discharge instructions?
4. How can there be assurance that Mr. Kong and/or his family understand the instructions?

given to both boys and girls. Some of these are Chue, Ka, Shua, Tong, and Yeng (Stratis Health, 2004).

Family Roles and Organization
Head of Household and Gender Roles

Hmong are organized into 18 clans, and each clan has a surname that all men and children use. Although wives and mothers usually retain the clan name with which they were born, they are still considered a member of their husband's clan. Hmong have no single leader, but each clan has leaders who are older males. Older males are the leaders in each family. If a husband dies, the oldest son is expected to make decisions for the family. The youngest son is expected to marry and bring his wife home to live with his parents. Older sons and their families leave the family home when the family increases in size. Daughters are expected to marry and to live with their husbands and in-laws. Traditionally, Hmong women marry young (13 to 15 years of age) and have assistance with childbearing from the extended family (Meyers, 1992).

The Hmong patrilineal and patriarchal family system has changed little since moving their culture to the Western world. Decisions about any family member of either gender are still passed down through the husband's family elders. Women still contribute a lot of effort to their families, only in different ways. Marriage is more modern in that women have a little more freedom in choosing their husband. However, the families of both the bride and the groom still have the final say in the match (Harrison, Pham Kim, & Kagawa-Singer, 2007). The median number of Hmong individuals in a household is 7 compared with the U.S. median of 2.6 individuals per household (U.S. Census Bureau, 2009).

A Hmong woman does not live outside the home before she is married to protect her reputation. Over time, the women of this group have lost some of their power or agency. The things they used to control have been stripped from them as they moved into the Western world and globalization consumed their lives. Hmong women no longer provide food for their families in the same way they once did, they no longer give birth to children in the traditional manner, standing or in a squatting position to facilitate a vertical delivery, and it is becoming increasingly more difficult for them to perform the ceremonies they find essential to life (Hang, 1997).

The Hmong community in the United States is well connected though telephone, email, and frequent family visits. Family "disgraces" are widely known even among Hmong who live in different parts of the United States. Things that might be considered disgraces are birth defects, opium addiction of a family member, or a divorce in the family. These are considered to reflect on every family member and may, for example, decrease the chances of making a good marriage.

Prescriptive, Restrictive, and Taboo Behaviors for Children and Adolescents

Single Hmong may find mates at the annual Hmong New Year celebrations held between Christmas and New Year's Day. Marriages are thought to be advantageous if they are between first cousins but not for those who retain the same last name. Hmong young women may be victims of a ritual called "capture bride," where a young girl is abducted from her home, taken to her future husband's home, and pronounced married. This process is being discouraged, however, because often the young woman manages to escape and reports the kidnapping to the police (Yang, 1994). Once a Hmong child is 5 years old, his or her behavior is expected to coincide with adult behavior (Johnson, 2009).

Hmong boys are not considered adults until they marry. Young girls are thought to be marriageable when they become "plump" or enter puberty. This results in young Hmong girls suddenly disappearing from schools because they have gotten married. Great social pressure exists for Hmong girls to marry in their early teens. These marriages are not legal marriages but traditional Hmong ceremonies; therefore, they do not break state laws. Although these girls may be in their early teens, their pregnancies tend to be very healthy, with few of the complications common to teenage pregnancies. These young families live with their in-laws, so child rearing becomes multigenerational. Hmong girls who go to college are sometimes thought to be "too old" to marry, and they have reduced choices of Hmong men to marry (Johnson, 2009).

Alternative Lifestyles

Plural marriages were common in Laos, and they persist today. Hmong men may marry as many women as they can afford to support. This is becoming less common with Hmong who no longer adhere to traditional beliefs. Same-sex relationships are not condoned and are a reflection on the entire family. Same-sex relationships should not be disclosed by health-care providers to family members or others in the community.

Workforce Issues
Culture in the Workplace

Hmong have the highest unemployment rate of all recent immigrants and have the lowest socioeconomic level of all Asians in the United States (U.S. Census Bureau, 2009). Employment for first-generation immigrants is difficult due to poor English-language skills and few workplace skills. Large family size results in low employment for women. Hmong men who gain sufficient English-language skills can find jobs in factories or agriculture (Johnson, 2009).

Issues Related to Autonomy

The Hmong's desire for social acceptance may result in them saying "yes" to questions regarding knowing how to perform something when they actually do not understand. Requesting demonstrations helps to assess knowledge so that better instructions can be given in the workplace. Young Hmong are rapidly achieving higher education and higher socioeconomic status, resulting in them helping other members of their family to live better lives and achieve higher education. Hmong are now in many professional roles and government service. They are hard workers and are loyal to their employers (Johnson, 2002).

Biocultural Ecology
Skin Color and Other Biological Variations

Recent immigrants tend to be shorter than European Americans; men average 5 feet 3 inches, and women average about 5 feet tall. Men may weigh 100 to 120 pounds and women 85 to 100 pounds. Since immigration, obesity is very common in children and adults. Skin color is light brown; faces are round, with almond-shaped eyes. A few Hmong have blond hair, light skin, and hazel eyes. In Laos, this variation was considered an aberration. Hmong children who are born in the United States are achieving greater heights, most likely due to improved nutrition (Johnson, 2009).

Diseases and Health Conditions

Many Hmong continue to have nightmares and flashbacks to the terrors they experienced in Laos. Type 2 diabetes and hypertension are common due to the rapidly increasing obesity of Hmong children and adults (Pinzon-Perez, 2006). Many Hmong settle in apartments and rely on public assistance. Their traditional hardworking agricultural lifestyle has been completely changed into a sedentary Western lifestyle.

Hmong of all ages in central California have a very high incidence of asthma (Johnson, 2002). Exacerbations are common when air quality is poor. Instructing the patients in the proper use of inhalers and other medications is important. Some older Hmong may have breathing difficulties due to paragonimiasis or opium addiction. Paragonimiasis is a parasite contracted in Southeast Asia. The parasites settle in the lungs, causing a diffuse infection. These patients need a correct diagnosis with appropriate treatment. The health-care provider should consider paragonimiasis when patients have pulmonary infections (Johnson, Falk, Iber, & Davies, 1982).

Recent immigrants have been diagnosed with tuberculosis at high rates; some were infected with drug-resistant tuberculosis. Hepatitis B occurs in high rates and tends to be present in all members of a family. Family members should be assisted to comply with public health monitoring, and all new immigrants should be screened for hepatitis B (Pinzon-Perez, 2006). *Helicobacter pylori* also occurs in high rates with peptic ulcers and adenocarcinoma of the gastrointestinal tract. Both hepatitis B and *H. pylori* transmission in families may be related to two factors: When eating, Hmong individuals often serve themselves from communal bowls, using the utensils they have been eating with. Also, traditional practices such as "cupping" or coin rubbing is practiced by pricking the skin to release blood; this is believed to release bad spirits (Pinzon-Perez, 2006). One method of releasing blood is using sewing needles that are not sterilized and thus may transmit hepatitis B (Johnson, 2009). Family members should be taught to sterilize needles and other sharp instruments.

An unexplained phenomenon among the Hmong is sudden unexplained death syndrome (SUDS) that has also been experienced among the Vietnamese in the United States. Nearly all of these deaths involve physically healthy, young, adult men who die at night or while sleeping. The Centers for Disease Control and Prevention (1990) reported 117 cases from 1981 to 1988 and suggested that a structural abnormality of the cardiac conduction system and stress may be risk factors for SUDS (Sheng-mei, 2005; Tobin & Friedman, 1983).

Variations in Drug Metabolism

No information on variations in drug metabolism could be found in the scholarly literature. Health-care providers may want to look at variations in drug metabolism among Chinese and Thais, whose dietary habits and genetic profiles are similar to the Hmong.

High-Risk Health Behaviors
Health-Care Practices

Opium was grown in Laos as a cash crop and was used by many older Hmong for their aging pains. In the

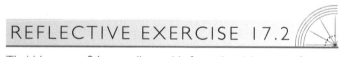

REFLECTIVE EXERCISE 17.2

Thai Hang, age 24 years, lives with five other Hmong refugees who came to the United States recently from a refugee camp in Thailand. They share living space in a two-bedroom apartment in Central Valley, California. They pool their money to pay for rent, utilities, food, and other household expenses. All of them are proud of their heritage but are eager to participate in American traditions. Thai has had some respiratory problems since he arrived and is seeking a traditional healer for assistance. They are taking English classes two evenings each week at a local church.

1. For what health conditions would Hmong refugees be screened?
2. What is the name for a Hmong traditional healer?
3. What conditions do traditional healers treat?
4. What is the training for a traditional healer?

United States, opium addiction persists, but it is rare and is considered disgraceful in the Hmong community. Individuals who smoke opium are usually very thin with a cyanotic skin color. They have generalized crackles throughout all lung fields and have frequent problems with lung infections such as bronchitis and pneumonia. Health-care providers should consider opium addiction with Hmong who are very thin with cyanosis and respiratory problems (Johnson, 2009).

Some newer immigrants have never heard of cancer, and some who know about it believe it is contagious. Many women have never heard of or had a Pap test. Many have never performed breast self-examination or had a mammogram. Encourage PAP smears as part of routine examinations, as well as other times when women are seen for health care (Johnson, 2009).

Many individuals do not know that cigarette smoking can cause cancer. Explain the adverse effects of cigarette smoking, and encourage cessation.

Nutrition
Meaning of Food
The rice and vegetables the Hmong worked so hard to grow are now easily available from grocery stores. They have also begun consuming American foods such as sugared soft drinks and high-sugar, high-fat pastries. When assessing nutrition, the health-care provider should ask what liquids the patient is consuming; this is often not revealed unless asked directly and may show a high consumption of sugared juices and drinks. Diet should not be taught using Western measuring amounts. Measured foods in cups and tablespoons may not be understood by Hmong patients because baking is uncommon in traditional Hmong households, and they may not possess these utensils. A "cup" may mean a drinking cup to the patient (Johnson, 2009).

Common Foods and Food Rituals
Hmong were primarily farmers, so many have developed small farms, where they sell fruits and vegetables. Even Hmong apartments have small plots for vegetables, and homes may have chickens in the backyard.

Rice is the primary staple of the Hmong diet. Vegetables, fish, chicken, and pork are consumed with the rice. Very hot peppers are made into a condiment that accompanies the meal. Occasionally a special dish called *laub* is made with raw pork and vegetables and spices. This increases the risk for *trichinosis*. Although this practice may not be common among Hmong in the United States, the practice continues among a few (Perez, Jula Moua, & Pinzon-Perez, 2006). Many younger Hmong prefer American diets such as hamburgers and other fast foods. Hmong eat two or three meals per day (Johnson, 2009).

Pregnancy and Childbearing Practices
Fertility Practices and Views Toward Pregnancy
Hmong families usually consist of many children, fulfilling several crucial purposes. First and foremost, it guarantees the continuation of the lineage and clan. In an agrarian society, lots of children provided helping hands for farm work, housework, and child care. Being able to produce many children also adds to a sense of importance for women, helping them feel a stronger sense of belonging within their clan. Children are also very highly celebrated in Hmong culture; a birth signifies the reincarnation of a soul in a new body. A new family member is cherished in a society in which family means everything (Quincy, 1995).

In the United States, most Hmong live with extended families—if not in the same household, then in the same apartment complex or neighborhood. Older adults often help take care of their grandchildren. Hmong women consider regular menstruation to be a sign of health and may not wish to use birth control that interferes with the regular menstrual cycle. Most women marry early and have pregnancies until menopause. Men tend to marry first when in their early 20s and 30s (Johnson, 2009; Quincy, 1995).

During pregnancy, women continue with their day-to-day responsibilities until the day they go into labor. A Hmong woman follows her food cravings to guarantee that her child will not be born with a deformity. Women are prohibited from drinking cold beverages and spicy foods during pregnancy (Johnson, 2009).

Prescriptive, Restrictive, and Taboo Practices in the Childbearing Family
The Hmong believe that a long labor can be eased by drinking water in which a key has been boiled to "unlock" the birth canal. Boiling a key is one example of the many sacred acts that are a part of Hmong religion performed before, during, or after childbirth (Fadiman, 1997). In the past, women had a strict postpartum diet that consisted solely of hot foods and drinks. Cold foods make the blood congeal in the womb instead of cleansing it by flowing freely (Fadiman, 1997; Johnson, 2009). Some Hmong may still follow these routines to ensure a woman's fertility.

Postpartum, white rice and chicken are the traditional diet for 1 month, and the mother may not have cold drinks. New mothers are expected to rest after delivery. The mother-in-law and husband help the new mother. New mothers may not want to eat hospital food, so the family should be permitted to bring traditional foods from home. Ask the mother what she prefers; many Hmong are now Christians and no longer adhere to traditional beliefs and practices (Johnson, 2009).

Death Rituals

Death Rituals and Expectations

Traditional Hmong view life as a continuous journey. Death is merely a phase people go through when passing from this plane of existence to the next. Many believe that people are destined to live to a certain age, and when that age is reached, the person departs but the spirit will reincarnate. Most Hmong believe in multiple souls that reincarnate—one that stays in the area of the body and another that stays in the present world, overlooking and caring for the family (Johnson, 2009; Stratis Health, n.d.).

Responses to Death and Grief

The deceased is dressed in fine Hmong clothes to demonstrate to all that the person has lived a good life, will be missed, and will make a proper entrance into the next world (Johnson, 2009; Stratis Health, n.d.).

Hmong funerals are distinctive with many rituals and may last many days to honor the deceased and their ancestors. The older or more revered the person, the longer the funeral. An animal sacrifice may be made to honor the deceased. The sacrificed animal is later used to provide food for the people present (Falk, 1996; Johnson, 2009; Stratis Health, n.d.). During the long funeral, family and friends tell stories and sing songs relating to the mountains from home (Falk, 1996).

Spirituality

Dominant Religion and Use of Prayer

Hmong who immigrated when young become more acculturated. Most older and more recent Hmong hold traditional animist beliefs where ancestors are revered, and they believe that spirits are widely distributed in the world and reside in many inanimate objects or places such as trees, rivers, and houses. Many believe that spirits can cause harm, misfortune, illness, or death, or can be helpful to protect or prevent bad events from occurring. Good spirits are thought to be ancestors who watch over and protect them (Plotnikoff, Numrich, Wu, Yang, & Ziong, 2002).

Meaning of Life and Individual Sources of Strength

The primary religious leader is the *shaman* (**tu txiv neeb**, pronounced "*too tse neng*"), who takes care of health and spiritual problems (Plotnikoff et al., 2002). Family, nuclear and extended, is a primary source of strength, followed by animistic beliefs for traditional Hmong. For acculturated Christian Hmong, family continues to be a primary source of strength and elements from their chosen new religion. The shaman may still be sought for help and advice with personal and health concerns.

Spiritual Beliefs and Health-Care Practices

Christian Hmong have beliefs and practices appropriate to their religion. Some may denounce animist beliefs and traditional Hmong beliefs such as soul loss and soul calling ceremonies by the shaman. Prayers and chants may be performed for healing (Johnson, 2002, 2009; Plotnikoff et al., 2002).

Health-Care Practices

Health-Seeking Beliefs and Behaviors

Although most Hmong in the United States readily access health care, they might first use traditional treatments and even combine them with Western medicine. Most Hmong foster the belief that American medicines are powerful, but they fear that serious side effects may accompany their use. American medicines are commonly diluted and/or blended with familiar indigenous herbs before use (Meyers, 1992). Additionally, there is suspicion among the Hmong that Western physicians experiment on people from different cultures. They believe surgery allows good spirits to leave and bad spirits to enter the body (Higgs & Rairdan, 1992; McInnes, 1991). Many distrust autopsies, dental fillings, and blood tests, believing that persons are reincarnated with a handicap if these procedures are performed (Cheon-Klessig, Camilleri, McElmurry, & Ohlson, 1988; Meyers, 1992). Despite this distrust of Western medical care, Southeast Asians seek treatment when their own indigenous practices are unsuccessful.

Responsibiity for Health Care

Most Hmong do not subscribe to preventative and health maintenance health-care practices. However, immunizations, which are needed for children to enter school, are accepted. The concept of germs and preventive asepsis may not be understood, especially among older adults. They generally do not subscribe to the importance of developmental stages and anticipatory guidance in young children (Johnson, 2009).

Folk and Traditional Practices

Diarrhea in Hmong children is traditionally treated with herbs and plants such as dry wood and plant roots, sida leaves, and herbs boiled with tea. For sprains and fractures, some steam leaves and wrap them around the ankle or wrist. Cords may be tied on the wrist and then massaged. In some cases, uncooked egg is rubbed on a child, as is blood or animal excrement, depending on the severity of the injury (Nuttall & Flores, 1997). Raw chicken chopped with herbs may be wrapped around a broken bone. Bone-twisting maneuvers are sometimes attempted to treat the sprain or set the bone. Home remedies include application of dung from black chickens to the broken bone (Nuttall & Flores, 1997). Studies have shown that these herbs may have pharmaceutical properties.

Ask patients about their use of herbs upon admission (Johnson, 2009).

Invasive procedures such as intravenous lines, injections, suturing, and casting are looked on skeptically. Most parents try herbal and traditional remedies first, using invasive procedures only if a favorable outcome is guaranteed. The Christian Hmong participant in one study believed that the outcome for congenital deformities should be "left to faith" (Johnson, 2009).

One cause of illness is thought to be loss of soul. It is believed that some individuals, such as babies and children, have souls that have difficulty staying in the body. If the soul leaves for too long, the baby can become ill or die. For this reason, parents may tie a string around the baby's neck or wrist soon after birth. Older children and adults may have strings tied around wrists, waists, or ankles. These must remain on until they fall off naturally, because removing them too soon can result in soul loss and illness or death (Johnson, 2009). Since immigrating to the United States, the strings have been replaced with gold necklaces and bracelets. Hmong who practice shaman ceremonies may have amulets in small bags around their neck or waist. These contain objects thought to be protective against evil spirits (Johnson, 2009). Do not remove strings, necklaces, bracelets, or amulets without the parents' or patient's permission.

Barriers to Health Care

The greatest barrier to adequate health care for the Hmong in the United States is accurate and culturally competent communication ensuring a correct diagnosis. For some, transportation and lack of finances can be significant barriers. The health-care provider must ensure the availability of interpreters at all times.

Cultural Responses to Health and Illness

Hmong seek Western medical care often; yet, they may also use traditional healers or shamans who perform rituals. They may seek herbalists and take multiple treatments for the same condition. Some practice home remedies such as coining or cupping. These traditional practices cause distinctive elongated or round bruises that are generally over the area where the problem is. For example, a sore throat will have bruises around the neck, and chest symptoms may have cupping over the front and back of the chest. Pricking the center of the bruise is done to release bad spirits; unsterilized sewing needles are generally used for this purpose (Johnson, 2009). The regular patterns of coining or cupping should not be mistaken for marks of abuse. Encourage sterilization of needles.

Blood Transfusions and Organ Donation

Traditionally, blood transfusions and organ donation are unacceptable to Hmong. Younger Hmong, however,

are more accepting of these medical procedures (Stratis Health, n.d.).

Health-Care Providers

Traditional Versus Biomedical Providers

Hmong cultural attitudes, values, and behaviors influence when, where, why, and with whom a Hmong person uses Western medicine. The foremost Hmong traditional healer is the shaman. There is no equivalent health professional in Western biomedicine. The scope of the shaman as a healer extends beyond the capacities and expertise of physicians (Plotnikoff et al., 2002).

Despite 25 years of Hmong acculturation in the United States and conversion to Christianity, Hmong shamanism maintains its traditional role in health and healing. Many Hmong who see physicians also rely on shamans for restoring health and balance to their body and soul. Thus, the Hmong shaman can be considered a powerful complement to Western health-care providers.

Shamans do not choose to become shamans; the occupation is considered a calling and is approved by the community (Plotnikoff et al., 2002). Shamans train for many years and learn as apprentices. Shaman ceremonies are conducted within the home with all the family present; they go into the spirit world to find out why the soul was lost or was taken to the spirit world.

Status of Health-Care Providers

The shaman is held in high regard because he or she is well known to the community and trusted. However, when traditional treatments do not work, Hmong do not hesitate to see Western health-care providers.

REFLECTIVE EXERCISE 17.3

A Hmong couple, Foua and Nao Xang, bring their 4-year-old daughter Mai to an urgent care clinic for infected puncture marks on her chest and back. The parents speak very little English, but the nurse understands by their demonstration that they were doing "some type" of traditional treatment.

1. What are some of the traditional treatments used by the Hmong?
2. What is the most likely cause of these infected puncture marks?
3. Should child protective officials be notified of possible child abuse? Why? Why not?
4. What advice should be given to the parents for the future?

REFERENCES

Caregiver Minnesota. (2006). *Education and resources for Hmong families.* Retrieved from http://www.caregivermn.org/hmong/h017carepage.htm

Carroll, E., & Uldova, V. (2005). Who is Hmong? *Hmong Studies Journal, 6,* 1–20.

Centers for Disease Control and Prevention. (1990). Update: Sudden unexplained death syndrome among Southeast Asian refugees—United States. *Journal of the American Medical Association, 260*(14), 2033.

Cheon-Klessig, Y., Camilleri, D.D., McElmurry, B.J., & Ohlson, V.M. (1988). Folk medicine in the health practice of Hmong refugees. *Western Journal of Nursing Research, 10,* 647–660.

Doctors Without Borders. (2008). Retrieved from http://www.doctorswithoutborders.org/news/article.cfm?id=2714

Duffy, J., Harmon, R., Ranard, D., Thao, B., & Yang, K. (2004). An introduction to their history and culture, *The Hmong Culture Profile No. 18,* Center for Applied Linguistics. Washington, DC.

Encarta® Online Encyclopedia. (2003). *Hmong.* Retrieved from http://autocww.colorado.edu/~toldy2/E64ContentFiles/AnthropologyAndCultures/Hmong.html

Fadiman, A. (1997). *The spirit catches you and you fall down: A Hmong child, her American doctors, and the collision of two cultures.* New York, NY: Farrar, Straus and Giroux.

Falk, C. (1996). Upon meeting the ancestors: The Hmong funeral ritual in Australia and Asia. *Hmong Studies Journal, 1*(1), 1–15.

Grigoleit, G. (2006). Coming home? The integration of Hmong refugees from Wat Tham Krabok, Thailand, into American society. *Hmong Studies Journal, 7,* 1–22.

Hang, Maykao Yangblongsua. (1997). Growing up Hmong American: Truancy policy and girls. *Hmong Studies Journal, 2,* 1–54.

Harrison, G., Pham Kim, L., & Kagawa-Singer, M. (2007). Perceptions of diet and physical activity among California Hmong adults and youths. *Preventing Chronic Disease, 4*(4), A93.

Higgs, Z., & Rairdan, B. (1992). When your patient is a Hmong refugee. *American Journal of Nursing, 92,* 52–55.

Johnson, S. (2002) Hmong health beliefs and experiences in the Western health care system. *Journal of Transcultural Nursing, (13)*2, 27–133.

Johnson, S. (2009). People of Hmong heritage. In L. Purnell (Ed.), *Guide to culturally competent health care* (pp. 202–214). Philadelphia, PA: F. A. Davis Co.

Johnson, J.R., Falk, A., Iber, C., & Davies, S. (1982). Paragonimiasis in the United States. A report of nine cases in Hmong immigrants. *Chest, 82*(2), 168–171.

Lindsay, J. (2010). Hmong life in America: A story of tragedy and hope. Retrieved from http://www.jefflindsay.com/Hmong_tragedy.html

McInnes, K. (1991). Ethnic-sensitive work with Hmong refugee children. *Child Welfare, 70*(5), 571–580.

Meyers, C. (1992). Hmong children and their families: Consideration of cultural influences in assessment. *American Journal of Occupational Therapy, 46,* 737–744.

Nuttall, P., & Flores, P.C. (1997). Hmong healing practices used for common childhood illnesses. *Pediatric Nursing, 23*(3), 247–251.

Perez, M.A., Julah Moua, L., & Pinzon-Perez. (2006). Food preparation practices and safety in the Hmong community. *Hmong Studies Journal, 7,* 1–24.

Pinzon-Perez, H. (2006). Health issues for the Hmong populations in the US: Issues for health educators. *International Electronic Journal for Health Education, 9,* 122–133.

Plotnikoff, G.A., Numrich, D., Wu, C., Yang, D., & Ziong, P. (2002). Hmong shamanism: Animist spiritual healing in Minnesota. *Minnesota Medicine, 85*(6), 29–34.

Quincy, K. (1995). *Hmong history of a people.* Cheney, WA: Eastern Washington University Press.

Samovar, L., Porter, R., & McDaniel, E. (2009). *Intercultural communication: A reader.* Boston: Wadsworth Cengage.

Sheng-mei, M. (2005). Hmong refugee's death fugue. *Hmong Studies Journal 6,* 1–36.

Stratis Health. (n.d.). Cultural Orientation Project. (2004). Retrieved April 28, 2011 from http://www.cal.org/co/hmong/hlaos.html

Tobin, J. J., & Friedman, J. (1983). Spirits, shamans, and nightmare death: Survivor stress in a Hmong refugee. *American Journal of Orthopsychiatry, 53*(3), 439–448.

U.S. Census Bureau. (2009). *Factfinder2. American community survey.* Retrieved from http://factfinder.census.gov/servlet/SAFFIteratedFacts?_event=&geo_id=01000US&_geoContext=01000US&_street=&_county=&_cityTown=&_state=&_zip=&_lang=en&_sse=on&ActiveGeoDiv=&_useEV=&pctxt=fph&pgsl=010&_submenuId=factsheet_2&ds_name=DEC_2000_SAFF&_ci_nbr=039&qr_name=DEC_2000_SAFF_R1010&reg=DEC_2000_SAFF_R1010%3A039&_keyword=&_industry=

Yang, J. (1994). Hmong marriage by capture: Case in Fresno, California. *Southern California Interdisciplinary Law Journal, 10,* 38–48.

Yau, J. (2005). *Migration information source.* Retrieved from http://www.migrationinformation.org/usfocus/display.cfm?ID=281

DavisPlus *For reflective exercises, review questions, and additional information, go to*

http://davisplus.fadavis.com

Chapter 18

People of Japanese Heritage

Misae Ito and Keiko Hattori

Overview, Inhabited Localities, and Topography

Overview

Nihon, or **Nippon**, as Japan is called in the Japanese language, is a 1200-mile chain of islands in the northwestern Pacific Ocean, slightly smaller than California, and one-quarter the size of the United States (*CIA World Factbook,* 2011). Japan's neighbors are Russia, Korea, and China, and its modern history has been shaped by conflict with these countries.

Japan's territory extends generally from northeast to southwest. The northern and westernmost areas have a climate similar to that of the northern United States, with some heavy snowfalls in the winter; the Ryukyu Islands in the south are subtropical. The climate of the Tokyo region, where most of the population is clustered, is similar to that of Washington, DC. Winters are moderate, with snows that seldom accumulate except in the north, whereas summers are hot and steamy.

The population of around 127 million resides mainly on the four largest islands (U.S. Department of State, 2010): Honshu, Kyushu, Hokkaido, and Shikoku. Tokyo, on Honshu Island, is the capital and largest city with 80 million people residing in its greater metropolitan area. The Japanese, who refer to themselves as **Nihonjin**, share a strong sense of nationalism and pride in ethnic purity. Japanese citizenship is not readily obtained, and currently there are over 2 million foreign residents in Japan, who are required to register as aliens. The inclusion of even third-generation Korean residents in the category of foreigners has received considerable adverse international press in recent decades. However, some changes are on the way as Japan has begun acknowledging that a long-revered sense of ethnic homogeneity may not be sustainable. Globalization, low birth rate, an aging population, and increasing labor shortages are causing the country to rethink its immigration policies. However, this has to be balanced against tensions arising from growing international terrorism, and therefore, stricter controls on immigration have been implemented (Kashiwazaki & Akaha, 2005).

Heritage and Residence

The original inhabitants of Japan most likely migrated from the Korean peninsula. The marked Chinese cultural influence began in the late 400s and included the Chinese system of writing, the calendar, Confucianism, Buddhism, and East Asian beliefs about health and illness. Following World War II, from 1945 to 1952, Japan was an occupied territory of the United States. As a bitter legacy of that war, the northernmost Kuril Islands are still claimed by Russia, and today, Japan still has U.S. military bases on its soil, in part to counteract perceived threats from neighboring countries.

Japanese citizens residing in North America have tended to locate in large commercial and educational centers. With the establishment or purchase of factories in the midwestern and southern states by Japanese companies, communities of Japanese expatriates can now be found in smaller cities as well.

Reasons for Migration and Associated Economic Factors

In the late 1800s, Japanese people began to migrate to the United States and Canada, and from 1891 to 1924, more than 250,000 Japanese immigrated, settling primarily in the Territory of Hawaii and along the Pacific coast (Yanagisako, 1985). By 2004, however, an estimated 369,639 Japanese nationals lived in the United States, of whom 240,000 were considered long-term and 129,600 permanent (UN Secretariat, 2005). Japanese love overseas travel, and in 2010 approximately 3.4 million of them visited the United States and spent dollars on goods and services (U.S. Commercial Service, 2011).

Educational Status and Occupations

Education is highly valued in Japan, where the illiteracy rate is only about 1 percent (U.S. Department of State, 2010). According to the Ministry of Education, Culture, Sports, Science, and Technology (2010a), in

Japan the ratio of completion of the 12th grade is about 98 percent, and those of young people ensure a highly competent workforce. For instance, calculus is part of the mandatory junior high school curriculum, and high school graduates complete 6 years of English instruction. In addition, activities are introduced in which English is spoken in elementary school.

Many youngsters prepare for high school or college entrance examinations by attending proprietary *juku*, or cram, schools in the evenings or on weekends, which creates enormous pressure on youth to succeed. Moreover, over 70 percent of high school graduates go on to higher education at over 2000 universities, junior colleges, and technical schools. Entrance examinations for high school and college are very competitive. Because the alumni network helps to provide job placements, the school that one attends determines to a great extent where one is employed after graduation. To gain higher education degrees, Japanese commonly study at the university where they earned their undergraduate degree rather than go to different universities like many of their American counterparts do.

Whereas the concept of adults returning to college is not common, self-improvement is a huge industry. Hobbies are taken very seriously and often entail formal study to seek mastery in a particular hobby. For example, the traditional Japanese arts, such as *chadō* or *sadō* (tea ceremony); *ikebana* (flower arranging); *bonsai*; *kimono* wearing; *shodo* (calligraphy); painting; wood carving; and even doll making, are studied diligently by large numbers of women and by some retired men.

Sales of books, periodicals, and daily newspapers in Japan are among the highest among industrialized nations, and there is an increasing love of *manga*, comics or print cartoons. In fact, almost half of all periodicals or books are *manga* (Japan Media Review, 2006). Popular *manga* are adopted into *anime* (or animation), and at any time of day, one can witness the very young to the middle-aged crowding train stations, bookstores, or convenience stores, voraciously reading their favorite comics, some with explicit sexual or violent content. This has a significant impact on the way in which messages are passed on culturally. Healthcare providers need to consider the use of *manga* and *anime* when promoting health education to Japanese patients. The national broadcasting system, NHK, offers high-quality radio and television news and entertainment, and cable TV is increasingly popular.

Although culture reflects Japan's recent agrarian past, at present few Japanese are engaged in agricultural occupations because a significant amount of foodstuffs are imported. In the United States, **issei** (first-generation immigrants) originally tended to work in agriculture or as small-business owners. More recent immigrants work in business, the professions, service industries, and manufacturing. Second- (**Nisei**) and third-generation (**sansei**) Japanese Americans tend to be highly educated professionals. Most Japanese nationals living in the United States are well-educated executives, visiting scholars, individuals with technical expertise, and students.

Communication

Dominant Language and Dialects

Japanese is the language of Japan, with the exception of the indigenous *Ainu* people (see biological variations later in this chapter). The Japanese spoken in Tokyo is the national standard heard in media broadcasts; however, regional variations to the language do exist. Because high school graduates in Japan complete 6 years of English instruction, even newer Japanese immigrants and sojourners can understand, read, and write the English language to some degree. The biggest problem, however, is conversational English; whereas many Japanese may have studied the language for many years, they often lack strong conversational skills and are frequently embarrassed to try their language ability with foreigners.

In the United States, *issei* vary widely in their English-language ability. *Nisei* and *sansei* have been educated under the American educational system to the extent that they were permitted; for example, educational access was limited or segregated during the World War II internment of American citizens of Japanese ancestry. Although the language barrier may be an obstacle to understanding verbal instructions or explanations in English-speaking health-care settings, Japanese patients are likely to use written materials effectively. More recent immigrants to the United States are likely to understand English but may need prompting in conversation skills.

Cultural Communication Patterns

Japanese society is both highly structured and traditional. Politeness, personal responsibility, loyalty, and people working collectively for the greater good of the group are very important. One complexity of the Japanese language is the customizing of speech according to relative social status and gender. The Japanese sensitivity to relative status and the need to constantly gauge one's behavior accordingly is one reason the circle of intimates with whom one can truly relax is quite limited. In addition, men tend to speak more coarsely and women with more gentility or refinement.

Light social banter and gentle joking are mainstays of group relations, serving to foster group cohesiveness. Polite discussion unrelated to business, often over *o-cha* (green tea), precedes business negotiations, and *sake* parties are common during the negotiation period. *Sake*, a fermented beverage with a history of over 2000 years in Japan, is integral to the culture and society. Relationship building and respect for personal privacy are important aspects of working relationships in all sectors.

In a densely populated society that values group harmony above all else, open communication is discouraged, making it difficult to learn what people think (Doi, 1971). In particular, among people of Japanese descent, saying no is considered extremely impolite; rather, one should let the matter drop.

A high value is placed on "face" and "saving face." Asking someone to do something that he or she cannot do induces loss of face or shame. Proving people wrong is deeply humiliating to them. People may feel shame for themselves and their group, but they are expected to bear that shame in stoic silence. In fact, Japan is considered to have a shame-based culture rather than a guilt-based culture (Leonardsen, 2004), unlike many Western cultures. Suicide over shame is a common theme in Japanese literature, lore, and media. Regular reports of suicides occur in the daily media, often mentioning the name of the suicidee who has committed the act after embarrassment, shameful deeds, allegations of corruption, or bullying in the workplace or at school. Because of ethnic homogeneity; an ingrained sensitivity to the feelings of others; and close contact with one's family, classmates, and work group, Japanese believe that vague, intuitive communication, called *hara wo yomu* (belly talk), is well understood by fellow group members. Nonverbal communication or innate harmonious relationship is also expressed *a-un no kokyu* or *a-un no kankei,* meaning people can communicate without gestures or words.

In Japan, presenting a person with choices is regarded as a burden, and it is a kindness to spare people the burden of decision making. For example, a hostess may serve drinks in glasses to spare her guests the burden of deciding what they would like to drink. Professors do not offer a choice of learning activities to their students; a teacher may arrange employment for a former student; and a physician will tell the patient what to do about a health problem. These actions are motivated by concern for the well-being of the person in one's care. Japanese society is sometimes described as a web of *giri* (mutual obligations) that serves to ensure societal integrity and harmony.

Etiquette and harmony are very important, and many Japanese people exhibit considerable control over body language. Anger or dismay may be quite difficult for Westerners to detect. Smiling and laughter are common shields for embarrassment or distress. However, one need only see tearful family partings at train stations to know that, contrary to Western assumptions, Japanese people do show their feelings but seldom hug or kiss one another at such partings, as is so common in many other cultures.

Prolonged eye contact is not polite even within families. Social touching occurs among group members but not among people who are less closely acquainted.

In general, body space is respected. Intimate behavior in the presence of others is taboo. When people greet one another, whether for the first time or for the first time on a given day, the traditional bow is performed. The depth of the bow, its duration, and the number of repetitions reflect the relative status of the parties involved and the formality of the occasion. An offer to shake hands by a Westerner is reciprocated graciously. With an introduction, *meishi* (business cards) are exchanged first, enabling the parties to assess their relative status.

Temporal Relationships

An awareness of Japanese history and legend, a high regard for older people, the value of family honor, and veneration of dead ancestors suggest a strong connection with the past. However, the overall orientation of the Japanese people, who are known for their postwar economic miracle, is toward the future. The population made huge sacrifices in the decades after the war for the good of the nation, enabling it to become a world power. Parents encourage their children to study hard so that their futures will be bright. Housewives are diligent savers for future family expenses. Companies plot their growth, and the government anticipates needs decades in advance. Whereas Zen calls its providers to attend to the here and now, this tenet actually has few adherents in Japan. Health-care providers may find that Japanese patients are astonishingly motivated in health-related decision making by considering their children's needs and the economic future for their family.

Punctuality is highly valued among the Japanese. Commuter trains run to split-second timing, and people are expected to be in attendance at the exact start of meetings. In an interesting contrast, the clinic system of health care pervades even the private sector in Japan. Clinic services are not expected to be efficient, and hospital stays are still longer than in many Western countries, although the average number of hospitalization bed-days per illness is falling, owing to economic problems and some shortages of qualified nurses.

Format for Names

In Japan, family names are stated first, followed by given names. Seki Noriko would be the name of a woman, Noriko, of the Seki family, and often women's names end with *-ko*. The family names of both men and women, married or single, are designated by the suffix *-san*, but one does not use that designation when referring to oneself. Women generally assume their husband's family name upon marriage. Schoolchildren may use given names when speaking to one another, also designated with *-san*. Work groups and business associates tend to use family names. Infants and young children are called by their first names followed by *-chan*. Schoolboys are usually referred to by

REFLECTIVE EXERCISE 18.1

Mr. and Mrs. Tanaka, a Japanese-*issei* couple in their 80s, come to day care at the local community center to attend the craft and art classes. Mrs. Tanaka always follows Mr. Tanaka, and he speaks with her in a strong tone. They have been feeling isolated and ashamed to talk to others. Their family members—their son, daughter-in-law, and grandchildren—are not able to spend much time with them because of work and school.

1. How can they be introduced to others?
2. How would the communication patterns of this couple be assessed?
3. What elements of communication might be important to make this couple feel welcome?
4. Is this communication style congruent with *issei*? With *nisei*? With *sansei*?

their first or last names followed by -*kun*, whereas schoolgirls' first names are usually followed by -*chan* or -*san*. Elders are referred to respectfully. The designation **sensei** (master) is a term of respect used with the names of physicians, teachers, bosses, or others in positions of authority.

Family Roles and Organization
Head of Household and Gender Roles

The predominant family structure among the Japanese is nuclear, accounting for 58 percent of families in 2005, with 30 percent of households composed of one person, and the number of these has been increasing (Ministry of Internal Affairs and Communications, 2010). This contributes to problems in social isolation, particularly among older people, because the number of households in which three generations are present is falling. In feudal Japan, a bride had very limited contact with her own family after marriage, and the mother-in-law dominated the household. Now, wives often determine the household budget, their husbands' pocket money, investments, family insurance, real-estate decisions, and all matters related to child rearing.

Even today, with higher education widely available to women, the role of wife and mother remains dominant. Young women in the workplace may have jobs with little substantive responsibility, even if they are college graduates, but matters are slowly changing. In 2009, the Ministry of Internal Affairs and Communications (2010) reported that the ages for first marriages are rising (30.4 years for men and 28.6 for women). Moreover, the natural increase rate per 1000 population showed –0.6; –0.2 (in 2005) was the first negative result recorded since statistics gathering began in its present form in 1899. With this knowledge, the government is attempting to reduce the strong social pressure confronting women who try to continue working after motherhood, primarily because of Japan's need for skilled workers.

International Longevity Center Japan (2006) described a new law in 2005 that gave workers the opportunity to take leave to care for sick children and other family members, developed corporate strategies to support workers or other family members who take care of children, permitted shorter working hours for workers who are raising a young child, and allowed more generous family-care provisions. The effects of this law are yet to be seen; it is still difficult for women to return to work after childbearing. An equal rights amendment has been part of Japan's constitution since the U.S. occupation of Japan. Whereas Japan has protected women's interests in matters such as property ownership and voting, women are treated far from equally in the workplace. Conversely, increasing numbers of child-care centers assist families in which both parents are working, and a few of the larger corporations have begun to offer child care. Daily newspapers are filled with discussions about how Japan can increase its birth rate, and any reforms to date have failed to stop the trend of increasing numbers of working women, women who choose not to marry, or couples who choose to have few or no children at all. The difficulty of paid employment or a career after motherhood and the desire for two incomes to maintain a middle-class lifestyle often cause couples to delay having a family.

Wives in Japan care for their husbands to a degree that many Western women would not tolerate. Japanese men are presumed not to be capable of managing day-to-day matters, and some *salarymen* (white-collar workers) or office workers may leave for work at 7 a.m. and return after 10 p.m., Monday through Saturday. On Sundays, men may be so exhausted that they sleep a good part of the day, or they may be obligated to socialize with colleagues. Wives and children often stay behind when husbands are transferred by their companies within Japan or overseas, leaving women to raise children singlehandedly. Not surprisingly, one focus of the Ministry of Health, Labour and Welfare (2011a) in addressing the low birth rate is to convince men to assume more responsibility for child care and housework and for companies to change policies to keep families from being separated.

The paramount family concern is for the children's education, and it is the mother's responsibility to oversee the completion and quality of homework. When the children grow up and leave home, women tend to become involved in volunteer activities, community groups, travel, arts, and the previously mentioned self-improvement classes.

Western observers would be wrong to presume that married Japanese couples do not love each other. But in Japan, love sometimes has not been valued highly as a prerequisite for a successful marriage, and men and women have tended to be more motivated by duty to fulfill societal expectations than by the desire for spousal companionship. Conversely, domestic violence has begun to be openly acknowledged. The Gender Equality Bureau (2010) explained that according to statistics provided by the National Policy Agency, the majority of the victims in arrest cases involving murder, injury, or violence inflicted by a spouse are females. The Law for the Prevention of Spousal Violence and the Protection of Victims was implemented in 2001 and then amended in 2004. Under this law, shelters for victims were established and counseling programs offered. Moreover, restraining orders and orders to vacate are now issued at a rate of about 100 a month. With this law, a number of public education programs are in place, and some women's shelters have opened. In a society marked by strict norms differentiating the public and the private realms, couples have lacked resources to learn how to deal with tension and conflict.

Health-care providers need to be aware of differences in spousal relationships when assessing the quality of family dynamics and communication, sexual health, and sensitivity to risk for sexually transmitted infections. Health-care providers who work with college-age and young adults may find that Japanese youth are less autonomous than their American counterparts. Conflicts between traditional and American values may arise among these young people and within their families.

Prescriptive, Restrictive, and Taboo Practices for Children and Adolescents

The primary relationship within a Japanese family is the mother–child relationship, particularly that of mothers and sons. It is customary for the mother, and sometimes both parents, to sleep with the youngest child on *futons*, or mattresses, on the floor or in adult beds (Fukumizu, Kaga, Kohyama, & Hayes, 2005) until a child is age 10 years or older. When a new baby is born, the older sibling may sleep with the father or a grandparent. A special child bed is used for neonates to prevent the parents rolling on the child during sleep. Fukumizu and colleagues (2005) found that 80 percent of Japanese parents sleep with their young infants and young children. The primacy of the mother–son relationship and the absence of fathers contribute to the known problem of mother–son incest. Father–daughter incest occurs, but a stronger taboo prohibits public discussion of it (Kanazumi, 1997), and so it is very difficult to find data on it. Despite the occasional occurrence of family dysfunction in this area, health-care providers working with childbearing couples and children need to be aware of Japanese family sleeping practices and refrain from judgment.

The maternal role is so important for women in Japan that it is not unusual for a young mother to spend hours watching her infant sleep. If she observes the reflexes of urination, she changes the diaper immediately. Babies are not allowed to cry; they are picked up instantly. Women constantly hold their babies in carriers on their chests and sleep with them (Sharts Engel, 1989). "Skinship" or direct contact, is a value to be desired.

Young Japanese children tend to be indulged, especially if they are single children. At the same time, they are socialized to study hard, make their best effort, and be good group members. They are taught to take care of one another, and self-expression is not highly valued.

Corporal punishment has been more accepted in Japan than in some Western cultures, and *shitsuke* (to discipline) has traditionally included it to instruct a child to follow a particular pattern of behavior. And the word *punishment*, for example, is often used in the daily English newspapers to describe actions to counteract the transgressions of government workers. Cases of punishment by school officials or *ijime* (bullying) by their peers at school have resulted in the suicide of young children recently—matters debated hotly in the local press. The fears are that bullying is reaching epidemic proportions. Children who are bullied by schoolmates typically have different appearances, interests, or family structures, and health-care providers need to be aware of this among Japanese American children.

In 2006, the Ministry of Education, Culture, Sports, Science, and Technology (2011b), under the directives of the new prime minister, Abe, has begun a review of school education across the country, intending to incorporate content on national values. The government has also begun to address ways for families and schools to more effectively foster the development of Japanese children. It has been a serious matter that has radically increased the reports of child abuse in recent years, most of which have involved violence and neglect. It is now mandatory for teachers and health professionals to report child abuse cases. The Equal Employment, Children and Families Bureau implements the support for abused children as well as the early detection of and the prevention of child abuse.

Despite strong social pressure to conform, many adolescents in Japan have their rebellious streaks and use popular music, pornography, unconventional clothing, and illicit drugs and alcohol to escape social restrictions. Increasing numbers of young people are expressing themselves through their clothing, hair, and makeup, but vandalism is a minimal concern in the country. Teenagers and college students in Japan generally do not date to the degree that Western youth do. They typically join clubs, membership in which is taken seriously; most social activities, such as ski trips, are club activities. However, sex education in school and/or university settings is minimal, despite teenagers having sexual encounters. The use of contraceptives as a preventive measure is not common among teenagers, and about 2 percent of Japanese girls have had abortions by the time they reach their late teens. The number of abortions in women in their early 20s continues to increase annually (Sato & Iwasawa, 2006). The HPV vaccine was first approved by the Ministry of Health, Labour, and Welfare (2011b) and domestically sold in 2009. The vaccine has been started at the governmental expense.

Japan, however, has one of the lowest incidences of births to teenagers in the world. American health-care providers cannot assume that dating holds the degree of concern for Japanese young people as it does for American teenagers, nor can they assume that Japanese youths are well informed about sexuality and sexual health risks.

Other health concerns among young people include the pressures to conform within a peer group and to perform well in school, pressures that may lead to depression and suicide (Takakura & Sakihara, 2000). Interest in studying eating disorders is increasing, although research indicates lower rates among Japanese youths than among U.S. youths and in college students rather than high school students in Japan (Makino, Hashizume, Yasushi, Tsuboi, & Dennerstein, 2006). One reason for this may be young students' increasing identification with very thin models from the West, increasingly portrayed in the media.

After graduation from high school or college, young adults are traditionally expected to be employed through their network of school contacts or family friends. Young women now typically live with their parents for many years after they finish school, whereas young men are likely to live in company housing until marriage, and even after.

Family Goals and Priorities

Promoting success in school is the mother's main focus in child rearing. Children compete for their junior and senior high school admission, and high schools vary in the caliber of universities to which their graduates are admitted. The schools from which individuals graduate determine such major issues as career prospects for men and the status of husbands with whom young women are likely to marry.

Children are highly valued, and motherhood traditionally has been revered in Japan. The recent extreme drop in the birth rate has taken the society by surprise, although in prior decades, the expense of rearing and educating children triggered its beginning. Nothing is permitted to interfere with child-rearing responsibilities. Japanese women may be less likely than North American women to engage in activities, including health-care appointments that require them to leave their children with babysitters.

The ideal of romantic love plays less of a role in marriage in Japan than in the United States, and the marriage rate in 2009 was 5.6 per 1000 population in Japan (Ministry of Internal Affairs and Communications, 2010), lower than in the United States, with 6.8 per 1000 population (Tejada-Vera & Sutton, 2010). Traditionally Japanese marriage has been arranged, often by employers or family friends. The *o-miai* is the ritual of the first arranged meeting between prospective partners. Although about 30 percent of marriages were arranged, the ratio of the marriages has been reduced.

As mentioned previously, Japanese couples are marrying later in life. The groom's goals for marrying focus on advancement of his career and a desire to be cared for. For the bride, economic security and child rearing are traditional goals. A "honeymoon baby" is becoming less common, and couples are delaying having a family early in the marriage. Few Japanese women bear children outside of marriage, and abortion is one of a number of contraceptive practices, with the use of condoms more prevalent than the use of the contraceptive pill.

Japanese couples place less emphasis on companionship and sexual fulfillment than do North American couples and are far less likely to live together without being married. The divorce rate has declined. In 2010, there were about 2 divorces in Japan per 1000 population (Ministry of Internal Affairs and Communications, 2010) compared with 3.4 in the United States (Tejada-Vera & Sutton, 2010).

The Japanese family (especially the eldest son, who has a sense of obligation to his parents) has traditionally cared for and respected older people and children. However, with the drift to living in urban areas in small apartments and with more couples working, it is increasingly difficult to care for older parents. Retirement and nursing homes are growing in number across the country, although many of the latter have a poor public image and are poorly regulated. With the longevity of its people, Japan is aging more rapidly than any other nation. The government has begun to address how to care for older people, who now account for 22 percent of the total population. North American health-care providers must be sensitive to Japanese patients' sense of obligation and commitment. Helping families network within the Japanese American community both for social support and for resources or good long-term-care facilities is a useful strategy.

Elements of social status include age, gender, educational background, and work group affiliation of oneself or one's husband. Though there is a peerage system, and some old families are known to be descendants of *samurai*, Japan is largely a meritocracy. Exceptions include Korean descendants or descendants of the burakumin, the untouchable caste (hereditary social class) who cared for the dead and tanned leather in feudal times. In this largely middle-class society, schoolchildren can reasonably expect to study hard and go on for higher education if that is the family goal.

Biases that may be evident among Japanese people who reside in North America are directed at minority groups such as African Americans, Jews, and individuals with limited education, as well as women in high-status positions. This prejudice is seldom overt, but it may threaten the comfort of Japanese people, who are likely to encounter such diversity among health-care providers in North America.

Alternative Lifestyles

In Japan, a small segment of women have long lived outside the usual constraints for their gender. Women of "the floating world," or the entertainment industry, enjoy a fair degree of autonomy. The most traditional of these, the *geisha*, live in all-female communal arrangements, but they are reducing in number annually. *Geisha* are not prostitutes but are considered highly skilled artists, and they are now recognized as a cultural treasure. However, other women in the entertainment industry fulfill men's need to relax in a society highly constrained by social norms; therefore, the sex trade is flourishing, and occasional mention is made of the sex slave trade in Japan. Hostesses at bars look after their male customers, pour their drinks, and listen to them. In earlier eras, concubines were accepted within families. Today, infidelity by married men is more tolerated than in North America, but much less so for married women.

An increasing number of the Japanese population remains single throughout life, and only a few men and women enter monastic life. The small proportions of heterosexual couples who live together outside of marriage find greater tolerance in urban settings in Japan. Marriage of a Japanese person to a foreigner is less tolerated than it is in the United States. The existence of a gay and lesbian social network and of cross-dressing clubs is evident in English-language publications in Tokyo.

The pornography industry thrives, and prostitution is big business. Rape and other sexual abuses are acknowledged in Japanese society and are now being more openly discussed. In fact, there have been a number of incidences since 2005 regarding harassment; rape and murder cases are on the increase. In Tokyo, commuter trains for women now run at night to combat sexual harassment. Health education about avoiding rape and inappropriate touching, when approached in a matter-of-fact way, is very appropriate for Japanese in North America.

Workforce Issues
Culture in the Workplace

Japanese employees in North American institutions need to be carefully oriented to the legal and professional requirements of patient autonomy and of accountability in reporting, solving, and documenting problems that occur. An overview of dominant American society values may prepare them for the directness of communication they will encounter.

Claims for medical malpractice are growing slowly in Japan but are far less common than in the United States; for example, in 2003 in Japan, only 1019 newly accepted lawsuits in the Supreme Court were associated with medical malpractice across the country (Ehara, 2005). American practices designed to avoid liability, such as informed consent, are not routinely implemented in Japanese health-care settings. Patient autonomy is recommended in health-care settings; however, the real priority in Japan is meeting dependency and recuperation needs, and a family has a crucial role in health-care decision making (Ito, Tanida, & Turale, 2010).

Like most Japanese workers, nurses in Japan work long hours, often between 8 and 10 hours per day, 5 days per week. Nurses often work extra time after their shift without pay. Their pay is low in relation to their cost of living compared with that of other health-care providers. With the advance of a university education, nursing is slowly becoming a respected profession. Staffing is complicated by federal restrictions on shift work among women, although change is underway because Japan, like North America, is experiencing a nursing shortage.

The mix of people providing nursing care in Japan represents many levels of educational preparation, and nurses may be prepared for registered nursing (RN) practice in a number of different ways. Baccalaureate degrees, representing 4 years of education at university, are growing. RNs are still being prepared in colleges of nursing and schools attached to hospitals offering diploma and associate degree programs. In the face of the nursing shortage and the growing

---

REFLECTIVE EXERCISE 18.2

Mrs. Ishikawa, a 34-year-old mother and housewife, has lived in the United States for almost 1 year. Her husband is a businessman and works hard away from the family home. Mrs. Ishikawa takes care of their 1- and 3-year-old sons. She has Japanese friends, and they exchange information and help one another. Mrs. Ishikawa brings her sons to a pediatric clinic. In a tearful voice, she tries to explain why she came to the clinic.

1. What cultural factors need to be considered in this situation?
2. How can the nurse help Mrs. Ishikawa to express her concerns?
3. What agencies or persons could be called for assistance?

health-care needs of a rapidly aging population, aides are likely to be used more extensively, and Japan is now actively seeking to recruit nurses from selected Asian countries, especially the Philippines and Indonesia. According to the Ministry of Health, Labour and Welfare (2011a), 15 Indonesians and 1 Filipino passed the national examination for nurses in 2011.

After RN preparation, an additional year of courses prepares individuals for certification as midwives or as public-health nurses. A recent nursing role is that of clinical specialist in a variety of settings. In addition, the number of master's and doctoral degree programs across the country has experienced a strong growth over the last decade. Like nursing students, medical students enter medical school immediately after high school, and after graduation, they complete a clinical residency.

Issues Related to Autonomy

Japanese workers are quite sensitive to the desires and expectations of colleagues and superiors. Because saying no or delivering bad news is extremely difficult, they may avoid issues or indicate that everything is fine rather than state the negative. Of course, sensitive Japanese workers who are attuned to nonverbal cues may understand the true situation. In addition, many Japanese workers tend not to leave work before their boss does, nor do they take their full complement of paid vacation time each year, which may contribute to worker stress and tiredness. North American employers should explicitly discuss expectations about starting and quitting times and vacation leave with Japanese employees. Japanese workers do not assert individual rights. Japanese health-care providers working in North America accept the need to assert themselves if it is presented within the context of legal and professional requirements to protect their patients.

Japanese nurses are less likely than North American nurses to confront or question physicians or to suggest strategies. Workers tend to do what the head of the group tells them to do and make every effort to do it very well. Japanese health-care providers seeking to practice in the United States have studied English from grade 7 throughout professional school, and will have passed an examination certifying minimal competency, but their verbal skills may still be weak. Specific approaches to documentation, such as problem-oriented record-keeping, are now being more widely taught and used in Japan. However, these may still be unfamiliar to some nurses and need to be addressed specifically in employees' orientation.

Biocultural Ecology

Skin Color and Other Biological Variations

Racial features of Japanese people include the epicanthal skin folds that create the distinctive appearance of Asian eyes, a broad and flat nose, and "yellow" skin that varies markedly in tone. Hair is straight and naturally black with differences in shade. Health-care providers who are not accustomed to assessing racially diverse patient groups may need to rely on color changes in the mucous membranes and sclerae to assess oxygenation and liver function in Japanese patients. The average stature of Japanese adults is smaller than that of Americans, although the gap has steadily decreased as national wealth has increased and a greater percentage of the population is able to improve their dietary practices.

The Ainu people of northern Japan, described earlier in this chapter, who number only about 23,000 in the Hokkaido area, are a fair-skinned people whose racial and linguistic origins are inconclusive. Estimates of ethnic Japanese with Ainu ancestry vary between 50,000 and 150,000. Recent genetic studies have suggested that the ancient Ainu may have been among the peoples who came from Asia to settle in North America. In previous centuries, the Ainu underwent significant discrimination (*New World Encyclopedia*, 2007). The Okinawa people of the Ryukyu Islands are darker-skinned than "mainlanders" and have a stockier build.

Diseases and Health Conditions

The three leading causes of death in Japan are malignant neoplasm, heart disease, and cerebrovascular diseases. These account for over 50 percent of deaths in both sexes. In descending order, other causes are pneumonia, accidents, traffic accidents, suicide, renal disease, liver disease, diabetes mellitus, hypertensive diseases, and tuberculosis (Ministry of Health, Labour and Welfare, 2011b). Moreover, men have a life expectancy of 78.9 years, whereas women have a life expectancy of 85.7 years, making the Japanese the longest-lived people in the world (*CIA World Factbook*, 2011). An increasing focus is on reducing suicide, particularly among depressed men, because Japan ranks ninth in the world for suicides (Nakao & Takeuchi, 2006). Asthma and other allergic reactions related to dust mites in the *tatami* (straw mats that cover floors in Japanese homes) are considered some of the few endemic diseases, along with illnesses related to air pollution in urban areas. In rural areas, allergic reactions to the pollen from numerous *sugi* (cedar) trees are a seasonal problem.

Variations in Drug Metabolism

In general, drug dosages may need to be adjusted for the physical stature of Japanese adults, and racially linked genetic differences in drug metabolism can be important. More Asians than whites are poor metabolizers of mephenytoin and related medications, potentially leading to increased intensity and duration of the drugs' effects (Levy, 1993). Asians tend to be more sensitive to the effects of some beta blockers, many psychotropic drugs, and alcohol. A greater proportion of Japanese people rapidly metabolize acetylate substances, which has an impact on the metabolism of tranquilizers, tuberculosis drugs, caffeine, and some cardiovascular agents. Asians often require lower doses of some benzodiazepines, such as diazepam, and neuroleptics. Opiates may be less effective analgesics, but gastrointestinal side effects may be greater than those among whites. Health-care providers need to take all patients' body mass into consideration in dosing; even with that precaution, patients' responses to drugs need to be monitored carefully.

High-Risk Behaviors

The smoking rate for Japanese men has declined since the mid-1990s to around 40 percent of all men aged over 20 years in 2009, but it is slightly decreasing in women (12 percent). Around 16 to 18 percent of women in the 20- to 39-year-old age group now smoke (Ministry of Health, Labour and Welfare, 2010a). Many restaurants, aware of the dangers of secondhand smoke, now offer nonsmoking areas, and plans are to make all restaurants smoking-free in the not too distant future. Public facilities, hospitals, schools, public transportation vehicles, and many offices prohibit smoking. Cigarettes are available at shops or in vending machines with a special card "Taspo" as *Tabako no Pasupoto* introduced in 2008 for sale to those over 20 years of age.

Alcohol has ritual significance. For example, in the marriage ceremony, the bride and groom drink *sake* or *miki* (rice wine), which is also an appropriate offering at **Shinto** shrines and at the *butsudan*, or household ancestral shrine. In addition, alcohol is part of many social rituals, such as picnics to celebrate cherry blossoms, autumn leaves, or moon viewing. Adults commonly drink beer and *sake* in the home, and college students drink beer when they socialize, although the legal age for drinking is 20 years.

The most serious concerns about alcohol use reflect the informal work requirement for men in Japan to socialize after hours or during weekends. Considerable alcohol may be consumed, and it is common to see intoxicated businessmen snoozing on the trains or stumbling home late in the evening. In part, this extensive use of alcohol reflects the stress of Japanese corporate life and the rigid protocols that dictate social interactions. Once alcohol is consumed, workers can relax and speak freely. This is called *bureiko*, which means a gathering at which a man can say whatever is on his mind; they are forgiven because the blame is placed on the alcohol. Although diminished in the recent economic downturn, entertaining is expected in the Japanese business culture, and drinking is tolerated as an obligation to one's company.

Public acknowledgment of alcoholism is limited, and alcoholism rates are very difficult to determine. According to the Ministry of Health, Labour and Welfare (2010a), the rate of customary alcohol drinking in male and female adults in 2009 was 36.4 percent and 6.9 percent, respectively. Higuchi (2009) reported that the annual average rate of alcohol consumption per person from 2000 to 2007 was about 7 to 8 liters, an increase from about 5 liters in 1963. The rate of youth abuse of alcohol is increasing (Tsuchiya & Takei, 2004). Over several decades, the Maryknoll Missionaries established alcohol treatment centers throughout the country and were among the first to publicize the problem of alcoholism among housewives, opening the first treatment center for women in the mid-1980s. Health-care providers need to be aware of the prevalence of smoking and heavy alcohol consumption among Japanese people, particularly men. An effective strategy for curtailing these abuses is to give individuals specific medical reasons why they must abstain, thus providing a socially acceptable excuse to do so.

Over the last few years, Japan has witnessed a soaring abuse of illicit drugs by young people, particularly in high-density urban districts. The drugs used are mostly narcotics and stimulants, which have caused an increase in mental health problems, school dropout rates, and drug-related crimes. The most serious is methamphetamine use, which has been increasing since the 1990s and is connected to mental illness. Distribution of methamphetamines is believed to be controlled by the *yakuza*, the Japanese mafia (Tsuchiya & Takei, 2004). Also increasing are serious crimes involving guns, which have often been smuggled into the country. The government instituted the Drug Abuse Prevention Center in 1987 and continued to implement the Third Five Year Drug Abuse Strategy in 2008. The government increased efforts to combat the smuggling of drugs and guns into the country by sea (Customs and Tariff Bureau, 2009). Punishment is harsh and swift, and there is no popular sentiment for liberalization. Despite such problems, the crime rate is quite low, and in most cities, the streets are safe at all hours.

Students and workers in Japan also make heavy use of over-the-counter stimulants. Students and young professionals are commonly seen consuming high-dosage caffeine drinks at train stations in the morning.

In Japan, as in a number of Western countries, the rate of new cases of HIV and AIDS is on the increase, and in 2008, the number of people living with **HIV** was twice as high as in 2000 (UNAIDS, 2010). This shows the great need for early-detection efforts and treatment and for education on prevention. Every health-care contact with Japanese businessmen and/or their wives should be considered an opportunity to inform them about infectious disease risks. The United States is perceived as a place with a high risk for contracting **HIV**, and concerns among Japanese who come to the United States tend to focus on casual contact as a possible modality.

Other growing concerns are the rise in inactivity and obesity levels of Japanese children. Success in the educational system demands long hours of study each day, thus reducing participation in physical activities, and this is compounded by the growth in the fast-food industry and the predilection for computer and electronic games usage among the young. Another problem is the prevalence of dental caries, which is high owing to unfluoridated water supplies across the country.

Health-Care Practices

Japanese people are likely to attribute their generally high level of well-being to the centuries-old tradition of the daily bath. The *o-furo* (Japanese bathtub) is deep enough for an adult to enjoy a leisurely soak in neck-deep water, and the temperature is typically set around 105°F. The purpose of the bath is relaxation. Scrubbing for cleanliness and thorough rinsing are done before climbing into the tub. Families share the same water; in fact, they may soak together in the bath. Bathwater may be reheated for several days before the tub is drained; depending on the type of bath, the water may be recycled for washing clothes or watering plants. Herbs or bath salts with therapeutic properties are sometimes added.

Young people in Japan do not drive until age 18, and an expensive and lengthy course of instruction is mandatory. Driving under the influence of alcohol or reckless operation of a vehicle carries stiff penalties. Rigorous inspection standards mean that people drive recent models of vehicles that are fully equipped with standard safety features. One major problem, however, is the rise in injury by rear seat passengers not using seat beats, a common feature in busy traffic, even though Japanese generally exhibit a high degree of public safety consciousness.

Traditional housing materials and the close proximity of buildings have made fire a common and large-scale hazard. Each neighborhood has modern fire stations. Japanese readily use public services. Explicit instructions for accessing the local police, fire station, paramedics, and an emergency medical facility in a given North American community may be necessary, as well as the circumstances under which access is appropriate.

Nutrition
Meaning of Food

Many Japanese social and business interactions begin or end (or both) with the serving of *o-cha* (green tea and sweets) or an *o-bento* (boxed lunch). Business entertaining can be lavish. Part of the atmosphere of congeniality depends on the artistic presentation of the food.

Common Foods and Food Rituals

In Japan, all food groups are well represented, even in small shops, and the national diet is steadily becoming more Western, particularly among young people. In a wealthy, cosmopolitan society in the big cities, one can find just about any food or drink in common use in North America and Europe.

Large-scale agricultural production within Japan provides rice, beef, poultry, pork, seafood, root vegetables, cabbage, persimmons, apples, and *mikan* (tangerines). Rice, or *gohan*, the mainstay of the traditional diet, is included in all three meals as well as snacks. The electric rice cooker is a household necessity.

A traditional breakfast includes fish, pickles, *nori* (a sheet of seaweed that is often used to wrap rice balls), a raw egg stirred into the hot rice, *miso* (soybean-based) soup, and green tea. Some people prefer a Western breakfast of toast or cold cereal and coffee.

Schoolchildren lunch on their *o-bento*, packed with rice, pickles, vegetables, and meat or fish. Elementary schools generally provide a school lunch for pupils. A popular lunch among working people is *o-bento*, which can be ordered to be delivered quite cheaply to workplaces, or cold noodles on a hot summer day. Instant broth, or instant noodles, though high in sodium, is another popular quick lunch.

A traditional dinner style would be *ichiju-nisai*: one bowl of soup, two kinds of entrees, and rice. In major cities, Japanese housewives and working people have easy access to an enormous range of take-out food or home-delivery service, including Japanese, Chinese, and Western selections. American or Japanese fast-food hamburger chains can be found in all cities. The daily intake of sweets can be high and often includes European-style desserts, sweet breads and cookies, sweet bean cakes, soft drinks, and heavily sweetened coffee, which may contribute to the high incidence of tooth decay.

For people in Japan, rice has a symbolic meaning related to the Shinto religion, analogous to the concept of the "bread of life" among Christians. One of the emperor's duties is to ceremonially plant the first rice in the spring and harvest the first rice in the late summer. A staple of schoolchildren's *o-bento* is a bed of white rice garnished with a red plum pickle,

REFLECTIVE EXERCISE 18.3

Mr. Murakami, a 54-year-old business executive, has led a very busy life. He traveled a lot inside and outside the country, worked long hours, and socialized frequently with his clients. He usually does not eat much dinner and drinks alcohol every night with his colleagues and clients. He has been diagnosed with diabetes mellitus at his health checkup.

1. What are the culturally sensitive elements to consider when advising Mr. Murakami about his alcohol consumption and diet?
2. Who needs to be involved in the decision making about a plan for his lifestyle changes?

reminiscent of the Japanese flag. Meals combine elements of land and sea.

Holidays and family celebrations are times for ritual use of food. *O-bon*, in the summer, is a holiday for remembering family members who have died and a time when many travel to their family home, causing transport congestion across the country. Vegetables, especially *daikon* (large white radishes), are carved into animals, which are said to carry dead ancestors back to the afterlife after the holiday. Likewise, the new year's festival, *O-shogatsu*, is a 3-day celebration with food that has been prepared in advance. Japanese may ring in the new year by standing in line at a Shinto shrine to ring a gong and then drinking a cup of warm *sake*. Another traditional new year's food is *mochi*, a ball of sticky rice dough that celebrants take turns pounding out with a heavy mallet. Red rice, or rice with red beans, is a celebratory food, as are various sweet bean desserts. A meal customarily begins with the simple grace, *Itadakimasu*, with the palms of hands facing together, and ends with the compliment "*Gochisosama deshita.*" Western food rituals, including birthday cakes, wedding cakes, Christmas cakes, Valentine's chocolates, and Halloween trick or treats, have been incorporated into Japanese life, no doubt spurred on by a consumer-driven market economy.

Dietary Practices for Health Promotion

Increasingly Westernized food tastes, resulting in higher fat and carbohydrate intake, have contributed to the rise in obesity, particularly in young children, in modern Japan as it has in many Western countries. These dietary changes and other lifestyle factors are causing great concern about an increase in conditions such as type 2 diabetes and heart disease (Urakami, Morimoto, Nitadori, Harada, Owada, & Kitagawa, 2007).

A huge Japanese diet industry has arisen that includes weight-loss clinics and programs and an amazing array of diet foods and medications in supermarkets and pharmacies. Public education programs continue to warn the public about the high sodium content of soups and the overuse of food additives, soy sauce, and table salt. General principles of nutrition are the same in America as in Japan, although the food preferences may differ significantly.

Green tea, although high in caffeine, is a good source of vitamin C. Garlic and various herbs are widely used for their medicinal properties. In larger cities, health-food stores offering organically grown produce are available. Sales in Japan's health food industry, including supplements, have grown to almost US$20 billion (Kenko Sangyo Shinbun, 2010).

Nutritional Deficiencies and Food Limitations

Although some Asian people, including the Japanese, may have difficulty digesting milk products owing to lactose intolerance, increasing amounts of dairy products, including milk, cream, cheese, butter, ice cream, and yogurt, are on sale throughout the country, although these are not used to the same extent as in Western diets. Reduced-lactose milk is now available, as are low-fat milks and cheeses. Calcium is supplied in other foods such as *tofu* (soybean curd) and small, fileted fish. Water supplies are not fluoridated, and dental caries continue to be widespread. Fluoridated dental products can be recommended to Japanese patients, with the rationale for their use provided. Iron deficiency anemia is a concern among young women and can be alleviated with dietary counseling or dietary supplements. *Nori* (seaweed) is a traditional food source for iron.

Pregnancy and Childbearing Practices

Fertility Practices and Views Toward Pregnancy

After a national debate that lasted nearly 40 years, oral contraceptives became legal in Japan in 1999, and shortly afterward, sildenafil citrate (Viagra) was quickly approved. The use of oral contraceptives, however, still remains fairly limited, and they are still not often used to treat menstrual cycle problems. In fact, Japan has managed to achieve a low birth rate without the major use of contraceptive pills. Condoms remain the most common contraceptive method used in Japan. Although the number of reported abortions has steadily declined each year in Japan (just over 240,000 in 2008), the incidence is the highest in the 20- to 30-year-old age group (Ministry of Health, Labour and Welfare, 2010). Some temples have *mizuko jizo* shrines where women give offerings of gifts and money to attendants who watch over aborted or miscarried fetuses (Orenstein, 2002), and often a woman or a couple will place *jizo* at a temple or shrine in memory of their aborted or miscarried fetus (Fig. 18-1).

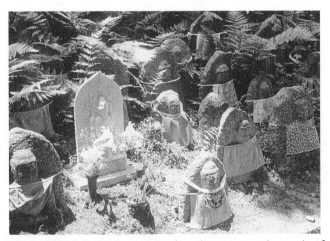

Figure 18-1 Misuko jizu are implored to protect the souls of aborted fetuses in the Japanese Buddhist tradition.

The decline in the Japanese birth rate, which was 1.3 in 2008, is regarded as a national crisis, and the economic implications are devastating as the country ages. An educated female population, in a society in which women are oppressed, has asserted itself in a way that has certainly caught the nation's attention. As a result, many social structures and policies regarding female labor laws and child-care and social support systems are under scrutiny. Japan's status as a low-birth-rate country has created great interest in assistive reproductive technology within the last few years, and the Ministry of Health, Labour and Welfare (2010b) supports a part of the costs for infertility treatments.

Within traditional Japanese culture, pregnancy is highly valued as a woman's fulfillment of her destiny. Women may enjoy attention and pampering that they get at no other time, and our observations are that they take their role as mother-to-be very seriously, including health and diet. When a pregnancy is first detected in Japan, it is registered with the local government office, which distributes a special mother/child handbook that becomes a comprehensive longitudinal health record for the child right up until kindergarten. Japanese nationals in the United States want to access the handbook (Nakamura, 2010).

Maternity clothes are now often very fashionable. Some believe that keeping one's feet warm will promote uterine health. Pregnant women may undergo a ceremony involving the wrapping of a *hara obi* (a bleached cotton abdomen sash) obtained and purified at a Shinto shrine. The sash is wrapped around the abdomen for protection as part of a small ceremony performed on the Day of the Dog in the 5th month of pregnancy (Ito & Sharts-Hopko, 2002). Because dogs give birth easily, the Chinese word for "dog" may be drawn on the *obi* by the obstetrician or midwife before they wrap it on the woman. Some women wear this sash throughout the rest of the pregnancy, but others may use a maternity girdle, a stomach band, or a special amulet to ensure a safe delivery.

Continuity of care throughout pregnancy is generally different in the United States and Japan. In Japan, a woman usually receives medical care and birthing support, including ultrasonography and physical examinations, from the same medical staff. In the United States, these may occur in different locations. Japanese women often return to their mother's home for the last 2 months of their pregnancy (called *satogaeri bunben*) and through the first 2 months postpartum. Alternatively, mothers may come to stay with their daughter during this period, even traveling abroad to be with her. American health-care providers should explore a Japanese woman's expectations during pregnancy and the possibility that she might return to Japan. Finding another Japanese woman who has experienced childbearing in the United States and who can share her experiences can provide support for the pregnant patient.

Prescriptive, Restrictive, and Taboo Practices in the Childbearing Family

Health teaching for pregnant women in Japan emphasizes rest and restraint from stressful activities. Women who are found working until late in their pregnancy are given special considerations in the workplace. Loud noises, such as trains or very loud music, are believed to be bad for the baby. Shinto shrines sell amulets for conception and easy delivery, and women may pray for their safe delivery at these shrines. Some women now attend exercise classes for pregnant women but are rarely accompanied by their husbands.

In the past, it was not so common for husbands to attend the births of their children; however, this is changing and varies considerably across Japan. Some hospitals still do not allow husbands to be present. Most Japanese women choose private obstetric care and give birth in 1 of the 2500 maternity hospitals in which most births occur with a physician delivering the baby. Certified nurse-midwives often give perinatal massages during childbirth. They may deliver the baby, sometimes observed by a physician who assists if complications occur. However, the strong tradition of local community-based midwifery, with independent midwives offering services at their own birthing houses, is regaining popularity. Currently, about 350 of these across the country cater to about 2 percent of the births. Birthing houses are quite separate from hospitals and are supported by the community. Birthing at home is quite rare in Japan.

Episiotomies may still be performed for first deliveries, but shaving and the use of enemas predelivery are not common in Japan. In addition, Japanese midwives often use perinatal massage. Oxytocics are common in the second stage of delivery if contractions are weak, and antibiotics are often prescribed after delivery even though there may be no sign of infection. Pregnant women are educated about balanced natural foods, and easily digested foods are preferred during the first stage of labor.

The differences in birthing procedures need to be explained to women giving birth in the United States, especially when they may have knowledge only of procedures in their home country. It is important for midwives and obstetricians in the United States to remember that Japanese families want the dried umbilical cord that falls from the newborn's abdomen, which they store in boxes made of *kiri* (paulownia) wood. This tradition comes from several cultural and regional beliefs. One of them is that its spiritual energy would protect the baby throughout his or her life.

Physicians are skilled at mid- and high-forceps deliveries because cesarean delivery is viewed as hard on the mother; such surgery is reserved for emergency cases. Vaginal deliveries are usually performed with minimal medication, and the mother tries to be very stoic, using the breathing exercises taught during pregnancy. Ito and Sharts-Hopko (2002) explained that Japanese women prefer nonpharmacological interventions such as the Lamaze method whenever possible. To give in to pain dishonors the husband's family, and mothers are said to appreciate their babies more if they suffer in childbirth.

Japan enjoys one of the lowest rates of infant and maternal mortality in the world. Maternal mortality, 4.8 per 10,000 births in 2009, is most commonly caused by hemorrhage and is associated with delivery in small, single-physician birthing hospitals (Ministry of Health, Labour and Welfare, 2010b).

Japanese women in the United States are not likely to have a birth plan when they are admitted to a health-care facility. They prefer natural methods of child delivery as they would in Japan and to avoid cesarean delivery and pain relief whenever possible. Their husbands may choose not to attend the actual delivery, in which case, women will need additional supportive nursing care.

In the postpartum period, time to recover from childbirth is taken seriously because *chi-no-michi* (pathway of blood) is believed to be an indication of the woman's health. In Japan, a woman may stay in the hospital 5 days to 1 week while learning to breastfeed and attending daily mother-care classes. Japanese hospitals vary about allowing rooming-in of babies. Culturally, postpartum women often do not wash their hair for a few days postpartum. Because the new mother often stays with her mother, the new father may not see his baby for a few months until he comes to take the mother and baby home from the grandmother's house. Because of the perceived risk of infections, it is unusual to see infants in public before the age of 3 months.

Mothers will often be asked about the feeding method they used for their baby—for example, on kindergarten admission forms. Maternal rest and relaxation are deemed essential for success. Lactation nurses are widely available, and breast massage is one of their strategies for promoting milk production and flow. A number of promotional campaigns have been held recently to encourage women to breastfeed, and concerns do exist about its decline when women choose to reenter the workforce.

Japanese women who give birth in the United States may resent the American expectation that they will resume self-care and child-care activities quickly, which they believe is harmful to them and their relationship with the baby. Although American health-care providers

cannot provide the length of hospital stay the women would have experienced in Japan, they can explain the expectations for postpartum care, exercise sensitivity, and help plan for assistance upon discharge.

Death Rituals

Death Rituals and Expectations

In Japan, death, serious illness, and mental illness are usually not common subjects for discussion, but recently, the daily media have begun to include more awareness and discussion about depression, and dementia. In the last decade, physicians are more commonly revealing diagnoses of cancer or other life-threatening illnesses to patients only when there is a clear family agreement to do so. In the past, patients were rarely told of the possibility of their impending death. This paternalistic approach was meant to relieve the patient of emotional suffering. In recent years, the biomedical literature has begun to reflect open discourse on pain management in terminal illness, the need for greater national investment in intensive-care services, the need to increase organ transplantation, and the need for end-of-life decision making.

The most extraordinary cultural differences between Japan and Western societies are the roles and responsibilities of family members for end-of-life decision making (Hattori, McCubbin, & Ishida, 2006). Currently families are expected to perform as reliable decision makers for a dying patient: however, analysts predict that the Japanese people will become more self-oriented rather than family-oriented in regard to their health decision making. Western individualism is expected to increase in the Japanese end-of-life health-care structure.

Responses to Death, Grief, and Suffering

When considering the death and grief reactions of Japanese, one must not neglect the close intertwining of Buddhist and Shinto beliefs at large in the population. In Shinto, death is believed to be impure and one should not spend time dwelling on it. According to the first Noble Truth of Buddhism, all human beings suffer. When a Japanese person is dying, the family should be notified of the impending death so they can be at the dying person's bedside. Traditionally, the eldest son has particular responsibility during this time.

Many homes have a Buddhist altar, *butsudan*, where deceased family members are honored and remembered. Photographs of the deceased are displayed, floral arrangements are placed within and outside of the home, and a special altar may be constructed when a person dies. An alternate version of this custom dictates that if the dead is satisfied with the amount of money, then the inheritance is freed for the survivors. Visitors bring gifts of money and food for the bereaved family. White flowers are the symbol of death in Japan and are used at funerals; therefore, these should not be sent to someone who is ill.

Modern corporate life in Japan does not allow for taking more than a few days off from work for official mourning. However, in terms of religious practice, the mourning period is 49 days, the end of which is marked by a family prayer service and the serving of special rice dishes. At this time, the departed has joined those already in the hereafter. Perpetual prayers may be donated through a gift to the temple. In addition, special prayer services can be conducted for the

1st, 3rd, 7th, 13th, and 17th anniversaries of the death. The common belief is that the dead need to be remembered, and failure to do so can lead the dead to rob the living of rest. Proper funeral rites and reassurance that they are remembered during temple and family prayers alleviate the agitation of the dead. In addition, it gives the family a sense of relief and protection from their ancestors.

Spirituality
Dominant Religion and Use of Prayer

Japan does not have a clearly articulated theology or religious belief system. Tradition holds that the Japanese people are descendants of the Sun goddess and that the emperor is a god (Keene, 1983), although the Occupation forces required Hirohito to publicly renounce this status after World War II ended. Some say that the demotion of the emperor from god to mortal has left the Japanese with a spiritual vacuum. Reischauer and Jansen (1995) believed this secularization of Japanese society began when Confucianism, imported during the 9th century, grew in influence during the 17th century. Confucian values, including faith in education, hard work, and the emphasis on interpersonal relationships and loyalty, continue to be important today.

Shinto, the indigenous religion, is the focus of joyful events such as marriage and birth. Many *matsuri* (festivals) are marked by offerings, parades through the streets, and a carnival on the grounds of the shrine. Buddhism, brought to Japan in the 6th century, has permeated Japanese artistic and intellectual life. Very few Japanese people regularly attend services, but most are registered temple members, if only to ensure a family burial plot. One percent of Japanese people are Christian (*CIA World Factbook,* 2011), and Christianity has been known, although at times not well tolerated, in Japan since the 16th century. Most Japanese do not identify themselves solely with one religion; even a baptized Christian might have a Shinto wedding and a Buddhist funeral. These days, some young people get married in a commercial-style chapel that looks like a Christian chapel but has nothing to do with religion.

Meaning of Life and Individual Sources of Strength

This crossover of Shinto and Buddhist beliefs and customs may be a surprise to visitors from overseas. Many Japanese believe in reincarnation, a Buddhist belief, and also accept the Shinto recognition of the eternal life of the soul, which needs purification in the earthly life. Ancestor worship is widespread, and many Japanese believe that their ancestors can be called back to earth. Such beliefs play a large part in mourning the dead. Other valid interpretations include honoring one's family and country, working

---

REFLECTIVE EXERCISE 18.5

Mr. Yamamoto is a 76-year-old Japanese man who has been living in the United States for 30 years. He became widowed 1 month ago. When his daughter visited him a week ago, he had fallen and had been on the floor, calling for help for several hours. She called a community health nurse for consultation. When the nurse visits Mr. Yamamoto, he seems depressed. He has been able to manage his daily life and has no cognitive impairment. He refuses to leave his home, which is full of happy memories.

1. In order to help Mr. Yamamoto to deal with his wife's death, what culturally congruent rituals could the nurse and the social worker suggest to assist him?
2. Who else might be called to help him?
3. What are some challenges the nurse might encounter while working with him?

hard, being a good group member, and joining one's deceased ancestors (Woss, 1992).

Spiritual Beliefs and Health-Care Practices

Japanese religions play a significant role in health-care practices. People or objects such as cars are taken to special shrines for purification from evil by priests. People often buy protective *omamori* (amulets) at shrines or temples for a wide variety of reasons. At the temple or shrine, a person might be seen scooping incense smoke onto an ailing body part or praying for good health. Prayer boards might bear requests for special healing. Gifts of toys or devices used in child care may be left with Buddha statues. Shichi-go-san (7-5-3) cerebration is a special family event to take newborns (about 1 month old) and children (3, 5, and/or 7 years old) to a shrine for blessings for their health and wisdom (Fig. 18-2). Visits to shrines and temples in Japan are social, recreational, and spiritual outings. Souvenirs and refreshments are usually available, and the hike into the prayer area provides exercise, with access to many temples or shrines involving a climb up steps (Shinto Online Network Association, 2006).

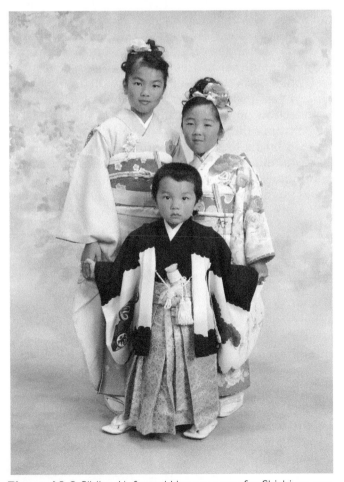

Figure 18-2 Siblings' informal kimono wear for Shichi-go-san (7-5-3) celebration.

Various types of diviners, soothsayers, and prophets may be present at shrines, temples, and even along the most fashionable streets in Tokyo. Statues depicting folktale heroes, often animals, are believed to bring luck. Americans may have difficulty understanding and accepting the reliance of sophisticated and well-educated people on what may be viewed as superstitions. But these measures appear to be more sources of comfort than deciding factors in health-care decision making. They should be accepted as a very important part of what it means to be Japanese.

Health-Care Practices

Health-Seeking Beliefs and Behaviors

The general health of the populations of Japan and the United States are similar, with a shift in leading causes of morbidity and mortality from infections to chronic illnesses and diseases. However, behaviors and underlying belief systems differ markedly between Japan and the United States. The Japanese are more tolerant of self-indulgence, even during minor illnesses. Because Japanese are less likely to express feelings verbally, this indulgence may be a way for people to affirm caring for one another nonverbally. Hypochondriasis among the Japanese has been described in the medical literature and is more tolerated. Bodily flaws—for example, birthmarks—are a source of concern, and body piercing is now becoming more fashionable in the young.

In Japan, people seem less inclined to seek correction of minor orthopedic and dental variations than those in middle-class American society, although immigrant families make full use of services offered in the United States. Health-care providers engaged in health promotion and screenings need to be aware of this difference. Function, rather than appearance, may be a more appropriate emphasis.

Humankind is a part of nature, subject to its forces, and a person is an integrated whole. Whereas Chinese tradition calls for a restoration of balance when one is ill, Shinto calls for purging and purification. Both influences operate in modern Japan. In the past, Shinto was the source of principles of prevention, whereas Buddhist priests healed the sick. Centuries before the germ theory was known, Shinto effectively distinguished between spaces and body parts that were dirty versus those that were clean and pure. For example, taking off one's shoes at the doorway keeps one's home clean, and people wear slippers inside. However, only socked or bare feet are used on grass matting or *tatami*. Family members will also change their slippers when entering bathroom or toilet areas. People with colds in Japan customarily wear disposable surgical masks in public to shield others from their infection.

Americans who visit Japanese homes should usually assume that outside shoes are taken off before entering the home, and the hostess will usually offer guests slippers to wear. The same thing may occur in special types of businesses, in some restaurants, or in areas in aged-care homes or special clinics.

Responsibility for Health Care

Newsstands and vending machines, particularly in commuter rail stations in Japan, provide large quantities of flavored caffeine elixirs, high-potency vitamin elixirs, and electrolyte replacement drinks. These products are promoted to give workers and students an edge in their daily work. Health-care providers need to ask specifically what remedies are being used and why. Japanese patients in North America find general principles of nutrition to be the same as those taught in Japan, although their food preferences may differ.

The health of pregnant and nursing mothers and of children has the highest priority in the Japanese health-care system, and all schoolchildren and workers have comprehensive annual checkups at the expense of their school system or employer. National insurance is available to all Japanese, including foreigners, for a sliding-scale fee and covers both medical and dental care. Treatment by osteopaths, chiropractors, and traditional providers is covered if patients have been referred by a physician. Generally, national insurance covers 80 percent of medical expenses for children under age 3, 70 percent for those ages 3 to 69 years, and 90 percent for those ages 70 years and over. Mothers can receive ¥350,000 (approximately US$3800) upon their delivery, because the medical costs regarding healthy natural delivery are not covered by such insurance. To respond to the growing need for nursing care for the elderly, a nursing care insurance fee is deducted from the salaries of working people age 40 to 64.

Japanese residents in the United States frequently carry Japanese health insurance. Japanese nationals working for American institutions or companies may be eligible for the same coverage as other employees, but they often need assistance in understanding how their benefits work. Students and others can continue their Japanese national health insurance while in America, but they may need assistance in seeking care and understanding the American billing and payment process.

Many American over-the-counter medications, or their Japanese equivalents, are widely available in Japanese pharmacies. In addition, many pharmacies stock *kampo* (traditional Chinese medicine) preparations, as well as a large amount of stomach preparations for gastric upset.

Japanese people make liberal use of both modern medical and traditional providers of health care. Influenced by German and American medical science, the Japanese health-care system incorporates local primary care, neighborhood hospitals, specialty clinics, academic medical centers, and national research institutes.

There is no similar concept with American GPs. The Japanese patients need to self-examine what is wrong on their body first. Then they are expected to find and make an appointment to see a specialist by themselves. Most hospital beds are found in tiny, unregulated, physician-owned neighborhood clinics, and it is not common for patients to have their own room, even if they have private insurance. A sophisticated public health system offers prenatal and well-child care, school health initiatives, visiting nursing services, home health services, senior centers, and health education at little or no cost to the public.

Japanese residents in the United States have Internet and mail order access to traditional medications, if they are not available locally. As with any patient population, a complete health assessment includes inquiry about home therapies. From the second generation of immigrants onward, the tendency is to rely fully on the American health-care system.

Folk and Traditional Practices

Morita therapy, one of the most popular indigenous models of psychotherapy in Japan, is used to address shinkei shitsu, excess sensitivity to the social and natural environment. Morita therapy focuses on constructive physical activities that help patients adjust to and accept the reality in their lives and the interconnectedness to others (Tamura & Lau, 1992). This form of psychotherapy is very different from Western psychotherapy in that it tries to avoid introspection and deep analysis of self in an individualistic sense. *Naikan* **therapy** is another indigenous psychotherapy of reflection on how much goodness and love is received from others and is very much focused on well-being in Japanese culture. A third indigenous therapy, **Shinryo Naika**, focuses on bodily illnesses that are emotionally induced.

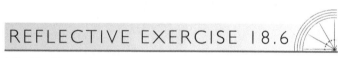

REFLECTIVE EXERCISE 18.6

Mika Tsuji is a 19-year-old Japanese international student studying at the local university. She has been referred to the mental health clinic by one of her tutors because she has been missing classes, appears not to be taking care of herself, and is withdrawn and uncommunicative. She would not visit the health center at the university or visit her local doctor. When the nurse meets her, it is clear that she seems depressed and unhappy, and she says she misses her family in Japan.

1. What specific cultural factors could be contributing to Mika's present state?
2. Why has she been reluctant to seek help?
3. How could the nurse provide education about depression to her in a culturally sensitive fashion?

Within the last several decades, Western-style psychiatry has been fully incorporated into Japanese health-care services. Indeed, psychiatric care in Japan in the early 1990s was predominantly given in overcrowded institutions. Today, it is moving toward a community-based emphasis. However, according to Tsuchiya and Takei (2004), substantial changes are needed in forensic psychiatry, child and adolescent psychiatry, substance misuse, and the naming of psychiatric disorders. One major problem is inadequate provision of mental health care for children and adolescents. Japan today has 351,762 psychiatric beds for a population of nearly 27 million people, approximately three times higher than the 10 psychiatric beds per 10,000 population in the United Kingdom in 2007 (Ministry of Health, Labour and Welfare, 2010c). Despite the greater availability of psychiatric inpatient care, increased stress and violent attacks in the community continue to fill the daily newspapers without any sign of improvement. This is of great concern to Japanese people at large, especially when Tsuchiya and Takei (2004) pointed out that there is no special provision for violent mentally ill offenders other than in regular psychiatric hospitals.

Health-care providers need to be sensitive to workplace or family issues that may underlie illnesses among Japanese patients, as among all patients. If a health-care provider believes that psychotherapy is indicated, the therapist must be someone familiar with the Japanese culture. Guidance in locating resources may be obtained through large academic medical centers or universities in coastal (particularly the Pacific coast) cities, as well as through professional associations, Japanese churches, or other religious organizations.

Health care is easily obtained in Japan. However, the system of referrals is unique. When a physician leaves medical school, she or he becomes part of that school's "family." She or he is unlikely to refer patients to specialists or hospitals outside the "family" of her or his fellow alumni or former professors. Personal acquaintance is essential for doing business in Japan, and it is also reflected in health-care practice.

Japanese people may be unlikely to assert themselves in American settings, and their efforts to do so may seem inappropriate to American health-care providers. Their high regard for the status of physicians decreases the likelihood of asking questions or making suggestions about their care. The idea that patients should be given care options may be alien to Japanese patients. Health-care providers need to provide ample opportunity for dialogue and explain the choices that are offered. Japanese and Japanese American health-care providers may be an important resource in bridging gaps in understanding.

Cultural Responses to Health and Illness

Pain, *itami*, may not be expressed, and bearing pain is considered a virtue and a matter of family honor.

Medications that specifically relieve pain, such as opioids, are used less frequently in Japan than in the United States. Addiction is a strong taboo in Japanese society. Around 90 percent of deaths in Japan occur in a hospital (Ministry of Health, Labour and Welfare, 2011c), compared with 60 percent in the Western society. There is a great need to increase an opportunity to access to palliative care in the Japanese community.

American health-care providers may use a schedule of analgesic administration rather than an as-requested or a patient-controlled approach to ensure adequate pain management. Japanese patients may respond positively to the information that physiological status and healing are actually enhanced by pain control.

Physically and intellectually handicapped children and adults are not commonly seen in public in Japan. In fact, most handicapped children, if they attend school, go to special schools rather than being integrated in the public school system. In addition, many public areas in Japan are not designed to cope with people with disabilities, making it very difficult for people who use wheelchairs or other assistive mobility devices. However, recently, the number of public toilets with facilities for handicapped people has increased. Many Japanese families hide knowledge of deformity or disability in family members because of shame, and there are still instances of people with physical handicaps—for example, cerebral palsy—being admitted to psychiatric hospitals owing to a lack of suitable facilities elsewhere. Japanese families residing in the United States need encouragement to avail themselves of community resources and to understand that shame associated with disability is not as prevalent in American society.

Assumption of the sick role is highly tolerated by families and colleagues, and a long recuperation period is encouraged by Japanese health-care providers. For example, in Japan, a patient with a myocardial infarction may be hospitalized for a month, with outcomes comparable with those found in the United States (Kinjo et al., 2004). However, changes to the national insurance system to extend care for rehabilitation, to shorten hospital stays, and to provide for more rehabilitation are now starting to have an effect, particularly in rehabilitation after stroke (Miyoshi, Teraoka, Date, Kim, Nguyen, & Miyoshi, 2005). Rehabilitation to achieve the full level of activities of daily living after serious illness or injury is less aggressive than in the United States. However, the number of higher-education programs to train occupational and rehabilitation specialists is slowly growing across the country, and the importance of rehabilitation is becoming more recognized and implemented.

Blood Transfusions and Organ Donations

Giving blood is encouraged in the Japanese culture. The Japanese Red Cross is a very active and highly respected organization that runs 92 Red Cross hospitals in the country and collects blood in 79 centers, using over 340 bloodmobiles, which travel around the country. Donors are not paid for their contributions. Blood usage is accounted for by 100 percent of domestic usage; however, 41 percent of albumin and 5 percent of immunoglobulin have to be imported (Japan Red Cross, 2010). People with negative blood types account for less than 1 percent of the population; therefore, RhoGam, used to protect an Rh-positive fetus from antibodies from an Rh-negative mother, is not commonly stocked in Japanese hospitals.

Under the Organ Transplant Law of 1997, organ transplant was not performed without having obtained the brain-dead patient's signature for the transplant in advance. In addition, children under the age of 15 were not permitted to donate organs. By March 2010, 374 transplants were conducted from 86 eligible donors (Japan Organ Transplant Network, 2010). In July 2009, the parliament passed a controversial bill that defines patients who are medically brain dead as legally dead and allowed to be a donor with family consent only, regardless of age. In addition, it allows children under 15 who are brain dead to become a donor with family consent. The first case of organ transplant between children occurred in April 2011. Such news was broadcasted nationwide.

Health-Care Providers

Traditional Versus Biomedical Providers

In modern Japan, physicians are clearly in charge of the health-care team. Some physicians may have a high degree of understanding of *kampo*, or Japanese herbal medicine, and may offer patients their choice of Western medicine, *kampo*, or a combination of both. More than 72 percent of physicians employ *kampo* in their daily practice. *Kampo* may be used in various symptoms, such as psychiatric care, bronchitis, constipation, dullness, irregular menstruation, and

REFLECTIVE EXERCISE 18.7

Yuji Nakata, age 10 years, was admitted to intensive care following a serious car accident in which he sustained ruptured kidneys as well as other injuries. He is currently on renal dialysis. His attending and other physicians believe he requires a kidney transplant. Yuji was on vacation in California with his Japanese parents when the accident happened.

1. Given that Yuji and his parents are Japanese, what are some cultural issues that may be involved in this case?
2. What specific information should be given to the parents about organ donation in the United States?
3. What may cause his parents to hesitate about approving a kidney transplant for their son?

more. Japanese health providers who come to the United States face a different type of health-care system, with greater diversity and autonomy for many professionals. The authority of insurers to dictate care is novel for them, as is the extent of concern for malpractice liability.

Status of Health-Care Providers

Physicians, referred to as *sensei*, are highly esteemed. Self-care as a philosophy is not evident in Japan. Being told what to do by the physician or *kampo* practitioner is expected, and his or her authority is not questioned. Physicians control most health-care delivery in Japan, running public and private hospitals and owning most private hospitals. Hospital administration is not an established field, and administrators in public hospitals are generally physicians elected to their post.

In Japan, females account for only about 15 percent of physicians, and male nurses account for about 6 percent. However, the professions and their interrelationships generally tend to reflect traditional gender roles. In the past, nurses were titled according to gender: *kango-shi* (士) if a male and *kango-fu* if a female. The former means approximately "Mr. Nurse," whereas the latter means "Ms. Nurse." Since 2002, the unified *kango-shi* (師), literally "person to be a nurse by profession," has started to be used.

Nurses in Japan today believe that nursing is still not highly regarded in Japanese society, but the raising of educational levels to a baccalaureate will undoubtedly change this, as has been the case in the United States. However, as noted previously, Japanese women do not hold high status in society, so this reflects strongly on the status of a largely feminine occupation. Japanese residents in the United States need considerable assistance in understanding how the health-care delivery systems work and the functions of the different health-care providers they encounter. In particular, they need to understand the autonomy of a diverse group of health professionals. Home care, and the orchestration of many community-based providers, may be overwhelming for Japanese residents who expect longer recuperations in the hospital.

Japanese health-care providers working in the United States need careful orientation to laws and institutional regulations about appropriate male–female interactions and professional requirements for accountability in communicating problems. Japanese residents seeking health care in America may be surprised by the assertiveness and autonomy of nonphysician professionals. An overview of the details of their care, and who will be doing various aspects of that care, can be helpful. Japanese residents in the United States may need assistance in seeking care. Their verbal English skills may be an impediment to making their needs known and to understanding the care they are offered, although their ability to understand written information is often very good. Japanese people tend to believe that they are physiologically different from non-Japanese people, and they may be skeptical of recommendations. The family members, including daughters-in-law, are expected to be involved in clinical decision making. Calling on the local Japanese community for support and encouragement may be a useful strategy with these patients.

REFERENCES

CIA World Factbook. (2011). *Japan.* Retrieved from https://www.cia.gov/library/publications/the-world-factbook/geos/ja.html

Customs and Tariff Bureau. (2009). *Trends in illicit drugs and firearms smuggling in Japan (2009 edition).* Retrieved from http://www.customs.go.jp/english/enforcement/report2009_e/index.htm

Doi, T. (1971). *The anatomy of dependence* (J. Bester, Trans.) Tokyo: Kodansha International Ltd.

Ehara, A. (2005). Lawsuits associated with medical malpractice in Japan [Letter to the editor]. *Pediatrics, 115*(6), 1792–1793.

Fukumizu, M., Kaga, M., Kohyama, J., & Hayes, M.J. (2005). Sleep-related nighttime crying (*yonaki*) in Japan. A community-based study. *Pediatrics, 115,* 217–224.

Gender Equality Bureau. (2011). *Women and men in Japan 2011.* Retrieved from http://www.gender.go.jp/english_contents/category/pub/pamphlet/women-and-men11/index.html

Hattori, K., McCubbin, A.M., & Ishida, N.D. (2006). Concept analysis of good death in the Japanese community. *Journal of Nursing Scholarship, 38*(2), 165–170.

Higuchi, S. (2009). The drinking realities and intervention for a large amount of drinking in Japan. Retrieved from http://www.mhlw.go.jp/topics/tobacco/houkoku/dl/100222f.pdf

International Longevity Center Japan. (2006). *The spread of corporate measures to support child care and family care. One dimension of action in response to the declining birth rate in Japan.* Retrieved from http://longevity.ilcjapan.org/f_issues/0605.html

Ito, M., & Sharts-Hopko, N. (2002). Japanese women's experience of childbirth in the United States. *Health Care for Women International, 23*(6–7), 666–677.

Ito, M., Tanida, N., & Turale, N. (2010). Perceptions of Japanese patients and their family about medical treatment decisions. *Nursing and Health Sciences, 12*(3), 314–321.

Japan Media Review. (2006). *Publishers push the return of the E-book.* Retrieved from http://ojr.org/japan/media/1082135229.php

Japan Organ Transplant Network. (2010). Newsletter, 14. Japan Organ Transplant Network.

Japan Red Cross. (2010). 2009 *business report (blood business).* Retrieved from http://www.jrc.or.jp/

Kanazumi, F. (1997). Interview. In S. Buckley (Ed.), *Broken silence: Voices of Japanese feminism* (pp. 70–81). Berkeley: University of California Press.

Kashiwazaki, C., & Akaha, T. (2005). *Japanese immigration policy: Responding to conflicting pressures.* Retrieved from http://www.migrationinformation.org/Profiles/display.cfm?ID=487

Keene, D. (1983). Ise. In D. Richie (Ed.), *Discover Japan: Vol. 2. Words, customs and concepts* (pp. 196–197). Tokyo: Kodansha International, Ltd.

Kenko Sangyo Shinbun. (2010). *Supplement market has been rapidly recovered by 1.8 trillion yen (sapri shijo 1chou 1800okuen kyukaihukuhe).* Retrieved from http://www.kenko-media.com/health_idst/006188.html

Kinjo, K., Sato, H., Nakatani, D., Mizuno, H., Shimizu, M., Hishida, E., Ezumi, A., Hoshida, S. Koretsune, Y., & Hori, M. (2004). Predictors of length of hospital stay after myocardial infarction in Japan. *Circulation Journal, 68*(9), 809–815.

Leonardsen, D. (2004). *Japan as a low-crime nation.* New York: Palgrave Macmillan.

Levy, R. A. (1993). Ethnic and racial differences in response to medicines: Preserving individualized therapy in managed pharmaceutical programmes. *Pharmaceutical Medicine, 7,* 139–165.

Makino, M., Hashizume, M., Yasushi, M., Tsuboi, K., & Dennerstein, L. (2006). Factors associated with abnormal eating attitudes among female college students in Japan. *Archives of Women's Mental Health, 9*(4), 203–208.

Ministry of Education, Culture, Sports, Science, and Technology in Japan. (2010). *School basic survey FY2010.* Retrieved from http://www.mext.go.jp/b_menu/toukei/chousa01/kihon/kekka/k_detail/1296403.htm (Japanese)

Ministry of Education, Culture, Sports, Science, and Technology. (2011). *Vital statistics tables 2005.* Retrieved from http://www.mhlw.go.jp/

Ministry of Health, Labour and Welfare (2010a). *Outline of National Health and Nourishment Investigation Results.* Retrieved from http://www.mhlw.go.jp/stf/houdou/2r9852000000xtwq.html

Ministry of Health, Labour and Welfare. (2010b). *Population movement status.* Retrieved from http://www.mhlw.go.jp/toukei/list/81-1.html

Ministry of Health, Labour and Welfare. (2010c). *Annual change in the number of hospitals with beds for psychiatric patients, the number of beds for psychiatric patients, the number of inpatients at month-end, and the rate of bed utilization at month-end.* Retrieved from http://www.mhlw.go.jp/english/wp/wp-hw3/dl/9-13.pdf

Ministry of Health, Labour and Welfare. (2011a). *Press release material on March 23, 2011.* Retrieved from http://www.mhlw.go.jp/stf/houdou/2r98520000016bot.html

Ministry of Health, Labour and Welfare. (2011b). *Vital statistics in Japan—_he latest trends.* Retrieved from http://www.mhlw.go.jp/english/database/db-hw/dl/81-1a2en.pdf

Ministry of Health, Labour and Welfare. (2011c). *Research on the palliative care program in the community.* Retrieved from http://www.mhlw.go.jp/seisaku/11e.html

Ministry of Internal Affairs and Communications. (2010). *The statistical handbook of Japan 2010.* Retrieved from http://www.stat.go.jp/English/data/handbook/c02cont.htm

Miyoshi, Y., Teraoka, J.K., Date, E.S., Kim, M.J., Nguyen, R.T., & Miyoshi, S. (2005). Changes in stroke rehabilitation outcomes after the implementation of Japan's long-term care insurance system: A hospital-based study. *American Journal of Physical Medical Rehabilitation, 84*(8), 613–619.

Nakamura, Y. (2010). Maternal and child health handbook in Japan. *JMAJ, 53*(4), 259–265.

Nakao, M., & Takeuchi, T. (2006). The suicide epidemic in Japan and strategies of depression screening for its prevention. *Bulletin of the World Health Organization, 84*(6), 492–493.

New World Encyclopedia. (2007). *Ainu.* Retrieved from http://www.newworldencyclopedia.org/entry/Ainu#Origins

Orenstein, P. (2002, April 21). Mourning my miscarriage. *New York Times.* Retrieved from http://www.nytimes.com

Reischauer, E.O., & Jansen, M. (1995). *The Japanese today.* New York. Longitude Books.

Sato, R., & Iwasawa, M. (2006). Contraceptive use and induced abortion in Japan: How is it so unique among developed countries? *The Japanese Journal of Population, 4*(1), 33–54.

Sharts Engel, N. (1989). An American experience of pregnancy and childbirth in Japan. *Birth, 16*(2), 81–86.

Shinto Online Network Association. (2006). Retrieved from http://www.jinja.or.jp/

Takakura, M., & Sakihara, S. (2000). Gender differences in the association between psychosocial factors and depressive symptoms in Japanese junior high school students. *Journal of Epidemiology, 10*(6), 383–391.

Tamura, T., & Lau, A. (1992). Connectedness versus separateness: Applicability of family therapy to Japanese families. *Family Process, 4,* 319.

Tejada-Vera, B., & Sutton, P.D. (2010). Births, marriages, divorces, and deaths: Provisional data for 2009. *National Vital Statistics Reports; Vol. 58, No. 25.* Hyattsville, MD: National Center for Health Statistics. 2010. Retrieved from http://www.cdc.gov/nchs/data/nvsr/nvsr58/nvsr58_25.pdf

Tsuchiya, K.J., & Takei, N. (2004). Mental health care in Japan: An overview. *The British Journal of Psychiatry, 184,* 88–92.

UNAIDS. (2010). *Japan—2010 country progress report.* Retrieved from http://www.unaids.org/en/dataanalysis/monitoringcountryprogress/2010progressreportssubmittedbycountries/japan_2010_country_progress_report_en.pdf#search='Country progress report: Japan

UN Secretariat. (2005). *Possibilities and limitations of Japanese migration policy in the context of economic partnership in East Asia.* Retrieved from http://www.un.org/esa/population/meetings/ittmigdev2005/P07-iguchi.pdf

Urakami, T., Morimoto, S., Nitadori, Y., Harada, K., Owada, M., & Kitagawa, T. (2007). Urine glucose screening program at schools in Japan to detect children with diabetes and its outcome-incidence and clinical characteristics of childhood Type 2 diabetes in Japan. *Pediatric Research, 61*(2), 141–145.

U.S. Commercial Service. (2011). *Japanese tourism marketing opportunities.* Retrieved from http://www.tourism.jp/english/statistics/outbound.php

U.S. Department of State. (2010). *Background note—Japan.* Retrieved from http://www.state.gov/r/pa/ei/bgn/4142.htm

Woss, F. (1992). When blossoms fall: Japanese attitudes towards death and the other world: Opinion polls 1953–1987. In R. Goodman & K. Refsing (Eds.), *Ideology and practice in modern Japan* (pp. 72–100). New York, NY: Routledge.

Yanagisako, S.J. (1985). *Transforming the past: Tradition and kinship among Japanese Americans.* Stanford, CA: Stanford University Press.

DavisPlus *For reflective exercises, review questions, and additional information, go to*

http://davisplus.fadavis.com

Chapter 19

People of Jewish Heritage

Janice Selekman

Overview, Inhabited Localities, and Topography

Overview

Being Jewish refers to both a people and a religion, not a race. Judaism is more than a religion; it is a people and a culture. Throughout history, the terms *Hebrew*, *Israelite*, and *Jew* have been used interchangeably. In the Bible, Abraham's grandson, Jacob, was renamed Israel. His 12 sons and their descendants became known as the children of Israel. The term *Jew* is derived from Judah, one of Jacob's sons. **Hebrew** is the official language of the state of Israel and is used for religious prayers by all Jews wherever they live. While the people are called Jewish, their faith is called Judaism, their religious language is Hebrew, and their 'homeland' is Israel, regardless of where their relatives were born.

The religion of **Judaism** is practiced along a wide continuum that includes liberal **Reform** with 28 percent, **Conservative** with 22 percent, **Reconstructionist** with 2 percent, and strict **Orthodox** with 9 percent. Another 39 percent just identify as Jewish without identifying their affiliation (American Jewish Committee, 2010). Reform Judaism maintains that traditions should be modernized and compatible with participation in the surrounding community, and Progressive Judaism, an umbrella term used by strands of Judaism, embrace pluralism, modernity, equality, and social justice as core values (Myers, 1988). Although Reform and Progressive Jews might not engage in any special daily practices, they still observe holidays, religious rites, and selected dietary or cultural customs. The traditional Orthodox Jew attempts to adhere to most of the religious laws. Ultra-Orthodox groups also exist. No caste system or social hierarchy exists within the Jewish community. However, instances occur within the ultra-Orthodox communities, where individuals cannot make life and health-related decisions without consulting their rabbis.

A significant issue within Orthodox communities in Israel, frequently debated in America is "Who is a Jew?" A child born to a Jewish mother is Jewish. As mixed marriages have increased, a debate over patrilineal descent has ensued. A child born from the union of a Jewish father and a non-Jewish mother is recognized as Jewish by those in more liberal branches of Judaism, especially if they are raised as a Jew, but not by those in the Orthodox movement (DeLange, 2010). Although Judaism does not actively proselytize, the vast majority welcome converts as full members of their community. Clergy offer preconversion classes for adults and perform conversions.

Whereas the goal of this chapter is to provide an understanding of all Jewish Americans, the focus is on the needs of the more traditional religious individuals and their families. These descriptions may vary somewhat for Jewish people according to variant characteristics of culture (see Chapter 1) and the other parts of the world where they live.

Heritage and Residence

The initial group of 23 Jews in North America arrived in 1624, having fled the Office of the Inquisition in Brazil. As a result of European immigrations, their numbers grew to between 1000 and 2500 individuals by the time of the American Revolution, when many fought for the colonial army. Haim Solomon, a banker, raised significant funds in Europe and the colonies and dedicated all his personal resources and finances to George Washington's army. Their numbers reached approximately 250,000 by the 1880s, close to 6 million a century later, and finally stabilized by 2002. According to American Jewish Demographics (2011), there are 5,275,000 Jews in the United States, accounting for 2.7 percent of the U.S. population. States with over 3 percent of their population being Jewish include New York (8.4 percent), New Jersey (5.5 percent), Massachusetts (4.3 percent), Maryland (4.2 percent), Florida (3.7 percent), and California (3.3 percent) (Jewish Virtual Library, 2011). Although many prefer to live in or within reach of large Jewish communities in order to have access to specific services, Jews make their homes in rural as well as urban centers in the United States. In comparison, 76 percent of the State of Israel is Jewish (Jewish Virtual Library, 2011).

Depending on how one defines being Jewish, a 2010 unpublished study by Saxe and his Brandeis researchers indicated that there may be as many as 6.5 million Jews in America (Beckerman, 2010). These are thought to be individuals who consider themselves Jewish by their culture but do not participate in the Jewish community or in Jewish life-cycle events.

Reasons for Migration and Associated Economic Factors

Migration of Jews from Europe began to increase in the mid-1800s, often because of religious persecution and economic opportunities. However, the greatest influx of immigrants occurred between 1880 and 1920. Many of these immigrants came from Russia and Eastern Europe after a wave of **pogroms**, anti-Jewish riots and murders (Jewish American Committee, 2011). Once in America, acculturation became their motivation to live in safety and practice their religion.

Most Jewish families in America today are descendants of these Eastern European and Russian immigrants. They are referred to as **Ashkenazi** Jews. Ashkenazi Jews make up more than 80 percent of the world's Jewish population (Hebrew University of Jerusalem, 2009). This becomes an important concept when exploring diseases prevalent among the Jewish population. Many American Jews of Ashkenazi descent have stories of how some members of their families escaped to America, whereas others had relatives who were part of more than the 6 million Jews killed in the pogroms and the Holocaust. Sephardic Jews, conversely, are originally from Spain, Portugal, the Mediterranean area, and North Africa. They represent a more diverse group. A *Sabra* is a Jew who was born in Israel.

In the 1980s and 1990s, a significant increase occurred in the number of Jewish immigrants from Russia. Because the practice of religion was illegal there for over half a century, these Jews often have a relatively relaxed connection to religious and cultural practices. The same was true of the **Falasha** Jewish community in 1984. These black Jews from Ethiopia participated in a mass exodus to Israel, and subsequently, a small number continued on to America.

Educational Status and Occupations

Despite bias against Jews in every century, they have made major contributions to society, across the arts and professions, including the fine arts, sciences, and health care. Throughout their history, they have placed a major emphasis on education and social justice through social action.

Continued learning is one of the most respected values of the Jewish people, who are often called the *People of the Book* (Diamant, 2007). Education is considered a lifelong obligation regardless of age or status. Whereas this usually refers to the study of Torah, it includes both Jewish and secular learning. Formal education is highly valued, and advanced degrees are respected. Overall, this population is well educated. Jews have won 22 percent of all Nobel Prizes awarded between 1901 and 2010. This includes 20 percent of the Nobel Prizes in chemistry, 25 percent in physics, 42 percent in economics, and 27 percent in physiology and medicine (Jewish Nobel Prize Winners, 2011).

Well-known American composers with Jewish ancestry include George Gershwin, Aaron Copland, Leonard Bernstein, Jerome Kern, Richard Rogers, Irving Berlin, and Stephen Sondheim; the American theater counts Arthur Miller as one of its most celebrated of playwrights, along with Woody Allen, Mel Brooks, Oscar Hammerstein II, Alan Lerner, and Neil Simon. The 20th century finally saw the first Jewish Supreme Court justices in Louis Brandeis and, most recently, Ruth Bader Ginsburg and Elena Kagan.

Because of their emphasis on education, a high percentage of Jewish Americans have succeeded in science, medicine, law, and dentistry. Thirty-nine percent of Jewish men and over 36 percent of Jewish women list their occupation as "professional," compared with only 15 percent of the American white population. With respect to higher education, over 10 percent of professors in American colleges and universities are Jewish; the majority of American Jews attend college (Diamant, 2007). Their traditional values of study and preserving life have contributed to directing many into the life sciences, medicine, and research.

In addition to receiving a regular elementary, secondary, and college education, many Jewish children are also provided a Jewish education. Many attend Hebrew school classes 1 or 2 days a week, as well as classes on Judaism, commonly referred to as Sunday School.

Throughout their history, Jews were repeatedly forbidden to own land, and the Christian Church barred its members from moneylending. As a result, since the early Middle Ages, Jews frequently became moneylenders, peddlers, and tailors because these were the only options available to them. The early Jews in America were businessmen and craftsmen (Center for Jewish History, 2007). They became well respected for their expertise in trade and commerce, and thus many went into banking or retail sales.

Social action, volunteerism, and involvement in helping others are common vocations or avocations. Health-care professions, social work, teaching, and the legal profession became other popular occupational pursuits. The term *tzedakah* (justice) is used to indicate charity or righteous giving, a central concept to Judaism. Jewish children are raised with the concept of giving *tzedakah* by sharing with others who have less than they do (Diamant, 2007).

Communication

Dominant Language and Dialects

English is the primary language of Jewish Americans. Although Hebrew is the official language of Israel and is used for prayers and is the language of the Torah, it is generally not used for conversation in the United States.

Many older Ashkenazi Jews who immigrated early in the 20th century or who are first-generation Americans speak **Yiddish**, a Judeo-German dialect. Many Yiddish terms have worked their way into the English language, including *kvetch* (to complain); *chutzpah* (clever audacity); *bagel* (a boiled roll with a hole in the middle); *challah* (a rich, braided white bread); *knish* (a dumpling with filling); *mitzvah* (a good deed); *nosh* (to snack); *zaftig* (plump); *tush, tushie,* or *tuchus* (buttocks); *ghetto* (a restricted area in which certain groups live); *klutz* (a clumsy person); *mentsch* or *mensh* (a respected person with dignity); *shlep* (to drag or carry); *kosher* (technically applying to food preparation, but idiomatically meaning legal; and *oy* or *oy vey* (oh my), and *oy veys mier* (woe is me).

Common Hebrew expressions include *"l'chaim"* (to life), which is said after blessing wine or giving a toast; *"shalom alechem"* (peace be with you), a traditional salutation; *"mazel tov"* (congratulations); and *"shabbat shalom"* (a good and peaceful Sabbath), which is said from Friday evening at sunset until Saturday at sunset.

Cultural Communication Patterns

No religious ban or ethnic characteristics prevent Jews from openly expressing their feelings. Communication practices are more related to their American upbringing than to their religious practices.

Humor is frequently used as a coping mechanism and as a way to communicate with others. However, jokes are considered to be insensitive when they reinforce mainstream stereotypes about Jews, such as implying that Jews are cheap or pampered (e.g., Jewish princess). Any jokes that refer to the Holocaust or concentration camps are also inappropriate. Jewish self-criticism through humor is acceptable, but it is usually expressed by insiders.

Modesty is a primary value in Orthodox Judaism. It is seen in the style of dress and in all behavior. Modesty involves humility. Jews are encouraged not to "show off" or try to impress others.

In **Hasidic** Judaism, the ultra-Orthodox fundamentalists, men are not permitted to touch a woman other than their wives. They often keep their hands in their pockets to avoid touch. They do not shake hands with women, and their failure to do so when one's hand is extended should not be interpreted as a sign of rudeness. Because women are considered seductive by nature, Hasidic men may not engage in idle talk with them or look directly at their faces. Non-Hasidic Jews may be much more informal and may use touch and short spatial distance when communicating. Healthcare providers should touch Hasidic men only when providing direct care. Hands-on "therapeutic touch," as in holding a patient's hand to give comfort, is not appropriate with these patients.

Temporal Relationships

Jews live with regard for, and in, the present, conscious of being a part of a long historical tradition and with both hope and a wary eye to the future. The last 2 millennia have seen a succession of struggles to survive external pressures, yet the tradition affirms their belief in survival and a better time to come. They are raised with stories of their past, including the relatively recent Holocaust. They are warned to "never forget," lest history be repeated. Therefore, their time orientation is simultaneously to the past, the present, and the future.

The Jewish calendar is based on both a lunar and a solar year, with each month beginning with the appearance of the new moon and lasting 29 to 30 days. The festivals and holidays are based on lunar phases, whereas the seasons are based on the solar year, which is 11 days longer than the lunar year. Therefore, an extra month is periodically added, usually during the end of winter (7 times in every 19 years). The Jewish day starts at sunset; therefore, all holidays, as well as the Sabbath, begin when the sun sets, usually identified as the evening before the date identified on a calendar. The basis for this practice is the line in Genesis "And there was evening and there was morning."

Format for Names

For secular use, the Jewish format for names follows the Western tradition. The given name comes first, followed by the family surname. Only the given name is used with friends and in informal situations. In more formal situations, the surname is preceded by the appropriate title of Mr., Miss, Ms., Mrs., Dr., and so on.

Babies may be named after someone who has died to keep their memory alive or after a living person to honor him or her (the latter only in Sephardic families). In ultra-Orthodox circles, children are not referred to by their names until after the *bris* or *brit milah* (circumcision). The biblical traditions are preserved for religious occasions. Infants are given a Hebrew name that is used when they are older and are called to read from the Torah at age 13 or older, following their bar or bat mitzvah). An example would be Ephraim ben Reuven (Frank, son of Robert). Although one's Hebrew name may be the same as one's birth certificate "official" name, parents may choose a non-Hebrew, main-culture name for the birth certificate that is entirely different or one that preserves the initial letter (i.e., Reuven could become Robert).

Family Roles and Organization
Head of Household and Gender Roles

The family is the core of Jewish society, and whereas the man is traditionally considered the breadwinner for the household and the woman is recognized for running the home and being responsible for the children, in recent times there is more flexibility for gender roles, even in very observant homes. According to Jewish law, the father has the legal obligation to educate his children in Judaism, to teach them right from wrong, to teach them to swim, and to teach his sons a trade (Cohn-Sherbok, 2010). He must provide his daughters with the means to make them marriageable. With acculturation, little difference is seen today between Jewish and non-Jewish white families with regard to gender roles. In most Jewish families, both parents share the responsibilities for supporting the home and raising the children. However, it is still common to find the mother lighting the Sabbath candles and the father blessing the wine (DeLange, 2010).

The Orthodox ideology puts increased responsibility on males to study the Torah and perform mitzvoth (religious commandments). While the reform movement embraces feminism, the orthodox movement is more skeptical. According to the Talmud, Jewish husbands are required to provide their wives with food, clothing, medical care, and conjugal relations, in addition to meeting other needs. The *ketubah*—marriage contract—usually includes wording that entitles the wife to the same dignity and social standing as her husband.

Although traditional Jewish law is clearly male-oriented, Jewish women have been at the forefront of activities to demand and protect all human rights, especially those of women. They were prominent in movements to gain women's suffrage, reproductive health-care rights, and equal rights for all segments of society. Women are now expected to achieve an optimal level of education and to seek gainful employment if they so desire. Both sexes are expected to give service to their community.

Prescriptive, Restrictive, and Taboo Behaviors for Children and Adolescents

Children are the most valued treasure of the Jewish people. They are considered a blessing and are to be treated with respect and provided with love. Jewish children are to be afforded an education, not only in studies that help them progress in society but also in studies that transmit their Jewish heritage and the laws. Jewish school-age children may attend Hebrew school as least two afternoons a week after public school throughout the school year. Children are welcomed and incorporated into most holiday celebrations and services.

Respecting and honoring one's parents is the fifth of the Ten Commandments. Children should be forever grateful to their parents for giving them the gift of life. Jewish parents are expected to be consistent and fair to all their children, avoiding favoritism. In addition, parents should not promise something to their children that they cannot deliver. They must be flexible and yet caring and attentive to discipline. The individuality of each child's special traits should be recognized.

In Judaism, the age of adulthood is 13 years and 1 day for a boy, and 12 years and 1 day for a girl (Cohn-Sherbok, 2010; Jacob & Zemer, 2006). At this age, children are deemed capable of differentiating right from wrong and capable of committing themselves to performing the commandments. Recognition of religious adulthood and assumption of its responsibilities occur during a religious ceremony called a *bar* or *bat mitzvah* (son or daughter of the commandment, respectively); during this ceremony, the child reads from the Torah and *Haftorah,* prophetic writings, for the first time (Kranson, 2010). None of the denominations require girls to have this ceremony, although with the feminist movement as impetus, it has increased in prevalence among modern Jews. In America, this rite of passage is usually accompanied by a family celebration. However, because sons and daughters are still teenagers living at home, it is recognized that they are still the responsibility of their parents. In Orthodox communities, boys who have reached their bar mitzvah are now responsible to perform the multiple religious rituals expected.

Family Goals and Priorities

The goal of the Orthodox family is to live their lives as prescribed by *halakhah*, which emphasizes maintaining health, promoting education, and helping others. In addition, each individual is considered unique and must maximize their potential. The family is central to Jewish life and essential to the continuation of Judaism from one generation to the next.

Marriage is considered the ideal human state for adults; it is considered a sacred bond between adults and a means of personal fulfillment (Cohn-Sherbok, 2010). The Bible states that man should not be alone. The goals of this union are to build a home, procreate, and provide companionship, allowing an individual to focus on another person. Marriages are monogamous, and limitations on whom one may marry exclude close blood relatives and—although this has changed considerably with the increase in interfaith unions—non-Jews.

Sexuality is a right of both men and women. The sex instinct is neither sinful nor shameful, but restraint is expected (Jacob & Zemer, 2006). In addition to procreation requirements, conjugal rights for women exist. Nonprocreative intercourse is required, if desired, for married women who may be pregnant or are unable to conceive, and after menopause as this is not considered "wasting seed" (Jacob & Zemer, 2006). Sexual intercourse is viewed as a pure and holy act when performed mutually within the relationship of marriage. With some exceptions, a husband's refusal to have sex with his wife is grounds for a divorce. However, the act of sex, if not performed with sobriety and modesty and the wife's willingness), is considered against Jewish values (DeLange, 2010). Premarital sex is not condoned.

Among the ultra-observant, women must physically separate themselves from all men during their menstrual periods and for 7 days after (DeLange, 2010). No man may touch a woman or sit where she just sat until she has been to the *mikveh*, a ritual bath, after her period is over. Sexual contact for this group may, therefore, occur only during 2 weeks of each month.

Judaism supports the need for sex education. The Jewish community sees this as its responsibility. This belief was reemphasized during the AIDS epidemic, with the goals of protecting the next generation and providing them with accurate information so they can make informed choices.

Whereas it is recognized that the later years are a time of physical decline, older people receive respect, especially for the wisdom they have to share. Old age is a state of mind rather than a chronological age; one may continue to "give" to society in a variety of ways other than employment. In addition, one may never "retire" from practicing the commandments.

Honoring one's parents is a lifelong endeavor and includes maintaining their dignity by feeding, clothing, and sheltering them, even if they suffer from senility. Respect for older people is essential even when their actions are irrational. The care of an older family member is the responsibility of the family; when the family is unable to provide care owing to physical, psychological, or financial reasons, the responsibility falls to the community. This role has always been a hallmark of Jewish communal life.

Few Jewish American families now have three generations living together. Older immigrants who experienced imprisonment in concentration camps during the Holocaust in the 1940s, or those more recently incarcerated in Russia, may refuse to enter long-term-care facilities for fear of returning to an institutional environment that robs them of their freedom (Martha Braverman, personal communication, 2007).

Alternative Lifestyles

The Jewish view on homosexuality varies with the branch of Judaism. As might be expected, the Orthodox are largely unanimous in scripture-based (Lev. 18:22) nonacceptance of same-sex unions. The Bible, especially as interpreted by the Orthodox, prohibits homosexual intercourse for men; it says nothing specifically about sex between lesbians (DeLange, 2010). Some of the objections to gay and lesbian lifestyles include the inability of these unions to fulfill the commandment of procreation and the possibility that acting on the recognition of one's homosexuality could ruin a marriage. The official position of the Conservative movement had sided with the Orthodox until as recently as 2006, when it revised its position to increase inclusivity of views within Jewish philosophy. They can now perform same-sex commitment ceremonies. They can also ordain gay and lesbian clergy. The liberal movement within Judaism, however, supports full legal and social equality for homosexuals (Cohn-Sherbok, 2010).

Workforce Issues

Culture in the Workplace

Specific workforce issues may occur, especially with Sabbath observance. Jews who observe the Sabbath must have Friday evenings and Saturdays off. They may work on Sundays. Supervisors must be sensitive to the needs of Jewish staff and recognize the holiness of the Sabbath. Jewish staff should be allowed to request time off for the major Jewish holidays. Remembering that all holidays begin the evening before, they must have off the evening shift before and the following day. Staff should not be penalized by having to use this time off as unpaid holidays or vacation time, but they should have the option to exchange for the Christmas and Easter holidays, time usually afforded to Christian staff.

Jewish health-care providers are fully acculturated into the American workforce. Judaism's beliefs are congruent with the values American society places on the individual and family. As English is the primary language for Jewish Americans, no language barriers to communicating in the workplace exist. For some newer Jewish immigrants (e.g., those from Russia), English may pose a challenge.

Issues Related to Autonomy

Jewish nurses have begun to speak out on their needs in the workplace. With the recent emphasis on cultural competence, including cultural sensitivity, many are now addressing this long-ignored area. In 1990, a National Nurses Council was established through Hadassah, the Zionist women's organization (Benson, 1994). This group promotes solidarity and empowerment to enhance sensitivity within the health-care community. Still proportionally underrepresented among American nurses, Jewish nurses have a higher percentage of advanced degrees and positions in management, education, and research (Benson, 2001).

Ways in which the professional nursing community demonstrates its insensitivity to Jewish nurses are by scheduling major nursing conferences during the High Holy Days in the fall or during Passover in the spring, by serving pork products during catered affairs, or reciting a prayer before the conference meal invoking the name of Jesus.

Biocultural Ecology

Skin Color and Other Biological Variations

According to DeLange (2010), "there are no racial characteristics that are shared by Jews and that distinguish them from non-Jews" (p. 3). Ashkenazi Jews have the same skin coloring as white Americans. They may range from fair skin and blonde hair to darker skin and brunette hair. Sephardic Jews have slightly darker skin tones and hair coloring, similar to those from the Mediterranean area and those who lived for centuries in nearby regions such as Yemen. There are also Jewish groups throughout Africa who are black, most notably the Jews originally from Ethiopia, known as *Falasha*.

Diseases and Health Conditions

Because Jews are integrated throughout the United States, no specific risk factors are based on topography. Genetic risk factors vary based on whether the family immigrated from Ashkenazi or Sephardic areas. There is a greater incidence of some genetic disorders among individuals of Jewish descent, especially those who are Ashkenazi. It is estimated that 1 in 16 to 1 in 110 Ashkenazi Jews carries one of these mutations (Hebrew University of Jerusalem, 2009). Most of these disorders are autosomal recessive, meaning that both parents carry the affected gene. Although the best known is Tay-Sachs disease, Gaucher's disease is more prevalent. Others include Canavan's disease, familial dysautonomia, torsion dystonia, Niemann-Pick disease, Bloom syndrome, Fanconi's anemia, and mucolipidosis IV (Center for Jewish Genetic Diseases, 2011).

Gaucher's disease is the most common genetic disease affecting Ashkenazi Jews, with 1 in 10 carrying the gene (Center for Jewish Genetic Diseases, 2011). Gaucher's disease is a lipid-storage disorder. This inborn error of metabolism results in a defective enzyme that normally breaks down glucocerebroside, a lipid by-product of erythrocytes. The glucocerebroside accumulates in the body, resulting in weakening and fracturing of the bones owing to infarctions, anemia, and platelet deficiencies. The spleen becomes painfully enlarged. There are 34 different genetic mutations of the disease; 4 of them account for 95 percent of cases in Ashkenazi Jews. The disorder can be detected by a blood test for both those affected and carriers. Gene therapy treatments are now being tested (National Gaucher Foundation, 2011).

The gene for Tay-Sachs disease (also called *infantile cerebromacular degeneration*) is carried by 1 in 25 to 1 in 30 Ashkenazi Jews and 1 in 250 Jews of Sephardic origin. This autosomal recessive condition is a lysosomal sphingolipid storage disorder caused by an absence of hexosaminidase A, resulting in an accumulation of a lipid called *GM2 ganglioside* in the neural cells. The onset of intellectual and developmental delay begins in the middle of the first year of life, with progressive deterioration, increasing seizure activity, blindness, deafness, and death by approximately age 4 (Center for Jewish Genetic Diseases, 2011). Because of the ease of testing for carriers as well as testing the fetus during pregnancy, and because of a concerted effort among the Jewish American community to provide testing, the incidence of Tay-Sachs disease has decreased significantly since the early 1980s. Because the ultra-Orthodox are opposed to abortion, this group recommends the testing only before marriage (Washofsky, 2000). It should be noted that because there are 50 different mutations, testing can only identify 95 percent of carriers with a Jewish background and 60 percent of non-Jewish individuals (Center for Jewish Genetic Diseases, 2011).

Canavan's disease is a rare, fatal, degenerative brain disease caused by a defective gene that impairs the formation of myelin in the brain. Approximately 1 in 40 Ashkenazi Jews carry the gene. The resulting symptoms begin in mid-infancy and include developmental delay, loss of vision, and a loss of reflexes resulting in death by the age of 10 years (Center for Jewish Genetic Diseases, 2011).

Familial dysautonomia, or Riley-Day syndrome, is also an autosomal recessive genetic disease, with the gene located on chromosome 9q31. It causes dysfunction of the autonomic and peripheral sensory nervous systems. Affected children have decreased myelinated fibers on nerves that lead to afferent impulses but maintain a normal intelligence. Symptoms include a decrease in the number of taste buds; altered pain sensation; increased salivation and sweating; abnormal sucking or swallowing difficulties and vomiting, resulting in failure to thrive; decreased tears, resulting in increased risk of corneal ulceration; and temperature and blood pressure fluctuations. Fifty percent of newly diagnosed infants will live to the age of 40. One in 27 Ashkenazi Jews is a carrier (Center for Jewish Genetic Diseases, 2011).

Other conditions that have a higher incidence among Ashkenazi Jews include the following:

- **Torsion dystonia**, an autosomal dominant condition, is carried by 1 in 1000 to 1 in 3000 Ashkenazi Jews in the United States. The disease leads to rapid progression in loss of motor control and twisting spasms of the limbs, resulting in contractures. Affected individuals lead a full life and have a normal intelligence.

- **Niemann-Pick disease type A** is an autosomal recessive severe neurodegenerative disorder that starts at 6 months of age. It involves an abnormal storage of sphingomyelin and cholesterol in organs caused by an enzyme deficiency and leads to central nervous system degeneration. Whereas those with type A usually die by age 3, those with type B survive into their 50s and have a milder presentation, with the sphingomyelin building up in their liver, spleen, lymph nodes, and brain. The gene for Type A is carried by 1 in 90 Ashkenazi Jews.
- **Bloom syndrome**, a rare genetic condition that results in abnormal breakage of chromosomes, results in respiratory and gastrointestinal infections, erythema, telangiectasia, photosensitivity, and dwarfism. Whereas the intelligence of those affected is usually normal, they face an increased risk of infertility, malignancy, and diabetes. The average age of death is 27; the gene is carried by 1:110 Ashkenazi Jews.
- **Fanconi's anemia** also results in chromosomal alterations. Symptoms include pancytopenia and an increased risk of cancer. Many die before early adulthood. Type C is found more frequently among Ashkenazi Jews; 1 in 89 are carriers.
- **Mucolipidosis IV** is found in 1 of 100 Ashkenazi Jews. This lipid-storage disease results in central nervous system deterioration during the first year with motor and mental retardation, as well as various eye disorders. The prognosis varies (Center for Jewish Genetic Diseases, 2011).

Orthodox rabbis usually do not support genetic testing because it might cause couples to refrain from marrying or having children, thus preventing them from fulfilling the *mitzvah* of procreation. The Reform movement supports a couple's right to make the decision as to whether or not to have the testing done. Because the knowledge is available, and for the emotional and psychological well-being of a couple, testing is allowed. Some Orthodox rabbis allow the practice of preimplantation screening of in vitro fertilized zygotes if both husband and wife are known carriers of Tay-Sachs and then to only use the healthy ones for implantation. "The discarding of the affected zygotes is not considered as abortion, since the status of a fetus or a potential life in Judaism applies only to a fetus implanted and growing in the mother's womb" (Jewish Virtual Library, 2011).

Other conditions with increased incidence in the Jewish population include inflammatory bowel disease (ulcerative colitis and Crohn's disease), which is seen 2 to 8 times more often in Ashkenazi Jews than in other ethnic groups; colorectal cancer occurs in 6 percent of Ashkenazi Jews; and the BRCA1 and BRCA2 genes that cause breast and ovarian cancer are found in 1 out of every 50 Jewish women of Ashkenazi background (Rosenberg, 2011).

Variations in Drug Metabolism

One of the few drugs found to have a higher rate of side effects in people of Ashkenazic ancestry is clozapine, used to treat schizophrenia. Twenty percent of Jewish patients taking this drug developed agranulocytosis, compared with about 1 percent of non-Jewish patients. A specific genetic haplotype has been identified to account for this finding (Schatzberg & Nemeroff, 2009). Thus, health-care providers must order testing for agranulocytosis when Jewish patients are prescribed clozapine.

High-Risk Behaviors

According to Jewish law, individuals may not intentionally damage their bodies or place themselves in danger. The basic philosophy is that the body must be protected from harm. To the religious, the body is viewed as belonging to God; therefore, it must be returned to Him intact when death occurs. Consequently, any substance or act that harms the body is not allowed. This includes smoking, suicide, taking nonprescription or illegal medications, and permanent tattooing (Jewish Virtual Library, 2011).

Alcohol, especially wine, is an essential part of religious holidays and festive occasions and is a traditional symbol of joy. The Jewish attitude toward wine is ambivalent. The Bible speaks of the undesirable effects of wine on the person, as well as its positive use as a medicine. Consequently, wine is appropriate and acceptable as long as it is used in moderation.

Health-Care Practices

Because of the respect afforded physicians and the emphasis on keeping the body and mind healthy, Jewish Americans are health conscious. Taking care of one's body is a mitzvah. In general, they practice preventive health care, with routine physical, dental, and vision screening. This is also a well-immunized population. Although the older generation is still more likely to defer to medical authority, Jewish adults tend to want to participate in health-care decision making.

Nutrition
Meaning of Food

Eating is important to Jews on many levels. Besides satisfying hunger and sustaining life, it also teaches discipline and reverence for life. For those who follow the dietary laws, a tremendous amount of attention is given to the slaughter, preparation, and consumption of food. In addition, the family dinner table is often the site for religious holiday celebrations and services, especially the Sabbath, Passover, Rosh Hashanah (Jewish New Year), and breaking the fast for Yom Kippur (Day of Atonement). Jewish dietary practices serve as a spiritually refining act of self-discipline and are a unifying factor in ethnic identity.

Common Foods and Food Rituals

Perhaps the food identified as "Jewish" that receives the most attention is chicken soup. This has frequently been referred to as *Jewish penicillin*, and it is often served with *knaidlach or matzoh balls* (dumplings made of matzoh meal). Although it has no intrinsic meaning or religious value, it is a staple in religious homes, especially on Friday evenings to usher in the Sabbath and during times of illness. It is frequently associated with a mother's warmth and love.

Other common foods include gefilte fish (ground karp molded into oblong balls, steamed, then served cold with horseradish), challah (a rich, braided white bread), kugel (noodle pudding, either sweet or savory), blintzes (crepes filled with a sweet cottage cheese), chopped liver (served cold), hamentashen (a triangular pastry with different types of filling), and Nova Scotia or "belly" lox (cold smoked salmon) served with cream cheese and salad vegetables on a bagel. Slow-cooked beef brisket is often the entrée at Rosh Hashanah (New Year) dinner.

The laws regarding food are found in Leviticus and Deuteronomy. They are commonly referred to as the laws of **kashrut**, or the laws that dictate which foods are permissible under religious law. The term **kosher** means "fit to eat" (Hoffman, 2008); it is not a brand or form of cooking. Whereas some believe that the mandatory statutes were developed and implemented for health reasons, religious scholars dispute this view, claiming that the only reason for following the laws is that they are mandatory commandments of God. Therefore, the laws are followed as a personal attachment to the religion and as a belief that God has mandated them. The laws' promotion of health is only a secondary gain. Kashruth issues may be a significant part of an inpatient stay, making it helpful to know what is and is not acceptable.

Foods are divided into those considered kosher (permitted or clean) and those considered ***treyf*** (forbidden or unclean). A permitted animal may become *treyf*, or forbidden, if it is not slaughtered, cooked, or served properly. Because life is sacred and animal cruelty is forbidden, kosher slaughter of animals must be done in a way that prevents undue cruelty to the animal and ensures the animal's health for the consumer. The jugular vein, carotid arteries, and vagus nerve must be severed in a single quick stroke with a sharp, smooth knife, causing the animal to die instantly. No sawing motion and no second stroke are permitted (DeLange, 2010). This also allows the maximal amount of blood to leave the body. Care must be taken that all blood is drained from the animal before it is eaten. Drinking of blood is prohibited. An animal that dies from old age or disease may not be eaten, nor may it be eaten if it meets a violent death or is killed by another animal. In addition, flesh cut from a live creature may not be eaten.

Milk and meat may not be mixed together in cooking, serving, or eating in order to respect the sensitivity of living creatures ("You must not boil a calf in its mother's milk" [Deut. 14:20]). To avoid mixing foods, utensils and plates used to serve them are separated. Religious Jews who follow the dietary laws have two sets of dishes, pots, and utensils: one set for milk products (*milchig* in Yiddish) and the other for meat (*fleishig*). Some homes have different sets of dish towels and even different sinks. Because glass is not absorbent, it can be used for either meat or milk products, although religious households still usually have two sets. Therefore, cheeseburgers, lasagna made with meat, and grated cheese on meatballs and spaghetti are unacceptable. Milk cannot be used in coffee if it is served with a meat meal. Nondairy creamers can be used instead, as long as they do not contain sodium caseinate, which is derived from milk. Thirty minutes is the minimum time between eating milk and meat products, but some families wait up to 6 hours, with the premise that food takes that long to digest from the stomach (Hoffman, 2008).

A number of foods are considered ***parve*** (neutral) and may be used with either dairy or meat dishes. These include fish, eggs, anything grown in the soil (vegetables, fruits, coffee, sugar, and spices), and chemically produced goods. Vegetables and fruits must be washed carefully to ensure that they are free of insects. A "U" with a circle around it is the seal of the Union of Orthodox Jewish Congregations of America and is used on food products to indicate that they are kosher. A circled "K" and other symbols may also be found on packaging to indicate that a product is kosher.

When working in a Jewish person's home, the health-care provider should not bring food into the house without knowing whether or not the patient adheres to kosher standards. If the patient keeps a kosher home, do not use any cooking items, dishes, or silverware without knowing which are used for meat and which for dairy products. Health-care providers must fully understand the dietary laws so they do not offend the patient, can advocate for kosher meals if they are requested, and can plan medication times accordingly.

Mammals are considered clean if they meet the other requirements for their slaughter and consumption and have split (cloven) hooves and chew their cud. These animals include buffalo, cattle, goat, deer, and sheep. The pig is an example of an animal that does not meet these criteria. Although liberal Jews decide for themselves which dietary laws they will follow, many still avoid pork and pork products out of a sense of tradition and symbolism. Serving pork

REFLECTIVE EXERCISE 19.1

Mr. Orr, an 80-year-old Jewish patient, originally from Eastern Europe, has heart disease and a pancreatic deficiency. He is being cared for in his home by visiting nurses. His wife of 55 years has some physical limitations but is self-sufficient to maintain her home. The visiting nurse discovers that Mr. Orr is not taking his pancreatic enzymes as ordered. He states that he found out that the enzymes are made of pork products, and he does not eat pork. The nurse may want to teach his wife how to make meals that will meet his health needs and enters the kitchen to obtain a measuring cup. Concerned because she has a kosher kitchen, Mrs. Orr starts yelling at the visiting nurse.

1. What options are available regarding pancreatic enzymes that do not contain pork?
2. What responses regarding his medication might be made to Mr. Orr?
3. What questions should the nurse ask Mrs. Orr about her degree of *kashrut* (keeping kosher)?
4. What might be an approach to planning kosher meals appropriate for someone with cardiac and pancreatic problems?
5. What needs to be known in advance before entering Mrs. Orr's kitchen?

products to a Jewish patient, unless specifically requested, is insensitive.

Birds of prey are considered "unclean" and unacceptable because they grab their food with their claws. Acceptable poultry are chicken, one of the most frequently consumed forms of protein; turkey; goose; and duck. Fish can be eaten if it has both fins and scales. Nothing that crawls on its belly is allowed, including clams, lobsters, and other shellfish; tortoises; and frogs (DeLange, 2010).

In religious homes, meat is prepared for cooking by soaking and salting to drain all the blood from the flesh. As increased residual salt may result, patients with sodium restrictions may need counseling to assist them in making dietary adjustments. Broiling is acceptable, especially for liver, because it drains the blood. Care must be taken in serving cheese to ensure that no animal substances are served at the same time. Breads and cakes made with lard are *treyf*, and breads made with milk or milk by-products (e.g., casein) cannot be served with meat meals. Eggs from nonkosher birds, milk from nonkosher animals, and oil from nonkosher fish are not permitted. Butter substitutes are used with meat meals. Honey is allowed.

Kosher meals are available in most hospitals or can be obtained from frozen food suppliers. They arrive on paper plates and with sealed plastic utensils. Health-care providers should not unwrap the utensils or change the foodstuffs to another serving dish.

Frozen kosher meals are available on a commercial basis. Help may be needed for a patient to choose from a facility's menu options. No milk or yogurt should be placed on a tray with meat, and butter cannot be served with bread. Even salad dressing needs to be made without dairy ingredients. If health-care providers have difficulty locating a supplier, they should contact a local rabbi. Determining a patient's dietary preferences and practices regarding dietary laws should be done during the admission assessment.

Dietary Practices for Health Promotion

Many Jewish dietary practices are thought to afford the secondary gain of preventing disease, their intention is for observance of a commandment. Many Jews understand the dietary laws as a guide to raising the act of eating to a spiritual level, which is also true of the practice of washing one's hands and praying before and after eating.

Nutritional Deficiencies and Food Limitations

No nutritional deficiencies are common to individuals of Jewish descent. As with any ethnic group, nutritional deficiencies may occur in individuals in lower socioeconomic groups because of the expense of certain foods.

In addition to the dietary laws discussed previously, other dietary laws are followed at specified times. For example, during the week of Passover, no bread or product with yeast may be eaten. Matzoh (unleavened bread) is eaten instead. Any product that is fermented or can cause fermentation may not be eaten (Hoffman, 2008). Rather than attend synagogue, the family conducts the service (*seder*) around the dinner table during the first 2 nights and incorporates dinner into a service that includes all participants in study, singing, and retelling the story of Moses and the Exodus from Egypt.

The Jewish calendar has a number of fast days. The most observed is the holiest day of the year, Yom Kippur. On this Day of Atonement, Jews abstain from food and drink as they pray to God for forgiveness for the sins they have committed during the past year. They eat an early dinner on the evening before the holiday begins and then fast until after sunset the following day. Ill people, older people, the young, pregnant or lactating mothers, and the physically incapacitated are absolved from fasting and may need to be reminded of this exception to Jewish law. Maintaining an ill person's health supersedes the act of fasting. If concerns arise, a consultation with the patient's rabbi may be necessary.

Pregnancy and Childbearing Practices

Fertility Practices and Views Toward Pregnancy

God's first commandment to humanity is "Be fruitful and multiply" (Genesis 1:28). Children are considered a gift and a duty, with men considered more important by the ultra-Orthodox because they can say **kaddish** (the prayer for the dead) for their parents. In other branches of Judaism, both sexes may recite the *kaddish*. Families are encouraged to have at least two children to fulfill the biblical commandment to propagate the people (Jacob & Zemer, 2006).

Couples who are unable to conceive should try all possible means to have children. This includes infertility counseling and interventions, comprising egg and sperm donation. In Orthodox communities, artificial insemination is usually allowed if the sperm and egg are from the married Jewish partners (Hoffman, 2008). If the source is other than the married couple, it could be considered incest or adultery. Others argue that it cannot be considered adultery if no sexual intercourse has occurred. When all natural attempts have been made, adoption may be pursued. Having children allows religious parents to fulfill many of the commandments.

The lower number of children born to Jewish Americans and the high interfaith marriage rate have resulted in a decreased Jewish population. While the average-size Jewish family in the United States is fewer than 2 children, in Israel, the average Jewish family in 2009 had 2.96 children (Jewish Virtual Library, 2011). Because one-third of all Jews were killed during the Holocaust, some believe that today's Jews have a moral obligation to bring one more child into the world than they would have normally.

Prevention of pregnancy in the more Orthodox view implies deferring the commandment to be fruitful and multiply. While birth control is not against religious law, birth suppression is (Jacob & Zemer, 2006). Unless pregnancy jeopardizes the life or health of the mother, contraception is not looked on favorably among the ultra-Orthodox (Hoffman, 2008). Liberal Judaism recognizes that children have the right to be wanted and that they should be born into homes in which their needs can be met. Therefore, the use of temporary birth control may be acceptable. Condom use is supported, especially if unprotected sexual intercourse would pose a medical risk to either spouse.

To the Orthodox, it is important to know the mechanism of action of the birth control. Coitus interruptus and masturbation (referred to as solitary sex) are not acceptable because they result in the needless expenditure of semen, although most Jews consider the former practice a normal, healthy activity. The ban on masturbation does not apply to women (DeLange, 2010). Barrier techniques are not acceptable because they interfere with the full mobility of the sperm in its natural course. The birth control pill does not result in any permanent sterilization, nor does it prevent semen from traveling its normal route. Therefore, use of this method is the least objectionable to most branches of Judaism (Hoffman, 2008). Some

Orthodox groups do allow the use of birth control once the mitzvah of having children is achieved (DeLange, 2010). Sterilization implies permanence, and Orthodox Jews generally oppose this practice, unless the life of the mother is in danger; vasectomy is regarded by the ultra-Orthodox as mutilation of the body and thus is not permitted (Hoffman, 2008). Reform Judaism leaves the choice of what to use and whether to use contraceptives up to the parents.

Recognizing that Judaism's primary focus is the sanctity of life, it is important to identify when life begins. The fetus is not considered a living soul or person until it has been born. Birth is determined when the head or "greater part" is born (Judaism 101, 2005). Until that time, it is merely part of the mother's body and has no independent identity. The unborn is not actually a person and has no independent life (Jacob & Zemer, 2006).

The mother and her health are paramount. If her physical or mental health is endangered by the fetus, all branches of Judaism consider the fetus the aggressor, which must be aborted (Hoffman, 2008). Therefore, any ban on abortion could be a violation of religious freedom. Whereas saving the mother's life is certainly grounds for abortion, random abortion is not permitted by the Orthodox branch because the fetus is part of the mother's body, and one must not do harm to one's body. Progressive Jews allow abortion, if the mother desires it, if there is physical or psychological danger to the mother or in the case of incest or rape (Jacob & Zemer, 2006).

Reform Judaism believes that a woman maintains control over her own body, and it is up to her whether to abort a fetus. Although no connotation of sin is attached to abortion, the decision is not to be made without serious deliberation. Most Jews favor a woman's right to choose regarding abortion.

Prescriptive, Restrictive, and Taboo Practices in the Childbearing Family

While pregnancy is an exciting time for parents, in religious Jewish homes, baby showers are not held and nothing is purchased for the potential child. Baby names are not discussed until after the child is born (Judaism 101, 2005). This is based on superstition that drawing attention to the pregnancy will result in bad luck for the child-to-be.

A Hasidic husband may not touch his wife during labor and may choose not to attend the delivery, because by Jewish law he is not permitted to view his wife's genitals. These behaviors should never be interpreted as insensitivity on the part of the husband. During the delivery of a child to an ultra-Orthodox family, these interventions should be initiated: The mother should be given hospital gowns that cover her in the front and back to the greatest extent possible. She may prefer to wear a surgical cap so that her hair remains covered. The father should be given the opportunity to leave during procedures and during the birth, or, if he chooses to stay, the mother can be draped so that the husband may sit by his wife without viewing her perineum, including by way of mirrors, in order to protect her dignity. Because he is not permitted to touch his wife, he may offer only verbal support. The female nurse may need to provide all of the physical care. Pain medication during delivery is acceptable.

For male infants, circumcision, which is both a medical procedure removing the foreskin and a religious rite, is performed. The origin of this ritual dates back to Abraham and Isaac in the Book of Genesis. A *brit milah* (sometimes referred to as a *bris*) symbolizes the covenant made between the Jewish people and God (Diamant, 2007). The procedure itself and the accompanying ceremony are performed on the 8th day of life by person called a **mohel**, an individual trained in the circumcision procedure, asepsis, and the religious ceremony. Although a rabbi is not necessary, it is also possible to have the procedure done by a physician with a rabbi present to say the blessings. Jewish parents who are not very observant and/or are unaffiliated may still opt for medical circumcision, illustrating how the power of this ritual endures over thousands of years.

Attending a *brit milah* is the only mitzvah for which religious Jews must violate the Sabbath so that the *brit* can be completed at the proper time (Diamant, 2007). The naming of the newborn son occurs during the *bris* ceremony (girls are named in the synagogue). The *brit milah* is a family festivity, and many relatives are invited. In most cases today, the ceremony is performed in the home; however, if the child is still in the hospital, it is important for the hospital to provide a room for a small private party to celebrate. Whereas the medical community sometimes debates the practice of circumcision, to even suggest to Jewish parents that the practice is "barbaric" is insensitive.

A circumcision may be delayed for medical reasons, including unstable condition owing to prematurity, life-threatening concerns during the early weeks after birth, bleeding problems, or a defect of the penis, which may require later surgery (Diamant, 2007). At birth, a child is free of all sin; failure to circumcise carries no eternal consequences should the child die. Although there is no rule against designating godparents for a newborn, it is considered a local, not traditional, custom.

Death Rituals

Death Rituals and Expectations

Death is an expected part of the life cycle. Yet, each day is to be appreciated and lived as fully as possible. Religious Jews start each day with a prayer of appreciation for having lived another day. The goal is to appreciate things and people while one still has them. Brain death as a criterion for organ donation remains controversial, with some sects agreeing to this criterion, while others do not (DeLange, 2010). Many also accept a flat electroencephalogram as a determination of death.

Traditional Judaism believes in an afterlife in which the soul continues to flourish, although many dispute this interpretation because it is not mentioned in the Torah. Most Jews do not dwell much on life after death and are unconcerned about it; their focus is on how to conduct one's present life.

Active euthanasia, in which something is given or done to result in death, is forbidden for religious Jews. One of the Ten Commandments is "Thou shalt not kill," and euthanasia is considered murder. A dying person is considered a living person in all respects. Sufficient pain control should be provided, even if it decreases the person's level of consciousness (Beitowitz, 2006). Withholding food from a deformed child to speed its death is considered active euthanasia and is forbidden.

Passive euthanasia may be allowed, depending on its interpretation. Nothing may be used or initiated that prevents a person from dying naturally or that prolongs the dying process. Therefore, anything that artificially prevents death (e.g., cardiopulmonary resuscitation, use of ventilators) may possibly be withheld, depending on the wishes of the patient and his or her religious views. Regardless of the decisions made, pain control must be maintained.

Taking one's own life is prohibited and is viewed as a criminal act and morally wrong because it is forbidden to harm any human being, including oneself. To the ultrareligious, suicide removes all possibility of repentance. Adult Jews who commit suicide, who are not mentally ill or depressed, and who belong to ultrareligious factions of Judaism are not afforded full burial honors. They are buried on the periphery of the Jewish cemetery, and mourning rites are not observed, unless the individual was not mentally competent. However, the more liberal view is to emphasize the needs of the survivors, and all burial and mourning activities proceed according to the usual traditional rites and wishes of the family. Children are never considered to have intentionally killed themselves and are afforded all burial rights.

The dying person should not be left alone. It is considered respectful to stay with a dying person, unless the visitor is physically ill or their emotions are out of control. Judaism does not have any ceremony similar to the Catholic sacrament of the sick. Any Jew may ask God's forgiveness for her or his sins; no confessor is needed. However, it is not commonly known that Jews have a personal confession called *Viddui*, which is recited when death is imminent. It may be said by the dying person or by somebody for her or him. Some

REFLECTIVE EXERCISE 19.2

Samuel is an older Jewish adult who is in the final stage of terminal cancer. His nurse has developed a close relationship with him, but has never discussed religion. Samuel states that he is not afraid of dying. The nurse asks him if he wants a clergy in order to make confession; he says no and appears annoyed. Samuel decides he wants to end all treatments, but the nurse tries to encourage him to continue the treatments in the hope that his cancer will enter remission. Then the nurse tells Samuel's wife, "God doesn't give you anything that you can't handle" and "This is your cross to bear." The nurse is perplexed as to why her well-intentioned comfort modalities are not effective with either the patient or his wife.

1. What does the nurse need to understand about a Jew's relationship with God?
2. What does the nurse need to understand about the Jewish view of death?
3. Why are the comments made to Samuel's wife inappropriate?
4. What interventions might be most helpful to the family in the final stage of life?

Jews feel solace in saying the *Shema* in Hebrew or English. This prayer confirms one's belief in one God.

At the time of death, the nearest relative can gently close the eyes and mouth; the face is covered with a sheet. The body is treated with respect and revered for the function it once filled. Health-care providers need to ask the closest relative of the deceased specifically about the practices to follow after death. Health-care providers who have acquired some familiarity with Jewish practices associated with death go a long way toward helping their patients and families. They are performing *mitzvot* (good deeds) with their informed presence that will continue to benefit all involved as the long process of integrating loss into their lives continues.

Ultra-Orthodox Jews follow a ritual that is not conducive to hospital protocols and is more commonly observed for those who die at home. After the body is wrapped, it is briefly placed on the floor with the feet pointing toward the door. A candle may be placed near the head (Cohn-Sherbok, 2010). However, this does not occur on the Sabbath or holy days. The dead body is not left alone from the time of death until the funeral, so as not to leave it defenseless (Diamant, 2007).

Autopsy is usually not permitted among religious Jews because it results in desecration of the body, and it is important that the body be interred whole (Hoffman, 2008). Allowing an autopsy might also delay the burial, something that is not recommended. Conversely, autopsy is allowed if its results would save the life of another patient (Diamant, 2007). Many branches of Judaism currently allow an autopsy if it is required by law; the deceased person has willed it; or it saves the life of another, especially an offspring (Diamant, 2007). The body must be treated with respect during the autopsy.

Any attempt to hasten or retard decomposition of the body is discouraged. Cremation is prohibited because it unnaturally speeds the disposal of the dead body (Hoffman, 2008). Embalming is prohibited because it preserves the dead. However, in circumstances in which the funeral must be delayed, some embalming may be approved. Cosmetic restoration for the funeral is discouraged.

Jewish funerals and burials follow certain practices; they usually occur within 24 to 48 hours after the death. The funeral service is directed at honoring the departed by speaking only well of him or her. It is *not* the practice to have flowers at either the funeral or at the cemetery; this was a Christian custom used to offset the odor of decaying bodies. A donation to a charity in the name of the deceased is a more meaningful tribute. The casket is often a simple pine box with no ornamentation. The body may be wrapped only in a shroud to ensure that the body and casket decay at the same rate. A wake or viewing is *not* part of a Jewish funeral. The prayer said for the dead, the *kaddish*, is usually not said alone, but is recited in and with the company of others. The prayer says nothing about death, but rather, it praises God and reaffirms one's own faith. A funeral according to *halachah* (Jewish law) emphasizes that death is death. Realism and simplicity are the characteristics of the Jewish burial.

After the funeral, mourners are welcomed at the home of the closest relative. Water to wash one's hands before entering is outside the front door, symbolic of cleansing the impurities associated with contact with the dead. The water is not passed from person to person, just as it is hoped that the tragedy is not passed. At the home, a meal is served to all the guests. This "meal of condolence" or "meal of consolation" is traditionally provided by the neighbors and friends; it frequently includes hard-boiled eggs to remind all of the continuing cycle of life (Diamant, 2007).

Shiva (Hebrew for "seven") is the 7-day period that begins with the burial. *Shiva* helps the surviving individuals face the actuality of the death of the loved one. During this period when the mourners are "sitting *shiva*," they do not work. When health-care providers are the ones experiencing the loss, it is important for supervisors to understand the mourning customs. In some homes, mirrors are covered to decrease the focus on one's appearance; no activity is permitted to divert attention from thinking about the deceased; and evening and morning services may be conducted in the closest relative's home. Condolence calls and the giving of consolation are appropriate during this time.

After *shiva*, the mourning period varies based on who has died. Mourning for a relative lasts 30 days, and for a parent, 1 year. Judaism does not support prolonged mourning. A tombstone is erected within 1 year of the death, at which time a graveside service is held. This is called an *unveiling*. According to the Jewish calendar, the anniversary of the death is called *yahrzeit*, and at this time, candles are lit and the *kaddish* is said.

Understanding some specific practices related to death and dying may have an impact on other aspects of health care, including the death of premature infants and the care of amputated limbs. Mourning is not required for a fetus that is miscarried or stillborn. This is also true of any premature infant who dies within 30 days of birth. However, parents are required to mourn for full-term infants who die at birth or shortly thereafter (Washofsky, 2000). Although the baby should be named, not all of the traditional burial customs are followed.

Within Orthodoxy, when a limb is amputated before death, the amputated limb and blood-soaked clothing are buried in the person's future gravesite. This custom might not be practiced by recent Russian immigrant Jews because they were not allowed to practice their faith under Communism and, therefore, lost many of the traditional practices. Because the blood and limb were part of the person, they are buried with the person. No mourning rites are required. In the case of an amputation, the health-care provider may need to assist with arrangements for burial of the body part.

When one visits a Jewish cemetery, one of the most noticeable differences is that small stones are left on the top of the gravestone. While the original reason for this practice is unknown, it is now used as a token to indicate that the grave has been visited and the person has not been forgotten (Diamant, 2007).

Responses to Death and Grief

The period following a death has discrete segments to assist mourners in their adjustment to the loss. The period of time between the death and the burial is short, and it is the time for the emotional reaction to the death. The burial may be delayed only if required by law, if relatives must travel great distances, or if it is the Sabbath or a holy day. Mourners are absolved from praying during this time. Crying, anger, and talking about the deceased person's life are acceptable. A common sign of grief is the tearing of the garment that one is wearing before the funeral service. In liberal congregations, a black ribbon with a tear in it is a symbolic representation of mourning (Diamant, 2007). During *shiva*, the mourner sets the tone and initiates the conversation. Because there are such discrete periods of mourning, Judaism tells the mourner that it is wrong to

mourn more than 30 days for a relative and 1 year for parents (Hoffman, 2008).

Spirituality
Dominant Religion and Use of Prayer

Judaism, one of the oldest monotheistic religions, is over 4000 years old (BBC Religions, 2011). Its early history and laws are chronicled in the **Torah**, called the *Old Testament* by Christians. Jews consider only the Torah as their Bible. They have a history of being singled out as a people and have often been persecuted, expelled from countries and forbidden to practice their religion; "black-balled" from jobs, housing, and admission to college; rounded up and killed; and mass-exterminated. Many Jews in America have immediate family members who were killed in the pogroms in Russia in the early 1900s and in the Holocaust in Eastern Europe. Yet, throughout this persecution, Judaism has lived and flourished.

Judaism is a monotheistic faith that believes in one God as the Creator of the universe. The watchword of the faith is found in Deuteronomy (6:4): "Hear O Israel, the Lord is our God, the Lord is One." No physical qualities are attributed to God, and making and praying to statues or graven images are forbidden by the second commandment.

The spiritual leader is the **rabbi** (teacher). He (or she, in liberal branches) is the interpreter of Jewish law. Rabbis are not considered to be any closer to God than common people are. All Jews pray directly to God. They do not need the rabbi to intercede, to hear confession, or to grant atonement. The following are some of the major principles that guide Judaic bioethics:

- Man's purpose on earth is to live according to certain God-given guidelines.
- Life possesses enormous intrinsic value, and its preservation is of great moral significance.
- All human lives are equal.
- Our lives are not our own exclusive private possessions (Perlin, 2006).

The first five books of the Bible, also known as the *five books of Moses*, are handwritten in Hebrew on parchment scrolls called *Torah*. These scrolls are kept in the "Holy Ark" within each synagogue under an "eternal light." The Torah directs Jews on how they should live their lives; it provides guidance on every aspect of human life. The rest of the Bible includes sacred writings and teachings of the prophets.

The 613 commandments within the Torah (also called *Mitzvot*) and the oral law derived from the biblical statutes determine Jewish law, or *halakhah*. These commandments ask for a commitment in behavior and also address ethical concerns. Thus, the commandments reflect the will of God, and religious Jews feel it is their duty to carry them out to fulfill their covenant with God. This makes Judaism not only a religion but also a way of life.

The current practice of Judaism in America spans a wide spectrum. Whereas there is only one religion, there are multiple branches or denominations of Judaism. The Orthodox are the most traditional. They adhere most strictly to the *halakhah* (Code of Jewish Law) of traditional Judaism and try to follow as many of the laws as possible while fitting into American society. They observe the Sabbath by attending the synagogue on Friday evening and Saturday morning and by abstaining from work, spending money, and driving on the Sabbath. Orthodox Jews observe the Jewish dietary laws; men wear a **yarmulke** or *kippah* (head covering) at all times in reverence to God, whereas women usually wear long sleeves and modest dress. In many Orthodox synagogues, the services are primarily in Hebrew, and men and women sit separately.

Orthodox Jews and some Conservative men and women use the *tefillin*, or phylacteries, during morning prayer services. These are two small black boxes, with parchment containing biblical passages, that are connected to long leather straps. These are wrapped around the arms and forehead as reminders of the laws of the Torah. The *tallis* (or *tallit*) is a rectangular prayer shawl with fringes. This is also used only during prayer but is frequently used by both Conservative and Orthodox Jews. Ultra-Orthodox men wear a special garment under their shirts year-round; the *tzitzit* has long fringes as a reminder of the laws of the Torah.

A *mezuzah* is a small elongated container with scripture inside and marked with a Hebrew letter on the outside that denotes God. Its origin was a sign ensuring God's protection; it serves as a reminder of the presence of God, His commandments, and a Jew's duties to Him. Jewish homes have a *mezuzah* on the doorframe of the house. A number of individuals also wear a *mezuzah* as a necklace. Other religious symbols include the *Star of David*, a six-pointed star that has been a symbol of the Jewish community since the 1350s, and the *menorah* (candelabrum).

The Conservative branch is not quite as strict in its traditions. Whereas Conservative Jews observe most of the *halakhah*, they do make concessions to modern society. According to DeLange (2010), "The aim of the founders [of Conservative Judaism] was to embrace the liberalism and pleuralism of American Reform while safeguarding traditional practice" (p. 13). Many drive to the synagogue on the Sabbath, and men and women sit together. Many keep a kosher home, but they may or may not follow all of the dietary laws outside the home. Women are ordained as rabbis and are counted in a *minyan*, the minimum number of 10 required for communal prayer. (These practices are unacceptable to the Orthodox.) Whereas

a yarmulke is required in the synagogue, it is optional outside of that environment.

The liberal or progressive movement is called *Reform* Judaism. Reform Jews claim that postbiblical law was only for the people of that time, and only the moral laws of the Torah are binding. They practice fewer rituals, although they frequently have a *mezuzah* for their homes, celebrate the holidays, and have a strong ethnic identity. They consider education and ethics of paramount importance in one's personal life and try to link Jewish religious values with American political liberalism. They may or may not follow the Jewish dietary laws, but they may have specific unacceptable foods (e.g., pork) that they abstain from eating. Men and women share full equality, and they engage in many social-action activities.

Of the many small groups of ultra-Orthodox fundamentalists, the **Hasidic** (or **Chasidic**) Jews are perhaps the most recognizable. They usually live, work, and study within a segregated area. They are visually identifiable by their full beards, uncut hair around the ears (*pais*), black hats or fur *streimels*, dark clothing, and no exposed extremities. Women, especially those who are married, also keep their extremities covered and may have shaved heads covered by a wig and often a hat as well.

A relatively new denomination, Reconstructionism is a mosaic of the three main branches. It views Judaism as an evolving religion of the Jewish people and seeks to adapt Jewish beliefs and practices to the needs of the contemporary world. It bridges the Conservative religious world with the secular world of Judaism.

"'Secular Jew' is a term that refers to Jews who have chosen to abandon the belief in God" (DeLange, 2010, p. 78). They have not rejected their Jewish identity or their attachment to the Jewish people. They remain very supportive to Jewish causes without a belief in a supernatural being. Many Jews, however, do not indicate any affiliation.

The Jewish house of prayer is called a **synagogue**, **temple**, or **shul**. It is never referred to as a *church*. Jews may pray alone or communally when 10 male Jews over the age of 13 who have had their *bar mitzvah* are gathered together for prayer. This group is called a *minyan*. Orthodox Jews pray three times a day: morning, late afternoon, and evening. They wash their hands and say a prayer on awakening in the morning and before meals. Reform and Reconstructionist groups may allow women to form a *minyan*.

Religious patients in hospitals may want their prayer items (*yarmulke* or *kippah*, *tallit*, *tzitzit*, *tefillin*) and may request a minyan. Hospital policies regarding the number of visitors in the sick person's room may have to be ignored in such instances.

One of the most common religious practices related to patients involves "visiting the sick" (*bikkur cholim*).

This commandment is one of the social obligations of Judaism and ensures that Jews look after the physical, emotional, psychological, and social well-being of others and provides hope as well as companionship. Moreover, one must consider the patient's welfare and not stay too long, tire the patient, or come only to satisfy one's own needs.

Meaning of Life and Individual Sources of Strength

The preservation of life is one of Judaism's greatest priorities. Even the laws that govern the Sabbath may be broken if one can help save a life. Health-care providers should do everything to save a life (Hoffman, 2008). Each individual is considered special, and the individuality of the human experience is one of the precepts of the faith. Good health is considered an asset.

Spiritual Beliefs and Health-Care Practices

The second of the Ten Commandments is to remember the Sabbath day and keep it holy. The Sabbath begins 18 minutes before sunset on Friday. Lighting candles, saying prayers over challah and wine, and participating in a festive Sabbath meal usher in this weekly holy day. It ends 42 minutes after sunset (or when three stars can be seen) on Saturday, with a service called *Havdalah*. The Sabbath serves as a release from weekday concerns and pressures. During this time, religious Jews engage in congregational study and do no manner of work, including answering the telephone, operating any electrical appliances, handling money, driving, or operating a call bell from a hospital bed.

If an Orthodox patient's condition is not life-threatening, medical and surgical procedures should not be performed on the Sabbath or holy days. However, extenuating circumstances such as illness or foul weather are legitimate reasons for not attending the services. Although the Sabbath is holy, and holidays that require fasting are part of Jewish law, matters involving human life take precedence over them.

Therefore, a gravely ill person and the work of those who need to save her or him are exempted from following the commandments regarding the Sabbath and fast days. This even includes eating nonkosher food if there is the slightest chance that human life will be saved (Jewish Virtual Library, 2011).

In addition to the Sabbath, a number of Jewish holidays are celebrated with special traditions. Rosh Hashanah (Jewish New Year) and Yom Kippur (Day of Atonement) are called the *High Holy Days*, and usually occur in September or early October. They mark a 10-day period of self-examination and repentance. This is a time when Jews apologize for wrongs they have committed knowingly or unknowingly against others (Cohn-Sherbok, 2010). According to tradition, during these 10 days, each person stands before God, and their fate for the coming year is determined. Thus, the greeting during this time is "May you be written into the book of life for a good year." As noted earlier, Yom Kippur is the most solemn of the Jewish holidays.

Rosh Hashanah is started by eating apples and honey to wish for a sweet year, and on Yom Kippur, one fasts for a day to cleanse and purify oneself. As noted before, fasting for Yom Kippur may be broken for reasons of critical illness or labor and delivery or for children under the age of 12. The holiday includes the blowing of the *shofar* (a ram's horn) that is to remind individuals to repent or atone for their sins.

Other major holidays include Passover, the Feast of the Unleavened Bread, which lasts 8 days and celebrates the Exodus from Egypt and freedom from slavery; Sukkot, a festival of the harvest in which individuals may live in temporary huts built outside their homes or synagogues for a week; and Shavuot, which celebrates the giving of the Ten Commandments. Minor holidays include Chanukah, an 8-day holiday, and Purim, both of which celebrate religious freedom. Table 19-1 provides a list of Jewish holidays for the years 2011 through 2017.

▶ Table 19-1   Jewish Holidays: 2011–2017

Holiday	2011–2012 (5772)*	2012–2013 (5773)*	2013–2014 (5774)*	2014–2015 (5775)*	2015–2016 (5776)*	2016–2017 (5777)*
Rosh Hashanah	9/29–9/30	9/17–9/18	9/5–9/6	9/25–9/26	9/14–9/15	10/3–10–/4
Yom Kippur	10/8	9/26	9/14	10/4	9/23	10/12
Sukkot	10/13–10/18	10/1–10/6	9/19–9/24	10/9–9/14	9/28–10/3	10/17–10/22
Chanukah	12/21–12/28	12/9–12/16	11/28–12/5	12/17–24	12/7–12/14	12/25–1/1
Purim	3/8	2/13	3/16	3/5	3/24	3/12
Passover	4/7–4/14	3/26–4/2	4/15–4/22	4/4–4/11	4/23–4/30	4/11–4/18
Shavuot	5/27–5/28	5/15–5/16	6/4–6/5	5/24–5/25	6/12–6/13	5/31–6/1

Note: Jewish holidays always begin at sundown the evening before the date recorded on this type of calendar; holidays end at sundown on the date shown.
*Dates on the Jewish calendar.

REFLECTIVE EXERCISE 19.3

Emma is 8 years old and hospitalized for an acute infection requiring a central line and antibiotics. It is December 24, and the hospital is decorated for Christmas. Multiple organizations have paraded through the unit with someone dressed as Santa Claus handing out presents. Emma thinks it is "neat" to get all these presents. However, when the staff ask her if she is excited that Santa Claus is there, she says "no." When they ask if she misses putting up a Christmas tree, she also says "no." The nurse is even more perplexed when she finds out that there are no decorations in the home at all, including a wreath on the door. The nurse asks if she wants to hang up a stocking, and she does not know what they are talking about. When Emma's mother hears the nurse telling her that this is the night to celebrate Jesus's birth, she becomes angry. When the mother explains that they do not believe in Jesus, the nurse responds, "I feel sorry for you."

1. What discussion could have been held with Emma's parents in the days before Christmas?
2. How might Emma still enjoy the "presents" without attaching it to religion?
3. How might the nurse have handled the situation better?
4. It is inappropriate to compare Christmas with Chanukah. How else might the nurse have recognized the assets of Judaism?

Health-Care Practices

Health-Seeking Beliefs and Behaviors

According to Jewish law, all people have a duty to keep themselves in good health. This encompasses physical and mental well-being and includes not only early treatment for illness but also prevention of illness. Judaism teaches its members to "choose life." To refuse lifesaving medical treatment is seen by some as committing suicide, as one is choosing death over life. All denominations recognize that religious requirements may be laid aside if a life is at stake or if an individual has a life-threatening illness. However, once it is clear that an individual is dying and that medical treatment is no longer working, individuals may choose not to interfere with death. Hospice care is fully consonant with Jewish beliefs.

In ultra-Orthodox denominations of Judaism, taking medication on the Sabbath that is not necessary to preserve life may be viewed as "work" (i.e., an action performed with the intention of bringing about a change in existing conditions) and is unacceptable. This belief may result in some people with conditions such as asthma not recognizing the severity of their condition; they may also be unaware of the laws that allow them to take their necessary medications. These patients need to be taught about the potential life-threatening sequelae of their condition as well as the exceptions to Jewish law that permit them to take their medications. In the Jewish faith, all individuals have value regardless of their condition. This includes individuals with developmental disabilities and AIDS.

Preventing disease, restoring health, and prolonging life are acceptable goals within Judaism. Therefore therapeutic genetic engineering via gene therapy is permitted if it prevents disease and disability in future generations (Solomon, 2006). Extending life gives more time for an individual to be involved in doing good deeds. Because genomics is the interaction between one's genes and the environment, improving the environment to improve healthy lives is also valued.

Responsibility for Health Care

Although it is the responsibility of health-care providers to heal, individuals must seek the services of the physician to ensure a healthy body. Once individuals have the knowledge necessary to effect their healing, it is their obligation to do so. To abstain from healing would be equivalent to murder. Jews believe that God provides human beings with "the tools and the knowledge to tamper with the Divine arrangement of the world" (Solomon, 2006, p. 134); it is up to them to use that wisdom to create a better world. This includes the discovery of new medications and treatments to eliminate or modify disease and suffering; therefore, man can help God heal and cure. Jews also believe that God gives humans freedom of choice.

Because the preservation of life is paramount, all ritual commandments are waived when danger to life exists. Physical and mental illnesses are legitimate reasons for not fulfilling some of the commandments. Because adult Jews are often well read, they may be interested in trying the newest available treatments. This could have both positive and negative consequences. The literature reveals no studies regarding Jews' self-medicating practices.

Folk and Traditional Practices

Jewish folk practices are historically and biblically based. Jews have adopted and adapted to customs from the cultures and countries in which they have lived during the centuries of the *diaspora*. Specific practices are explained in the sections of this chapter on Nutrition and Spiritual Beliefs and Health-Care Practices.

Barriers to Health Care

Aside from the unavailability of health insurance for some people, or being underinsured secondary to economic situations, no major barriers to health care for Jews in contemporary America exist. The Jewish community helps those in need, including new immigrants, and assists fellow Jews in becoming self-sufficient. Community organizations, especially the Jewish Federation in each state, include programs to help the needy; these agencies are ubiquitous today wherever Jews live in the United States.

Cultural Responses to Health and Illness

The verbalization of pain is acceptable and common. Individuals want to know the reason for the pain, which they consider just as important as obtaining relief from it. The sick role for Jews is highly individualized and may vary among individuals according to the severity of symptoms. As prescribed in the *halakhah*, the family is central to Jewish life; therefore, family members share the emphasis on maintaining health and assisting with individual responsibilities during times of illness.

Many Jews have become physicians, psychoanalysts, psychiatrists, and psychologists. In addition, many of their patients are Jewish. The maintenance of one's mental health is considered just as important as the maintenance of one's physical health. This designation includes psychiatric conditions. However, requirements for those who are rational but have cognitive deficiencies are decided on an individual basis. According to Jewish law, individuals must be taught the Torah regardless of their age or level of disability; this speaks to the unique value of each individual.

Blood Transfusions and Organ Donation

Jewish law views organ transplants from four perspectives: the recipient, the living donor, the cadaver donor, and the dying donor. Because life is sacred, if the recipient's life can be prolonged without considerable risk, then transplant is favorably viewed. For a living donor to be approved, the risk to the life of the donor must be considered. One is not obligated to donate a body part unless the risk is small. Examples include kidney and bone marrow donations (Lamm, 2000). If there is more than a 50 percent chance of either the patient or the donor dying, the organ donation is not permitted (Hoffman, 2008). The action of donating an organ to save another is considered a great *mitzvah*.

Conservative and Reform Judaism approve using the flat EEG as the determination of death so that organs, such as the heart, can be viable for transplant. Burial may be delayed if organ harvesting is the cause of the delay. However, among other groups, this definition of death remains controversial (Beitowitz, 2006). Health-care providers may need to assist Jewish patients to obtain a rabbi when they are making a decision regarding organ donation or transplant.

The use of a cadaver for transplant is generally approved if it is to save a life. No one may derive economic benefit from the corpse. Although desecration of the dead body is considered purposeless mutilation, this does not apply to the removal of organs for transplant. Use of skin for burns is also acceptable.

Health-Care Providers

The ancient Hebrews are credited with promoting hygiene and sanitation practices and basic principles for public health care. From the religious mandate of visiting the sick and the desire to initiate measures to prevent the spread of disease, Lillian Wald, a well-known Jewish nurse, developed the Henry Street Settlement in New York City as a prototype of public health nursing for those in need and initiated the idea of school nursing. Jewish physicians have made significant contributions, ranging from development of immunizations (Baruch Blumberg [hepatitis B] and Jonas Salk and Albert Sabin [polio]) to psychotherapy (Aaron Beck [cognitive therapy] and Sigmund Freud [psychoanalysis]).

Status of Health-Care Providers

Physicians are held in high regard. Whereas physicians must do everything in their power to preserve life, they are prohibited from initiating measures that prolong the act of dying (Hoffman, 2008). Once standard therapy has failed, or if additional treatments are unavailable, the physician's role changes from that of curer to providing supportive care, such as food and water, good nursing care, and optimal psychosocial support.

REFERENCES

American Jewish Committee. (2010). Retrieved from http://www.ajc.org/site/apps/nlnet/content3.aspx?c=ijITI2PHKoG&b=846741&ct=8801845

American Jewish Demographics. (2011). Retrieved from http://www.jewishvirtuallibrary.org/jsource/US-Israel/jewdemotoc.html

Beckerman, G. (December 22, 2010). New study finds more Jews in the United States than previously thought. Forward.com. Retrieved from www.forward.com/articles/134138

Beitowitz, Y.A. (2006). Brain death controversy in Jewish Law. Retrieved from http://www.jlaw.com/Articles/brain.html

Benson, E. (1994). Jewish nurses: A multicultural perspective. *Journal of the New York State Nurses Association, 25*(2), 8–10.

Benson, E. (2001). *As we see ourselves: Jewish women in nursing.* Indianapolis, IN: Center Nursing Publishing.

British Broadcasting Company. (2011). *Religions.* Retrieved from http://www.bbc.co.uk/religion/religions/judaism/

Center for Jewish Genetic Diseases. (2011). Retrieved from http://www.mssm.edu/research/programs/jewish-genetics-disease-center/screening-program/current-screenings

Center for Jewish History. (2007). Retrieved from www.cjh.org/

Cohn-Sherbok, D. (2010). *Judaism today.* London: Continuum International.

DeLange, N. (2010). *An introduction to Judaism.* Cambridge, UK: Cambridge University Press.

Diamant, A. (2007). *Living a Jewish life.* New York, NY: Harper.

Hebrew University of Jerusalem. (2009). *Ashkenazi Jews.* Retrieved from http://hugr.huji.ac.il/AshkenaziJews.aspx

Hoffman, C. (2008). *Judaism.* London: McGraw-Hill.

Jacob, W., & Zemer, M. (2006). *Sexual issues in Jewish law.* Pittsburgh, PA: Rodef Shalom Press.

Jewish Nobel Prize Winners. (2011). Retrieved from http://www.jinfo.org/Nobel_Prizes.html

Jewish Virtual Library. (2011). *Jewish population of the United States by state.* Retrieved from http://www.jewishvirtuallibrary.org/index.html

Judaism 101. (2005). *Birth and the first month of life.* Retrieved from www.jewfaq.org/birth.htm

Kranson, R. (2010). More bar than mitzvah: Anxieties over bar mitzvah receptions in postwar America. In L. Greenspoon (Ed.), *Rites of passage* (pp. 9–23). West Lafayette, IN: Purdue University Press.

Lamm, M. (2000). *The Jewish way in death and in mourning.* Middle Village, NY: Jonathan David.

Myers, M. (1988). *Response to modernity: A history of the reform movement in Judaism.* New York: Oxford University Press.

National Gaucher Foundation. (2011). Retrieved from http://www.gaucherdisease.org

Perlin, E. (2006). Jewish bioethics and medical genetics. *Journal of Religion and Health, 33*(4), 333–340.

Rosenberg, Y. (2011). *Jewish genetic diseases.* Retrieved from www.mazornet.com/genetics/index.htm

Schatzberg, A., & Nemeroff, C. (2009). *Textbook of psychopharmacology.* Arlington VA: The American Psychiatric Publishing.

Solomon, L. (2006). The quest for designer children. In W. Jacob & M. Zemer (Eds.), *Sexual issues in Jewish law.* Pittsburgh, PA: Rodef Shalom Press.

Washofsky, M. (2000). *Jewish living: A guide to contemporary reform Jewish practice.* New York: Union of American Hebrew Congregations Press (UAHC).

DavisPlus *For case studies, review questions, and additional information, go to*
http://davisplus.fadavis.com

Chapter 20

People of Korean Heritage

Eun-Ok Im

Overview, Inhabited Localities, and Topography

Overview

This chapter focuses on the commonalities among people of Korean heritage, with historical reference to the mother country, South Korea. The word *Korea* limitedly refers to the Republic of Korea. Because some information may not be pertinent to every Korean, this chapter serves as a guide for health-care providers rather than as a mandate of facts. Differences in beliefs and practices among Koreans in Korea, the United States, and other countries vary according to variant cultural characteristics as presented in Chapter 1. An understanding of Korean culture and history gives health providers the insight needed to perform culturally appropriate assessments, plan effective care and follow-up, and work effectively with Koreans in the workforce.

South Korea is a peninsula separated by North Korea to the north at the 38th parallel and surrounded by the former Soviet Union to the northeast, the Yellow Sea to the west, and the East Sea to the east. South Korea has a landmass of 98,480 square kilometers (38,031 square miles), which is about the size of the state of Indiana, and a population of 48 million (*CIA World Factbook,* 2010). South Korea has 1 percent of the landmass of the United States, but has one-sixth as many people, making it 16 times more densely populated than the United States (Kohls, 2001). The mega-modern metropolitan area of Seoul, the capital, has a population of 10.3 million people (Asianinfo, 2010a). A new international state-of-the-art airport is located in Incheon, 60 kilometers from the center of Seoul. Other large cities are Busan (Pusan) and Daegu (Taegu). Planes, trains, and buses link all South Korean major cities, making travel easy and efficient. With the recent increase in the number of automobiles and the construction of highways, motorways are becoming more congested. Major industries are electronics, telecommunications, automobile production, chemicals, shipbuilding, and steel (*CIA World Factbook,* 2010). South Korea is now well known as riding on the "*hallyu* movement" or the "Korean wave," which is the globalization of Korean dramas throughout Singapore, Malaysia, Japan, China, and the United States. Since the 1990s, the entertainment industry of South Korea has grown explosively, producing Asia-wide successes in music, television, and film (Asianinfo, 2010b).

The continental and monsoon climate of Korea is fairly consistent throughout the peninsula, except during the winter months. North Korea has cold, snowy winters, with an average temperature in January of 17°F. South Korea is milder, with an average January temperature of 23°F. During the summer months, the monsoon winds create an average temperature of 80°F, with high humidity throughout the peninsula. August is the hottest month of the year, when temperatures reach over 100°F in many areas. Precipitation occurs mostly during the summer months and is heavier in the south. The peninsula is mountainous; only 20 percent of the terrain is located in lowlands. Such topography encourages the development of concentrated living areas. Most cities and residential areas are located along the coastal plains and the inland valleys opening to the west coast.

Heritage and Residence

Korea is one of the two oldest continuous civilizations in the world, second only to China. Koreans trace their heritage to 2333 B.C. In the 1st century A.D., tribes from central and northern Asia banded together to form this "Hermit Kingdom," littering the countryside with palaces, pagodas, and gardens. Over the ensuing centuries, Mongols, Japanese, and Chinese invaded the Korean peninsula. Japan forcibly annexed Korea in the early 20th century, ruling it harshly and leaving ill will that persists to this day. As a result of the Potsdam Conference after World War II, the United States took over the occupation of South Korea, with the USSR occupying North Korea. By 1948, Korea's new government was recognized by the United Nations, only to be followed by the North Korean Communist forces invading South Korea in 1950. The result was the Korean War, which lasted until 1953 and caused mass devastation, from which the country has made a remarkable recovery. Open aggression between North and South Korea again occurred in 1998 and 1999. In 2000, the two Koreas signed a vague, yet hopeful, agreement that the two countries would be reunited. However, North Korea's recent resumption of its nuclear weapons program has set its neighbors and much of the rest of the world on edge (CNN, 2010).

In 1988, the year Seoul hosted the Olympic Games, elections were held, and relations were reestablished with China and the Soviet Union. Intermittent corruption among political officials has continued to surface, threatening internal relationships and the economy. In 1997, South Korea's economy tumbled dramatically, resulting in economic and democratic reforms. With unwavering persistence, Koreans have rebuilt their major world economy, reflecting a 4 to 5 percent annual growth rate with moderate inflation from 2003 to 2007 but decreased to .2 percent in 2009 (*CIA World Factbook,* 2010). The United States continues to maintain a strong military presence throughout South Korea (Fig. 20-1).

Reasons for Migration and Associated Economic Factors

Koreans are one of the most rapidly increasing immigrant groups in the United States (Migration Information Source, 2010). The first major immigration from Korea to the United States occurred between 1903 and 1905, when the Korean government prohibited further emigration; about 10,000 Koreans had entered Hawaii, and 1000 reached the U.S. mainland. The U.S. Immigration Act of 1924 practically closed the door to Japanese and Koreans. During the civil rights movements of the 1950s and 1960s, new immigration laws repealed the earlier limitations on Asian immigration. Koreans continue to immigrate to America to pursue the American dream, to increase socioeconomic opportunities, and to attend colleges and universities. In addition, many Koreans and Americans marry, making both Korea and America their homes. In a 2005 U.S. Census Bureau survey, an estimated 432,907 Koreans in the United States were native-born Americans, 1 million were foreign-born Korean, and more than 57 percent were women (U.S. Census Bureau, 2006).

Most of the population pursues higher education, and South Korea has more citizens with PhDs per capita than any other country in the world. Owing to Confucian cultural influence, education is emphasized as a virtue of human beings (all human beings should be educated) and is highly valued in the Korean culture (Im, 2002).

Before the late 19th century, education was primarily for those who could afford it. State schools educated the youth from the *yangban* (upper class), focusing on Chinese classics in the belief that these contained the tools of Confucian morality and philosophy that also apply in politics. In the late 1800s, the state schools were opened to all citizens. Early Christian missionary work introduced the Western style of modern education to Korea. Initially, many Koreans were skeptical of the radical curriculum and instruction for females, but the popularity of this style grew rapidly.

After the takeover of Korea by the Japanese in 1910, two types of schools emerged—one for Japanese and another for Koreans. The Korean schools focused on vocational training, which prepared Koreans for only lower-level positions. Japanese colonial education was designed to keep Koreans subordinate to ethnic Japanese in all ways (Sorensen, 1994). In 1949, South Korea allowed for the implementation of an educational system similar to that of the United States. This 6–3–3–4 ladder (6 years in elementary school, 3 years in junior high, 3 years in high school, and 4 years in college) continues today in contemporary South Korea. Anti-Communism and morality are taught throughout elementary and secondary schools.

In the United States, many Koreans own their own small businesses, which vary from mom-and-pop stores and gas stations to grocery stores and real estate agencies to retail shops. Their reputation for hard work, independence, and self-motivation has given them the label "the model minority." However, this has caused a backlash in some communities, such as Washington, DC, where they have been compared with other minority groups. The message has become "If the Koreans can do it, why not other groups?" The turmoil and riots that took place in Los Angeles in April 1992 between the African American community and the Korean American merchants are examples of conflicts that arise from such labeling.

Many Korean small businesses are located in African American neighborhoods because of low capital investment requirements and limited resources of the owners. Korean merchants begin dealing in inexpensive consumer goods as a practical way to start a business in a capitalistic society. Koreans often assist each other in establishing businesses by pooling their

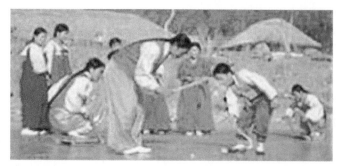

Figure 20-1 Traditional Korean games that are played in the beginning of a new year.

money and taking turns with rotating credit associations to provide each family with the opportunity for financial success.

Communication

Dominant Language and Dialects

The dominant language in Korea is *Korean*, or *han'gul*, which originated in the 15th century with King Se Jong, and is believed to be the first phonetic alphabet in East Asia. Several dialects exist in the Korean language, called *saturi* in Korean (Korean Language, 2010). The Korean standard language in South Korea is based on the dialect of the area around *Seoul*, and the Korean standard language in North Korea is based on the dialect of the area around *Pyongyang*. All the dialects of Koreans are similar to one another except that of Jeju Island (Korean Language, 2010). The most notable difference among dialects is the accent. For example, the Korean standard language has a very flat intonation, while the Gyeongsang dialect has a very strong accent and intonation (Korean Language, 2010).

The Korean language has four levels of speech that are determined based on the degree of intimacy between speakers. These varying levels reflect inequalities in social status based on gender, age, and social positions. Use of an inappropriate sociolinguistic level of speech is unacceptable and is normally interpreted as intended formality to, disrespect for, or contempt to a social superior.

Chinese and Japanese have influenced the Korean language. Before the Japanese occupation in Korea, highly educated Koreans used Chinese characters, and Chinese characters were taught in Korean traditional schools. Then, during the Japanese occupation in the early 20th century, the Japanese forbade public use of the Korean language, requiring the use of the Japanese written and spoken language, which introduced some Japanese terms and words into contemporary Korean language.

Most Koreans in the United States can speak, read, write, and understand English to some degree. However, some Americans may have difficulty understanding the English spoken by Koreans, especially those who learned English from Koreans who spoke with their native intonations and pronunciations.

Cultural Communication Patterns

Sharing thoughts, feelings, and ideas is very much based on age, gender, and status in Korean society. Traditionally, the Korean community values the group over the individual, men over women, and age over youth. Those holding the dominant position are the decision makers who share thoughts and ideas on issues.

Koreans prefer indirect communication because they perceive direct communication as an indication of intention or opinions as rude. Moreover, Koreans may agree with the health-care provider in order to avoid conflict or hurting someone's feelings, even if something is impossible (Im, 2002). Thus, it is important to read between the lines when working with these families and remember those growing up in the United States may adopt the dominant American communication style.

Koreans tend to avoid eye contact, especially with older people, perceived authorities (e.g., health-care providers), and strangers. Avoiding direct eye contact with older people and perceived authorities indicates respect, and women's avoiding direct eye contact with men shows modesty. Younger generations of Koreans educated in the United States may adopt the dominant communication style of eye contact. Koreans are usually comfortable with silence owing to the Confucian teaching "Silence is golden." Silence was traditionally emphasized as a virtue of educated people. Even among Korean Americans, people who are silent, especially men, are viewed as humble and well educated. However, the social fabric and cultural norms of Koreans are changing as they interact with Western societies and culture. Younger generations of Koreans, even in South Korea, are noted as being very sociable and kind to visitors (Asianinfo, 2010a).

Close personal space (less than a foot) is shared with family members and close friends, but it is inappropriate for strangers to step into "intimate space" unless needed for health care (Im, 2002). Visitors from America may be uncomfortable with Koreans' spatial distancing in public spaces. Koreans stand close to one another and do not excuse themselves if they bump into someone on the street. This may be due to the high population density in the metropolitan areas of South Korea and Koreans' cultural attitudes toward strangers (e.g., they usually do not speak with strangers). Among family members and close friends, touching, friendly pushing, and hugging are accepted. However, among strangers, touching is considered disrespectful unless needed for care. Also, touching among friends and social equals of the same sex is common and does not carry a homosexual connotation as it might in Western societies. However, more social etiquette rules apply when it comes to touching older family members or those of higher social status. Hugging and kissing recently have become common among parents and young children, as well as among young children and aunts or uncles.

Feelings are infrequently communicated in facial expressions. Smiling a lot shows a lack of intellect and disrespect. One would not smile at a stranger on the street or joke around during a serious conversation. Joking and amusement have their designated times. In Korea, men frequent bars after work and may express their sense of humor in this setting. Men and women alike appreciate and encourage jokes and laughter in appropriate settings. Koreans generally do not express their emotions directly or in public; expressing emotions in front of others, including family members, is regarded as shameful, especially among men (Im, 2002). A common Korean belief related to men's emotions is that men should cry only three times in their lives: when they are born, when their parents die, and when their country perishes (Im, 2002). Given these cultural communication patterns, health-care providers should not interpret these nonverbal behaviors as meaning that Korean patients are not interested in, or do not care about, information presented during health teaching and health promotion interventions.

Temporal Relationships

Traditional Koreans are past oriented. Much attention is paid to the ancestry of a family. Yearly, during the Harvest Moon in Korea, *chusok* (respect) is paid to ancestors by bringing fresh fruits from the autumn harvest, dry fish, and rice wine to gravesites. However, the younger and more educated generation is more futuristic and achievement oriented.

In Korea, Korean traditional shamans (called *modang* and/or *jumjangi*) are visited to determine the best home to purchase, the best date for having a wedding, and the best time to start a new business. The busiest time of the year for the shaman is just before the Chinese New Year. Koreans are eager to know their fortune for the coming year. Many believe that misfortunes occur because ancestors are unhappy. During these times, families show respect to ancestors by more frequent visits to their gravesites in the hope of appeasing the spirits. Shamans, who may be used by Koreans of all socioeconomic levels, are also used in Korea to rid homes and new places of business of spirits. The Korean concept of time depends on the circumstances. Koreans embrace the Western respect

for time for important appointments, transportation connections, and working hours, all of which are recognized as situations in which punctuality is necessary. Yet, socially, Korean Americans arrive at parties and visit family and friends up to 30 minutes later (and sometimes 1 to 2 hours later) than the agreed-upon time. This is socially acceptable when the person or family is waiting at home. If the social meeting is being held in a public setting, a half-hour time span for arrival at the meetingplace can be expected.

Format for Names

The number of surnames in Korea is limited, with the most common ones being Kim, Lee, Park, Rhee or Yi, Choi or Choe, and Chung or Jung. Korean names contain two Chinese characters, one of which describes the generation and the other the person's given name. The surname comes first; however, because this may be confusing to many Americans, some Koreans in the United States follow the Western tradition of using the given name first, followed by the surname. Adults are not addressed by their given names unless they are on friendly terms; individuals should be addressed by their surname with the title Mr., Mrs., Ms., Dr., or Minister.

Given the diversity and acculturation of Korean Americans, health-care providers need to determine the Korean patient's language ability, comfort level with silence, and spatial-distancing characteristics. In addition, Koreans should be addressed formally until they indicate otherwise.

Family Roles and Organization
Head of Household and Gender Roles

Fundamental ideas about morality and the proper ordering of human relationships among Koreans are closely associated with kinship values derived mainly from Confucian concepts of filial piety, ancestor worship, funerary rites, position of women, the institution of marriage, kinship groups, social status and rank, and respect for scholars and political officials. Although constitutional law in South Korea declares equality for all citizens, not all aspects of society have accepted this. Korean culture is largely based on patriarchal and Confucian norms that subordinate women (Im, 2002). In Confucian traditional Korean families, the father was always the head of the family; he had power to control the family, and the family had to obey any order from the father. Wives did not share household tasks with their husbands, so they tended to be physically overloaded and psychologically distressed. Wives' exploitation was hidden under Confucian norms that praised women who sacrifice themselves for their families and nation (Im & Meleis, 2001). Also, the wife was confined to the home and bore the major responsibility for household tasks; the husband was the breadwinner.

REFLECTIVE EXERCISE 20.1

Lisa, a school nurse, is examining Mina Lee, who was referred by her teacher because of her reluctance to speak in class. Mina Lee is a first-grader whose family has recently immigrated from South Korea. She is the second child of her family, and she is living with her mother, father, and brother who do not speak English fluently.

1. What should the nurse to do assess Mina's reluctance to speak in class?
2. Could language be a possible barrier?
3. What cultural barriers besides language might explain Mina's silence in class?
4. What are the traditional Korean cultural attitudes and values related to silence and teacher–student relationships?
5. What are some implications for nursing practices for children who recently immigrated from Korean culture?

Nowadays, this typical family structure has been changed, especially among younger generations. Many women and men remain single until their 30s and 40s. Even when they marry, they sometimes do not have a child; they choose to enjoy their lives rather than raise the next generation.

Among Korean immigrants in the United States, women hold the family together and play a vital role in building an economic base for the family and community, often sacrificing themselves in the immigration process. The Korean immigrant woman may have started as a cleaning woman or seamstress, then worked at a fast-food restaurant, and then in a small shop owned with her husband. However, the women's financial contributions to the family usually do not change the gender roles; their husbands still occupy center stage, exercise the authority, and make the major family decisions (Im & Meleis, 2001).

Prescriptive, Restrictive, and Taboo Behaviors for Children and Adolescents

In contrast to the Western culture in which mothering is individually fashioned and relies on the expertise of health-care providers, in the highly ritualistic Korean culture mothering is molded by societal rules and information is less frequently sought from health-care providers. In this context, mothers tend to view infants as passive and dependent, and they seek guidance from folklore and the extended family (Choi, 1995). In Korea, children over the age of 5 years are expected to be well behaved because the whole family is disgraced if a child acts in an embarrassing manner. Most children are not encouraged to state their opinions. Parents usually make the decisions.

Korean families have high standards and expectations for their children, and "giving a whip to a beloved child" is the basis for discipline of children (Im, 2002). Thus, the pressure of high performance in school and entering a highly ranked university is prevalent among Korean children and adolescents (Im, 2002). Usually, Koreans are not happy with very masculine girls or very feminine boys (Im, 2002).

"Teaching to the test" is also common in Korea, but the role of teachers is also to encourage self-study. The future of Korean students is determined by their teachers' recommendations, and this pressure can be extremely intense for students who are not doing well. The teaching style is one in which students listen and learn what is being taught. Regardless of private doubts, a student rarely questions a teacher's authority. Korean children in America must be taught the teaching style in American schools, in which questioning is positive and is valued as class participation. Even if Korean American students understand the style of teaching, it can be difficult to know the appropriate timing for asking questions.

The pressure of doing well in school and attending a university of high quality leaves Korean adolescents little room for social interactions. Activities that interfere with one's education are considered taboo for adolescents. In Korea, students frequently attend study groups after school or special tutoring sessions paid for by their families in preparation for examinations to enter a university. Short coffee breaks or snacks at local coffee shops or noodle houses are permissible, but then it is "back to the books."

Dating is now common among high school students in South Korea. Even an elementary student would say that she or he has a boyfriend or a girlfriend. Yet, adolescent girls are usually not allowed to spend the night at their friends' houses, virginity is emphasized, and sexual activities and pregnancy at puberty stigmatize the family across social classes. Although talking about sexuality, contraception, or pregnancy in public is taboo, close girlfriends or boyfriends exchange information on these topics or get their information from women's magazines. Neither the school system nor the family assumes responsibility for sex education. Girls in elementary school are given a class regarding their menstrual cycle, but no information is given about sexual relations.

Once young adults have entered a university, they receive their freedom and are then permitted to make their own decisions about personal and study time. Group outings are common for meeting the opposite sex. Dating may occur from these group meetings and consists of movies, dinner, and walks in the park.

Issues arise between the first-generation Korean immigrant parents and the second-generation children in relation to conflicting values and communication. With rapid acculturation, the second generation often takes on the values of the dominant society or culture. Thus, parents who are of the first generation in most cases are challenged when their second-generation children do not accept traditional values and ideals that they may still hold dear. The different cultures between the first-generation parents and the second-generation children are sometimes the cause of domestic violence. Most of the first generation of Korean immigrants were educated in Korea, and they have a strong stereotype of Korean patriarchal culture. However, because the second generation is educated in the United States (some of them never visited Korea), most second-generation individuals feel a spirit of insubordination and often quarrel. For some, physical abuse might be involved if they do not follow orders (Kim, Cain, & McCubbin, 2006; Kim & Chung, 2003; Park, 2001).

Family Goals and Priorities

In a Korean traditional family, family members have specific rights and duties within their family. For example, the first son inherits all the properties of his parents and has the duty of caring for his elderly parents until they die. A family member replaces the roles of another family member who dies. Thus, if the first son dies, the second son is in charge of all the duties of the first son. However, this traditional family system is dissolving among both Koreans and Korean Americans. Usually in Korean Americans, both parents work to provide every opportunity possible for their family. As each family member learns to adjust to the changing roles in the new country, conflict can result. Children adapt most easily to the new culture and may even take on the dominant culture's values.

Lee and Lee (1990) studied the adjustment of Korean immigrant families in the United States in relation to roles, values, and living conditions between husbands and wives, and parents and children. The findings showed a transition from an independent family structure, in which the woman had little knowledge of the man's activities outside the home, to a joint family structure. Many activities were carried out together with an interchange of roles at home. Conflict centered on undefined role expectations. In Korea, the roles of men and women were very clear. However, upon immigrating to the United States, men and women were faced with conflicting roles in the new culture and had to struggle to redefine them. Other conflict areas were the couple's ability to speak English, the woman's inability to drive, the degree of acculturation, the limited social contact, and the stressors of living in a new culture.

In Korea, education is a family priority. The outcome of having a highly educated child was a secure old age for the parents. Because of the dependent relationship between parents and their children, parents were more willing to make drastic sacrifices for the advancement of their children's education. Today, status is achieved rather than inherited in Korea. Education in Korea is a determinant of status, independent of its contribution to economic success.

Traditionally in Korea, parents expected their children to care for them in old age. *Hyo* (filial piety), which is the obligation to respect and obey parents, care for them in old age, give them a good funeral, and worship them after death, was a core value of Korean ethics. The obligation to care for one's parents is written into civil code in Korea. The burden was on the eldest son, who was obliged to reside with his parents and carry on the family line. Such an arrangement made the generations dependent on each other. The son felt obligated to care for his parents because of the sacrifices they made for him. Similarly, he made the same sacrifices for his children and expected them to provide for him and his wife in their old age. Many of these traditions in Korea have changed. Some of the eldest children emigrated, leaving the responsibility for their parents to the siblings who remained in Korea.

Some older Koreans were brought to the United States without their friends and with minimal or no English skills. They often felt obligated to assist the family in any way possible by preparing meals or taking care of the children when the parents were not home. Decision making for older people was hampered in their new culture. Korean older people were frequently consulted on important family matters as a sign of respect for their life experiences. Older people's roles as decision makers in the United States have shifted with the younger generation of Korean Americans wanting the final decision-making authority in their young families.

Traditionally, Koreans give great respect to their elders. Old age begins when one reaches the age of 60 years, with an impressive celebration prepared for the occasion. The historical significance of this celebration is related to the Chinese lunar calendar. The lunar calendar has 60 cycles, each with a different name. At the age of 60, the person is starting the calendar cycle over again. This is called **hwangap**. This celebration was more significant in the past when life expectancy in Korea was much lower than it is today. Despite a change in the direct role of older people in their families, older Koreans are socially well respected in Korea. In public, an older woman is called *Halmoni* (grandmother), and those who are not blood relatives call an older man *Harabuji* (grandfather). Older people are offered seats on buses out of respect and honor. However, recent changes in Korean culture have made this tradition change as well. Sometimes quarrels between older people and young people, usually about respect, are reported in the daily news in South Korea.

Traditionally, the extended Korean family played an important role in supporting its members throughout the life span. With the breakup of the extended family, Korean Americans support one another through secondary organizations such as the church. The church assists new immigrants with the transition to life in the United States. The church is a resource for information about child care, language classes, and social activities (Im & Yang, 2006). Korean Americans without family support may seek other Korean Americans who live in the area. With Korean Americans dispersed throughout the United States, this task can be difficult.

Whereas some Koreans inherit social status, many have the ability to change their status through their education and professions. Traditional Korean culture espouses respect not only for older people but also for those of valued professions. In modern Korea, professors, bureaucrats, business executives, physicians, and attorneys receive a high level of respect. Historically, those with the highest education were handsomely paid. Even though the salary differences between university professors and other professions have narrowed significantly in recent years in Korea, the status of the intellectual remains high. Similarly, the bureaucratic officer has a high social status, wielding much respect and influence.

Alternative Lifestyles

Alternative lifestyles are usually frowned upon in Korean culture. Women who divorce suffer social stigma, the degree of which depends on the situation. However, recent changes in the Family Law in South Korea now permit women to head a household, recognize a wife's right to a portion of the couple's property, and allow a woman to maintain greater contact with her children after a divorce. South Korea now has one of the highest divorce rates in the world; Korea has the highest divorce rate among 33 Organization for Economic Cooperation and Development (OECD) countries (OECD, 2010). Yet, the stigma of divorce remains strong among Koreans in both South Korea and the United States, and there is little government or private assistance for divorced women in South Korea. Mixed marriages, between a Korean and a non-Korean, are highly disregarded by some, and the Korean government makes it very difficult for these marriages to occur. Korean women who have married American servicemen are often the objects of Korean jokes and are ridiculed by some.

Living together before marriage is not customary in Korea. If pregnancy occurs outside marriage, it may be taken care of quietly and without family and friends being aware of the situation. However, with recent changes in Korean culture, some celebrities began to announce their pregnancies before marriage, and a pregnancy right before marriage is not looked upon as harshly as in the past. In the United States, pregnancy outside of marriage may not carry such a great stigma among the more acculturated.

As in other Asian cultures, homosexuality has not been accepted in Korean culture (Kimmel & Yi, 2004). Also, Korean's understanding and knowledge of homosexuality are ambiguous and limited (Kim & Hahn, 2006). Koreans believe that homosexuality is an abnormal and impure modern phenomenon. Despite the recent coming out of several Korean homosexual entertainers in South Korea, those who have relations with a person of the same sex still remain "in the closet." Personal disclosure to friends and family usually jeopardizes the family name and may lead to ostracism. The community may stigmatize both the family and the individual, making it difficult to conduct their personal lives.

Workforce Issues

Culture in the Workplace

Korean Americans come from a culture that places a high value on education. Many Korean immigrants are college educated and held white-collar jobs in Korea. Moreover, it is difficult for Korean immigrants to obtain work in the United States commensurate with their experience because of language difficulties, restricted access to corporate America, and unfamiliarity with American culture (Im & Meleis, 2001). The skills and work experiences they had in Korea are often not accepted by American businesses, forcing them to take jobs in which they may be over skilled while they save money to start their own businesses. Korean American women frequently need to find jobs to assist the family financially, which may cause role conflicts between more traditional husbands and wives.

Korean Americans have a strong work ethic. They work long hours each week for the advancement of family opportunities. Family is the priority for Korean Americans, but on the surface this may not always be apparent when long hours are devoted to work. The goal is to save money for education and other opportunities so the family can provide for their children in the future.

The number of Korean medical personnel working in the American health-care system is unknown. Significant numbers of Korean nurses and physicians are practicing in the United States and Canada; many have received part or all of their education in the United States. Yi and Jezewski's study (2000) of 12 Korean nurses' adjustment to hospitals in the United States identified five phases of adjustment. The first three phases—relieving psychological stress, overcoming language barriers, and accepting American nursing practices—take 2 to 3 years. The remaining two phases—adopting the styles of American problem-solving strategies and adopting the styles of American interpersonal relationships—take an additional 5 to 10 years. Accordingly, orientation programs need to address language skills, practice differences, and communication and interpersonal relationships to help Koreans adjust to the American workforce. These same phases may occur with other Korean health-care providers.

Issues Related to Autonomy

Those in supervisory positions need to recognize the roles and relationships that exist between Koreans and their employers. A supervisor is treated with much respect in work and in social settings. Informalities and small talk may be difficult for Korean immigrants. For an employee to refuse an employer's request is unacceptable, even if the employee does not want or feel qualified to complete the request. Supervisors should make an effort to promote open conversation and the expression of ideas among Korean Americans. Asking Korean employees to demonstrate procedures is better than asking them whether they know how to perform them. Those who have adjusted to the American business style may be more assertive in their positions, but an understanding of this work role gives supervisors the tools to more readily use Korean Americans' skills and knowledge.

As with any new language, it is often difficult to understand American slang and colloquial language. Employers and other employees should be clear in their communication style and be understanding of miscommunications. Ethnic biases are often directed at Korean Americans who speak English with an accent. Employers' and coworkers' preconceived notions of immigrants can also be a deterrent to Korean Americans in the workforce.

Biocultural Ecology

Skin Color and Other Biological Variations

Koreans are an ethnically homogeneous Mongoloid people who have shared a common history, language, and culture since the 7th century A.D. when the peninsula was first united. Common physical characteristics include dark hair and dark eyes, with variations in skin color and degree of hair darkness. Skin color ranges from fair to light brown. Epicanthal skin folds create the distinctive appearance of Asian eyes. With the popularity of drastic plastic surgeries in recent years, Koreans' typical facial characteristics might not be easily found in some cases.

Diseases and Health Conditions

Schistosomiasis and other parasitic diseases are endemic to certain regions of Korea, and Koreans love sushi and *sashimi* (raw fish). Therefore, health-care providers should consider parasite screening with Korean immigrants, when appropriate. South Korea continues to manufacture and use asbestos-containing products and has not taken the precautions necessary to adequately protect employees and meet international standards. Thus, Korean immigrants to the United States need to be assessed for asbestos-related health problems (Johanning, Goldberg, & Kim, 1994).

The high prevalence of stomach and liver cancer, tuberculosis, hepatitis, and hypertension in South Korea predispose recent immigrants to these conditions. High rates of hypertension lead to an increase in cardiovascular accidents and renal failure. The high incidence of stomach cancer is associated with environmental risks, such as diet and infection (*Helicobacter pylori*), and in some cases, genetic predisposition (Kim, 2003). As with other Asians, a high occurrence of lactose intolerance exists among people of Korean ancestry. Dental hygiene and preventive dentistry have recently been emphasized in health promotion in South Korea. Because of the high incidence of gum disease and oral problems, however, these conditions deserve attention.

Variations in Drug Metabolism

Growing research in the field of pharmacogenetics has found variations in drug metabolism among ethnic groups. Studies suggest that Asian populations require lower dosages of psychotropic drugs (Levy, 1993). Other studies have shown variations in drug metabolism and interaction with propranolol, isoniazid, and diazepam among Asians in comparison with those of European Americans and other ethnic groups (Meyer, 1992). Although these studies primarily focus on people of Chinese and Japanese heritage, health-care providers should be aware and attentive to the possibility of drug metabolism variations among Korean Americans (Munoz & Hilgenberg, 2005).

High-Risk Behaviors

Because Koreans place great emphasis on education, many subject their children to intense pressure to do well in school. A national survey conducted among 80,000 middle and high school students in South Korea demonstrated such pressures: 1 out of 20 Korean youths attempted suicide, and a major reason was their lack of success in school (The Hankyoreh, 2007). Similar pressures have been seen in the United States, where suicide has occurred in Korean high school and college students because of intense pressure to do well in school.

Korea has a high incidence of alcohol consumption, up from 7.0 liters in 1980 to 8.1 liters per adult per capita, which is similar to that of the United States and Ireland at 7.8 liters per adult per capita (World Health Organization, 2004). Korean business transactions commonly occur after the decision makers have had several drinks. Koreans believe that people let their masks down when they drink and that they truly get to know someone after they have had a few drinks. Socioeconomic changes in Korea have resulted in differences in alcohol-related social and health problems, with a change from drinking mild fermented beverages with meals to drinking distilled liquors without meals.

REFLECTIVE EXERCISE 20.2

Laurie, a nurse working at a local clinic, is assessing Young Kim, who is a high school senior entering college in the coming fall. Born in South Korea, he was 4 years old when his family emigrated from South Korea. His mother accompanied him to the clinic to get his immunization records cleared for his entrance to college. All immunization records were adequately documented in his medical records, but there was an issue related to his tuberculosis (TB) immunization because his TB skin test was positive. His mother claimed that he received the Bacille Calmette Guerin (BCG) vaccination.

1. What might explain Young's positive TB skin test?
2. Most Korean immigrants have BCG immunization records and subsequent positive TB skin tests. What are the pros and cons of BCG vaccination, subsequent positive TB skin tests, x-rays for verifying TB status, and taking preventive medications?
3. Besides tuberculosis, what are some other prevalent infectious diseases among Koreans?

In Korea, women drink far less than men. Sons' drinking patterns are similar to their fathers' patterns. A substantial generational difference exists among females, with daughters abstaining from alcohol less frequently than their mothers and drinking more, and more often, than their mothers (Weatherspoon, Park, & Johnson, 2001). In the United States and South Korea, drinking and vehicular accidents among Koreans and Korean Americans are a cause for concern.

In a study by Lew and colleagues (2001), about 39 percent of Korean American men and 6 percent of Korean American women were current smokers. Lee, Sobal, and Frongillo (2000) also found that bicultural Korean men were least likely to smoke, whereas acculturated and bicultural women were more likely than traditional women to smoke. In Korea, a few women do smoke, and for those who do, smoking in public, such as on the street, is considered taboo.

Cho and Faulkner (1993) studied the cultural conceptions of alcoholism among Korean and American university students. Students had to decide whether the person described in a vignette was an "alcoholic" or not and why. The results showed that American-born students tended to define alcoholism in terms of social and interpersonal problems related to drinking, whereas Korean-born students defined alcoholism in terms of physical degeneration and physiological addiction. The authors caution against the misuse of American concepts and diagnostic scales in the cross-cultural arena. Cultural factors should be examined closely in relation to the study, diagnosis, and treatment of alcohol problems. Nakashima and Wong (2000) also reported alcohol misuse among Korean American adolescents and concluded that alcohol misuse among Korean American adolescents is influenced by the social variables found to affect the use among other ethnic groups, such as psychological variables (depression, self-esteem), perceived prejudice, and feeling safe where one lives.

Health-Care Practices

Seat belts are infrequently worn in South Korea, although seat belts are now mandatory (U.S. Department of State, 2010). Korean Americans understand the legal mandates in the United States and comply with seat belt and child-restraint laws.

Hobbies such as hiking and golf are enjoyed in South Korea. Korean Americans do not identify hiking as a frequent pastime, either because of environmental constraints or because of living situations. Golf remains a significant activity among those Korean Americans who are financially able to play the sport.

Nutrition

Meaning of Food

Food takes on a significant meaning when one has been without food. Many Koreans over the age of 60 who lived during the Korean War experienced a time when their next meal was not guaranteed. Because of a devastated economy and agricultural base, barley and *kimchee*, a spicy pickled cabbage, were dietary staples during the war. Koreans are taught to respect and not waste food.

Common Foods and Food Rituals

Korean food is flavorful and spicy. Rice is served with 3 to 5 (and sometimes up to 20) small side dishes of mostly vegetables and some fish and meats. Seasonings in Korean cooking include red and black pepper, garlic, green onion, ginger, soy sauce, and sesame seed oil. The traditional Korean diet includes steamed rice; hot soup; *kimchee*; and side dishes of fish, meat, or vegetables served in some variation for breakfast, lunch, and dinner. Breakfast is traditionally considered the most important meal.

Kimchee is made from a variety of vegetables but is primarily made from a Chinese, or Napa, cabbage (Fig. 20-2). Spices and herbs are added to the previously salted cabbage, which is allowed to ferment over time and is served with every meal in a variety of forms. Some common Korean American dishes include the following:

- *Beebimbap* is a combination of rice, finely chopped mixed vegetables, and a fried egg served in a hot pottery bowl. Hot pepper paste is usually added.
- *Bulgolgi* is thinly sliced pieces of beef marinated in soy sauce, sesame oil, green onions, garlic, and sugar, which is then barbecued.
- *Chopchae* are clear noodles mixed with lightly stir-fried vegetables and meats.

Rice is usually served in individual bowls, set to the left of the diner. Soup is served in another bowl, placed to the right of the rice. Chopsticks and large soupspoons are used at all meals. Korean Americans

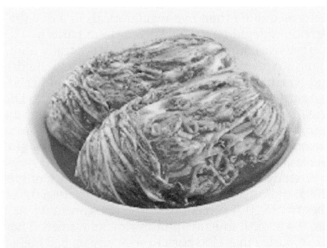

Figure 20-2 Kimchee, a spicy pickled cabbage that is a staple of the Korean diet.

may use forks and knives, depending on their degree of assimilation into American culture. Meals are frequently eaten in silence, using this opportunity to enjoy the food. When Koreans migrate to the United States, they increase their consumption of beef, dairy products, coffee, soda, and bread, as well as decrease their intake of fish, rice, and other grains. However, incorporating a larger quantity of Western foods does not make a less healthy diet. They consume diets consistent with their traditional Korean food patterns, with 60 percent of calories coming from carbohydrates and 16 percent of calories from fat (Kim, Yu, Chen, Cross, & Kim, 2000). To increase compliance with dietary prescriptions, health teaching should be geared to the unique Korean American food choices and practices.

Understanding the ritual offering of food and drink to guests is important. Koreans offer a guest a drink on first arriving at their home. The guest declines courteously. The host offers the drink again and the guest again declines. This ritual can occur three to five times before the guest accepts the offer. This interaction is done out of respect for the hosts and their generosity to share with their guest and to express an unwillingness to impose on the hosts. Accepting an offer when first asked is considered rude and selfish.

Dietary Practices for Health Promotion

Most dietary practices for health promotion apply to pregnancy, discussed later in this chapter. Someone suffering from the common cold is served soup made from bean sprouts. Dried anchovies, garlic, and other hot spices are added to the hot soup, which assists in clearing a congested nose.

Nutritional Deficiencies and Food Limitations

Lee, Lee, Kim, and Han (2009) conducted an in-depth assessment of the nutritional status of 202 Korean American elderly in a metropolitan city on the East Coast and reported that the Korean American elderly consumed more than two regular meals in a day that were considered part of a Korean food pattern. The average consumption of nutrients was generally lower than in Americans reported in the National Health and Nutrition Examination Survey III, except carbohydrates, vegetable protein, and sodium intake. The researchers noted inadequate intake of calcium, dietary fiber, and folate, and suggested that health-care providers consider ways to lower sodium intake and increase fruit and vegetable consumption.

A study by Park, Murphy, Sharma, and Kolonel (2005) indicated that the proportion of overweight or obesity was 31.4 percent in U.S.-born Korean women and 9.4 percent in Korean-born Korean women. They also reported that U.S.-born Korean women had higher intakes of total fat and fat as a percentage of energy and lower intakes of sodium, vitamin C, beta-carotene,

and carbohydrate as a percentage of energy than Korean-born women. In addition, Cho and Juon (2006) reported that of 492 Korean American respondents, 38 percent were overweight and 8 percent were obese according to the World Health Organization for Asian populations. These findings suggest that acculturation of Korean immigrants affects dietary intakes in ways that may alter their risks of several chronic diseases.

Korean Americans, as with most other Asians, are at a high risk for lactose intolerance. Thus, milk and other dairy products are not part of the traditional Korean diet, emphasizing the need to assess them for calcium deficiencies.

Korean Americans living in or near large metropolitan cities have access to Korean markets and restaurants. When no Korean stores are available, Chinese or Japanese markets may contain some of the foods Koreans enjoy. When no Asian markets are available, the American grocery store suffices.

Pregnancy and Childbearing Practices

Fertility Practices and Views Toward Pregnancy

To curtail population growth in Korea, the government promotes the concept of two children per household. The government supported the use of contraception when a 10-year family planning program was adopted in the early 1960s, resulting in a mass public education program on contraception. When contraceptive devices became easily available in Korea, fertility control spread widely among married women. Contraceptive devices are covered by the present national health insurance of Korea. Recently, South Korea's fertility rate fell to a new record low in 2007 as more women engaged in economic activities and got married at older ages (*The Korean Times,* 2007). The average number of babies per woman of childbearing age was 1.19 as of the end of 2006, which is much lower than the average 2.56 for the UN member countries (*The Korean Times,* 2007).

Induced abortion only with legally acceptable rationales is allowed in South Korea, yet there is an unspoken acceptance of the practice. The legally acceptable reasons for induced abortion include genetic defects, communicable diseases, pregnancy due to rape, pregnancy by family members or close relatives, and pregnancy that threatens the mother's health.

Pritham and Sammons (1993) investigated Korean women's attitudes toward pregnancy and prenatal care with regard to their beliefs and interactions with health-care providers from the United States. The survey was conducted with 40 unemployed Korean women between the ages of 18 and 35 at an American military medical-care facility in a major metropolitan area of Korea. Attitudes toward childbearing practices and relationships with health-care providers were elicited. The results indicated that these women were happy about their pregnancies. Only one-third of the respondents agreed with the traditional preference for a male child. About 40 percent of the women reinforced strong food taboos and restrictions and acknowledged the need to avoid certain foods during pregnancy. Twenty percent disagreed with the use of prenatal vitamins, and 25 percent indicated needing only a 10- to 15-pound weight gain in pregnancy. The women generally had sound health habits in relation to physical activity and recognized the harm of smoking while pregnant. The study sample was homogeneous and small, limiting the ability to generalize about the findings.

Pregnancy in the Korean culture is traditionally a highly protected time for women. Both the pregnancy and the postpartum period have been ritualized by the culture. A pregnancy begins with the ***tae-mong***, a dream of the conception of pregnancy. Once a woman is pregnant, she starts practicing ***tae-kyo***, which literally means "fetus education." The objective of *tae-kyo* is to promote the health and well-being of the fetus and the mother by having the mother focus on art and beautiful objects. Some beliefs include the following:

- If the pregnant woman handles unclean objects or kills a living creature, a difficult birth can ensue (Howard & Barbiglia, 1997).
- Some women wear tight abdominal binders beginning at 20 weeks gestation or work physically hard toward the end of the pregnancy to increase the chances of having a small baby (Howard & Barbiglia, 1997).
- In addition, expectant mothers should avoid duck, chicken, fish with scales, squid, or crab because eating these foods may affect the child's appearance. For example, eating duck may cause the baby to be born with webbed feet (Howard & Barbiglia, 1997).

REFLECTIVE EXERCISE 20.3

Alex, a nurse working at a prenatal clinic in a hospital, is assessing Sook Park, who is 12 weeks pregnant. Sook was raised and educated in South Korea; recently married Robert Kim, a Korean American; and moved to the United States early in her pregnancy. Alex found that Sook lost 5 pounds since her last visit.

1. From a cultural standpoint, what might explain Sook's recent loss of weight?
2. Identify Koreans' cultural beliefs, attitudes, and practices related to foods during pregnancy.
3. What Korean cultural beliefs, attitudes, and practices related to foods during pregnancy might explain Sook's weight loss?
4. What are some immigration and acculturation issues that might influence Sook's nutrition?

Prescriptive, Restrictive, and Taboo Practices in the Childbearing Family

Ludman, Kang, and Lynn's study (1992) explored the food beliefs and diets of 200 pregnant Korean American women. The food items most frequently consumed were *kimchee* (82.5 percent), rice or noodles (81.5 percent), and fresh fruit (79 percent). Foods avoided during pregnancy included coffee (19.8 percent), spicy foods (9.9 percent), chicken (6.9 percent), and crab (6.9 percent). A list of 20 food items was then given to the women, who were asked to respond whether they consumed the food or not and, if not, to indicate their reasons. A number of respondents indicated that they did not eat rabbit (91.5 percent), sparrow (91.5 percent), duck (89.5 percent), goat (84 percent), or blemished fruit (63 percent) because of dislike or lack of availability. The reason most frequently given for not eating blemished fruit was that it might produce a skin disease on the infant or cause an unpleasant face. The study showed that although many Korean American women were aware of traditionally taboo foods, they did not avoid consuming them. An awareness of these beliefs can give health providers a basis for nutritional education for Korean American women.

Birthing practices among both Koreans and Korean Americans are highly influenced by Western methods. Women commonly labor and deliver in the supine position. After the delivery, women are traditionally served seaweed soup, a rich source of iron, which is believed to facilitate lactation and to promote healing of the mother. Bed rest is encouraged after pregnancy for 7 to 90 days. Women are also encouraged to keep warm by avoiding showers, baths, and cold fluids or foods.

The postpartum period is seen as the time when women undergo profound physiological, psychological, and sociological changes; this period is known as the *Sanhujori* belief system. In this dynamic process, postpartum women should care for their bodies by augmenting heat and avoiding cold, resting without working, eating well, protecting the body from harmful strains, and keeping clean (Howard & Barbiglia, 1997). In Western society in which they may lack extended family members from whom to seek assistance, Korean women may be faced with a cultural dilemma.

Park and Peterson (1991) studied Korean American women's health beliefs, practices, and experiences in relation to childbirth. Using structured questions, they interviewed in Korean a nonrandom sample of 20 female volunteers. Those interviewed subscribed to a holistic view, which emphasized both emotional and physical health. Only one-half of the women interviewed rated themselves healthy. The authors related this to the stresses of immigration and pregnancy. Preventive practices were not found among members of this group. Only one woman regularly received Pap smears and did breast self-examinations. A common finding was that most women participated in a significant rest period during puerperium. Those who did not rest lacked help for the home. All the women ate brown seaweed soup and steamed rice for about 20 days after childbirth to cleanse the blood and to assist in milk production. Because pregnancy is a hot condition and heat is lost during labor and delivery, some women avoided cold foods and water after childbirth to prevent chronic illnesses such as arthritis. The baby should be wrapped in warm blankets to prevent harm from cold winds. Herbal medicines are also used during puerperium to promote healing and health (Howard & Barbiglia, 1997).

Health-care providers can improve the health of Korean American women by providing factual information about Pap smears and teaching breast self-examination. Pregnant Korean American women should be asked about their use of herbal medicine during pregnancy so that harmless practices can be incorporated into biomedical care. Recommendations for improving postpartum care among Korean American women include (1) developing an assessment tool that health-care providers can use to identify traditional beliefs early in a pregnancy, (2) developing a bilingual dictionary of common foods, (3) developing pamphlets with medical terms used in the U.S. health-care system, and (4) providing time for practicing English skills (Park & Peterson, 1991).

Death Rituals

Death Rituals and Expectations

Traditionally in Korea, it was important for Koreans to die at home. Bringing a dead body home if the person died in the hospital was considered bad luck. Consequently, viewing of the deceased occurred at home if the individual died at home and at the hospital if the person died at the hospital. Several days or more were set aside for the viewing, depending on the status of the deceased. The eldest son was expected to sit by the body of the parent during the viewing (Martinson, 1998). Friends and relatives paid their respects by bowing to a photograph of the deceased placed in the same room in which the body rested. The guests were then offered the favorite foods of the deceased. Today, most Korean Americans are not accustomed to viewing the body of the deceased. More commonly, relatives and friends come to pay their respects by viewing photographs of the deceased.

Although Korean Americans view life support more positively than European Americans, the majority in one study did not want such technology (Blackhall et al., 1999). In addition, they were less likely to have made a prior decision about life support. Older and more educated Koreans were less likely to favor telling patients the truth, believing that patients should not be told that they have a terminal illness.

An ancestral burial ceremony follows, with the body being placed in the ground facing south or north. Both the place and the position of the deceased are important for the future fortune of the living relatives. Koreans believe that if the spirit is content, good fortune will be awarded to the family. Unlike Western graves, a mound of dirt covers the gravesite of the deceased in Korea.

Cremation is an individual and family choice and is practiced more commonly in Korea for those who have no family or die at a young age. For example, when unmarried people die without any children to perform ancestral ceremonies, they are often cremated and their ashes scattered over a body of water.

Rice wine is traditionally sprinkled around the grave. Korean families bow two to four times in respect at the gravesite, and then the men, in descending order from the eldest to the youngest, drink rice wine. Some Korean Americans dedicate a corner of their home to honor their ancestors because they cannot go to the gravesite.

Circumstances in which "do not resuscitate" orders are an issue need to be addressed cautiously. Families trust physicians and may not question other options. Because death and dying are fairly well accepted in the Korean culture, prolonging life may not be highly regarded in the face of modern technology. Korean hospitals focus on acute care. Families are expected to stay with family members to assist in feeding and personal care around the clock. Thus, many Korean Americans may expect to care for their hospitalized family members in health-care facilities.

Responses to Death and Grief

Mourning rituals, with crying and open displays of grief, are commonly practiced and socially accepted at funerals, and they signify the utmost respect for the dead. The eldest son or male family member who sits by the deceased sometimes holds a cane and makes a moaning noise to display his grief. The cane is a symbol of needing support. Health-care providers may need to provide a private setting for Korean Americans to be able to grieve in culturally congruent ways.

Spirituality

Dominant Religion and Use of Prayer

Confucianism was the official religion of Korea from the 14th to the 20th centuries. Buddhism, Confucianism, Christianity, shamanism, and **Chondo-Kyo** are practiced in Korea today. *Chondo-Kyo* (religion of the Heavenly Way) is a nationalistic religion founded in the 19th century that combines Confucianism, Buddhism, and Daoism. Among Koreans in South Korea, the most recent estimates of organized religions include no affiliation, 49 percent; Christianity, 26 percent; Buddhism, 23 percent; and other and unknown, 2 percent (*CIA World Factbook*, 2010). In the United States, the church acts as a powerful social support group for Korean immigrants (Im & Yang, 2006). Jo, Maxwell, Yang, and Bastani (2010) even suggest that Korean churches have a high potential to serve an important role in the health of Korean Americans.

Koreans in America might not pray in the same fashion as Westerners, but for many people, the spirits demand homage. Korean churches often have prayer meetings several times a week, some with early-morning prayers. Buddhist temples have spirit rooms attached to them. Although Buddhists believe the spirit enters a new life, the beliefs of the shamans are so strong that the Buddhist church incorporated an area of their church for those who believe that ancestral spirits need honoring and homage. With such a variety of spiritual beliefs, caregivers must assess each Korean patient individually for religious beliefs and prayer practices.

Meaning of Life and Individual Sources of Strength

Family and education are central themes that give meaning to life for Korean Americans. The nuclear and extended families are primary sources of strength for Korean Americans in their daily lives. These concepts were covered earlier under Family Roles and Organization and Educational Status and Occupations.

Spiritual Beliefs and Health-Care Practices

Shamanism is a powerful belief in natural spirits. All parts of nature contain spirits: rivers, animals, and even inanimate objects. The many religions of Koreans create numerous ideologies about what happens with the spirits of the deceased. Christians believe the spirit goes to heaven; Buddhists believe the spirit starts a new life as a person or an animal; and shamanists believe the spirit stays with the family to watch over them and guide their actions and fortunes. Such a variety of faith systems provide a great diversity in beliefs of the Korean people. Given this diversity of spiritual beliefs among Koreans, each patient needs an individual assessment with regard to spiritual and health-care practices.

Health-Care Practices

Health-Seeking Beliefs and Behaviors

Beliefs that influence health-care practices include religious beliefs (see Dominant Religion and Use of Prayer) and dietary practices (see Nutrition). Health-care providers need to be aware that the theme dominating these beliefs is a holistic approach, which emphasizes both emotional and physical health.

Health-care practices among Koreans in America are primarily focused on curative rather than preventive measures. Health promotion in Korea is a relatively new public-health focus. In Korea, education on dental hygiene, sanitation, environmental issues, and other preventive health measures is being encouraged. Visits to the physician for an annual physical examination, Pap smears, and mammograms are uncommon. Among Koreans, traditional patterns of health promotion include harmony with nature and the universe, activity and rest, diet, sexual life, covetousness, temperament, and apprehension (Lee, 1993).

Responsibility for Health Care

One American study reported that only 13.5 percent of Korean American men and 11.3 percent of Korean American women had a digital rectal examination (DRE) for occult blood. Regression analysis indicated that gender, education, knowledge of the warning signs of cancer, and length of residence in the United States were significantly related to having undergone DRE. The researchers determined that this group of Korean Americans did not see health-care providers or health brochures as valuable sources of information, and to target this group, efforts should be coordinated with church and community leaders (Jo et al., 2010).

Because of women's modesty during physical examinations and their preferences that women perform intimate examinations, many Korean women defer having Pap tests or breast cancer screening tests (Lee, Fogg, & Sadler, 2006). A recent study among Korean immigrant women reported that 78 percent of the participants had gotten a mammogram at some point in their lives and that 38.6 percent had gotten one in the previous year (Lee et al., 2006). The reluctance for undergoing Pap tests directly relates to cervical cancer's rating as the number one female cancer diagnosed among women in Korea (Lee, 2000). Modesty has also been associated with low rates of mammography among Korean Americans (Lee, Kim, & Han, 2009), as well as limited knowledge about breast self-examination and causes of breast cancer (Han, Williams, & Harrison, 2000).

Recent Korean immigrants come from a country in which universal health insurance was implemented in the late 1980s. A government mandate established employer-based health insurance for medium and large firms. Regional health insurance systems, subsidized by the government, were later established for small firms, farmers, and the self-employed. Ryu, Young, and Park (2001) reported that health insurance coverage was the strongest predictor of Korean Americans' utilization of health-care services and that uninsured Korean Americans have less access regardless of their health-care needs.

The use and availability of over-the-counter medications vary tremendously between the United States and Korea. Many prescription drugs in the United States such as antibiotics, anti-inflammatory and cardiac medications, and certain pain control medications can be purchased over-the-counter in Korea at any *yak bang* (pharmacy). For example, when feeling "tired" or "fatigued," older people in Korea may perform home infusions of dextrose and water or albumin.

Self-medication with herbal remedies is also practiced. Ginseng is a root used for anything from a remedy for the common cold to an aphrodisiac. Seaweed soup is used as a medicine. Chinese traditional herbs are used to control the degree of "wind" that may be in the body. Other herbal medications are taken for preventive or restorative purposes. Accordingly, health-care providers should query their patients about their use of traditional Korean medicine and must be aware that herbal medicine may be used in conjunction with Western biomedicine.

Folk and Traditional Practices

Hanyak, traditional herbal medicine used for creating harmony between oneself and the larger cosmology, is a healing method for the body and soul. *Hanbang*, the traditional Korean medical-care system, works on the principle of a disturbed state of *ki*, cosmological vital energy. Symptoms are often interpreted in terms of a psychological base. Treatments include acupuncture, acumassage, acupressure, herbal medicines, and moxibustion therapy. The therapeutic relationship between *hanui* (oriental medicine) doctors and their patients is genuine, spontaneous, and harmonious. Patients who use both Western and traditional Korean practitioners may experience conflicts because of the lack of cooperation between *hanui* and biomedical health-care providers. Even Korean Americans are known to use both *hanui* and biomedical health-care providers.

Shamans are used in healing rituals to ward off restless spirits. Shamans originated with the religious belief of shamanism, the belief that all things possess spirits. A shaman, *mundang*, is usually a woman who has special abilities for communicating with spirits. The shaman is used to treat illnesses after other means of treatment are exhausted. The shaman performs a *kut*, a shamanistic ceremony to eliminate the evil spirits causing the illness. Such a ceremony may take place when a young person dies to prevent his or her spirit from staying tied to the earth. Others believe a shaman can eliminate evil spirits that may be causing difficulty with financial transactions. Although shamans have been around for many years, Koreans consider them part of the lowest class. Health-care providers need to determine whether Koreans in America are using folk therapies and should include nonharmful practices with biomedical therapies and prescriptions.

Barriers to Health Care

Because many Korean Americans use various options for healing, Western medical practices may be used in conjunction with acupressure, acupuncture, and herbal medicine. Barriers for Koreans in America may result from the expense of non-Western therapies, because many insurance companies do not cover alternative therapies.

As for many other American residents, the lack of insurance creates barriers to health care. Paying for health care out-of-pocket is expensive and not feasible for many Korean American families. Language, modesty, cultural attitudes toward certain illnesses, and communication problems also serve as impediments for access to health care.

Cultural Responses to Health and Illness

Perceptions of pain vary widely among Koreans. Some Koreans are stoic and are slow to express emotional distress from pain. Others are expressive and discuss their smallest discomforts. Family and friends are useful resources for learning some of the historical coping mechanisms of sick individuals. Nonverbal cues and facial expressions must be monitored for those who are stoic rather than expressive. Pain assessments should be conducted regularly, and education may be necessary for stoic individuals.

Mental illness is stigmatized in the Korean culture. Bernstein (2007) conducted a study of Korean American women and their reluctance to use mental health providers in the United States. Her study concluded that most of the participants acknowledged the need for mental health services but did not seek professional help and coped with the stressors of immigrant life by endurance, patience, and religion. Pang (1990) explored the cultural construction of *hwa-byung* among a group of Korean immigrant women in the United States, using a convenience sample. *Hwa-byung*, a traditional Korean illness, results from the suppression of anger or other emotions (Donnelly, 2001). *Hwa* means "fire and anger," and *byung* means "illness." All the women in the study knew the meaning of *hwa-byung*, and 80 percent

---

REFLECTIVE EXERCISE 20.4

Maria, a nurse working in an in-patient oncology unit, is assessing Jong Kim, age 72 years, who was recently diagnosed with lung cancer. Jong Kim emigrated from South Korea about 40 years ago and has smoked since he was in his early 20s. Although Jong does not request pain medication, his facial expressions show that he is obviously in significant pain.

1. What should the nurse do to adequately assess Jong's pain level?
2. What are some Korean cultural beliefs, attitudes, and practices related to cancer?
3. What Korean cultural beliefs, attitudes, and practices related to cancer might influence Jong's pain management?
4. What are some Korean cultural beliefs, attitudes, and practices related to pain and pain medication?

reported having experienced it. The emotions they reported suppressing were sadness, depression, worry, anger, fright, and fear. Most of the emotions described were related to conflicts with close relatives or family, such as sons and daughters or significant others. These were expressed as physical complaints, ranging from headaches and poor appetites to insomnia and lack of energy. The complaints were chronic in nature, and a variety of remedies were used to alleviate the symptoms. Most of the women suggested that *hwa-byung* was difficult to cure and accepted the symptoms as inevitable. For these older Korean women, *hwa-byung* was a mode for constructing illness as a personal, social, and cultural adaptive response (Pang, 1990). These women expressed life's hardships by channeling their emotional illnesses into physical symptoms.

A community study of Korean Americans addressed the prevalence, clinical significance, and meaning of *hwa-byung* (Lin, Lau, Yamamoto, Zheng, & Kim, 1992). The results indicated a high percentage of Korean Americans (11.9 percent) who identified themselves as suffering from *hwa-byung*. A strong association was shown between *hwa-byung* and major depressive disorders. Although *hwa-byung* is found predominantly among older Korean women with little education, this study's findings did not support this conclusion. The ability to generalize these findings, however, is limited because assignment to the study groups was not completely random and because the sample size was small.

Historically, the area of special education has not been well studied or researched in Korea. Families who have children with mental or physical disabilities often question what they have done wrong to make their ancestors angry. Families feel stigmatized for such a misfortune and cannot accept their children's disfigurement or low intellect. Korea lacks social support to assist families in caring for children with mental or physical disabilities. Some families abandon these children in their desperate need for support with long-term care and expenses. Other children are kept from the public eye in the hope of saving the family from stigmatization.

The estimated rate of students with a disability receiving special education in South Korea was about 85 percent in 2007, and about 10,000 students with disabilities were neglected in the Korean education system (Munhwa, 2007). Also, it was estimated in 2007 that the number of students with a disability in South Korea was 77,452 and that 65,940 of them attended either a specialized or regular school, in either special or normal education. In other words, 11,512 students with a disability were not receiving any education at all. These statistics may reflect negative attitudes toward people with a disability among Koreans, which may influence the idea of mainstreaming students with a mild disability in South Korea. Korean Americans may hold these same views regarding people with mental and physical disabilities and need special support in obtaining assistance.

In Korea, once hospitalized people are physically stable, they are discharged to their homes to be with the family. Bowel training and physical therapy activities are not the responsibility of the hospital. The families must care for family members at home. Long-term care for chronic problems or for rehabilitation is rare in Korea. Thus, Korean Americans are familiar with the concept of family home care. Depending on their adaptation to the American health-care system, and families' contact with American health-care providers, some Korean Americans adjust their ideologies on the sick role.

Blood Transfusions and Organ Donation

No beliefs held by Korean Americans prevent the acceptance of blood transfusions. Organ donation and organ transplantation are rare, reflecting traditional attitudes toward integrity and purity. These issues need to be approached sensitively with Korean Americans because they may be influenced by the individual's religious beliefs.

Health-Care Providers
Traditional Versus Biomedical Providers

In general, no taboos exist that prevent health-care providers from delivering care to the opposite gender. Female physicians are definitely preferred for maternity care and female problems because women feel more comfortable discussing gynecological and obstetric issues with female physicians. However, more traditional Koreans frequently prefer health-care providers who speak Korean, are older, and are of the same gender, although many will seek health care from others who do not meet these requirements if their preferred care provider is not available. Miller (1990) studied the use of traditional health practitioners, acupuncturists, and herbalists among a group of 102 Korean immigrants. The findings indicated that Korean immigrants with higher incomes were more likely to use traditional Korean practitioners.

The area of social work is new in Korea. The hospitals have no positions for such a role. A few educational programs exist in Korea for social workers, but much development is needed in the area of social support. Because these roles may be new to many Koreans, health-care providers may need to encourage Korean Americans to use these services.

Status of Health-Care Providers

Because traditional Korean culture accords high respect to men, older people, and physicians, the ideal physician is an older man with gray hair. This shows that he has experience and wisdom and is able to make the best decisions. With such a high status in Korea, physicians expect respect from all other health-care providers. Usually, nurses are expected to carry out physicians' orders explicitly. This is not to say that the nurse cannot question orders, but great time and effort are spent consulting other nurses before questioning physicians in the most respectful way. However, as nurses are becoming more educated in Korea, they are becoming more assertive and more closely mirror Western practice patterns.

With an emphasis on increasing the educational level of nurses, they too are gaining stature and respect in Korean culture. Baccalaureate, masters, and doctoral programs are available for nurses in Korea, although exact numbers are not available.

REFERENCES

Asianinfo. (2010a). *General information—Seoul.* Retrieved from http://www.asianinfo.org/asianinfo/seoul/general_information.htm

Asianinfo. (2010b). *Korean drama.* Retrieved from http://www.asianinfo.org/asianinfo/korea/about_korea.htm

Bernstein, K.S. (2007). Mental health issues among urban Korean American immigrants. *Journal of Transcultural Nursing, 18*(2), 175–180.

Blackhall, L., Frank, G., Murphy, S., Michel, V., Palmer, J., Azen, S., et al. (1999). Ethnicity and attitudes toward life sustaining technology. *Social Science Medicine, 48*(12), 1779–1789.

Cho, J., & Juon, H.S. (2006). Assessing overweight and obesity risk among Korean Americans in California using World Health Organization body mass index criteria for Asians. *Prevention of Chronic Disease, 3*(3), A79.

Cho, Y.I., & Faulkner, W.R. (1993). Conception of alcoholism among Koreans and Americans. *International Journal of the Addictions, 28*(8), 681–694.

Choi, E. (1995). A contrast of mothering behaviors in women from Korea and the United States. *Journal of Obstetric, Gynecologic, and Neonatal Nursing, 24*(4), 363–369.

CIA World FactBook. (2010). *Korea.* Retrieved from https://www.cia.gov/library/publications/the-world-factbook/geos/ks.html

CNN. (2010). *Complete coverage on North Korea.* Retrieved from http://topics.cnn.com/topics/north_korea

Donnelly, P.L. (2001). Korean American family experiences of caregiving for their mentally ill adult children: An interpretative study. *Journal of Transcultural Nursing, 12*(4), 292–301.

Han, Y., Williams, R., & Harrison, R. (2000). Breast cancer screening knowledge, attitudes, and practices among Korean-American women. *Oncology Nursing Forum, 27*(10), 1589–1591.

Howard, J., & Barbiglia, V. (1997). Caring for childbearing Korean women. *Journal of Obstetric, Gynecologic, and Neonatal Nursing, 26*(6), 665–671.

Im, E.O. (2002). Korean culture. In P.S. St. Hill, J. Lipson, & A.I. Meleis (Eds.), *Caring for women cross-culturally: A portable guide.* Philadelphia: F.A. Davis Company.

Im, E.O., & Meleis, A.I. (2001). Women's work and symptoms during menopausal transition: Korean immigrant women. *Women and Health, 33*(1/2), 83–103.

Im, E.O., & Yang, K. (2006). Theories on immigrant women's health. *Health Care Women International, 27*(8), 666–681.

Jo, A.M., Maxwell, A.E., Yang, B., & Bastani, R. (2010). Conducting health research in Korean American churches: Perspectives from church leaders. *Journal of Community Health, 35*(2), 156–164.

Johanning, E., Goldberg, M., & Kim, R. (1994). Asbestos hazard evaluation in South Korean textile production. *International Journal of Health Services, 24*(1), 131–144.

Kim, E., Cain, K., & McCubbin, M. (2006). Maternal and paternal parenting, acculturation, and young adolescents' psychological adjustment in Korean American families. *Journal of Child Adolescent Psychiatric Nursing, 19*(3), 112–129.

Kim, K.E. (2003). Gastric cancer in Korean Americans: Risks and reductions. *Korean American Studies Bulletin, 13*(1/2), 84–90.

Kim, H., & Chung, R.H. (2003). Relationship of recalled parenting style to self-perception in Korean American college students. *Journal of Genetic Psychology, 164*(4), 481–492.

Kim, K.K., Yu, E.S., Chen, E.H., Cross, N., & Kim, J. (2000). Nutritional status of Korean Americans: Implications for cancer risk. *Oncology Nursing Forum, 27*(10), 1573–1583.

Kim, Y.G., & Hahn, S.J. (2006). Homosexuality in ancient and modern Korea. *Culture Health and Sex, 8*(1), 59–65.

Kimmel, D.C., & Yi, H. (2004). Characteristics of gay, lesbian, and bisexual Asians, Asian Americans, and immigrants from Asia to the U.S.A. *Journal of Homosexuality, 47*(2), 143–172.

Kohls, R.L. (2001). *Learning to think Korean.* Yarmouth, ME: Intercultural Press.

Korean Language. (2010). *Dialects.* Retrieved from http://www.korean-language.org/korean/dialects.asp

Migration Information Source. (2010). *Korean immigrants in the United States.* Retrieved from http://www.migrationinformation.org/USfocus/display.cfm?ID=793

Lee, Y. (1993). Health promotion: Patterns of traditional health promotion in Korea. *Kanhohak Tamgu, 2*(2), 21–36.

Lee, M. (2000). Knowledge, barriers, and motivators related to cervical cancer screening among Korean-American women. A focus group approach. *Cancer Nursing, 23*(3), 168–175.

Lee, E. E., Fogg, L. F., & Sadler, G. R. (2006). Factors of breast cancer screening among Korean immigrants in the United States. *Journal of Immigrant and Minority Health, 8*(3), 223–233.

Lee, H., Kim, J., & Han, H. R. (2009). Do cultural factors predict mammography behaviour among Korean immigrants in the USA? *Journal of Advanced Nursing, 65*(12), 2574–2584.

Lee, D. C., & Lee, E. H. (1990). Korean immigrant families in America: Role and value conflicts. In H. C. Kim & E. H. Lee (Eds.), *Koreans in America: Dreams and realities* (pp. 165–177). Seoul: Institute of Korean Studies.

Lee, Y.H., Lee, J., Kim, M. T., & Han, H.R. (2009), In-depth assessment of the nutritional status of Korean American elderly. *Geriatric Nursing, 30*(5), 304–311.

Lee, S., Sobal, J., & Frongillo, E. (2000). Acculturation and health in Korean Americans. *Social Science Medicine, 51*(2), 159–173.

Levy, R. (1993). Ethnic and racial differences in response to medicines: Preserving individualized therapy in managed pharmaceutical programmes. *Pharmaceutical Medicine, 7*, 139–165.

Lew, R., Moskowitz, J.M., Wismer, B.A., Min, K., Kang, S.H., Chen, A.M., & Tager, I.B. (2001). Correlates of cigarette smoking among Korean American adults in Alameda County, California. *Asian American Pacific Islander Journal of Health, 9*(1), 49–60.

Lin, K., Lau, J.K., Yamamoto, J., Zheng, Y.P., & Kim, K.H. (1992). Hwa-Byung: A community study of Korean Americans. *Journal of Nervous and Mental Disease, 180*(6), 386–391.

Ludman, E.K., Kang, K.J., & Lynn, L.L. (1992). Food beliefs and diets of pregnant Korean American women. *Journal of the American Dietetic Association, 92*(12), 1519–1520.

Martinson, I.M. (1998). Funeral rituals in Taiwan and Korea. *Oncology Nursing Forum, 25*(10), 1756–1760.

Meyer, U. (1992). Drugs in special patient groups: Clinical importance of genetics in drug effects. In M. Melmon & T. Morrelli (Eds.), *Clinical pharmacology: Basic principles in therapeutics* (8th ed., pp. 62–83). New York: Pergamon Press.

Miller, J. (1990). Use of traditional Korean health care by Korean immigrants to the United States. *Sociology and Social Research, 75*(1), 38–48.

Munhwa. (2007). *About 10,000 disabled students neglected in education system.* Retrieved from http://www.munhwa.com/news/view.html?no=2007100601030527097070010

Munoz, C., & Hilgenberg, C. (2005). Ethnopharmacology. *American Journal of Nursing, 105*(8), 40–49.

Nakashima, J., & Wong, M.M. (2000). Characteristics of alcohol consumption, correlates of alcohol misuse among Korean American adolescents. *Journal of Drug Education, 30*(3), 343–359.

Organization for Economic Cooperation and Development (OECD). (2010). *Marriage and divorce rates.* Retrieved from http://www.oecd.org/dataoecd/4/19/40321815.pdf

Pang, K.Y. (1990). Hwa-Byung: The construction of a Korean popular illness among Korean elderly immigrant women in the United States. *Culture, Medicine, and Psychiatry, 14,* 495–512.

Park, M.S. (2001). The factors of child physical abuse in Korean immigrant families. *Child Abuse Neglect, 25*(7), 945–958.

Park, S.Y., Murphy, S.P., Sharma, S., & Kolonel, L.N. (2005). Dietary intakes and health-related behaviours of Korean American women born in the USA and Korea: The multiethnic cohort study. *Public Health Nutrition, 8*(7), 904–911.

Park, S., Oh, S., & Lee, M. (1998). Korean Status of alcoholics and alcohol-related health problems. *Alcohol and Clinical Expression Research, 22*(3, Suppl), 170S–172S.

Park, K.Y., & Peterson, L.M. (1991). Beliefs, practices, and experiences of Korean women in relation to childbirth. *Health Care for Women International, 12*(2), 261–269.

Pritham, U.A., & Sammons, L.N. (1993). Korean women's attitudes toward pregnancy and prenatal care. *Health Care for Women International, 14,* 145–153.

Ryu, H., Young, W.B., & Park, C. (2001). Korean American health insurance and health services utilization. *Research and Nursing Health, 24*(6), 494–505.

Sorensen, C.W. (1994). Success and education in South Korea. *Comparative Education Review, 38*(1), 10–35.

The Hankyoreh. (2007). *1 out of 20 Korean youths attempts suicide: Study.* Retrieved from http://english.hani.co.kr/arti/english_edition/e_national/199975.html

The Korean Times. (2007). *South Korea has 4th lowest birth rate.* Retrieved from http://www.koreantimes.co.kr/www/news/nation/2007/06/117_5515.html

U.S. Census Bureau. (2006). *2005 American community survey.* Minneapolis, MN: Minnesota Population Center.

U.S. Department of State. (2010). *Korea, Republic of Country Specific Information.* Retrieved from http://travel.state.gov/travel/cis_pa_tw/cis/cis_1018.html#safety

Weatherspoon, A., Park, J., & Johnson, R. (2001). A family study of homeland Korean alcohol use. *Addictive Behavior, 26*(1), 101–113.

World Health Organization. (2004). Alcohol consumption among adults. Retrieved from http://www.nationsencyclopedia.com/WorldStats/WHO-alcohol-consumption-adults.html

Yi, M., & Jezewski, M. (2000). Korean nurses' adjustment to hospitals in the United States of America. *Journal of Advanced Nursing, 32*(3), 721–729.

DavisPlus *For case studies, review questions, and additional information, go to*

http://davisplus.fadavis.com

Chapter 21

People of Mexican Heritage

Rick Zoucha and Cecilia A. Zamarripa

Overview, Inhabited Localities, and Topography

Overview

People of Mexican heritage are a very diverse group geographically, historically, and culturally and are not easy to describe. Although no specific set of characteristics can fully describe people of Mexican heritage, some commonalities distinguish them as an ethnic group, with many regional variations that reflect subcultures in Mexico and in the United States. A common term used to describe Spanish-speaking populations in the United States, including people of Mexican heritage, is **Hispanic**. However, the term can be misleading and can encompass many different people clustered together owing to a common heritage and lineage from Spain. Many Hispanic people prefer to be identified by descriptors more specific to their cultural heritage, such as Mexican, Mexican American, Latin American, Spanish American, Chicano, Latino, or Ladino. Therefore, when referring to Mexican Americans, use that phrase instead of Hispanic or Latino (Vázquez, 2004). As a broad ethnic group, people of Mexican heritage often refer to themselves as *la raza*, which means "the race." The Spanish word for race has a different meaning than the American interpretation of race. The concept of *la raza* has brought people together from separate worlds to make families and is about inclusion (Vázquez, 2000).

Heritage and Residence

Mexico, with an estimated population of 113,724,226 (*CIA World Factbook,* 2011), is inhabited by white Spanish, Indians, American Indians, Middle Easterns, and Africans. Mexican Americans are descendants of Spanish and other European whites; Aztec, Mayan, and other Central American Indians; and Inca and other South American Indians, as well as people from Africa (Schmal & Madrer, 2007). Some individuals can trace their heritage to North American Indian tribes in the southwestern part of the United States.

Mexico City, one of the largest cities in the world, has a population of over 20 million. Mexico is undergoing rapid changes in business and health-care practices. Undoubtedly, these changes have accelerated and will continue to accelerate since the passage of the North American Free Trade Agreement as people are more able to move across the border to seek employment and educational opportunities.

Historically, for generations, people of Mexican heritage lived on the land that is now known as the southwestern United States, long before the first white settlers came to the territory. By 1853, approximately 80,000 Spanish-speaking settlers lived in the area lost by Mexico during the Texas Rebellion, the Mexican War, and the Gadsden Purchase. After the northern part of Mexico was annexed to the United States, the settlers were not officially considered immigrants but were often viewed as foreigners by incoming white Americans. By 1900, Mexican Americans numbered approximately 200,000. However, during the "Great Migration" between 1900 and 1930, an additional 1 million Mexicans entered the United States. This may have been the greatest immigration of people in the history of humanity (Library of Congress, 2005).

Hispanics, the fastest-growing ethnic population in the United States, include over 44.3 million people (U.S. Census Bureau, 2008). Sixty-six percent of all Hispanics are of Mexican heritage (U.S. Census Bureau, 2010). Mexican Americans reside predominantly in California, Texas, Illinois, Arizona, Florida, New Mexico, and Colorado. However, the major concentration of Mexican Americans, totaling over 19 million, is found in the southern and western portions of the United States (U.S. Census Bureau, 2010). Ninety percent of Mexican Americans live in urban areas such as San Diego, Los Angeles, New York City, Chicago, and Houston, whereas less than 10 percent reside in rural areas.

Reasons for Migration and Associated Economic Factors

Historically, many Mexicans left Mexico during the Mexican Revolution to seek political, religious, and economic freedoms (Casa Historia, 2011). Following the Mexican Revolution, strict limits were placed on the Catholic Church, and, until recently, clerics were not allowed to wear their church garb in public. For many, this restricted the expression of faith and was a minor factor in their immigration north to the United States (Meyer & Beezley, 2000). Since the "Great Migration," the limited employment opportunities in Mexico, especially in rural areas, have encouraged Mexicans to migrate to the United States as sojourners or immigrants or with undocumented status; the latter are often derogatorily referred to as *wetbacks* (*majodos*) by the white and Mexican American populations.

Of the undocumented immigrants in the United States, an estimated 6 million are from Mexico (Van Hook, Bean, & Passel, 2005). Before the Immigration Reform and Control Act of 1986, hundreds of thousands of Mexicans crossed the border, found jobs, and settled in the United States. Although the numbers have decreased since 1986, border towns in Texas and California still experience large influxes of Mexicans seeking improved employment and educational opportunities. The tide of illegal immigration to the United States has decreased from 2008, at which time it was over 7 million. In 2010, that number decreased to 6,640,000 (Department of Homeland Security, 2011). Illegal immigration and what can or should be done to control it, especially in border states with Mexico, continue to be hotly debated issues. Annually, many migrants die trying to illegally emigrate. Solutions to U.S. citizens' concerns are not forthcoming in the near future. Even though the economy of Mexico has grown, the buying power of the peso has decreased, and inflation rates have increased faster than wages; thus, 47 percent of the population continues to live in poverty (*CIA World Factbook,* 2011). Recent Mexican immigrants are more likely to live in poverty, are more pessimistic about their future, and are less educated than previous immigrants. Many Mexicans are among the very poor, with little hope of improving their economic status. Between the years 1999 and 2000 in the United States, the poverty rate for Hispanics was 33.1 percent (U.S. Census Bureau, 2009).

Educational Status and Occupations

Many second- and third-generation Mexican Americans have significant job skills and education. By contrast, many, especially newer immigrants from rural areas, have poor educational backgrounds and may place little value on education because it is not needed to obtain jobs in Mexico. Once in the United States, they initially find work similar to that which they did in their native land, including farming, ranching, mining, oil production, construction, landscaping, and domestic jobs in homes, restaurants, and hotels and motels. Economic and educational opportunities in the United States are attainable, which allows immigrants to pursue the great American dream of a perceived better life (Kemp, 2001). Many Mexicans and Mexican Americans work as seasonal migrant workers and may relocate several times each year as they "follow the sun." Sometimes their unwillingness or inability to learn English is related to their intent to return to Mexico; however, this may hinder their ability to obtain better-paying jobs (Fig. 21-1).

The mean educational level in Mexico is 5 years. Until 1992, Mexican children were required to attend school through the sixth grade, but since the Mexican School Reform Act of 1992, a ninth-grade education is required. However, great strides have been made in educational standards in Mexico, which now reports an 86.1 percent literacy rate among its population (*CIA World Factbook,* 2011). A common practice among parents in poor rural villages is to educate their children in what they need to know. This group often finds immigration to the United States to be their most attractive option. For many Mexicans, high school and a university education are neither available nor attainable.

Hispanics are the most undereducated ethnic group in the United States, with only 45 percent aged 25 years or older having a high school education, compared with 90 percent for non-Hispanic whites. However, the number of Hispanics who completed 4 years of college has increased to 7.3 percent of the total Hispanic population, up from 6.4 percent in 2000 (U.S. Census Bureau, 2011). As second- and third-generation Mexican Americans acculturate and improve their socioeconomic status, these percentages are likely to increase the same as they have for

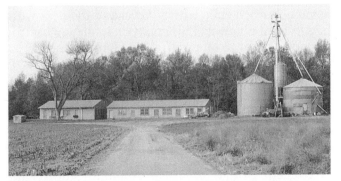

Figure 21-1 A migrant worker camp on Maryland's eastern shore. The Sanchez family (discussed in the case study on DavisPlus) lives in such a camp, as do many Mexican American farm workers in the United States.

immigrants from European countries in previous centuries.

Communication

Dominant Language and Dialects

Mexico is one of the largest Spanish-speaking countries in the world, with over 80 million speaking the language. The dominant language of Mexicans and Mexican Americans is Spanish. However, Mexico has 54 indigenous languages and more than 500 different dialects (Spanish Language, 2007). Knowing the region from which a Mexican American originates may help to identify the language or dialect the individual speaks. For example, major indigenous languages besides Spanish include Nahuatl and Otami, spoken in central Mexico; Mayan, in the Yucatan peninsula; Maya-Quiche, in the state of Chiapas; Zapotec and Mixtec, in the valley of Oaxaca; Tarascan, in the state of Michoacan; and Totonaco, in the state of Veracruz. Many of the Spanish dialects spoken by Mexican Americans have similar word meanings, but the dialects spoken by other groups may not. Because of the rural isolationist nature of many ethnic groups and the influence of native Indian languages, the dialects are so diverse in selected regions that it may be difficult to understand the language, regardless of the degree of fluency in Spanish.

Radio and television programs broadcasting in Spanish in both the United States and Mexico have helped to standardize Spanish. For the most part, public broadcast communication is primarily derived from Castilian Spanish. This standardization reduces the difficulties experienced by subcultures with multiple dialects. When speaking in a nonnative language, health-care providers must select words that have relatively pure meanings in the language and avoid the use of regional slang.

Contextual speech patterns among Mexican Americans may include a high-pitched, loud voice and a rate that seems extremely fast to the untrained ear. The language uses **apocopation**, which accounts for this rapid speech pattern. An apocopation occurs when one word ends with a vowel and the next word begins with a vowel. This creates a tendency to drop the vowel ending of the first word and results in an abbreviated, rapid-sounding form. For example, in the Spanish phrase for "How are you?," *¿Cómo está usted?* may become *¿Comestusted?*. The last word, *usted*, is frequently dropped. Some may find this fast speech difficult to understand. However, if one asks the individual to enunciate slowly, the effect of the apocopation or truncation is less pronounced.

To help bridge potential communication gaps, health-care providers need to watch the patient for cues, paraphrase words with multiple meanings, use simple sentences, repeat phrases for clarity, avoid the use of regional idiomatic phrases and expressions, and ask the patient to repeat instructions to ensure accuracy. Approaching the Mexican American patient with respect and ***personalismo*** (behaving like a friend) and directing questions to the dominant member of a group (usually the man) may help to facilitate more open communication. Zoucha and Husted (2002) found that becoming personal with the patient or family is essential to building confidence and promoting health. The concept of *personalismo* may be difficult for some health-care providers because they are socialized to form rigid boundaries between the caregiver and the patient and family.

Cultural Communication Patterns

Whereas some topics, such as income, salary, or investments, are taboo, Mexican Americans generally like to express their inner beliefs, feelings, and emotions once they get to know and trust a person. Meaningful conversations are important, often become loud, and seem disorganized. To the outsider, the situation may seem stressful or hostile, but this intense emotion means the conversants are having a good time and enjoying one another's company. Within the context of *personalismo* and ***respeto***—respect—health-care providers can encourage open communication and sharing and develop the patient's sense of trust by inquiring about family members before proceeding with the usual business. It is important for health-care providers to engage in "small talk" before addressing the actual health-care concern with the patient and family (Zoucha & Reeves, 1999).

Mexican Americans place great value on closeness and togetherness, including when they are in an inpatient facility. They frequently touch and embrace and like to see relatives and significant others. Touch between men and women, between men, and between women is acceptable. To demonstrate respect, compassion, and understanding, health-care providers should greet the Mexican American patient with a handshake. Once rapport is established, providers may further demonstrate approval and respect through backslapping, smiling, and affirmatively nodding the head. Given the diversity of dialects and the nuances of language, culturally congruent use of humor is difficult to accomplish and, therefore, should be avoided unless health-care providers are absolutely sure there is no chance of misinterpretation. Otherwise, inappropriate humor may jeopardize the therapeutic relationship and opportunities for health teaching and health promotion.

Mexican Americans consider sustained eye contact when speaking directly to an older person to be rude. Direct eye contact with teachers or superiors may be interpreted as insolence. Avoiding direct eye contact with superiors is a sign of respect. This practice may or may not be seen with second- or third-generation

Mexican Americans. Health-care providers must take cues from the patient and family.

Temporal Relationships

Many Mexican Americans, especially those from lower socioeconomic groups, are necessarily present oriented. Many individuals do not consider it important or have the income to plan ahead financially. The trend is to live in the "more important" here and now, because *mañana* (tomorrow) cannot be predicted. With this emphasis on living in the present, preventive health care and immunizations may not be a priority. *Mañana* may or may not really mean tomorrow; it often means "not today" or "later."

Some Mexicans and Mexican Americans perceive time as relative rather than categorically imperative. Deadlines and commitments are flexible, not firm. Punctuality is generally relaxed, especially in social situations. This concept of time is innate in the Spanish language. For example, one cannot be late for an appointment; one can only arrive late. In addition, immigrants from rural environments where adhering to a strict schedule is not important may not own a clock or even be able to tell time.

Because of their more relaxed concept of time, Mexican Americans may arrive late for appointments, although the current trend is toward greater punctuality. Health-care facilities that use an appointment system for patients may need to make special provisions to see patients whenever they arrive. Health-care providers must carefully listen for clues when discussing appointments. Disagreeing with health-care providers who set the appointment may be viewed as rude or impolite. Therefore, some Mexican Americans will not tell you directly that they cannot make the appointment. In the context of the discussion, they may say something like "My husband goes to work at 8:00 a.m., and the children are off to school, and then I have to do the dishes. . . ." The health-care provider should ask, "Is 8:30 a.m. on Thursday okay for you?" The person might say yes, but the health-care provider must still intently listen to the conversation and then possibly negotiate a new time for the appointment. In the conversation, the patient may just give clues that he or she will not arrive on time, because it is important to save face and avoid being rude by saying that outright.

Format for Names

Names in most Spanish-speaking populations seem complex to those unfamiliar with the culture. A typical name is La Señorita Olga Gaborra de Rodriguez. Gaborra is the name of Olga's father, and Rodriguez is her mother's surname. When she marries a man with the surname Guiterrez, she becomes La Señora (denotes a married woman) Olga Guiterrez de Gaborra y Rodriguez. The word *de* is used to express possession, and the father's name, which is considered more important than the mother's, comes first. However, this full name is rarely used except on formal documents and for recording the name in the family Bible. Out of respect, most Mexican Americans are more formal when addressing nonfamily members. Thus, the best way to address Olga is not by her first name but rather as Señora Guiterrez. Titles such as *Don* and *Doña* for older respected members of the community and family should remain—not all members are respected so not all would have the title *Don* or *Doña*. If using English while communicating with people older than the nurse or health-care provider, use titles such as Mr., Ms., Miss, or Mrs., as a sign of respect.

Health-care providers must understand the role of older people when providing care to people of Mexican heritage. To develop confidence and *personalismo*, an element of formality must exist between health-care providers and older people. Becoming overly familiar by using physical touch or addressing them by first names may not be appreciated early in a relationship (Kemp, 2001). As the health-care provider develops confidence in the relationship, becoming familiar may be less of a concern. However, using the first name of an older patient may never be appropriate (Zoucha & Husted, 2000).

Family Roles and Organization

Head of Household and Gender Roles

The typical family dominance pattern in traditional Mexican American families is patriarchal, with evidence of slow change toward a more egalitarian pattern in recent years (Grothaus, 1996). Change to a more egalitarian decision-making pattern is primarily identified with more educated and higher socioeconomic families. **Machismo** in the Mexican culture sees men as having strength, valor, and self-confidence, which are valued traits among many. Men are seen as wiser, braver, stronger, and more knowledgeable regarding sexual matters. The female takes responsibility for decisions within the home and for maintaining the family's health. *Machismo* assists in sustaining and maintaining health not only for the man but also with implications for the health and well-being of the family (Sobralske, 2006).

Prescriptive, Restrictive, and Taboo Behaviors for Children and Adolescents

Children are highly valued because they ensure the continuation of the family and cultural values (Locke, 1998). They are closely protected and not encouraged to leave home. Even *compadres* (godparents) are included in the care of the young. Each child must have godparents in case something interferes with the parents' ability to fulfill their child-rearing responsibilities. Children are taught at an early age to respect parents and older family members, especially grandparents.

Physical punishment is often used as a way of maintaining discipline and is sometimes considered child abuse in the United States. Using children as interpreters in the health-care setting is discouraged owing to the restrictive nature of discussing gender-specific health assessments.

Family Goals and Priorities

The concept of *familism* is an all-encompassing value among Mexicans, for whom the traditional family is still the foundation of society. Family takes precedence over work and all other aspects of life. In many Mexican families, it is often said "God first, then family." The dominant Western health-care culture stresses including both the patient and the family in the plan of care. Mexicans are strong proponents of this family care concept, which includes the extended family. By including all family members, health-care providers can build greater trust and confidence and, in turn, increase adherence to health-care regimens and prescriptions (Wells, Cagle, & Bradley, 2006).

REFLECTIVE EXERCISE 21.1

Mrs. Garcia is a 55-year-old Mexican American woman recently diagnosed with blockages in her coronary vessels, and as a result, she will undergo a coronary artery bypass graft. Mrs. Garcia is recently widowed and is grieving for her husband of 39 years. She has 7 children (3 sons aged 39, 34, and 31; 4 daughters aged 37, 35, 33, and 29) and 20 grandchildren. The youngest son lives at home with his mother along with his wife and 5 children. The other children live within 10 blocks. Mrs. Garcia spends a lot of time helping to care for the grandchildren while her children work. The five youngest members of the family were born in the United States, and the rest of the family was born in Oaxaca, Mexico. Mrs. Garcia has never worked outside of the home and receives survivor benefits from her husband's pension. The only job she has ever done is house cleaning and other domestic help for her husband's previous work acquaintances. Mrs. Garcia has one living brother who lives 8 miles away and a sister who died of heart disease 5 years ago.

The Garcia family members are Catholics. Mrs. Garcia is a very devout Catholic and attends Mass daily at the church three blocks away. The children attend Mass with the family on occasional Sundays. Mrs. Garcia prays the rosary and novenas so that God will take care of her and her family. Mrs. Garcia is a good cook and prepares dinner every evening for one of her sons and his family. The daughter-in-law helps cook the meals even after a full day of work. Mrs. Garcia and her family live in a three-bedroom wood frame house. The home is located in a Mexican American neighborhood 2 miles from the Mexican border in Reynosa, Texas.

Mrs. Garcia does not have any work experience and is grateful her husband left a small but substantial life insurance

policy. Mrs. Garcia receives help with shopping and rides to the doctor from her youngest daughter and many *comadres*. One of her *comadres* is a *curandera* who has been offering Mrs. Lopez herbs and teas to help healing. Mrs. Garcia enjoys making tamales and *menudo* in her kitchen along with her family and *comadres*. All of the Garcia children and *comadres* have committed to help Mrs. Garcia during and after her surgery.

1. When the home health nurse comes to assess Mrs. Garcia's incision and teaches about wound care, who should be included in the teaching and why?
2. Explain the importance of *familism* to the Garcia family.
3. Mrs. Garcia has been offered herbal tea by the *curandera* while the home nurse is making a visit. Should the nurse intervene to stop this practice? Please provide rationale for your answer.
4. The nurse is making a visit when the family is praying the rosary together for the health of Mrs. Garcia. The nurse is invited to join. What should the nurse do in this situation?

Blended communal families are almost the norm in lower socioeconomic groups and in migrant-worker camps. Single, divorced, and never-married male and female children usually live with their parents or extended families, regardless of economics. Extended kinship is common through *padrinos*: godparents who may be close friends and are considered the same as family (Zoucha & Zamarripa, 1997). Thus, the words *brother, sister, aunt,* and *uncle* do not necessarily mean that they are related by blood. For many men, having children is evidence of their virility and a sign of *machismo*.

When grandparents and older parents are unable to live on their own, they generally move in with their children. The extended family structure and the Mexicans' obligation to visit sick friends and relatives encourage large numbers to visit hospitalized family members and friends. This practice may necessitate that health-care providers relax strict visiting policies in health-care facilities.

Social status is highly valued among Mexican Americans, and a person who holds an academic degree or position with an impressive title commands great respect and admiration from family, friends, and the community. Good manners, a family, and family lineage, as indicated by extensive family names, also confer high status for Mexicans.

Alternative Lifestyles

Twenty-three percent of Mexican families in the United States live in poverty, and many are headed by a single female parent. This percentage is lower than that for other minority groups in the United States (U.S. Census Bureau, 2010). Because the Hispanic cultural norm is for a pregnant woman to marry, Mexicans are more likely to marry at a young age. Yet,

REFLECTIVE EXERCISE 21.2

Mr. Rodriguez is an 80-year-old Mexican American man who was recently diagnosed with bladder and prostate cancer. Mr. Rodriquez has been married for 60 years and has 8 adult children (3 daughters aged 57, 51, and 40; 5 sons aged 55, 53, 44, 43, and 42), 19 grandchildren, and 4 great-grandchildren. Mr. Rodriquez's youngest son and his family live with Mr. and Mrs. Rodriguez. The other Rodriquez children, except the second-oldest daughter, live within 3 to 10 miles from their parents. The second-oldest daughter is a teacher and lives out of state. All members of the family except for Mr. Rodriquez were born in the United States. He was born in Guanajuato, Mexico, and immigrated to the United States at the age of 16 in order to work and send money back to the family in Mexico. Mr. Rodriguez has returned to Mexico throughout the years to visit and has lived in California ever since. Mr. Rodriguez is retired from work as a carpet layer. Mr. Rodriquez has one living older brother who lives within 15 miles. All members of the family speak Spanish and English fluently.

The Rodriguez family is Catholic, as evidenced by the religious items hanging on the wall and prayer books and rosary on the coffee table. Statues of St. Jude and Our Lady of Guadalupe are on the living room table. Mr. and Mrs. Rodriguez have made many mandas (bequests) to pray for the health of the family, including one to thank God for the healthy birth of all the children, especially after the doctor had discouraged them from having any children after the complicated birth of their first child. The family attends Mass together every Sunday morning and then meets for breakfast *chorizo* at a local restaurant frequented by many of their church's other parishioner families. Mr. Rodriguez believes his health and the health of his family are in the hands of God.

The Rodriguez family lives in a modest three-bedroom ranch home they bought 52 years ago. The home is located in a predominantly Mexican American neighborhood located in the El Norte section of town. Mr. and Mrs. Rodriguez have been active in the church and neighborhood community until recently when Mr. Rodriguez had been experiencing abdominal pain and difficulty urinating. The Rodriguez home is usually occupied by many people and has always been the gathering place for the family.

During his years of employment, Mr. Rodriguez was the major provider for the family and now receives Social Security checks and a pension. Mrs. Rodriguez is also retired and receives a small pension for a short work period as a nurse's aide. Mr. and Mrs. Rodriguez count on their nursing student granddaughter to guide them and advise on their health care. Mr. Rodriguez visits a *curandero* for medicinal folk remedies. Mrs. Rodriguez is the provider of spiritual, physical, and emotional care for the family. In addition, their nursing student granddaughter is always present during any major surgeries or procedures. Mrs. Rodriguez, the eldest daughter, and her granddaughter (the nursing student) will be caring for Mr. Rodriguez during his procedure for a TURBT (transurethreal resection of bladder tumor) as well as radiation therapy.

1. Explain the significance of family and kinship for the Rodriguez family.
2. Describe the importance of religion and God for the Rodriguez family.
3. Identify two stereotypes about Mexican Americans that were dispelled in this case with the Rodriguez family.
4. What is the role of Mrs. Rodriguez in this family?

common-law marriages (*unidos*) are frequently practiced and readily accepted, with many couples living together their entire lives.

Although homosexual behavior occurs in every society, The Williams Project reported that five states—California, Texas, New York, Florida, and Illinois—have the highest number of same-sex Latino couples, totaling 100,796, living together in the United States (Gates, Lau, & Sears, 2006). Newspapers from Houston, Texas; Washington, DC; and Chicago, Illinois, report on the efforts of Hispanic lesbian and gay organizations in the areas of HIV and AIDS (*La SIDA* in Spanish) and life partner benefits. In Mexico, homosexuality is not a crime, but antihate groups raised serious concerns about killings of homosexual men, causing many to remain closeted (RefWorld, 2011). In Mexico, *machismo* plays a large part in the phobic attitudes toward gay behavior. Larger cities in the United States may have *Ellas*, a support group for Latina lesbians; El Hotline of Hola Gay, which provides referrals and information in Spanish; or Dignity, for gay Catholics. Health-care providers who wish to refer gay and lesbian patients to a support group may use such agencies.

Workforce Issues
Culture in the Workplace
In the United States, Hispanics are the most underrepresented minority group in the health-care workforce. Although more than 13 percent of the American population is of Hispanic origin, only 3.6 percent of registered nurses are from Hispanic heritage (U.S. Department of Health and Human Services Health Resources and Services Administration, 2010). Cultural differences that influence workforce issues include values regarding family, pedagogical approach to education, emotional sensitivity, views toward status, aesthetics, ethics, balance of work and leisure, attitudes toward direction and delegation, sense of control, views about competition, and time.

People educated in Mexico are likely to have been exposed to pedagogical approaches that include rote memorization and an emphasis on theory with little practical application taught within a rigid, broad curriculum. American educational systems usually emphasize an analytical approach, practical applications, and a narrow, in-depth specialization. Thus, additional training may be needed for some Mexicans when they come to the United States.

Because family is a first priority for most Mexicans, activities that involve family members usually take priority over work issues. Putting up a tough business front may be seen as a weakness in the Mexican culture. Because of this separation of work from emotions in American culture, most Mexican Americans tend to shun confrontation for fear of losing face. Many are very sensitive to differences of opinion, which are perceived as disrupting harmony in the workplace. People of Mexican heritage find it important to keep peace in relationships in the workplace.

For many Mexicans, truth is tempered by diplomacy and tact. When a service is promised for tomorrow, even when they know the service will not be completed tomorrow, it is promised to please, not to deceive. Thus, for many Mexicans, truth is seen as a relative concept, whereas for most European Americans, truth is an absolute value, and people are expected to give direct yes and no answers. These conflicting perspectives about truth can complicate treatment regimens and commitment to the completion of work assignments. Intentions must be clarified and, at times, altered to meet the needs of the changing and multicultural workforce.

For most Mexicans, work is viewed as a necessity for survival and may not be highly valued in itself, whereas money is for enjoying life. Most Mexican Americans place a higher value on other life activities. Material objects are usually necessities and not ends in themselves. The concept of responsibility is based on values related to attending to the immediate needs of family and friends rather than on the work ethic. For most Mexicans, titles and positions may be more important than money.

Many Mexicans believe that time is relative and elastic, with flexible deadlines, rather than stressing punctuality and timeliness. In Mexico, shop hours may be posted but not rigidly respected. A business that is supposed to open at 8:00 a.m. opens when the owner arrives; a posted time of 8:00 a.m. may mean the business will open at 8:30 a.m., later, or not at all. The same attitude toward time is evidenced in reporting to work and in keeping social engagements and medical appointments. If people believe that an exact time is truly important, such as the time an airplane leaves, then they may keep to a schedule. The real challenge for employers is to stress the importance and necessity of work schedules and punctuality in the American workforce.

Issues Related to Autonomy

Many Mexican Americans respond to direction and delegation differently from European Americans. Many newer immigrants are used to having traditional autocratic managers who assign tasks but not authority, although this practice is beginning to change with more American-managed companies relocating to Mexico. A Mexican worker who is not accustomed to responsibility may have difficulty assuming accountability for decisions. The individual may be sensitive to the American practice of checking on employees' work.

Mexicans who were born and educated in the United States usually have no difficulty communicating with others in the workplace. When better-educated Mexican immigrants arrive in the United States, they usually speak some English. Newer immigrants from lower socioeconomic groups have the most difficulty acculturating in the workplace and may have greater difficulty with the English language.

Biocultural Ecology
Skin Color and Other Biological Variations

Because Mexican Americans draw their heritage from Spanish and French peoples and various North American and Central American Indian tribes and Africans, few physical characteristics give this group a distinct identity. Some individuals with a predominant Spanish background might have light-colored skin, blond hair, and blue eyes, whereas people from indigenous Indian backgrounds may have black hair, dark eyes, and cinnamon-colored skin. Intermarriages among these groups have created a diverse gene pool and have not produced a typical-appearing Mexican.

Cyanosis and decreased hemoglobin levels are more difficult to detect in dark-skinned people, whose skin appears ashen instead of the bluish color seen in light-skinned people. To observe for these conditions in dark-skinned Mexicans, the health-care provider must examine the sclera, conjunctiva, buccal mucosa, tongue, lips, nailbeds, palms of the hands, and soles of the feet. Jaundice, likewise, is more difficult to detect in darker-skinned people. Thus, the health-care provider needs to observe the conjunctiva and the buccal mucosa for patches of bilirubin pigment in dark-skinned Mexicans.

Diseases and Health Conditions

Common health problems most consistently documented in the literature for both people from Mexico and Mexican Americans are difficulty in assessing and utilizing health care, malnutrition, malaria (in some places), cancer, alcoholism, drug abuse, obesity, hypertension, diabetes, heart disease, adolescent pregnancy, dental disease, and HIV and AIDS (Kemp, 2001). In Mexican American migrant-worker populations, infectious, communicable, and parasitic diseases continue to be major health risks. Substandard housing conditions and employment in low-paying jobs have perpetuated higher rates of tuberculosis in Mexican Americans. Intestinal parasitosis, amoebic dysentery, and bacterial diarrhea (*Shigella*) are common among Mexican immigrants (Kim-Godwin, Alexander, Felton, Mackey, & Kasakoff, 2006).

Newer Mexican immigrants from coastal lowland swamp areas and from some mountainous areas where mosquitoes are more prevalent may also have a higher incidence of malaria. People from high mountain terrains may have increased red blood cell counts on immigration to the United States (Centers for Disease Control and Prevention [CDC], 2006). Healthcare providers must take these topographic factors into consideration when performing health screening for symptoms of anemia, lassitude, failure to thrive, and weight loss among Mexican immigrants.

Cardiovascular disease is the leading cause of death and disability in minority populations, including Mexican Americans (Kurian & Cardarelli, 2007). However, current research shows that despite the adverse cardiovascular risk profile, including the incidence of obesity, diabetes, and untreated hypertension, Mexican Americans have a lower rate of coronary heart disease mortality than non-white Hispanics (Pandey, Labarthe, Goff, Chan, & Nichaman, 2001). Cardiovascular risk factors are influenced by behavioral, cultural, and social factors. Mexican Americans have the highest prevalence of no leisure time physical activity (Kurian & Cardarelli, 2007). In addition, poor health, low social support, lack of educational and occupational opportunities, low access to health care, and discrimination contribute to the risk factors associated with cardiovascular disease (Kemp, 2001).

Mexican Americans have five times the rate of diabetes mellitus, with an increased incidence of related complications, as that in European American cohort groups. In addition, health-care providers working with Mexican immigrants and Mexican Americans should offer screening and teach patients preventive measures regarding pesticides and communicable and infectious diseases because many of these people work with chemicals and live in crowded housing conditions.

Variations in Drug Metabolism

Because of the mixed heritage of many Mexican Americans, it may be more difficult to determine a therapeutic dose of selected drugs. Several studies report differences in absorption, distribution, metabolism, and excretion of drugs, including alcohol, in some Hispanic populations. The mixed heritage of Mexican Americans makes it more difficult to generalize drug metabolism. Few studies include only one subgroup of Hispanics; therefore, health-care providers need to consider some notable differences when prescribing medications. Hispanics require lower doses of antidepressants and experience greater side effects than non-Hispanic whites.

High-Risk Behaviors

Alcohol plays an important part in the Mexican culture. Many of this group's colorful lifestyle celebrations include alcohol consumption. Men overall drink in greater proportion than women, but this trend is changing owing to acculturation. Mexican American women are consuming more alcohol than their mothers or grandmothers (Stanley Bunting, 2011).

Because of these drinking patterns, alcoholism represents a crucial health problem for many Mexicans. More acculturated Hispanics consume more alcoholic beverages than non-Hispanic whites, possibly expecting alcohol to make them more socially acceptable and extroverted. Low acculturation and distorted self-image problems have special implications for nursing and health care.

Marijuana is the number-two drug used by Mexican Americans because it is readily available in their native land and easily accessible from people who work in farming and ranching occupations. Some adults who can afford drugs use cocaine and heroin, and the younger population uses inhalants (Stanley Bunting, 2011).

The trend toward decreasing cigarette smoking in the United States is extending to the Mexican American culture, in which cigarette smoking rates have steadily declined for both men and women between 1990 and 2009 (CDC, 2011). However, the reported decrease in cigarette smoking rates for Mexican American men and women should not promote a sense of complacency for nurses and health-care providers.

Health-Care Practices

Responsibility for health promotion and safety may be a major threat for those of Mexican heritage accustomed to depending on the family unit and traditional means of providing health care. Continuing disparities in health and health-seeking behaviors have been reported in several studies. Lower socioeconomic conditions and acculturation are responsible for Latina women being overweight, exhibiting hypertension, experiencing high cholesterol levels, and having increased smoking behaviors (Kemp, 2001). Latino men are less likely to have cancer screening or physical examinations than their non-Latino white counterparts. High-risk health behaviors such as drinking and driving, cigarette smoking, sedentary lifestyle, and nonuse of seat belts increase with fewer years of educational attainment. Through educational programs and enforcement of state laws, more Mexicans are beginning to use seat belts; however, it is still common to see their children traveling unrestrained in automobiles.

Nutrition
Meaning of Food

As in many other ethnic groups, Mexicans and Mexican Americans celebrate with food. Mexican foods are rich in color, flavor, texture, and spiciness. Any occasion—births, birthdays, Sundays, religious holidays, official and unofficial holidays, and anniversaries of deaths—is seen as a time to celebrate with food and enjoy the companionship of family and friends. Because food is a primary form of socialization in the Mexican culture, Mexican Americans may have difficulty adhering to a prescribed diet for illnesses such as diabetes mellitus and cardiovascular disease. Health-care providers must seek creative alternatives and negotiate types of foods consumed with individuals and families in relation to these concerns.

Common Foods and Food Rituals

The Mexican American diet is extremely varied and may depend on the individual's region of origin in Mexico. Thus, one needs to ask the individual specifically about his or her dietary habits. The staples of the Mexican American diet are rice (*arroz*), beans, and tortillas, which are made from corn (*maíz*) treated with calcium carbonate. However, in many parts of the United States, only flour tortillas are available. Even though the diet is low in calcium derived from milk and milk products, tortillas treated with calcium carbonate provide essential dietary calcium. Popular Mexican American foods are eggs (*huevos*), pork (*puerco*), chicken (*pollo*), sausage (*chorizo*), lard (*lardo*), mint (*menta*), chili peppers (*chile*), onions (*cebollas*), tomatoes (*tomates*), squash (*calabaza*), canned fruit (*fruta de lata*), mint tea (*hierbabuena*), chamomile tea (*té de camomile* or *manzanilla*), carbonated beverages (*bebidas de gaseosa*), beer (*cerveza*), cola-flavored soft drinks, sweetened packaged drink mixes (*agua fresa*) that are high in sugar (*azucar*), sweetened breakfast cereals (*cereales de desayuno*), potatoes (*papas*), bread (*pan*), corn (*maíz*), gelatin (*gelatina*), custard (*flan*), and other sweets (*dulces*). Other common dishes include chili, enchiladas, tamales, tostadas, chicken mole, arroz con pollo, refried beans, tacos, tripe soup (*Menudo*), and other soups (*caldos*). *Caldos* are varied in nature and may include chicken, beef, and pork with vegetables.

Mealtimes vary among different subgroups of Mexican Americans. Whereas many individuals adopt North American schedules and eating habits, many continue their native practices, especially those in rural settings and migrant-worker camps. For these groups, breakfast is usually fruit, perhaps cheese, or bread alone or in some combination. A snack may be taken in midmorning before the main meal of the day, which is eaten from 2 to 3 p.m. and, in rural areas especially, may last for 2 hours or more. Mealtime is an occasion for socialization and keeping family members informed about one another. The evening meal is usually late and is taken between 9 and 9:30 p.m. Health-care providers must consider Mexican Americans' mealtimes when teaching patients about medication and dietary regimens related to diabetes mellitus and other illnesses.

Dietary Practices for Health Promotion

A dominant health-care practice for Mexicans and many Mexican Americans is the hot-and-cold theory of food selection. This theory is a major aspect of health promotion and illness, and disease prevention and treatment. According to this theory, illness or trauma may require adjustments in the hot-and-cold balance of foods to restore body equilibrium. The hot-and-cold theory of foods is described under Health-Care Practices, later in this chapter.

Nutritional Deficiencies and Food Limitations

In lower socioeconomic groups, wide-scale vitamin A deficiency and iron deficiency anemia exist (Mendoza, Ventura, Saldivar, Baisden, & Martorell, 1992). Some Mexican and Mexican Americans have lactose intolerance, which may cause problems for schools and health-care organizations that provide milk in the diet because of its high calcium content.

Because major Mexican foods and their ingredients are available throughout the United States, native food practices may not change much when Mexicans immigrate. Of course, Mexican foods are extremely popular throughout the United States and are eaten by many Americans because of the strong flavors, spiciness, and color. Table 21-1 lists the Mexican names of popular foods, their description, and ingredients. Individual adaptations to these preparations commonly occur.

Pregnancy and Childbearing Practices

Fertility Practices and Views Toward Pregnancy

Mexican American birth rates were 722,055, or 24.3 percent, live births in 2007; the number of births has continued to rise every year since 1989 (Martin et al., 2010). Multiple births are common, especially in the economically disadvantaged groups. Men view a large number of children as proof of their virility. The optimal childbearing age for Mexican women is between 19 and 24 years. Fertility practices of Mexican Americans are connected with their predominantly Catholic religious beliefs and their tendency to be modest. Some women practice the belief that prolonged infant breastfeeding is a method of birth control. Abortion in many communities is considered morally wrong and is practiced (theoretically) only in extreme circumstances to keep the mother's life intact. However, legal and illegal abortions are common in some parts of Mexico and the United States. Despite the strong influence of the Catholic Church over fertility practices, being Catholic does not prevent some Mexican American women from using contraceptives, sterilization, or abortion for unwanted pregnancies.

Diaphragms, foams, and creams are not commonly used for birth control practice, mostly because they are

❚❙❘ Table 21-1   Mexican Foods

Common Name	Description	Ingredients
Arroz con pollo	Chicken with rice	Chicken baked, boiled, or fried and served over boiled or fried rice
Chili	Chili	Same as the United States but tends to be more spicy
Chili con carne	Chili with meat	Chili with beef or pork
Chili con salsa	Chili with sauce	Chili with a sauce that contains no meat
Dulces	Sweets	Candy and desserts usually high in sugar, lard, and eggs
Enchiladas	Enchiladas	Tortilla rolled and stuffed with meat or cheese and a spicy sauce
Papas fritas	Fried potatoes	Potatoes usually fried in lard
Flan	Flan	Popular dessert made of egg custard; may be filled with fruit or cheese
Gelatina	Gelatin	Popular dessert made with sugar, eggs, and jelly
Pollo con molé	Chicken molé	Chicken with a sauce made of hot spices, chocolate, and chili
Salchica or chorizo	Sausage	Sausage almost always made with pork and spices
Tacos	Tacos	Tortilla folded around meat or cheese
Tamales	Tamales	Fried or boiled chopped meat, peppers, cornmeal, and hot spices
Tortilla	Tortilla	A thin unleavened bread made with cornmeal and treated with lime (calcium carbonate)
Tostadas	Tostadas	Toast that may have a spicy sauce

not approved by Catholic doctrine and partly because of the belief that women are not supposed to touch their genitals. Birth control pills are unacceptable because they are an artificial means of birth control. Physicians' offices and clinics that see large numbers of migrant workers on the Delmarva Peninsula on the U.S. East Coast report that many younger female patients are using Norplant (levonorgestrel; a long-term contraceptive system) for birth control. Men are reluctant to use condoms because they are associated with prostitutes and because of the belief that they should be used only for disease control. A woman may reject the use of a condom and find it offensive because it means that she is "dirty." Family planning is one area in which health-care providers can help the family to identify more realistic outcomes consistent with current economic resources and family goals.

Foreign-born Mexicans are less likely to give birth to low-birth-weight babies than U.S.-born Mexican women, even though U.S.-born mothers are usually of higher socioeconomic status and receive more prenatal care. Research suggests that better nutritional intake and lower prevalence of smoking and alcohol use are some reasons for these protective outcomes (American Public Health Association, 2002).

Because pregnancy among Mexican Americans is viewed as natural and desirable, many women do not seek prenatal evaluations. In addition, because prenatal care is not available to every woman in Mexico, some women do not know about the need for prenatal care. With the extended family network and the woman's role of maintaining the health status of family members, many pregnant women seek family advice before seeking medical care. Thus, *familism* may deter and hinder early prenatal checkups. To encourage prenatal checkups, health-care providers can encourage female relatives and husbands to accompany the pregnant woman for health screening and incorporate advice from family members into health teaching and preventive care services. Using videos with Spanish-speaking Mexican Americans is one culturally effective way for incorporating health education, especially for those patients who have a limited understanding of English. In addition, incorporating cultural brokers known to the Mexican American family may help to empower patients and reduce conflict for Mexicans and Mexican Americans.

Prescriptive, Restrictive, and Taboo Practices in the Childbearing Family

Beliefs related to the hot-and-cold theory of disease prevention and health maintenance influence conception, pregnancy, and postpartum rituals. For instance, during pregnancy, a woman is more likely to favor hot foods, which are believed to provide warmth for the fetus and enable the baby to be born into a warm and loving environment (Eggenberger, Grassley, & Restrepo, 2006). Cold foods and environments are preferred during the menstrual cycle and in the immediate postdelivery period. Many pregnant women sleep on their backs to protect the infant from harm, keep the vaginal canal well lubricated by having frequent intercourse to facilitate an easier birth, and keep active to ensure a smaller baby and to prevent a decrease in the amount of amniotic fluid (Burk, Wieser, & Keegan, 1995). An important activity restriction is that pregnant women should not walk in the moonlight because it might cause a birth deformity. To prevent birth deformities, pregnant women may wear a safety pin, metal key, or some other metal object on their abdomen (Villarruel & Ortiz de Montellano, 1992). Other beliefs include avoiding cold air, not reaching over the head in order to prevent the baby's cord from wrapping around its neck, and avoiding lunar eclipses because they may result in deformities.

In more traditional Mexican families, the father is not included in the delivery experience and should not see the mother or baby until after both have been cleaned and dressed. This practice is based on the fear that harm may come to the mother, baby, or both. Integrating men into the birthing of a child is a process that requires changing social habits in relation to cultural aspects of life and gender roles. For many, the presence of men during delivery is considered an uninvited intrusion into the Mexican culture. Among less traditional and more acculturated Mexican Americans, men participate in prenatal classes and assist in the delivery room. However, based on personal experiences, men who provide support during delivery may receive friendly gibing from their male counterparts for taking the role of the wife's mother (personal communication, Larry Purnell, 2010). In any event, health-care providers must respect Mexicans' decision to not have men in the delivery room.

During labor, traditional Mexican women may be quite vocal and are taught to avoid breathing air in through the mouth because it can cause the uterus to rise up. Immediately after birth, they may place their legs together to prevent air from entering the womb (Olds, London, & Ladewig, 2000). Health-care providers can help the Mexican pregnant woman have a better delivery by encouraging attendance at prenatal classes.

The postpartum preference for a warm environment may restrict postpartum women from bathing or washing their hair for up to 40 days. Although postpartum women may not take showers or sit in a bathtub, this does not mean that they do not bathe. They take "sitz" baths, wash their hair with a washcloth, and take sponge baths. Other postpartum practices include wearing a heavy cotton abdominal binder, cord, or girdle to prevent air from entering the uterus; covering one's ears, head, shoulders, and feet to prevent blindness, mastitis, frigidity, or sterility; and avoiding acidic foods to protect the baby from harm (Olds, London, & Ladewig, 2000).

When the baby is born, special attention is given to the umbilicus; the mother may place a belt around the umbilicus (*ombliguero*) to prevent the navel from popping out when the child cries. Cutting the baby's nails in the first 3 months is thought to cause blindness and deafness.

Health-care providers need to make special provisions to provide culturally congruent health teaching for lactating women who work with or are exposed to pesticides, such as dichlorodiphenyldichlorothene (DDE), the most stable derivative from the pesticide DDT. High DDE levels among lactating women have a direct correlation with a decrease in lactation and increase in breast cancer, especially in women who have had more than one pregnancy and previous lactation (Gladen & Rogan, 1995). Education level and degree of acculturation are key issues when developing health education and interventions for risk reduction.

Death Rituals

Death Rituals and Expectations

Mexicans often have a stoic acceptance of the way things are and view death as a natural part of life and the will of God (Eggenberger et al., 2006). Death practices are primarily an adaptation of their religion. Family members may arrive in large numbers at the hospital or home in times of illness or an approaching death. In more traditional families, family members may take turns sitting vigil over the sick or dying person. Autopsy is acceptable as long as the body is treated with respect. Burial is the common practice; cremation is an individual choice.

Responses to Death and Grief

When a person dies, the word travels rapidly, and family and friends travel from long distances to get to the funeral. They may gather for a **velorio**, a festive watch over the body of the deceased person before burial. Some Mexican Americans bury the body within 24 hours, which is required by law in Mexico.

More traditional grieving families may engage in protection of the dying and bereaved, such as small children who have difficulty dealing with the death (Andrews & Boyle, 2008). Mexican Americans encourage expressions of feeling during the grieving process. In these cases, health-care providers can assist the person by providing support and privacy during the bereavement.

Spirituality

Dominant Religion and Use of Prayer

The predominant religion of most Mexicans and Mexican Americans is Catholicism. The major religions in Mexico are Roman Catholic with 76.5 percent; Protestant with 5.2 percent; Pentecostal with 1.4 percent; unspecified with 13.1 percent; Jehovah's Witness, 1.1 percent; other 0.3 percent; and 3.1 percent identified with no religion. Since the mid-1980s, other religious groups such as Mormons, Jehovah's Witnesses, Seventh Day Adventists, Presbyterians, and Baptists have been gaining in popularity in Mexico (*CIA World Factbook*, 2012). Although many Mexicans and Mexican Americans may not appear to be practicing their faith on a daily basis, they may still consider themselves devout Catholics, and their religion has a major influence on health-care practices and beliefs. For many, Catholic religious practices are influenced by indigenous Indian practices.

Newer immigrant Mexican Americans may continue their traditional practice of having two marriage ceremonies, especially in lower socioeconomic groups. A civil ceremony is performed whenever two people decide to make a union. When the family gets enough money for a religious ceremony, they schedule an elaborate celebration within the church. Common practice, especially in rural Mexican villages and some rural villages in the southwestern United States, is to post a handwritten sign on the local church announcing the marriage, with an invitation for all to attend.

Frequency of prayer is highly individualized for most Mexican Americans. Even though some do not attend church on a regular basis, they may have an altar in their homes and say prayers several times each day, a practice more common among rural isolationists.

Meaning of Life and Individual Sources of Strength

The family is foremost to most Mexicans, and individuals get strength from family ties and relationships. Individuals may speak in terms of a person's soul or spirit (*alma* or *espiritu*) when they refer to one's inner qualities. These inner qualities represent the person's dignity and must be protected at all costs in times of both wellness and illness. In addition, Mexicans derive great pride and strength from their nationality, which embraces a long and rich history of traditions.

Leisure is considered essential for a full life, and work is a necessity to make money for enjoying life. Mexican Americans pride themselves on good manners, etiquette, and grooming as signs of respect. Because the overall outlook for many Mexicans is one of fatalism, pride may be taken in stoic acceptance of life's adversities.

Spiritual Beliefs and Health-Care Practices

Most Mexicans enjoy talking about their soul or spirit, especially in times of illness, whereas many health-care providers may feel uncomfortable talking about spirituality. This tendency may communicate to Mexicans that the health-care provider has suspect intentions, is insensitive, and is not really interested in them as individuals. It may be common for a person needing care in the home or hospital to have a statue of a patron saint or a candle with a picture of the saint. Rosaries may be present, and at times, the family may pray as a group. Depending on the confidence maintained with the family and client, a health-care provider may be asked to join in the prayer. If time permits, it is very appropriate to pray with the family, even if only for a few minutes. This action promotes confidence in the relationship and can have a positive impact on the health and well-being of the patient and family (Zoucha, 2007).

Health-Care Practices

Health-Seeking Beliefs and Behaviors

The family is the most credible source of health information and the most significant impediment to positive health-seeking behavior. Mexican Americans' fatalistic worldview and external locus of control are closely tied to health-seeking behaviors. Because expressions of negative feelings are considered impolite, Mexicans may be reluctant to complain about health problems or to place blame on the individual for poor health. If a person becomes seriously ill, that is just the way things are; all events are acts of God (Eggenberger et al., 2006). This belief system may impair the dominant view of communications and hinder health teaching, health promotion, and disease-prevention practices. Therefore, it is imperative for health-care providers to plan health-promoting activities and teaching that are consistent with this belief but encourage health. For instance, if a person believes that the illness is due to a punishment from God, it may be possible to ask to be forgiven by God, thereby restoring health. This may be an opportune time to call a priest or minister for official recognition of forgiveness.

Responsibility for Health Care

To many Mexicans, good health may mean the ability to keep working and have a general feeling of well-being (Zoucha, 2011). Illness may occur when the person can no longer work or take care of the family. Therefore, many Mexicans may not seek health care until they are incapacitated and unable to go about the activities of daily living. Unfortunately, many people of Mexican heritage may not know and understand the occupational dangers inherent in their daily work. Migrant workers are often unaware of the dangers of pesticides and the potentially dangerous agricultural machinery. Health-care providers must serve as advocates for these people regarding occupational safety. Often, the companies do not tell the workers of the dangers of the work, or the workers may not understand owing to the inability of the company officials to speak the language of the workers.

The use of over-the-counter medicine may pose a significant health problem related to self-care for many Mexican Americans. In part, this is a carryover from Mexico's practice of allowing over-the-counter purchases of antibiotics, intramuscular injections, intravenous fluids, birth control pills, and other medications that require a prescription in the United States. Often, Mexican immigrants bring these medications across the border and share them with friends. In addition, friends and relatives in Mexico send drugs through the mail. To protect patients from contradictory or potentiating effects of prescribed treatments, health-care providers need to ask patients about prescription and nonprescription medications they may be taking.

Folk and Traditional Practices

Mexican Americans engage in folk medicine practices and use a variety of prayers, herbal teas, and poultices to treat illnesses. Many of these practices are regionally specific and vary between and among families.

The Mexican *Ministerio de Salud Publica y Asistencia Social* (Ministry of Public Health and Social Assistance) publishes an extensive manual on herbal medicines that are readily available in Mexico. Lower socioeconomic groups and well-educated upper- and middle-socioeconomic Mexicans to some degree practice traditional and folk medicine. Many of these practices are harmless, but some may contradict or potentiate therapeutic interventions. Thus, as with the use of other prescription and nonprescription drugs discussed earlier, it is essential for health-care providers to be aware of these practices and to take them into consideration when providing treatments (Rivera, Anaya, & Meza, 2003). The provider must ask the Mexican American patient specifically whether she or he is using folk medicine.

To provide culturally competent care, health-care providers must be aware of the hot-and-cold theory of disease when prescribing treatment modalities and when providing health teaching. According to this theory, many diseases are caused by a disruption in the hot-and-cold balance of the body. Thus, eating foods of the opposite variety may either cure or prevent specific hot-and-cold illnesses and conditions. Physical or mental illness may be attributed to an imbalance between the person and the environment. Influences include emotional, spiritual, and social state, as well as physical factors such as humoral imbalance expressed as either too much hot or cold. As health-care providers, it is important to understand that if people of Mexican heritage believe in the hot-and-cold theory, it means that they do not believe or use professional Western practices (Spector, 2008). Unless a level of trust and confidence is maintained, Mexicans who follow these beliefs may not express them to health-care providers (Zoucha, 2011).

Hot and cold are viewed as specific properties of various substances and conditions, and sometimes opinions differ about what is hot and what is cold in the Mexican community. In general, cold diseases or conditions are characterized by vasoconstriction and a lower metabolic rate. Cold diseases or conditions include menstrual cramps, *frio de la matriz*, rhinitis (*coryza*), pneumonia, *empacho*, cancer, malaria, earaches, arthritis, pneumonia and other pulmonary conditions, headaches, and musculoskeletal conditions and colic. Common hot foods used to treat cold diseases and conditions include cheeses, liquor, beef, pork, spicy foods, eggs, grains other than barley, vitamins, tobacco, and onions (Neff, 2011).

Hot diseases and conditions may be characterized by vasodilation and a higher metabolic rate. Pregnancy, hypertension, diabetes, acid indigestion, *susto*, *mal de ojo* (bad eye or evil eye), *bilis* (imbalance of bile, which runs into the bloodstream), infection, diarrhea, sore throats, stomach ulcers, liver conditions, kidney problems, and fever may be examples of hot conditions.

Common cold foods used to treat hot diseases and conditions include fresh fruits and vegetables, dairy products (even though fresh fruits and dairy products may cause diarrhea), barley water, fish, chicken, goat meat, and dried fruits (Neff, 2011).

Folk practitioners are consulted for several notable conditions. *Mal de ojo* is a folk illness that occurs when one person (usually older) looks at another (usually a child) in an admiring fashion. Another example of *mal de ojo* is if a person admires something about a baby or child, such as beautiful eyes or hair. Such eye contact can be either voluntary or involuntary. Symptoms are numerous, ranging from fever, anorexia, and vomiting to irritability. The spell can be broken if the person doing the admiring touches the person admired while it is happening. Children are more susceptible to this condition than women, and women are more susceptible than men. To prevent *mal de ojo*, the child wears a bracelet with a seed (*ojo de venado*) or a bag of seeds pinned to the clothes (Kemp, 2001).

Another childhood condition often treated by folk practitioners is **caida de la mollera** (fallen fontanel). The condition has numerous causes, which may include removing the nursing infant too harshly from the nipple or handling an infant too roughly. Symptoms range from irritability to failure to thrive. To cure the condition, the child is held upside down by the legs.

Susto (magical fright or soul loss) is associated with epilepsy, tuberculosis, and other infectious diseases and is caused by the loss of spirit from the body. The illness is also believed to be caused by a fright or by the soul being frightened out of the person. This culture-bound disorder may be psychological, physical, or physiological in nature. Symptoms may include anxiety, depression, loss of appetite, excessive sleep, bad dreams, feelings of sadness, and lack of motivation. Treatment sometimes includes elaborate ceremonies at a crossroads with herbs and holy water to return the spirit to the body (R. Zamarripa, personal communication, 2010).

Empacho (blocked intestines) may result from an incorrect balance of hot and cold foods, causing a lump of food to stick in the gastrointestinal tract. To make the diagnosis, the healer may place a fresh egg on the abdomen. If the egg appears to stick to a particular area, this confirms the diagnosis. Older women usually treat the condition in children by massaging their stomach and back to dislodge the food bolus and to promote its continued passage through the body.

Health-care providers are cautioned against diagnosing psychiatric illnesses too readily in the Mexican population. The syndromes **mal ojo** and *susto* are culture-bound and are potential sources of diagnostic bias. The potential culture-bound mental illness must be understood in the context of the culture and the unique symptoms that accompany each illness.

Barriers to Health Care

Thirty-five percent of Mexican Americans, compared with 17 percent of the U.S. population in general, do not have health insurance (CDC, 2011). A number of factors may account for this high percentage of uninsured individuals. First, many Mexican Americans constitute the working poor and are unable to purchase insurance. Second, many are migratory and do not qualify for Medicaid. Third, many have an undocumented status and are afraid to apply for health insurance. Fourth, even though insurance is available in their native homeland, it is very expensive and not part of the culture.

Whereas wealthier Mexican Americans have little difficulty accessing health care in the United States, lower socioeconomic groups may experience significant barriers, including inadequate financial resources, lack of insurance and transportation, limited knowledge regarding available services, language difficulties, and the culture of health-care organizations. Like many other immigrant groups who lack a primary provider, Mexican Americans may use emergency rooms for minor illnesses. Health-care providers have the opportunity to improve the care of Mexican Americans by explaining the health-care system, incorporating a primary-care provider whenever possible, using an interpreter of the same gender, securing a cultural broker, and assisting patients in locating culturally specific mental health programs (Zoucha & Husted, 2002).

Cultural Responses to Health and Illness

Good health to many Mexican Americans is to be free of pain, able to work, and spend time with the family. In addition, good health is a gift from God and from living a good life (Zoucha, 2011).

Mexicans and Mexican Americans tend to perceive pain as a necessary part of life, and enduring the pain is often viewed as a sign of strength. Men commonly tolerate pain until it becomes extreme (Luckmann, 1999). Often, pain is viewed as the will of God and is tolerated as long as the person can work and care for the family. These attitudes toward pain delay seeking treatment; many hope that the pain will simply go away. Research has shown that many Mexican Americans experience more pain than other ethnic groups but that they report the occurrence of pain less frequently and endure pain longer (Sobralske & Katz, 2005). Six themes have emerged that describe culturally specific attributes of Mexican Americans experiencing pain:

1. Mexicans accept and anticipate pain as a necessary part of life.
2. They are obligated to endure pain in the performance of duties.
3. The ability to endure pain and to suffer stoically is valued.
4. The type and amount of pain a person experiences are divinely predetermined.
5. Pain and suffering are a consequence of immoral behavior.
6. Methods to alleviate pain are directed toward maintaining balance within the person and the surrounding environment (Villarruel & Ortiz de Montellano, 1992).

By using these themes, health-care providers can evaluate Mexicans experiencing pain within their cultural framework and provide culturally specific interventions.

Because long-term-care facilities in Mexico are rare and tend to be crowded, understaffed, and expensive, many Mexican Americans may not consider long-term care as a viable option for a family member. In addition, because of the importance of extended family, Mexican Americans may prefer to care for their family members with mental illness, physical handicaps, and extended physical illnesses at home. In Mexican American culture, someone with a mental illness is not looked on with scorn or blamed for his or her condition because mental illness, like physical illness, is viewed as God's will. It is common to accept those with mental illness and care for them in the context of the family until the illness is so bad that they cannot be managed in the home (Zoucha & Husted, 2000).

Mexicans can readily enter the sick role without personal feelings of inadequacy or blame. A person can enter the sick role with any acceptable excuse and be relieved of life's responsibilities. Other family members willingly take over the sick person's obligations during his or her time of illness.

Blood Transfusions and Organ Donation

Extraordinary means to preserve life are frowned on in the Mexican and Mexican American culture, and ordinary means are commonly used to preserve life. Extraordinary means are defined and determined by the individual, taking into account such factors as finances, education, and availability of services.

Blood transfusions are acceptable if the individual and the family agree that the transfusion is necessary. Organ donation, although not deemed morally wrong, is not a common practice and is usually restricted to cadaver donations, because donating an organ while the person is still alive means that the body is not whole. Acceptance of organ transplant as a treatment option is seen primarily among more educated people. One reason that organ transplant is unacceptable to some groups is the belief that *mal aire* (bad air) enters the body if it is left open too long during surgery and increases the potential for the development of cancer.

Health-Care Providers

Traditional Versus Biomedical Providers

Educated physicians and nurses are often seen as outsiders, especially among newer immigrants. However, health-care providers are viewed as knowledgeable and respected because of their education (Zoucha & Husted, 2002). To overcome this initial awkwardness, health-care providers should attempt to get to know the patient on a more personal level and gain confidence before initiating treatment regimens. Engaging in small talk unrelated to the health-care encounter before obtaining a health history or providing health education is advised. Health-care providers must respect this cultural practice to achieve an optimal outcome from the encounter.

Folk practitioners, who are usually well known by the family, are usually consulted before and during biomedical treatment. Numerous illnesses and conditions are caused by witchcraft. Specific rituals are carried out to eliminate the evils from the body. Lower socioeconomic and newer immigrants are more likely to use folk practitioners, but well-educated upper- and middle-class people also visit folk practitioners and *brujas* (witches) on a regular basis (Torres, 2001). Although often no contradictions or contraindications to folk remedies exist, health-care providers must always consider patients' use of these practitioners to prevent conflicting treatment regimens.

Even though the Catholic Church preaches against some types of folk practitioners, they are common and meet yearly for several days in Catemaco, Veracruz. Folk practitioners include the ***curandero***, who may receive her or his talents from God or serve an apprenticeship with an established practitioner. The *curandero* has great respect from the community, accepts no monetary payment (but may accept gifts), is usually a member of the extended family, and treats many traditional illnesses. A *curandero* does not usually treat illnesses caused by witchcraft.

The ***yerbero*** (also spelled ***jerbero***) is a folk healer with specialized training in growing herbs, teas, and roots and who prescribes these remedies for prevention and cure of illnesses. A *yerbero* may suggest that the person go to a ***botanica*** (herb shop) for specific herbs. In addition, these folk practitioners frequently prescribe the use of laxatives.

A ***sobador*** subscribes to treatment methods similar to those of a Western chiropractor. The *sobador* treats illnesses, primarily affecting the joints and musculoskeletal system, with massage and manipulation.

Even though Mexicans like closeness and touch within the context of family, most tend to be modest in other settings. Women are not supposed to expose their bodies to men or even to other women. Female patients may experience embarrassment when it is necessary to touch their genitals or may refuse to have pelvic examinations as a routine part of a health assessment. Men may have strong feelings about modesty as well, especially in front of women, and may be reluctant to disrobe completely for an examination. Mexican Americans often desire that members of the same gender provide intimate care (C. Zamarripa, personal communication, 2011). Health-care providers must keep in mind patients' need for modesty when disrobing or being examined. Thus, only the body part being examined should be exposed, and direct care should be provided in private. Whenever possible, a same-gender caregiver should be assigned to Mexican Americans.

Status of Health-Care Providers

Mexican American patients have great respect for health-care providers because of their training and experience. They expect health-care providers to project a professional image and be well groomed and dressed in attire that reflects their professional status (Zoucha & Husted, 2002). Whereas they have great respect for health-care providers, some Mexican Americans may distrust them out of fear that they will disclose their undocumented status. Health-care providers who incorporate folk practitioners, the concept of *personalismo*, and respect into their approaches to care of Mexican American patients will gain their patients' confidence and be able to obtain more thorough assessments.

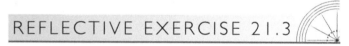

REFLECTIVE EXERCISE 21.3

Vicente Rios is a 25-year-old Mexican man who was recently diagnosed with a right radial bone fracture after a work-related injury. An emergency room physician has recommended surgery and physical therapy. Vicente is unmarried and is a recent immigrant from Mexico City, Mexico. He is an undocumented worker and has been working for a construction company doing roofing and bricklaying. Vicente's family resides in Mexico. His parents, maternal grandparents, five sisters, and two brothers live in a small two-bedroom stone home in the Colonia region of Mexico City. Vicente is the oldest of the children and has come to the United States to work and send money back to the family. Vicente's dad is being treated for colon cancer and needs money to pay for health care. Vicente is also trying to earn enough money to bring his dad to the United States for further cancer treatment. Vicente speaks mainly Spanish, with limited ability in English.

Vicente is a devout Catholic who attends Mass weekly and prays the rosary to *La Virgen de Guadalupe* daily. Vicente often blesses himself with holy water he brought from San Juan de Los Lagos. Vicente believes that God will heal him and that his health is in the hands of God.

Vicente is sharing the rent on a two-bedroom apartment with three other migrant workers from Mexico. The apartment is located 15 miles from his job where new homes are being built outside the city. Vicente usually takes two buses to work. One of the migrant workers has an uncle who helped secure the jobs for them. Vicente and his coworkers cook and eat dinner together most evenings and enjoy drinking *cervezas* (beer) on the weekends.

Vicente has saved money from working over the past 18 months but is worried about health-care coverage. He usually goes to a local clinic for his health-care needs. His friends suggested that he should visit a *bruja* because he might have had a spell cast upon him. He and his friends believe that the *bruja* can rid him of the spell and heal him. Vicente's friends are able to help take care of him on weekends only because of their weekday 12-hour work schedules. Vicente has an uncle from Mexico who is trying to get money together for a trip up to help Vicente as he recovers. Vicente will require home physical therapy and nursing care after his surgery. He will also be unable to work for 6 to 8 weeks.

1. The home-care case manager, a registered nurse, is sending a physical therapist to the home. What should the nurse consider?
2. What does the nurse need to know about what part of Mexico Vicente and his family are from?
3. Identify potential communication needs of Vicente, his friends, and his visiting family.
4. Vicente is concerned about letting his boss down because of his illness. Why is Vicente concerned about this with his boss?

Health-care providers can demonstrate respect for Mexican American patients by greeting the patient with a handshake, touching the person, or holding the person's hand, all of which help to build trust in the therapeutic relationship. Providing information and involving the family in decisions regarding health; listening to the individual's concerns; and treating the individual with *personalismo*, which stresses warmth and personal relationships, also foster trust.

REFERENCES

American Public Health Association. (2002). *Maternal health risks of immigrant women from Latin America.* Retrieved from http://www.apha.org

Andrews, M., & Boyle, J. (2008). *Transcultural concepts in nursing care* (5th ed.). Philadelphia: Lippincott.

Burk, M.E., Wieser, P.C., & Keegan, L. (1995). Cultural beliefs and health behaviors of pregnant Mexican-American women: Implications for primary care. *Advances in Nursing Science, 17*(4), 37–52.

Casa Historia. (2011, February 23). Mexican revolution and beyond. Retrieved from http://www.casahistoria.net/mexicorevolution.htm

Centers for Disease Control and Prevention (CDC). (2006). *Regional malaria information.* Retrieved from http://www.cdc.gov/travel/regionalmalaria/camerica.htm

Centers for Disease Control and Prevention (CDC). (2011). *Health of Mexican American population.* Retrieved from http://www.cdc.gov/nchs/fastats/mexican_health.htm

CIA World Factbook. (2012). Retrieved from https://www.cia.gov/library/publications/the-world-factbook/geos/mx.html URL remains the same even though the date changed.

Department of Homeland Security. (2011). *Estimates of the unauthorized immigrant population residing in the United States.* Retrieved from http://www.dhs.gov/xlibrary/assets/statistics/publications/ois_ill_pe_2010.pdf

Eggenberger, S.K., Grassley, J., & Restrepo, E. (2006). Culturally competent nursing care: Listening to the voices of Mexican-American women. *Online Journal of Issues in Nursing, 11*(3), 7.

Gates, G., Lau, H., & Sears, B. (2006). *Race and ethnicity of same-sex couples in California*: The Williams Project on Sexual Orientation Law and Public Policy UCLA School of Law. Los Angeles, CA: UCLA.

Gladen, B., & Rogan, W. (1995). DDE and shortened duration of lactation in a northern Mexican town. *American Journal of Public Health, 85*(4), 504–508.

Grothaus, K.L. (1996). Family dynamics and family therapy with Mexican Americans. *Journal of Psychosocial Nursing and Mental Health Services, 34*(2), 31–37.

Kemp, C. (2001). Hispanic health beliefs and practices: Mexican and Mexican-Americans (clinical notes) [Electronic version]. Retrieved from http://www3.baylor.edu/~Charles_Kemp/hispanic_health.htm

Kim-Godwin, Y.S., Alexander, J.W., Felton, G., Mackey, M.C., & Kasakoff, A. (2006). Prerequisites to providing culturally competent care to Mexican migrant farmworkers: A Delphi study. *Journal of Cultural Diversity, 13*(1), 27–33.

Kurian, A.K., & Cardarelli, K.M. (2007). Racial and ethnic differences in cardiovascular disease risk factors: A systematic review. *Ethnic Diseases, 17*(1), 143–152.

Library of Congress. (2005, April, 20). *Immigration: Mexican.* Retrieved from http://novaonline.nvcc.edu/eli/evans/his135/Events/Mexico/Mexico.html

Locke, D. (1998). *Increasing multicultural understanding: A comprehensive model* (2nd ed.). Newbury Park, CA: Sage.

Luckmann, J. (1999). *Transcultural communication in nursing.* Albany, NY: Delmar.

Martin, J.A., Hamilton, B.E., Sutton, P.D., Ventura, S.J., Mathews, T.J., Kirmeyer, & S. Osterman, J.K. (2010). Division of vital statistics, births: Final data for 2007. *National Vital Statistics Report, 58*(4). Retrieved from http://www.cdc.gov/nchs/data/nvsr/nvsr58/nvsr58_24.pdf

Mendoza, F.S., Ventura S., Saldivar L., Baisden K., & Martorell R. (1992). In A. Furino (Ed.), *Health policy and the Hispanic* (pp. 97–115). Boulder, CO: Westview Press.

Meyer, M., & Beezley, W. (2000). *The Oxford history of Mexico.* Oxford: Oxford University Press.

Neff, N. (2011). *Folk medicine in Hispanics in the southwestern United States.* Retrieved from http://www.rice.edu/projects/HispanicHealth/Courses/mod7/mod7.html

Olds, S., London, M., & Ladewig, P. (2000). *Maternal newborn nursing: A family-centered approach* (5th ed.). Redwood City, CA: Addison Wesley.

Pandey, D.K., Labarthe, D.R., Goff, D.C., Chan, W., & Nichaman, M.Z. (2001). Community-wide coronary heart disease mortality in Mexican Americans equals or exceeds that in non-Hispanic whites: The Corpus Christi Heart Project. *American Journal of Medicine, 110*(2), 81–87.

RefWorld. (2011). *Mexico: Treatment of homosexuals and availability of state protection.* Retrieved from http://www.asylumlaw.org/docs/sexualminorities/MexicoUNHCRRefworld061507.pdf

Rivera, J.O., Anaya, J.P., & Meza, A. (2003). Herbal product use in Mexican-Americans. *American Journal of Health-System Pharmacy, 60*(12), 1281–1282.

Schmal, J., & Madrer, J. (2007). Ethnic diversity in Mexico [Electronic version]. *Mexico Connect*. Retrieved from http://www.mexconnect.com/mex_/feature/ethnic/ethnicindex.html#imm

Sobralske, M. (2006). Machismo sustains health and illness beliefs of Mexican American men. *Journal of American Academy of Nurse Practitioners, 18*(8), 348–350.

Sobralske, M., & Katz, J. (2005). Culturally competent care of patients with acute chest pain. *Journal of American Academy of Nurse Practitioners, 17*(9), 342–349.

Spanish Language. (2007). *Fact, figures and statistics about Spanish*. Retrieved from http://spanish.about.com/library/weekly/aa070300a.htm

Spector, R. (2008). *Cultural diversity in health and illness* (7th ed.). Upper Saddle River, NJ: Pearson.

Stanley Bunting, J. (2011). Chemical dependency within the Hispanic population: Considerations for diagnosis and treatment. In G. Lawson & A. Lawson (2nd ed.), *Alcoholism and substance abuse in diverse populations* (pp. 227–242). Austin, TX: Pro-Ed.

Torres, E. (2001). *The folk healer: The Mexican American tradition of* curanderismo. Albuquerque, NM: Nieves Press.

U.S. Census Bureau. (2001). *Census 2000 briefs and special reports*. Retrieved from http://www.census.gov/population/www/cen2000/briefs.html

U.S. Census Bureau. (2008). *Population estimates, July 1, 2000, to July 1, 2006*. Retrieved from http://www.census.gov/population/www/socdemo/hispanic/hispanic_pop_presentation.html

U.S. Census Bureau. (2009). *Income, poverty, and health insurance coverage in the United States*. Report P60, n. 238, pp. 62–67.

U.S. Census Bureau. (2010). *Facts for features*. Retrieved from http://www.census.gov/newsroom/releases/archives/facts_for_features_special_editions/cb10-ff08.html

U.S. Department of Health and Human Services Health Resources and Services Administration. (2010, September). *The registered nurse population: Findings from the 2008 national sample survey of registered nurses*. Retrieved from http://bhpr.hrsa.gov/healthworkforce/rnsurveys/rnsurveyfinal.pdf

Van Hook, J., Bean, F., & Passel, J. (2005, September). Unauthorized migrants living in the United States: A mid-decade portrait. *Migration Information Source*. Retrievedfrom http://www.migrationinformation.org/Feature/display.cfm?ID=329

Vázquez, R. (2000). Is the phrase "La raza" racist? [Electronic version]. *Las Culturas*. Retrieved from http://www.lasculturas.com/aa/aa031200a.htm

Vázquez, R. (2004). Hispanic or Latino? [Electronic version]. *Las Culturas*. Retrieved from http://www.lasculturas.com/aa/aa070501a.htm

Villarruel, A.M., & Ortiz de Montellano, B. (1992). Culture and pain: A Mesoamerican perspective. *Advances in Nursing Science, 15*(1), 21–32.

Wells, J.N., Cagle, C.S., & Bradley, P.J. (2006). Building on Mexican-American cultural values. *Nursing, 36*(7), 20–21.

Zoucha, R. (2007). *Understanding* confianza *(confidence) in the nursing relationship with Mexican Americans*. Pittsburgh: Duquesne University School of Nursing.

Zoucha, R. (2011). *Understanding the meaning of* confianza *in the context of health for Mexicans in an urban community: A focused ethnography*. Pittsburgh: Duquesne University School of Nursing.

Zoucha, R., & Husted, G.L. (2000). The ethical dimensions of delivering culturally congruent nursing and health care. *Issues in Mental Health Nursing, 21*(3), 325–340.

Zoucha, R., & Husted, G.L. (2002). The ethical dimensions of delivering culturally congruent nursing and health care. *Review Series in Psychiatry, 3*, 10–11.

Zoucha, R.D., & Reeves, J. (1999). A view of professional caring as personal for Mexican Americans. *International Journal for Human Caring, 3*(3), 14–20.

Zoucha, R., & Zamarripa, C. (1997). The significance of culture in the care of the client with an ostomy. *Journal of Wound, Ostomy, and Continence Nursing, 24*(5), 270–276.

DavisPlus *For case studies, review questions, and additional information, go to*

http://davisplus.fadavis.com

Chapter 22

People of Polish Heritage

Larry Purnell

The author would like to thank Henry M. Plawecki, Lawrence H. Plawecki, Judith A. Plawecki, and Martin H. Plawecki for their contributions to this chapter in the 3rd edition.

Overview, Inhabited Localities, and Topography

Overview

Almost 9.9 million people in the United States (U.S. Census Bureau, 2011) and over 8 million people in Canada identify their ancestry as Polish (Statistics Canada, 2010). Poland—officially the *Republic of Poland*—occupies 120,727 square miles (312,683 square kilometers), which is slightly smaller than the state of New Mexico (*CIA World Factbook,* 2011). The capital of Poland is Warsaw. Located in Central Europe, Poland, with a population of about 38,111,000, is the eighth largest country in Europe. The life expectancy in Poland 72.1 years for men and 80.25 years for women (*CIA World Factbook,* 2011). Poland shares its western border with Germany, and to the south, it is bordered by Slovakia and the Czech Republic. Ukraine, Belarus, Lithuania, and Russia all share eastern and northeastern borders with Poland. The Baltic Sea borders the majority of the northernmost part of the country.

Poland is an ancient nation that was conceived near the middle of the 10th century. Its golden age occurred in the 16th century. During the following century, the strengthening of the gentry and internal disorders weakened the nation. In a series of agreements between 1772 and 1795, Russia, Prussia, and Austria partitioned Poland among themselves. Poland regained its independence in 1918, only to be overrun by Germany and the Soviet Union in World War II. It became a Soviet satellite state following the war, but its government was comparatively tolerant and progressive. Labor turmoil in 1980 led to the formation of the first independent free trade union in Eastern Europe, *Solidarnosc* (Solidarity) that over time became a political force and by 1990 had swept parliamentary elections and the presidency. A "shock therapy" program during the early 1990s enabled the country to transform its economy into one of the most robust in Central Europe, but Poland still faces the lingering challenges of high unemployment, underdeveloped and dilapidated infrastructure, and a poor rural underclass. Poland joined NATO in 1999 and the European Union in 2004. With its transformation to a democratic, market-oriented country largely completed, Poland is an increasingly active member of Euro-Atlantic organizations (*CIA World Factbook,* 2011).

In 1947, elections officially brought the Communist Party to power. The Stalinist model was implemented until 1956. After Stalin's death, Polish Communism vacillated between repression and liberalization until about 1970. Poland's resistance to Communist rule began in 1970 with the emergence of Lech Walesa, the leader of a strike in the Gdansk shipyards. Walesa headed Solidarity , which was created because of the Communists' violent repression of the workmen of Radom in 1976 and a second strike at the Gdansk shipyards in 1980, the result of the government's raising food prices (Gdansk, 2008).

The 1978 election of a Polish cardinal, Karol Wojtyla, as Pope John Paul II led to unprecedented social and political changes in Poland. The 1980 emergence of Solidarity and the election of a Polish pope rekindled a religious rebirth in the Poles, an increased sense of self, social identity, and the realization of their collective strength. Solidarity became a major social movement and phenomenon unheard of within the Soviet bloc's political system. Despite negotiations, confrontations, and, ultimately, repressive military operations by the ruling Polish Communist Party, the Solidarity movement survived as its influential unofficial opposition. Ultimately, the Polish Communist Party recognized that the people's massive opposition reduced their ability to govern. In 1988, formal negotiations between the Polish Communist Party leaders and the unofficial opposition, called the "Round Table talks," resulted in partially free Parliamentary elections. Solidarity won a landslide victory in the

June 1989 elections. In July 1989, the newly elected Parliament changed the country's name and constitution, establishing the Third Republic of Poland and a democratic system of government (von Geldern & Siegelbaum, 2003).

Polish immigrants and their descendants who immigrated to America for many generations have maintained their ethnic heritage by promoting their culture, attending Catholic churches, attending parades and festivals, maintaining ethnic food traditions, speaking the Polish language, and promoting interest in their home country through media events as well as economic and political channels. For newer immigrant Poles, maintaining ethnic heritage means learning English and obtaining a good job (Erdmans, 1998). Newer immigrants are less concerned with raising consciousness over Polish American issues than they are with financially helping families who remain in Poland and raising concerns over the political and economic climate in their homeland.

Heritage and Residence

The first contribution of the Poles to the development of American democracy occurred during the American Revolutionary War. Two prominent Poles who assisted the colonists in their fight for independence were Count Kazimierz (Casimir) Pulaski and Tadeusz Kosciusko. General Pulaski, a valiant cavalryman, led soldiers by courage and example. His many heroic actions on behalf of the colonists lead to naming him the "Father of the American Cavalry" (Polish American Center, 1997). Many American towns, counties, parks, and other memorials bear the names of these Polish heroes.

The Poles' dedication to the welfare of the United States was summarized by the motto of the first Polish American political club, the Kosciuszko Club, established in 1871, which states, "A good Pole is a good American citizen" (Jarczak, n.d.). Immigrants, regardless of their country of origin, leave their homeland for a variety of reasons that include avoiding ethnic, religious, and political persecution; seeking a better lifestyle; and providing a means of support for family and relatives who remained in the homeland. Like any other group who perceives themselves as unaccepted, displaced, and different, the Polish immigrants established a geographically and socially segregated area called a **Polonia**, the medieval name for Poland. Polonia allowed members of the immigrant group to experience social comfort, speak their native language, and openly practice the customs of their homeland.

The initial migration of about 2000 Polish immigrants occurred between 1800 and 1860. This group consisted of intellectuals and nobles who were motivated by political insurrections. The first substantive Polish settlement in America was founded in 1854 by Father Leopold Moczygemba and 100 Polish immigrant families in Panna Maria, Texas (Panna Maria, 2006). Even though most Poles preferred living in agrarian communities, they gravitated to cities where work for laborers was plentiful.

Between the early 1800s and the beginning of World War II, over 5 million Polish immigrants came to the United States. Many of these immigrants perceived America only as a temporary home. This first major immigrant group was called *za chlebem*, or "for-bread" immigrants. These immigrants came to earn money and then return to Poland. Polish immigration to America continues today. A new generation of immigrants recently freed from foreign domination have recently been coming to the United States seeking better lives (Library of Congress, 2004).

At the peak of Polish migration, Chicago was considered the most well-developed Polish community in the United States (Pacyga, 2004). The first Polish immigrants to Chicago were primarily nobles who fled Poland after the Polish-Russian war of 1830 to 1831. They came with plans of establishing a Polonia in Illinois (Pacyga, 2004). Chicago's Polish community grew rapidly after 1850. Peter Kiolbassa, who served as a captain in the Sixth Colored Cavalry during the Civil War, emerged as a local leader. Kiolbassa organized the first Polish Society of St. Stanislaus Kostka in 1864. This organization prepared the community for the development of the city's first Polish Roman Catholic parish. Located along the north branch of the Chicago River, the residents of Polonia initially attended a German parish church. Facing hostility from some of the Germans, who discouraged their priest from ministering to the Polish religious needs, the Polish community established its own Roman Catholic parish, St. Stanislaus Kostka. The parish was central to the creation of Polonia, because the establishment of ethnic Catholic parishes provided the community with a stable institutional base and served as a status symbol for the new immigrant colony.

The Polish community's development allowed them to actively participate in the labor movement, which, along with their involvement with fraternal groups, led to the development of neighborhood organizations. By 1980, Hispanics and African Americans had largely replaced Poles in the inner-city core neighborhoods. Polish Chicagoans left the old neighborhoods and moved to the suburbs. Chicago's Polonia played a crucial role in the political, religious, educational, business, institutional, and cultural life of Chicago.

Polonia was also the name given to Polish communities found in northeastern and midwestern cities after 1945 (Best, 2004). Members of these communities kept Polish nationalism alive by speaking their native language, preserving customs, and attending the local Catholic church run by Polish clergy and the Felician Sisters. Because Poland was partitioned until 1919, Poles coming to America during the 1800s and early

1900s were unable to report Poland as their emigrating country, but they tenaciously worked to ensure the survival of the Polish culture. Over time, the 120-year partition of Poland and its absence from the world map significantly reduced the number of immigrants who could identify Poland as their emigrating country. Therefore, the partition ultimately led to an undercount of the actual number of Americans with Polish ancestry.

For many older Poles, the neighborhood is their community. Polonias, especially in urban ethnic communities, provide a sense of belonging, reduce alienation, and enhance people's ability to solve problems and maintain the motivation to address modern-day frustrations. Plawecki (2000) states, "The assumption of voluntary Americanization continues to exist in spite of the behaviors of past generations who resisted the assimilation process and have, in fact, reestablished their pre-immigration cultures in multiple voluntarily segregated ethnic enclaves/communities" (p. 7). Consequently, the segregated group develops communication styles, cultural beliefs, and interactive behaviors that are socially accepted within their community but are different from those expected by the general populace (Plawecki, 1992).

Poles are a heterogeneous group. As such, they were slow to assimilate into multicultural America. Much of the variation within this ethnic group is due to variant cultural characteristics (see Chapter 1).

Polish Americans were well represented in the WWII war effort of the United States. Significant numbers of Polish Americans, both native and immigrant, joined the U.S. military. Even after displaying that sense of duty, honor, and patriotism, Polish Americans often experienced discrimination during and after the war. Poles were passed over for jobs because they had difficulties speaking English and their names were difficult to pronounce or spell. As a reaction to this discrimination, name changes became common for upwardly mobile Polish Americans. The shortening and changing of names were intended to decrease discrimination and promote greater acceptability in the job market as well as increase social acceptance. Many Polish Americans still experience discrimination and ridicule through ethnic Polish jokes, which are similar in scope to those about Irish, Italian, Mexican Americans, and other ethnic groups.

Reasons for Migration and Associated Economic Factors

Polish immigration to the United States occurred in three major waves. The first wave of immigrants, arriving in the early 1800s through 1914, came to America primarily for economic, political, and religious reasons. Many immigrants were illiterates, peasants, or unskilled laborers (Grocholska, 1999). They took low-paying jobs and lived in crowded dwellings just to make a meager living.

The second major wave of immigration occurred after World War II. During the war, Poland lost over 6 million of its 35 million people (Brogan, 1990). The nearly complete destruction of Poland prompted the post-WWII wave of Polish immigrants to come to America. This group primarily included political prisoners, dissidents, and intellectuals from refugee camps all over Europe. These immigrants, who were both educated and had a basic knowledge of English, assimilated more easily into American culture than those from the first wave. They consciously separated from Polonia and aligned themselves with other middle-class and professional groups in America. The upwardly mobile and middle-class aspirations of this group differed from the working-class orientation of the first- and second-generation descendants of the first wave (Grocholska, 1999).

The current third wave of immigrants, often called the *Solidarity immigrants*, began arriving in 1978 (Grocholska, 1999). These Solidarity immigrants reflect the ideologies of the first two waves—that is, they want to work and to speak freely about political and intellectual issues. Two types of third-wave immigrants came to America. The first came to work without any initial interest in permanently relocating. They entered this country on a visitor's visa and left their families in Poland. These immigrants frequently lived in low-income housing, shared rooms with other immigrants, and worked hard to send money to their families in Poland. Networking with other Poles was their primary source of job contacts. They quickly took any job available, particularly as laborers, domestics, and unskilled farm workers. Because many of these immigrants were sending money to their families in Poland, they often overstayed their visitor visas.

The second type of third-wave Polish immigrants chose to come to America for political and economic reasons. This group typically consists of well-educated professionals and small-business owners. They consciously decided to leave Poland forever and bring their families with them. This group epitomizes the Polish characteristics of hard work, determination, and frugality. Although many in this group are underemployed, they actively use English and integrate into their new country, recognizing that this may be a necessary first step to assimilation.

Many second- and third-wave immigrants avoid Polish communities because they believe that American ethnic Polonias are different from those in Poland. The concerns and issues of political representation and discrimination of established immigrants living in America are irrelevant to this wave of immigrant Poles. In addition, many older Polonias are located in diverse, changing, inner-city neighborhoods, and the upwardly mobile

Polish Americans, like other successful groups, have begun to leave the cities for the suburbs.

Educational Status and Occupations

Educational priorities and their desire to assimilate into American culture vary widely among Polish immigrants. The educational status, socioeconomic levels, and cultural philosophy often depend on the time frame when the family emigrated from Poland.

Until the 1950s and 1960s, many Polish families were slow to recognize the value of education for their children. Before WWII, most Polish children went to Catholic schools, where they learned about their culture, its language, and Catholicism. After WWII, parents felt an acute responsibility to have their children learn English. Subsequently, the Polish language was eliminated from the curriculum of many schools, and its use was restricted to the home.

The second wave of Polish immigrants placed a high value on education and culture. Educated, cultured Poles were expected to read widely and speak several languages. Cultured Poles have great pride and respect for Poland's most famous people, such as composer Frederic Chopin, two-time Nobel laureate scientist Marie Curie, novelist Joseph Conrad, astronomer Nicolaus Copernicus, and Karol Wojtyla, better known as Pope John Paul II. Poles are known for epic works in prose and poetry. Major themes in Polish literature are nationality, freedom, exile, and oppression.

After World War II, many Polish Catholics were blue-collar workers who perceived hard work as honorable. Many feared that education and its resultant mobility were a threat to their family, religious, and community life. For women, education was seen as even less necessary because of the value placed upon their staying at home and raising their children. Television helped change the character of ethnic communities forever as it brought the outside world into both the community and the home. The descendants of immigrants who did go to college valued obedience and self-control, respected authority, and exhibited determination (Bukowczyk, 1987).

Communication

Dominant Language and Dialects

The Polish language was influenced by the countries surrounding Poland and by the Latin of 11th- and 12th-century kings. Depending on the regional and cultural background of the speaker, Polish may sound German, Russian, or French. The Polish language has a lyrical quality that is pleasant to the ear, even if one has difficulty understanding the words. Poles are an animated group, and facial expressions generally convey the tone of the conversation.

The dominant language of people living in Poland is Polish, although there are some regional dialects and differences. Generally, most Polish-speaking people can communicate with one another. Recently, a resurgence of interest in learning to speak the Polish language has occurred among Polish Americans. Both adults and children are learning Polish in church-affiliated language schools, cultural centers, and colleges. Polish radio stations help keep an ongoing interest in the language, music, and culture.

Cultural Communication Patterns

Poles use touch as a form of personal expression of caring. Touch is common among family members and friends, but Poles may be quite formal with strangers and health-care providers. Handshaking is considered polite. In fact, failing to shake hands with everyone present may be considered rude. Most Poles feel comfortable with close personal space, but distances increase when interacting with strangers.

First-generation Poles and other people from Eastern European countries commonly kiss "Polish style"—that is, once on each cheek and then once again. For Poles, kissing the hand is considered appropriate if the woman extends it. Two women may walk together arm in arm, or two men may greet each other with an embrace, a hug, and a kiss on both cheeks.

To Poles, love is expressed through covert actions and displayed easily in the form of tenderness to children. However, loving phrases are uncommon among adult Polish Americans. Poles praise others' deeds and good works, but they may be reluctant to acknowledge how they feel about one another. These behavioral variations may have persevered through generations of assimilated Poles.

Acknowledging the hostess is important when Poles visit one another's homes; bringing flowers or candy is always in good taste. Normally, guests are discouraged from assisting the hostess in the kitchen or with cleanup after meals. After the event, thank-you letters and greeting cards should be sent to demonstrate an appreciation for the host's hospitality.

Many Polish Americans consider the use of spoken second-person familiarity rude. Polish people speak in the third person. For example, they might ask, "Would Martin like some coffee?" rather than "Would you like some coffee?" Although the first expression might sound awkward, the latter expression may be considered impolite and too informal, especially if the person being asked is older. Many Polish names are difficult to pronounce. Even though a name may be mispronounced, a high value is placed on the attempt to pronounce it correctly.

When interacting with others, Poles consider age, gender, and title. For example, when a group is walking through a door, an unspoken hierarchy requires the person of lower standing to hold the door for a woman or those of a higher title. To many Americans, this behavior may seem excessive, but for Poles, it shows respect and courtesy. Polish Americans also use direct eye contact when interacting with others. Many Americans may feel uncomfortable with this sustained eye contact and feel it is quite close to staring, but to Poles, it is considered ordinary.

Most Poles enjoy a robust conversation and have a keen sense of humor. Polish humor sometimes has an openness and bawdiness that may be unnerving to those unaccustomed to it. Cultural nuances may make it difficult to understand the underlying meaning of some transactions or exchanges. Because Poles in Poland have been censored for centuries, they have raised satire and political savvy to an art form.

Poles, as a group, tend to share thoughts and ideas freely, particularly as part of their hospitality. A guest in a Polish home is warmly welcomed and may be overwhelmed by the outpouring of generosity. Americans talk of sports, whereas Poles speak of their personal life, their jobs, families, spouse, aspirations, and misfortunes.

Temporal Relationships

Punctuality is important to Polish Americans. Being late is a sign of bad manners. Depending on the status of the person for whom they are waiting, Poles may be intolerant of lateness. Even in social situations, people are expected to arrive on time and stay late.

Polish Americans are both past and future oriented. The past is very much a part of Polish culture, with the families passing on their memories of WWII, which still haunt them in some way. A strong work ethic encourages Poles to plan for the future. Polish parents very much want their children to have a better life than the one they have experienced.

Format for Names

Many Polish peasants did not have surnames until the 1600s. The use of surnames appeared in the first half of the 18th century. After 1850, the practice of creating surnames was no longer used. Traditional Polish names are often a description of a person (e.g., John Wysocki, meaning "John the tailor"), a profession (e.g., the surname Recznik, meaning "butcher"), a place (e.g., Sokolowski, meaning "one came from a town named Sokoly or Sokolka"), or even a thing. Many factors caused this rather logical process to become somewhat confusing. Historical, linguistic, and political factors also directly affected the structure of Polish surnames. First of all, the partition of Poland for almost 120 years made it impossible for any emigrant at that time to claim Poland as their homeland. Consequently, names may have been "adjusted" to sound more like those of the dominant ethnic group (e.g., Russian, Prussian, or Austrian) controlling that part of Poland at the time. Second, changes in surnames may have been made during the country's record-keeping process or during the immigration processing on Ellis Island.

REFLECTIVE EXERCISE 22.1

Casimir Wronska, a 62-year-old Polish man, has been in the United States for 19 years. A colleague with whom he works at a construction site brought him to the Emergency Department (ED) because he had a severe laceration from a circular saw on his thigh. In broken English, he described what happened. After 2 hours in the ED, suturing was complete, and he was discharged to home with complex instructions on how to care for the wound and when he should return for follow-up. He was also given a prescription for antibiotics and pain pills. He accepted the prescription for antibiotics but refused the prescription for pain pills.

Mr. Wronska listened attentively as the nurse gave him his discharge instructions. He maintained rather intense eye contact and nodded frequently. When the nurse, Mark Babinska, asked him to repeat the instructions, he folded the instructions and put them in his pocket, telling Mark that his wife would take care of him. The nurse asked him to read the instructions back to him. He told the nurse that he left his glasses at home and would read the instructions later.

1. What statements by Mr. Wronska indicate that he might not understand the discharge instructions?
2. What should the nurse do to ensure that Mr. Wronska understands the instructions?
3. Is maintaining intense eye contact with the nurse culturally congruent with Polish nonverbal communication?
4. What are some possibilities as to why Mr. Wronska accepted the prescription for antibiotics but refused the prescription for pain pills?

The transfer of information from emigrant to official records was highly dependent on the pronunciation, spelling, and writing skills of both the recorder and the applicant (Generations Network, 2007).

Some examples of common Polish names include *Kowal* meaning "blacksmith." Numerous suffixes, such as "icz," "czyk," "iak," and "czak," which mean "son of," can be added. The most common suffixes are "ski" for males and "ska" for females, which originally were added to many names because they were associated with nobility. The suffix "cki" became the phonetic version of "ski." Surnames ending in "y," "ow," "owo," and "owa" are usually derived from names of places. The "ak" suffix is typical of western Poland, whereas "uk" is found in the east.

Family Roles and Organization
Head of Household and Gender Roles

Life in the Polish culture centers on family. Each family member has a certain position, role, and related responsibilities. All members are expected to work, make contributions, and strive to enhance the entire family's reputation and social and economic position.

Individual concerns and personal fulfillment are afforded little consideration, and sacrifices for the betterment of the family are expected. The family structure is interwoven with strong beliefs and traditions. In the United States, the Polish family has maintained itself as a strong economic unit.

In most Polish families, the father is perceived as the head of the household. Depending on the degree of assimilation, the father may rule with absolute authority in first-, second-, and even third-generation Polish American families. Depending on circumstances, only the Church may have greater authority than the father. For example, if a child wants to leave home and attend college, the priest may help in convincing the family that it is an appropriate thing to do. However, among some third- and fourth-generation Polish Americans and second- and third-wave immigrants, more egalitarian gender roles are becoming the norm. In addition, the father, as head of the house, worked as many hours a day in a mine or a factory as was permitted. He assumed responsibility of finding jobs for both offspring and newly immigrated friends and relatives.

Historically, large families were expected and commonplace among Poles. Polish women who followed the Church's teachings had many children, often experiencing between 5 and 10 pregnancies. Although women were pregnant a good deal of their early married lives, the wife began the workday well before dawn, and her responsibilities included cooking, caring for the children, laundering the clothes, and cleaning the house. If necessary, the wife also worked outside the home for additional income. Although the husband was the final authority in most matters, it was the woman who ran the house, disciplined the children, and cared for elderly family members.

Szaflarski used data from the *Polish General Social Survey* to estimate the structural and psychosocial effects on self-reported health, risk behaviors, and social participation between the genders. Employment status was identified as improving the health of men, whereas marital happiness increased the probability of better health for women. Marital status was identified to influence social interactions. Married women were found to socialize less than unmarried women, whereas marital status had no effect on men's socialization. Smoking was found to decline with the educational level among men but not among women, whereas excessive drinking increased for unhappily married men. Religiosity was determined to enhance and protect the health of both men and women (Szaflarski, 2001). The degree of religiosity may apply to Poles in the United States, especially among newer immigrants.

Prescriptive, Restrictive, and Taboo Behaviors for Children and Adolescents

The most valued behavior for Polish American children is obedience. Taboo child behaviors include anything that undermines parental authority. Parents are quite demonstrative with young children, but they resist showing much affection toward them once they are older than toddler age. This is the parents' way of teaching children to be strong and resilient. Many parents praise children for self-control and completing chores. Little sympathy is wasted on failure, but doing well is openly praised. Children are taught to resist feelings of helplessness, fragility, or dependence.

Family Goals and Priorities

Traditional family values and loyalty are strong in most Polish households. Children are valued in the Polish American family. For many first-wave immigrants, marriage is an institution of respect and economic solidarity and may not necessarily include romance. In the past, husbands owed their wives loyalty, fidelity, and financial support, whereas wives owed their husbands fidelity and obedience. Children owed their parents emotional and financial support before and after marriage. An important family priority for many is to maintain the honor of the family in the larger society, have a good job, and be a good Catholic.

The elderly are highly respected in most Polish families. They attend church regularly and carry on Polish traditions. The Polish ethic of contributing to the family and enhancing its status extends to the aged as well. The elderly play an active role in helping grandchildren learn Polish customs and in assisting adult children in their daily routine with families. For some families, one of the worst disgraces, as seen through the eyes of the Polish community, is to put an aged family member in a nursing home. Third- and fourth-generation Polish Americans may consider an extended-care or assisted-living facility because of work schedules and demands of care, but first-generation immigrants rarely perceive this as an option. If Polish people are to assimilate into a nursing home, the use of the Polish language and rituals may be crucial. Thus, health-care providers should assist patients in organizing these types of events for their family members or should help them select nursing homes that offer these cultural advantages.

The quality of life for elderly immigrants is an excellent area for research (Berdes & Zych, 2000). Immigrants who arrived before the age of 21 adjusted to aging much better than their elderly counterparts who arrived in America well into maturity. If the elderly Pole moved to America and was actively embraced by family and friends, adjusting to old age in America was less difficult. However, if the move to America was a forced choice, the adjustment was more difficult.

Extended family, consisting of aunts, uncles, and godparents, is very important to Poles. Longtime friends become aunts or uncles to Polish children. Numerous family rituals surround holidays, and family gatherings—such as for births, marriages, and name dates (calendar date of the patron saint for whom one is named)—are times to socialize and solidify relationships.

The goals of the family are to work, make economic contributions, and strive to enhance the position of the family in the community. The family unit comes together to help deter behaviors that might cause them shame or lower prestige in the eyes of the community. As Poles assimilate into the culture, the American value of success may prevail. Most Poles expect their children to have an education and a well-paying job and to provide for them in their old age.

Alternative Lifestyles

Alternative lifestyles are seen as part of assimilation into the blended American culture. Same-sex couples are frowned upon and may even be ostracized, depending on the level of assimilation. Older second- and third-generation Poles have one of the lowest divorce rates of ethnic groups (Lopata, 1994), but patterns are changing with succeeding generations as they assimilate into the American lifestyle. Marital problems do exist, but the Polish value for family solidarity is strong and divorce is seen as truly a last resort. When divorce does result, single heads of households are accepted in the Polish American community.

Workforce Issues

Culture in the Workplace

Most Polish Americans are more socially segregated than other ethnic groups. In the past, many Poles never rose above the level of foreman or supervisor. Polish American immigrants of the 1800s maintained group solidarity and could always be counted on to help their families. Because men were semiliterate and had low-level skills, they gravitated to industrial cities, such as Chicago, where they could work long hours as laborers and earn overtime pay. Because Poles were active in trade unions and maintained a sense of loyalty to the group, they were strong.

Polish Americans have extensive social networks, and their strong work ethic enables them to gain employment and assimilate easily into the workforce. It is still possible to spend one's entire life in the same house, be employed in the same factory, and have the majority of your social contacts inside the boundaries of Polonia. Whereas this may have helped immigrants in the past, it now acts as a deterrent to assimilation. The cultural tradition of hard work has caused employers to take advantage of this attitude.

Issues Related to Autonomy

Some Poles entering America are underemployed and may have difficulty working with authority figures who are less educated. Poles quietly comment that they are disrespected for their educational background

and that they must endure decreased status to stay in America (Lopata, 1994). Poles are usually quick learners and work hard to do a job well. The Polish characteristic of praising people for their work makes Poles strong managers, but some lack sensitivity in their quest to complete tasks.

Even though nursing in Poland is considered a profession, newer immigrants may be unprepared for the level of sophistication and autonomy of American nurses. Only since the 1980s has nursing entered the university setting in Poland. Most Polish nursing education is still completed in 1- to 2-year postsecondary education programs. As with many other professionals coming to America, if Polish nurses are willing to complete the extra courses to become registered or practical nurses, their employment as a nurse can be continued. A problem for many foreign nurses is that they may not receive credit for their work experiences in their home country. A nurse with 10 years of foreign nursing experience may have to start with the schedule, salary, and status of a new graduate. Poland's nursing students express fundamental values that are significantly influenced by a society characterized by strong religious conviction (Wronska, 2002). In the United States, nursing education's multireligious attitudes defer any discussion of religious beliefs.

Because Poles learn deference to authority at home, in the church, and in parochial schools, some may be less well suited for the rigors of a highly individualistic, competitive market. For Poles living in a country with a strong religious tradition, the American work culture may be very difficult for them to understand. Nevertheless, the strong Polish work ethic, exhibited as volunteering for overtime, being punctual, and rarely taking sick days, is valued by employers.

Native-born Polish Americans have little, if any, difficulty with the English language. Foreign-born Poles frequently have some difficulty understanding the subtle nuances of humor. Less-educated Poles tend to seek jobs as domestics or choose to perform manual labor because they are reluctant to rely on their English language and communication skills. Recent Polish immigrants, who had experience working under a Communist bureaucratic hierarchy, may have some difficulty with the structure, subtleties, and culture of the American workplace. New-wave Poles may be very naive in acclimating to the American work culture and, therefore, may become frustrated with what is considered an acceptable work ethic.

Biocultural Ecology

Skin Color and Other Biological Variations

Most Poles are of medium height with a medium to large bone structure. As a result of foreign invasions over the centuries, Polish people may be dark and Mongol-looking or fair with delicate features, blue eyes, and blonde hair. Those with fair complexions are predisposed to skin cancer and other illnesses related to exposure to environmental elements. Health-care providers must be aware of these conditions when assessing Polish patients and providing health teaching.

Diseases and Health Conditions

Poles consider themselves to be a tough people with an ability to tolerate pain from injuries, illness, and disease. Poles believe that suffering hardens individuals; therefore, they value that experience and perceive it to be good. In the Polish culture, a common belief is that enduring pain without complaining or asking for relief demonstrates virility in men and self-control in women. Young boys are taught at an early age that they can control illness, pain, or discomfort without the help of medicine and, thus, improve their inner strength. Another cultural belief is that taking medications weakens the entire system, which results in the decrease in family status. Fathers live vicariously through their children, especially their sons, and any weakness in the child is believed to reflect directly on them.

Risk factors for newer Polish immigrants are connected with their employment in industries in their homeland. Heavy industry in Poland produced prolonged, significant air pollution and environmental neglect. Living in polluted environments led to an increase in premature deliveries, low-birth-weight children, diseases of the pulmonary and circulatory systems, and various forms of cancer. The problem of occupational lead poisoning from 1970 to 1996 in Poland was documented by Szeszenia-Dabrowska and Wilczynka in 1998. Between 1972 and 1976, 8414 cases of lead poisoning, an occupational disease, were registered. A diminishing number of occupational lead poisoning cases were observed in the 1990s (Szeszenia-Dabrowska & Wilczynka, 1998). Trzcinka-Ochocka, Jakubowski, and Razniewska (2005) studied occupational exposure to lead and evaluated the competence of laboratories responsible for the monitoring and analysis of health risks in workers exposed to lead. The data indicated that occupational exposure to lead is still a problem and that neither the recommendations of 1996, reinforced by the Minister of Health in 2004, nor the European Union directive is universally followed. The Minister of Health mandated accreditation of all laboratories by January 1, 2008.

In Poland, air pollution remains a serious problem because of sulfur dioxide emissions from coal-fired power plants. In addition to the air pollution problems, Poles have had a long history of excessive smoking. Zatorski (2003) states, "At the end of the 1980s, Poland had the highest cigarette consumption in the world" (p. 97). In 1990, the Cancer Center and Institute, under the honorary patronage of Lech Walesa and in collaboration with the International Union Against Cancer and the American Cancer Society, hosted the conference "A Tobacco-Free New Europe." Public-health leaders from Eastern Europe were targeted; the participants heard comprehensive scientific evidence on the magnitude of health damage caused by cigarette smoking in the region. Ultimately, this conference provided the basis for health-related tobacco control legislation, which dramatically reduced the consumption of cigarettes (Zatorski, 2003).

Obviously, miners and workers in heavy industry are at an increased risk for the development of pulmonary diseases. Water pollution from industrial and municipal sources and disposal from industrial waste have also become environmental problems. Once these industrial establishments comply with the current European Union codes, the pollution levels should decrease (*CIA World Factbook,* 2011). The factors cited previously have contributed to the significant incidence of respiratory disease and lung and other cancers.

In 1986, the Chernobyl incident in Russia contaminated the land and water systems of eastern Poland. The full impact of this disaster on the incidence of cancer in Poland, as well as for Poles emigrating to other parts of the world, remains unknown.

The long-term effects of hypertension in the Polish population need to be addressed, and awareness needs to be increased through patient education efforts (Niewada, Skowronska, Ryglewicz, Kaminski, & Czlonkowska, 2006). Zdrojewski and colleagues (2006) examined high blood pressure, overweight and obesity, and smoking as risk factors from those attending the Polish Hygiene Society Congress. The results were presented to the participants, and the cumulative results were compared with the nation's current epidemiological burden caused by CVD (Zdrojewski et al., 2006). This strategy appears to be an effective way of impressing on the leaders the importance of these risk factors and improving the awareness, education, and lobbying efforts needed to establish a long-term educational program aimed at reducing the incidence of CVD risk factors.

Variations in Drug Metabolism

Documentation on the pharmacodynamics of drug metabolism in Polish individuals is limited. The health-care literature has yet to report any pharmacological studies specific to people of Polish descent.

High-Risk Behaviors

Alcohol abuse, with its subsequent physiological, psychological, and sociological effects and its related financial impact, continues to be an ongoing concern among Polish Americans. Manwell, Czabala, Ignaczak, and Munt (2002) found high rates of depression among heavy drinkers in the primary-care population. In addition, Cherpitel, Moskalewicz, and Swiatkiewicz (2004) reported that drinking patterns and subsequent injuries among males affected the number of emergency services used, suggesting a high recidivism for alcohol-related injuries. These results suggest that the patient's acknowledgment of the role of alcohol in the injury may be an important factor used in developing individualized intervention strategies.

In Poland, a high rate of alcoholic psychosis, cirrhosis of the liver, and acute alcohol poisoning exists. Other alcohol-related illnesses include cancer of the gastrointestinal tract, peptic ulcers, accidents, and suicide. An estimated 1 million Poles are dependent on alcohol, and another 3 million are alcohol abusers. Cumulatively, 4 million of Poland's estimated 38 million people are either alcohol-dependent or abusers (Manwell, Ignaczak, & Czabala, 2002). Alcohol abuse is an important part of the history of Poland. For some immigrants, alcohol was a way of relieving boredom, frustrations, and severe hardships. For other immigrants, alcohol was a way of mitigating the painful memories of WWII and reducing depression and the symptoms of post-traumatic stress syndrome. Alcohol still influences family patterns of behavior for many Polish immigrants.

Because Poles place a high value on hospitality in both Poland and America, drinking among Poles is an accepted part of the culture. Part of being a good hostess or host is to have enough alcohol for every guest. For newer immigrants and older Polish Americans, vodka is the alcohol of choice. Upper socioeconomic groups drink wine, whereas beer is consumed by all socioeconomic levels. In a study on drinking patterns of American and Polish college students, Polish students drank more than their American counterparts (Eng, Slawinska, & Hanson, 1991). Wine was the preferred drink of Polish students, and beer the preferred drink of American students.

Because alcohol use and cigarette smoking are prevalent among many Poles, health-care providers must assess individual patients for abuse and provide counseling and referral for those who express an interest. Children of immigrants should especially be targeted for counseling regarding the health effects of smoking and alcohol consumption.

Health-Care Practices

As with their U.S. counterparts, the behaviors of the Polish immigrants are directly associated with their level of education, income, and lifestyle. Those with higher levels of education are very interested in weight control, preventive health behaviors, and exercise. Health-care providers need to include interventions specific to the individual's social environment (Stelmach, Kaczmarczyk-Chalas, Bielecki, & Drygas, 2005).

Health-care providers should carefully screen Polish immigrants for diseases common in their home country. Hypertension, CVDs, respiratory conditions, alcoholism, cancer (particularly leukemia), and thyroid disorders are endemic diseases of Poland that are also found in the United States. Culturally congruent health teaching strategies associated with the risk factors for these diseases must be implemented when working with this population.

Nutrition
Meaning of Food

Another rather common depiction of cultural values is sometimes displayed on a wall hanging in a Polish home. The wall hanging often features a likeness of God with the inscription *Gosc W Dom, Bog W Dom*, which means "Guest in the House, God in the House."

Most Poles extend the sharing of food and drink to guests entering their homes. Eating and/or drinking with the host is perceived as social acceptance. Three important considerations influence Poles regarding food. First, Poland is primarily a land-based country with short summers and very cold winters. Thus, the major agricultural products in Poland include potatoes, vegetables, wheat, poultry, eggs, pork, and dairy products (*CIA World Factbook*, 2011). Second, the cold weather discourages outdoor activities, while also creating a craving for hot stews, soups, and foods that produce a feeling of satiety. Unfortunately, these foods are high in carbohydrates, fat, and sodium. Meats and vegetables are cooked for a very long time, resulting in the destruction of B and other vitamins. Third, the strong Catholic influence is evidenced by attending many food-laden celebrations, festivals, and rituals, each of which has its own traditional high-calorie foods. Many Poles continue these routine dietary practices after emigrating. Health-care providers need to assess how the Polish patients' dietary habits influence their weight, blood pressure, and overall health status and then structure a diet that is culturally acceptable, promotes healthy food choices, and is sustainable.

Common Foods and Food Rituals

Polish foods and cooking are similar to German, Russian, and Jewish practices. Staples of the diet are millet, barley, potatoes, onions, radishes, turnips, beets, beans, cabbage, carrots, cucumbers, tomatoes, apples, and wild mushrooms. Common meats are chicken, beef, and pork. Traditional high-fat entrees include pigs' knuckles and organ meats such as liver, tripe, and tongue. *Kapusta* (sauerkraut), *golabki* (stuffed cabbage), *babka* (coffee cake), *pierogi* (dumplings), and *chrusciki* (deep-fried bowtie pastries) are common ethnic foods. As mentioned previously, hot soups and stews are favored during the bitterly cold winters, and cold soups are preferred during the summer.

The meal plan for many Poles consists of a hearty breakfast of coffee, bread, cheese, sausage, and eggs. A midmorning snack is usually a sandwich and tea or coffee. The main meal in midafternoon includes soup, meat, potatoes, a hot vegetable, and dessert. In the evening, cold cuts, eggs, butter, sour cream, bread, and grains are common. This diet is modified depending on the availability of the food, the growing season, and the family's finances. Dill, paprika, garlic, and marjoram (used in *kielbasa*) are common herbs. Many foods may be pickled or canned for storage, which also increases their sodium content. Table 22-1 lists a variety of traditional Polish foods.

Dietary Practices for Health Promotion

The Polish American diet is frequently high in carbohydrates, sodium, and saturated fat. Assessing patients for increased blood sugar and cholesterol levels and high blood pressure should be routine. Interventions that require significant dietary modifications to their culturally based menus may be difficult.

Like many other economically developing countries, Poland's efforts to examine the health status of its citizens have become increasingly important. One disease with dramatic long-term consequences is insulin-dependent diabetes. Over the years, an increased incidence of this disease in Poles has been documented. Sobel-Maruniak, Grzywa, Oriowska-Florek, and Staniszewski (2006) compared the long-term trend in the incidence of insulin-dependent diabetes over a 20-year period (1980–1999). Their results showed a significant growth in the incidence of insulin-dependent diabetes among people aged birth to 29 years in the Rzeszow Province. Health-care providers should be especially alert to the symptoms of diabetes in younger Polish immigrants.

Nutritional Deficiencies and Food Limitations

Unfortunately, most of the land and water in Poland contains low levels of iodine. Iodine does not develop naturally in specific foods unless it is present in the soil or water. Iodine penetrates the foods that are grown in the soil, and their ingestion supplies it to the consumer. Ocean water also contains adequate amounts of iodine; thus, eating fish or other nutrients from the sea is likely to furnish sufficient amounts. Unfortunately, consuming fish on a regular basis has failed to become a part of the traditional diet in Poland.

Except for individuals living near the Baltic Sea in northern Poland, who consume fish regularly, Poles are in danger of developing nutritional problems related to the lack of iodine in their diet. Iodine is an essential component for the thyroid's hormonal function, and its deficiency results in the underproduction of thyroxine and triiodothyronine. Disorders related to the inadequate production of these hormones may include mental retardation, neurological system defects, goiters (e.g., enlarged thyroid), sluggishness, growth retardation, reproductive failure, and increased childhood mortality. Fortunately, this nutritional problem is being monitored and addressed.

Pregnancy and Childbearing Practices

Fertility Practices and Views Toward Pregnancy

Because family is very important, most Poles want children. In an agrarian society, and for early immigrants, children were considered important because they brought happiness and status to the family and were an economic necessity. In Poland, the Catholic Church strongly opposes abortion, which is the prevailing attitude of many Poles in America. However, during the years of war, poverty, and Communist rule, abortion and child spacing were considered necessities. For Poles, fertility practices are balanced between the needs of the family and the laws of the Church.

Prescriptive, Restrictive, and Taboo Practices in the Childbearing Family

Pregnant Polish Americans are expected to seek preventive health care, eat well, and get adequate rest to ensure a healthy pregnancy and baby. Immigrant families who have experienced poverty, famine, and inadequate health care are more likely to pay attention to prenatal care. The emphasis on food and "eating for two" is a common philosophy. Health-care providers must pay special attention to ensure that pregnant Polish American women restrict their weight gain during pregnancy.

Because the process of childbirth was poorly understood by an undereducated society, folk beliefs, magico-religious explanations, and taboos continue to surround the process. Many consider it bad luck to have a baby shower, and even now, many Polish grandmothers may be reluctant to give gifts until after the baby is born. Birthing is typically done in the hospital.

▐▌ Table 22-1	Polish Foods	
Common Name	Description	Ingredients
Babka	Coffee cake	Yeast bread
Barszcz	Beet soup	Served plain or with sour cream
Bigos	Hunter's stew	Stew with game, sausage, sauerkraut
Chrusciki	Polish bowties	Fried egg dough
Golabki	Cabbage rolls	Cooked cabbage stuffed with chopped meat and rice in tomato sauce
Kielbasa	Sausage	Sausage
Ogorki smietanie	Sour cream cucumbers	Sour cream, cucumbers
Pierogi	Boiled dumplings	Dumplings filled with potatoes, cheese, or sauerkraut
Sledzie	Herring	Pickled fish

Midwives may be used if there is a community feeling that they are "just as good as the doctor."

Pregnant women usually follow the physician's orders carefully. In America, Polish women seek prenatal clinics when they are unable to afford private fees. The birthing process is considered the domain of women. Newer Polish immigrants may feel uncomfortable with men in the birthing area or with family-centered care.

Women are expected to rest for the first few weeks after delivery. For many, breastfeeding is important. Health-care providers may need to provide active lactation counseling and education about appropriate care during breastfeeding (e.g., proper techniques) and to help the woman understand the balance among diet, rest, and exercise after delivery.

Death Rituals

Death Rituals and Expectations

Most Poles have a stoic acceptance of death as part of the life process and a strong sense of loyalty and respect for their loved ones. Family and friends stay with the dying person to negate any feelings of abandonment. The Polish ethic of demonstrating caring by doing something means bringing food to share, caring for children, and assisting with household chores.

Most Polish women are quick to help with the physical needs of the dying. Home hospice care is acceptable to most Poles. Health-care providers may encounter difficulty in convincing the family that the dying member may choose to refuse food as a result of the illness rather than because of stubbornness or the caretaker's cooking. Polish women may tend to hover. Health-care providers need to help families understand that it is important for the dying person to conserve energy.

Responses to Death and Grief

In early Poland, individuals were buried within 24 hours of their deaths. Historically, immigrant Poles continued the practice of burying the deceased from the home and having home burial ceremonies, which included a wake or vigil in which family members prayed and repeated the rosary over the dead person. Today, Polish American family members follow a funeral custom of having a wake for 1 to 3 days, followed by a Mass and religious burial. Most Poles honor their dead by attending Mass and making special offerings to the Church on All Saints' Day, November 1. Families may continue tending the gravesite for years.

Spirituality

Dominant Religion and Use of Prayer

The Catholic Church, with its required attendance at Mass on Sundays and holy days, is an integral part of the lives of most Polish people. There are holy days in almost every month of the year, in addition to the rituals of baptism, confirmation, marriage, sacrament of the sick, and burial. Christmas and Easter are the two most important holidays, requiring both special foods and rituals. On Christmas Eve, depending on the affluence of the family, up to 13 meatless dishes are served with the *oplatek* (similar to a large communion wafer) that everyone shares at the table. On Christmas Day, the main meal consists of *kielbasa*, goose, ham, or turkey. The Easter holiday may begin with women bringing food to the church on Easter Saturday to be blessed by the priest. On Easter Sunday, lamb or *kielbasa* and boiled eggs are served. A table ornament, usually a lamb made of salt or butter, is often displayed. Like many Americans of various ethnic backgrounds, Polish Americans have had a renewed interest in their ethnic roots. For example, their attendance at language classes, festivals, and Polish Catholic churches has become very widespread.

Religious ceremonies are a major part of maintaining Polish culture. Poles are very concerned that churches continue to act as a vehicle of Polish culture. Birthdays and name days are important religious and family events for Poles. One very popular expression is **Sto lat,** which conveys wishes that the celebrant live 100 years. Polish weddings are legendary. This is the time when family and friends get together and two families unite. One folk practice is to bring *chlebem i sola* (bread and salt) as a symbol of hospitality. Guests always receive plenty of food and drink, listen to music, and dance. In America, Polish weddings may last only 1 day, but plenty of food and alcoholic beverages are considered essential to the joyous occasion.

Primary spiritual sources are God and Jesus Christ, with many Polish immigrants praying to the Virgin Mary, saints, and angels to ward off evil and danger. Honor and special attention are paid to the Black Madonna or Our Lady of Czestachowa (Fig. 22-1). Czestachowa, a town in central Poland, displays a picture of the Virgin Mary with two scratch marks on her darkened face. Every year, many Poles join a walking pilgrimage to see the Madonna. During times of illness and serious family concerns, one might hear a Pole evoking *Matka Boska*, which literally translated means "Mother of God."

Many older Polish people believe in the special properties of prayer books, rosary beads, medals, and consecrated objects. Polish Americans commonly exhibit devotions to God, such as crucifixes and pictures of the Virgin Mary, the Black Madonna, and Pope John Paul II, in their homes.

Meaning of Life and Individual Sources of Strength

Most Polish Americans have a strong work ethic and pride themselves on being fastidious and punctual. They are loyal to friends and family, have a strong sense of Catholic ideals, are self-disciplined, and are

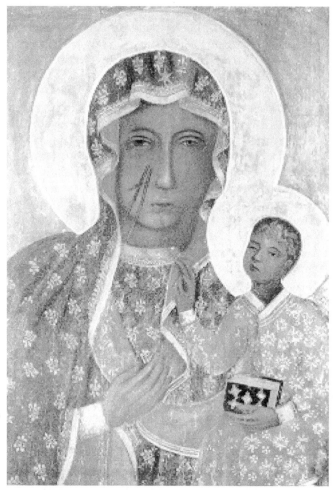

Figure 22-1 The Black Madonna or Our Lady of Czestachowa is an object of devotion to millions of native and immigrant Polish people. *(From The Marian Library/International Marian Research Institute, Dayton, OH; http://www.udayton.edu/mary/resources/blackm/blackm03.html)*

concerned about respect and honor. Most Polish Americans enjoy music, such as the works of Chopin and other classical composers, and dancing, including the jovial Polish polka, the waltz, or polonaise. Liturgical music may be important to older and more religious Poles.

After years of living under Communist censorship, newer immigrants value freedom, independence, being respected for their work, and having status in the community. Most Polish Americans find meaning in family loyalty and show great generosity to friends and extended family. Like all cultural groups, Polish Americans want to be shown respect.

Spiritual Beliefs and Health-Care Practices

Among the early immigrants, religion had both a folk tradition and a formal Catholic element. Most believed in mythological beings, water spirits, and house ghosts. Killing or any useless slaughter of animals was condemned. All life had meaning, and if an experience

---

REFLECTIVE EXERCISE 22.2

Lorenz and Ludwika Slawinska, ages 49 and 47 years, respectively, came to the United States with their son Christopher 25 years ago shortly after the Chernobyl nuclear accident. Lorenz is a physicist, and Ludwika is an elementary school teacher. Christopher is now 27 years old. He had great difficulty in elementary and high school but was able to complete them. Because he was overweight in school, the other children made fun of him. For the last 5 years he has successfully held a job as a janitor in a local factory. He and his fiancée of 3 years are planning their wedding, which is 3 months away. They both are only children and want to have a large family. Christopher's parents, who are devout Catholics, are not encouraging the marriage, mostly because they believe he should not have children.

1. What health problems can result from the Chernobyl nuclear accident?
2. Are potential health problems greater for adults or children?
3. Are the Slawinska family's views on marriage and children consistent with Polish Catholic ideology?
4. What community resources might the Slawinska family access for emotional support?
5. Would you support Christopher's desire to marry and have a large family? Why? Why not?

was unexplainable, mysterious, or magical, folk beliefs and/or religion provided the answer.

Health-Care Practices

Health-Seeking Beliefs and Behaviors

Most Poles put a high value on stoicism and doing what needs to be done. Many go to health-care providers only when symptoms interfere with function; then they may carefully consider the advice provided before complying. Describing anxiety and expecting nurturance are uncharacteristic of most Polish adults and children. Many Poles are reluctant to discuss their treatment options and concerns with physicians and routinely accept the proposed care plan. If Poles believe they are unable to pay the medical bill, they may refuse treatment unless the condition is life-threatening. Many have a strong fear of becoming dependent and resist relying on charity. Because many Poles consider Medicare, Medicaid, and managed care as forms of social charity, they are reluctant to apply for them. Any action that lowers their social status in their community is generally considered unacceptable. The health-care provider must describe the intent of these financial programs carefully, or Poles may perceive them as charity and, therefore, unacceptable options.

Poles usually look for a physical cause of disease before considering a mental disorder. If mental health problems exist, home visits are preferred. Talk-oriented interventions and therapies without pharmaceutical or suitable psychosocial strategies are dismissed unless interventions are action oriented. In addition, Poles consult other family members and the community to assess the appropriateness of treatments. Polish Americans often seek self-help groups such as Alcoholics Anonymous before seeing a health-care provider. Assimilated Poles respect the health-care system and tend to seek specialized care when necessary.

To many immigrant Poles, the U.S. health-care system is complex, confusing, and overpriced. They perceive access to health care as difficult, and many people who can afford to pay higher fees to see a private physician are unaware of how to gain access. Some Poles return to Poland to have medical or surgical procedures performed because these are more understandable, available, and/or affordable in their homeland.

Responsibility for Health Care

Given the continuation of limited access to care and the strong work ethic of this cultural group, health promotion practices are often undervalued by Polish Americans. In fact, older Polish Americans and newer immigrants commonly smoke and drink, engage in limited physical exercise outside of work, and receive poor dental care. Partial and complete dentures are common in older Poles. A number of secondary teeth are often found missing in Polish American immigrant children. This frequently surprises nurses who may be unaware of the limited number of dentists in Poland.

Attention to health promotion practices among women may be complicated by Polish American women's sense of modesty and religious background. Breast self-examination and Pap smear tests are poorly understood by many women. Health promotion practices vary greatly and are dependent on the woman's assimilation into American culture.

The Polish ethic of stoicism discourages the use of over-the-counter medications unless a symptom persists. Most Poles refuse to take time off from work to see a health-care provider until self-help measures have proved ineffective. Few Poles use vitamins unless these are suggested by a physician or a trusted family member, but even then, their extrinsic value is compared with the cost.

Folk and Traditional Practices

Many Poles continue their established health-related activities after immigration. For Poles just entering the United States, obtaining medical benefits has often been confusing and information facilitating access to the health-care system limited. This frequently resulted in Polish people treating themselves, delivering babies at home using a lay midwife, taking folk medicines and herbal remedies, and even setting their own broken bones when necessary. In addition, Polish Americans may use certain remedies to cure an illness, such as tea with honey and spirits to "sweat out" a cold. Herbs and rubbing compounds may also be used for problems associated with aches, pains, and inflammation from overworked joints and muscles. Because of individual differences, every patient must be assessed personally and asked specifically about his or her use of home remedies and over-the-counter medications.

The mother's or grandmother's responsibility was to know how to care for the family and their medical problems. Some additional common cultural practices included treating the symptoms of colds with herbs or poultices made from goose grease or fat. Gunpowder was ingested to promote emesis for an upset stomach. A boil was healed by soaking the heel of a loaf of white bread in milk and then placing it on the boil to draw out the core. Poor circulation or back pain was relieved by placing heated, alcohol-swabbed shot glasses, called *banki*, on the affected area. The heated *banki* were placed on the back or over the painful areas, causing circular, swollen areas on the skin. The Poles believed that this painless, raised area increased the circulation and reduced overall pain. Therefore, the health-care provider obviously needs to individually assess the cultural health behaviors of their Polish patients.

When a Pole is asked to undress for a physical examination, the health-care provider should pay special attention to any medals pinned to the patient's undergarments. Most of these medals have special religious significance to the wearer and should, if possible, remain on the garment.

Barriers to Health Care

Being unable to speak and understand English and the cost of health care and its complexity are the greatest barriers to health care for Polish immigrants. In addition to overcoming the language barrier, health-care providers need to understand Polish family values. Health-care providers also must consider that Poles often filter information through the extended family and neighborhood before accepting the recommended health-care regimen. Polish Americans who have learned English as a second language may have some difficulty with the nuances of health-care jargon and terminology. Inadequate or poor communication can result in tragic consequences for the patient.

Poles are polite to authority figures and avoid offending a health-care worker by disagreeing with them. Thus, they may be reluctant to ask for clarifications on questionable issues. In addition, many Poles are primarily concerned about how a disease affects daily functioning rather than about individual survival rates.

Cultural Responses to Health and Illness

Owing to their strong sense of stoicism and fear of being dependent on others, many Polish Americans use inadequate pain medication and choose distraction as a means of coping with pain and discomfort. When asked, many Poles either deny or minimize their pain or level of discomfort. Poles with chronic illnesses may have similar attitudes; thus, persevering with pain is common. The health-care provider should use a visual analog scale to assess pain, assist patients with distraction techniques, and help Poles to accept pain medication when needed.

Premigration stresses (e.g., losses, catastrophic experiences, anxiety, and internment) may be combined with postmigration stressors (e.g., language difficulty, loss of relationships, cultural pride, lack of support systems) to cause mental health problems (Fenta, Hyman & Noh, 2004). Social and geographic isolation within one's own ethnic neighborhood are common, albeit somewhat restrictive, reactions to this situation. Many immigrants are able to overcome the initial shock of moving to a foreign country, but they fail to have adequate coping skills to get through the stressors of total adjustment. Lack of language skills, feelings of unfamilarity, and fear of the unknown are some of the reasons given by those who fail to leave their Polonia. In these self-segregated cultural communities, children often become the go-betweens for their parents and the larger community. As children mature, they leave their parents and the Polonia to start their own families. Thus, the parents' avoidance of the acculturation process, even 25 years later, creates stressors leading to feelings of abandonment, loneliness, and displacement. These feelings may become significant and lead to major physical and/or mental illnesses.

Few Poles turn to psychiatrists or mental health providers for help. Those who seek help from mental health providers do so as a last resort. Many individuals choose their priest or seek assistance from a Polish volunteer-run agency before going to a health provider for psychiatric help.

Immigration to America failed to change the Pole's concerns about the delivery of appropriate health care. Immigrants are taught from infancy to resist asking for help or assistance from others but to bear the burdens of life independently.

Successful adaptation to the new homeland requires the immigrant to voluntarily progress through the process of assimilation and acculturation. Assimilation requires the individual to gradually adopt and incorporate the characteristics of the prevailing culture into their own lives. Acculturation mandates that the immigrants willingly modify their own culture as an accommodation to their transition to accepting the general values and attitudes of their new culture and homeland. The process of acculturation may affect the association between migration and health. The bidimensional approach describes acculturation as a process of adaptation to the mainstream culture while maintaining the inherited ethnic identity (Ryder, Alden, & Paulhus, 2000).

Aroian (1992) described three types of social support needed by Polish immigrants. During the first 3 years, immigrants need help finding housing and jobs and information about getting through the system—that is, learning English, buying groceries, and learning American customs. During the next 3 to 10 years, help is required to secure credit, obtain loans, and assimilate into American life. Finally, immigrants who have been in America for more than 10 years need support in honoring their Polish heritage through networks of other immigrants while maintaining an American support system. After immigrants are comfortable with resettlement, feelings of grief and loss begin to be acknowledged. Aroian (1990) states, "The psychological adaptation to migration and resettlement requires the dual task of mastering resettlement demands and grieving and removing the losses left in the homeland" (p. 8).

Blood Transfusions and Organ Donation

The ethic of being useful, independent, and a good Catholic influences one to refrain from using extraordinary means to keep people alive. The individual or family determines what means are considered extraordinary. Receiving blood transfusions or undergoing

REFLECTIVE EXERCISE 22.3

Mrs. Rutkowski is a 49-year-old second-generation Polish woman who has lived in a Polonia on Long Island, New York, her entire life. She has non-insulin-dependent diabetes mellitus and is borderline obese. Currently she has an open wound on her left ankle, which she has been treating with herbs and a homemade salve instead of the expensive prescription medicine recommended by her nurse practitioner. The nurse practitioner has recommended that she lose weight to help control her diabetes mellitus. The nurse is making a home visit for follow-up care.

1. What is a Polonia?
2. What is the first step in assessing Mrs. Rutkowski's nutritional needs?
3. Should the nurse actively discourage Mrs. Rutkowski from using her traditional treatments and rely solely on the prescription medications? What might the consequences be if the nurse does so?
4. Should the nurse recommend the use of a *banki*? Why? Why not?

organ transplantation is acceptable. However, it is important for a family to know the extent to which a patient will be able to function following organ transplantation. Cost is always an important consideration. Most Poles resist becoming a burden on their family's physical or financial resources and may attempt to convince the family that the procedure is too costly. Poles do consider it their duty to care for a sick member at home.

Health-Care Providers

Traditional Versus Biomedical Providers

Immigrant Poles often assess health-care providers by their demeanor, warmth, and show of respect. Health advice may be sought from chiropractors and local pharmacists as well as neighbors and extended family. Generally, professional biomedical advice is sought when a symptom persists and interferes with daily life.

Newer immigrants may fail to realize that many patients are discharged from the hospital before they have totally healed and are fully recovered. Poles may assume this practice is related to charity care, disrespect, or their financial status. Early discharges should be explained to the patient and family.

Status of Health-Care Providers

When caring for Polish patients, particularly older adults, all health-care providers should make every attempt to address individuals by their surname. Although this may be difficult, many names can be phonetically pronounced. Attempting to pronounce the names demonstrates respect for the patient. As a group, Poles are fiercely independent, relying on themselves or family members for almost every aspect of their social status, health, and livelihood. Nurses need to focus on the Polish patient's background and upbringing and take into consideration how health care becomes accepted or rejected. Illness or being sick is considered weakness for male family members. Polish women consider it their role to care for the family members without asking for help. It is also important to consider that Polish women are modest and self-conscious and may refuse health care when asked to disrobe in front of a male health-care provider. In some cases, it may be critical to request a female provider.

When it becomes evident that only professional help will resolve a problem, the affirmative act of seeking assistance is a major decision. Communication, consideration, displaying respect, and demonstrating cultural sensitivity will help to improve the Poles' attitudes toward the health-care provider. The health-care provider will need to introduce changes in ways that are appropriate and acceptable and can be integrated into an established, culturally dominated lifestyle.

Nurses will need to understand their own cultural values, beliefs, and practices in order to avoid or prevent alienating the Polish patient and family about the difficulty, complexity, and consequences of any recommended interventions. Using an authoritarian approach to gain compliance will cause conflict. Based upon their history, Poles have a tradition of survival, sometimes through stubbornness, pride, warmth, or genuineness. Therefore, being perceived as an amiable, respectful, and knowledgeable provider is integral in teaching health promotion and wellness; prevention of illness, disease, and injury; and health restoration. Communicating through the use of a bilingual family member as a liaison and finding agreements on cultural health beliefs and practices may be the best initial strategy for change when dealing with older immigrants or more traditional Polish Americans. However, when assessing intimate personal health information, an interpreter unknown to the family should be used.

A person's culture influences his or her perceptions of health and illness. How a patient accepts help or allows care to be rendered depends on her or his previous experiences, understanding, and trust in the provider. Respect, patience, and acceptance are important components of health care. Thus, health-care providers need to communicate compassionately with their patients through their professional appearance, words, actions, gestures, inflections, and postures. Patients of Polish descent interact with health-care providers, whom they perceive as authority figures, in very distinctive ways. Polite listening may determine how adherent a patient may be to the recommended regimen. Often the tone, how something is said, and the body language that accompanies it communicate whether the health-care provider respects the patient. Being culturally sensitive to the Polish American patient will be accepted as a gift from a stranger and will be reciprocated with appreciation, genuineness, and respect.

Physicians are held in high regard in Polish communities. Poles typically follow medical orders carefully. Poles may change physicians if they believe their recovery is too slow or if a second opinion is needed. Educated Poles are more willing than those less educated to follow medical orders and continue with prescribed treatment. Poles with less education tend to change physicians if the disease fails to subside quickly enough. Poles respect physicians but need to understand the purpose of the medical treatment.

Poles expect health-care providers to appear neat and clean, provide treatments as scheduled, administer medications on time, and enjoy their work. Immigrant Poles may be unfamiliar with the advanced roles of the American nurses, who are expected to know about, plan, and be directly involved in the patients' care. Thus, many Poles may still want only the physician to explain all aspects of their care.

REFERENCES

Aroian, K.J. (1990). A model of psychological adaptation to migration and resettlement. *Nursing Research, 39*(1), 5–10.

Aroian, K.J. (1992). Sources of social support and conflict for Polish immigrants. *Qualitative Health Research, 2*(2), 178–207.

Berdes, C., & Zych, A.A. (2000). Subjective quality of life of Polish, Polish-immigrant and Polish American elderly. *International Journal of Aging and Human Development, 50*(4), 385–395.

Best, W. (2004). *Polonia.* Retrieved from http://www.encyclopedia.chicagohistory.org/pages/992.html

Brogan, P. (1990). *The captive nations of Eastern Europe: 1945–1990.* New York: Avon Books.

Bukowczyk, J.J. (1987). *And my children did not know me: A history of Polish Americans.* Bloomington, IN: Indiana University Press.

Cherpitel, C.J., Moskalewicz, J., & Swiatkiewicz, G. (2004). Drinking patterns and problems in emergency services in Poland. *Alcohol and Alcoholism, 39*(3), 256–261.

CIA World Factbook. (2011). *Poland.* Retrieved from https://www.cia.gov/library/publications/the-world-factbook/geos/pl.html

Eng, R., Slawinska, J.B., & Hanson, D.J. (1991). The drinking patterns of American and Polish university students: A cross national study. *Drug and Alcohol Dependence, 27*, 167–174.

Erdmans, M.P. (1998). *Opposite Poles.* University Park, PA: Pennsylvania State University Press.

Fenta, H., Hyman, I., & Noh, S. (2004). Determinants of depression among Ethiopian immigrants and refugees in Toronto. *Journal of Nervous and Mental Disease, 192*(5), 363–372.

Gdansk. (2008). *Freedom broke out in Gdansk: History of August, 1980.* Retrieved from http://www.en.gdansk.gda.pl/about,2,20.html

Generations Network. (2011). *Learning: Polish names.* Retrieved from http://freepages.genealogy.rootsweb.com/~atpc/learn/tools/surname-origins.html

Grocholska, J. (1999). *Polish immigration to the US.* Retrieved from www.poloniatoday.com

Jarczak, C.R. (2012). *Polish-American contributions to our nation.* Retrieved from http://www.msu.edu/user/jarczakc/polesinus.html

Library of Congress. (2004). *Immigration: Polish/Russian: The Nation of Polonia.* Retrieved from http://memory.loc.gov/learn/features/immig/polish4.html

Lopata, H.Z. (1994) *Polish Americans* (2nd ed.). New Brunswick, NJ: Transaction.

Manwell, L.B., Czabala, J.C., Ignaczak, M., & Mundt, M.P. (2004). Correlates of depression among heavy drinkers in Polish primary care clinics. *International Journal of Psychiatry in Medicine, 34*(2), 165–178.

Manwell, L.B., Ignaczak, M., & Czabala, J.C. (2002). Prevalence of tobacco and alcohol use disorders in Polish primary care settings. *European Journal of Public Health, 12*(2), 139–144.

Niewada, M., Skowronska, M., Ryglewicz, D., Kaminski, B., & Czlonkowska, A. (2006). Acute ischemic stroke care and outcome in centers participating in the Polish National Stroke Prevention and Treatment Registry. *Stroke, 37*, 1837–1843.

Panna Maria, Texas: The oldest permanent Polish settlement in the USA. (2006). Retrieved from www.pannamariatexas.com

Pacyga, D.A. (2004). *Poles.* Retrieved from http://www.encyclopedia.chicagohistory.org/pages/982.html

Plawecki, H.M. (1992). Cultural considerations. *Journal of Holistic Nursing, 10*(7), 4–5.

Plawecki, H.M. (2000). The elderly immigrant: An isolated experience. *Journal of Gerontological Nursing, 26*(2), 6–7.

Polish American Center. (1997). *General Casimir Pulaski (1747–1779).* Retrieved from http://www.polishamericancenter.org/Pulaski.htm

Ryder, A.G., Alden, L.E., & Paulhus, D.L. (2000). Is acculturation unidimensional or bidimensional? A head-to-head comparison in the prediction of personality, self-identity and and adjustment. *Journal of Personality and Social Psychology, 79*(1), 49–65.

Sobel-Maruniak, A., Grzywa, M., Oriowska-Florek, R., & Staniszewski, A. (2006). The rising incidence of type 1 diabetes in south-eastern Poland. A study of the 0–29-year-old age group, 1980–1999. *Endokrynologia Polska, 57*(2), 127–130. Retrieved from http://www.ncbi.nlm.nih.gov/entrez/query.fcgi?db=pubmed&cmd=Retrieve&dopt=AbstractPlus&list_uids=16773587&query_hl=1&itool=pubmed_docsum

Statistics Canada. (2010). *Selected ethnic origins for Canada, provinces and territories.* Retrieved from www.statcan.gc.ca

Stelmach, W., Kaczmarczyk-Chalas, K., Bielecki, W., & Drygas, W. (2005). How education, income, control over life and life style contribute to risk factors for cardiovascular disease among adults in a post-communist country. *Public Health, 119*, 498–508.

Szaflarski, M. (2001). Gender, self-reported health and health-related lifestyles in Poland. *Health Care for Women International, 22*, 207–227.

Szeszenia-Dabrowska, N., & Wilczynska, U. (1998). Occupational lead poisoning in Poland. *Medycyna Pracy, 49*(23), 217–222. Retrieved from http://www.ncbi.nlm.nih.gov/entrez/query.fcgi?db=pubmed&cmd=Retrieve&dopt=AbstractPlus&list_uids=9760431&query_hl=4&itool=pubmed_DocSum

Trzcinka-Ochocka, M., Jakubowski, N., & Razniewska, G. (2005). Assessment of occupational exposure to lead in Poland. *Meycyna Pracy, 56*(5), 395–404. Retrieved from http://www.ncbi.nlm.nih.gov/entrez/query.fcgi?db=pubmed&cmd=Retrieve&dopt=AbstractPlus&list_uids=16483011&query_hl=2&itool=pubmed_docsum

U.S. Census Bureau. (2011). *Population by selected ancestry.* Retrieved from http://www.census.gov/compendia/statab/2011/tables/11s0052.pdf

von Geldern, J., & Siegelbaum, L. (2003). Solidarity and the Soviet Union. Retrieved from http://www.soviethistory.org/index.php?action=L2&SubjectID=1980solidarity&Year=1980

Wronska, I. (2002). The fundamental values of nurses in Poland. *Nursing Ethics, 9*(1), 92–100.

Zatorski, W. (2003). Democracy and health: Tobacco control in Poland. In J. deBeyer & L. Waverley (Eds.), *Tobacco control policy: Strategies, successes & setbacks* (pp. 97–120). Washington, DC: RITC and The World Bank.

Zdrojewski, T., Babinska, Z., Katol, M., Januszko, W., Rutkowski, M., Bandosz, P., et al. (2006). How to improve cooperation with political leaders and other decision-makers to improve prevention of cardiovascular disease: Lessons from Poland. *European Journal of Cardiovascular Prevention and Rehabilitation, 13*, 319–324.

DavisPlus For case studies, review questions, and additional information, go to
http://davisplus.fadavis.com

Chapter 23

People of Puerto Rican Heritage

Larry D. Purnell

The author would like to thank Josue Toro Navarro for contributing the Reflective Exercises in this chapter.

Overview, Inhabited Localities, and Topography

Overview

The island of Puerto Rico, located between the Caribbean Sea and the North Atlantic Ocean, is an important location along the Mona Passage, a key shipping lane to the Panama Canal. The capital, San Juan, is one of the biggest and best natural harbors in the Caribbean. The country's many small rivers and high central mountains ensure that the land is well watered, the south coast is relatively dry, and the north has a fertile coastal plain belt.

Populated for centuries by aboriginal peoples, Puerto Rico was claimed by the Spanish Crown in 1493 following Columbus's second voyage to the Americas. In 1898, after 400 years of colonial rule that saw the indigenous population nearly exterminated and African slave labor introduced, Puerto Rico was ceded to the United States as a result of the Spanish-American War (*CIA World Factbook,* 2011a).

Puerto Ricans are the third largest Hispanic cultural subgroup, with over 3 million living in the continental United States, compared with over 3.9 million residents in Puerto Rico, of whom 76.2 percent are white; 6.9 percent are black; and the rest are Amerindian, Asian, mixed, or other (*CIA World Factbook,* 2011b). Most Puerto Ricans on the mainland live in metropolitan areas, such as in Connecticut, Florida, Illinois, and New York. Puerto Ricans have a unique pride in their country, culture, and music. They self-identify as *Puertorriqueños* or **Boricuans** (Taíno Indian word for Puerto Rican) or **Niuyoricans**, for those born in New York.

In 2010, the mean annual income for Puerto Ricans was $16,000 (*CIA World Factbook,* 2011b), compared with the overall U.S. mean annual income of $47,400 (*CIA World Factbook,* 2011a). The percentage of Puerto Rican families living below the poverty level is greater than other Hispanic/Latino populations in the United States (National Center for Health Statistics, 2011).

Heritage and Residence

In 1917, Puerto Ricans were granted U.S. citizenship through the Jones Act; in 1952, Puerto Rico became a Commonwealth. This Commonwealth "status question" is a sensitive topic for most Puerto Ricans. From the *jíbaros* (peasants) to educated political leaders, the perception of many is that the *Americanos* (European Americans), their culture, and their politics are a potential threat to the Puerto Rican culture, language, and political future.

Reasons for Immigration and Associated Economic Factors

Puerto Ricans have been migrating to the United States for decades to seek employment, education, and a better quality of life. Initially, the Puerto Rican migration was fostered by a need for manual labor in the United States. More recently, Puerto Rican physicians, lawyers, and other professionals have migrated to enhance their educational status, social mobility, and employment opportunities.

Puerto Ricans select geographic areas where they can preserve their cultural, social, and familial wealth; enhance their assimilation into the U.S. culture; and increase their opportunities for employment and social support. For Puerto Ricans, citizenship status has created a controversial *Va y Ven* (go and come) circular migration in which individuals and families are often caught in a reverse cycle of immigration, alternately living a few months or years in the United States and then returning to Puerto Rico.

Educational Status and Occupations

Education is greatly respected among Puerto Ricans. Children are praised and encouraged to become educated to improve their opportunities for the future.

The educational system in Puerto Rico is similar to the system in the mainland United States for all educational levels. Nevertheless, when children migrate from Puerto Rico to the mainland, many educational organizations place them one grade below their previous academic year, mainly as a result of language barriers.

The literacy level in Puerto Rico is 94 percent and is about the same for both men and women (*CIA World Factbook,* 2011a). Puerto Rico boasts five well-developed and sophisticated public and private universities, plus three medical schools accredited locally and by the United States. However, on the mainland, Puerto Ricans have high secondary school dropout rates (National Center for Education Statistics, 2011). Historically, many Puerto Ricans have valued private rather than public education. Many parents make great financial sacrifices to enable their children to attend private educational organizations, most often Catholic schools. Private schools are often referred to as *colegios* (colleges), creating confusion with the American English translation of undergraduate institutions and the Central American term for college education. Instead of "college," the term *universidad* (university) is most commonly used to refer to 4-year college institutions in Puerto Rico, where bachelor's and master's degrees equate to those on the mainland.

Many Puerto Ricans who migrated before the 1970s had less than a fifth-grade education. Most were farmers who worked on rice, sugar cane, and coffee plantations and in the garment and manufacturing industries in northeastern and midwestern cities. However, since the mid-1970s, this pattern has begun to change as more educated Puerto Ricans migrate to the United States. After 1970, thousands of Puerto Ricans lost their jobs, suddenly finding themselves without the necessary education or training to find employment. Unemployment resulted in an increase in alcoholism, drug abuse, street crime, and family disruption and conflict.

Puerto Rico has one of the most dynamic economies in the Caribbean region. A diverse industrial sector has far surpassed agriculture as the primary locus of economic activity and income. Encouraged by duty-free access to the United States and by tax incentives, U.S. firms have invested heavily in Puerto Rico, where U.S. minimum wage laws apply, since the 1950s (*CIA World Factbook,* 2011b). Sugar production has lost out to dairy production and other livestock products as the main source of income in the agricultural sector. Tourism has traditionally been an important source of income (*CIA World Factbook,* 2011a). Even though many Puerto Ricans value education, high school completion rates are only 76.6 percent and a college degree is held by only 16.5 percent (U.S. Census Bureau, 2009).

Modest advances have been made in the educational status of Puerto Ricans, but the unemployment status remains a challenge. Among Hispanics, Puerto Ricans have the highest unemployment rate at 12 percent (*CIA World Factbook,* 2011b).

Communication

Dominant Language and Dialects

Until recently, Puerto Rico was the only Spanish-speaking Latin American country in which children, beginning in kindergarten, learned to read and write English and Spanish. The issue of two official languages, English and Spanish, is a sensitive one for some Puerto Ricans who, after the U.S. occupation in 1898, were forced to learn English. At that time, many could not read and write in Spanish. This sensitivity results from the fear that speaking English would eventually replace speaking Spanish and affect Puerto Rican culture, traditions, and practices. For Puerto Ricans, language is a political issue. With each government change since the early 1980s, the official prevailing language has been disputed and debated. Spanish is spoken at home, in schools, in businesses, and in the media. However, people from the metropolitan cities are more likely to read, write, and speak some English.

Puerto Ricans use the standard form of Spanish, speaking with no dialects or indigenous languages. Puerto Ricans frequently use the phrase "*!Ay bendito!*" to express astonishment, surprise, lament, or pain. Some contextual differences occur, mainly in pronunciation by people from rural areas. Rural dwellers may substitute the sound of *e* for *i* and often drop the last letters of words. For example, *después* (after) may be pronounced as *dispu*, and *para donde vas* (where are you going?) may be pronounced as *pa'onde vas*. In addition, most Puerto Ricans exchange the letter *r* for the letter *l*; for example, *animar* (encouragement) may be pronounced as *animal*, sounding like "animal." Some use a rolling *r*, a pharyngeal pronunciation that uses double *r*, such as *arroz* (rice) and *perro* (dog). Puerto Ricans speak with a melodic, high-pitched, fast rhythm that may leave non–Puerto Rican health-care providers confused. This pitch and these inflections are maintained when speaking English. Because some Puerto Ricans feel uncomfortable or even insulted if people comment on their accent, the health-care provider should avoid making comments about accent, use caution when interpreting voice pitch, and seek clarification when in doubt about the content and nature of a conversation that may seem confrontational.

Cultural Communication Patterns

Puerto Ricans are known for their hospitality and the value placed on interpersonal interaction such as **simpatia**, a cultural script in which an individual is perceived as likeable, attractive, and fun-loving. Puerto Ricans enjoy conversing with friends and sharing information about their families, heritage, thoughts, and feelings. They often expect the health-care provider to exchange personal information when beginning a professional relationship. The health-care provider may wish to set boundaries with discretion and *personalismo*, emphasizing personal rather than impersonal and bureaucratic relationships.

Most Puerto Ricans readily express their physical ailments and discomforts to health-care providers, with the exception of taboo issues such as sexuality. If *confianza* (trust) is established, health-care providers can establish open communication channels with individuals and family.

Spatial distancing among Puerto Ricans in the United States varies with age, gender, generation, and acculturation. Personal space may be a significant issue for some older women, particularly those from rural areas of Puerto Rico, who may prefer to maintain a greater distance from men. However, Puerto Ricans born on the mainland may be less self-conscious about personal space. Young Puerto Rican women may take offense to verbal and nonverbal communications that portray women as nonassertive and passive. Thus, health-care providers must carefully assess each individual's perception of distance and space.

Most Puerto Ricans are very expressive, using many body movements to convey their messages. During conversations, hand, leg, head, and body gestures are commonly used to augment messages expressed by words. Puerto Ricans express feelings and emotions through touch and are *cariñosos* (loving and caring) in verbal and nonverbal ways. Greeting Puerto Ricans with a friendly handshake is acceptable. Once trust is established, a patient might greet the health-care provider with a friendly hug. During conversations, they are likely to touch with love and affection, including a gentle hand stroke on the shoulder. Puerto Rican women greet one another with a strong familiar hug, and if among family or close friends, a kiss is included. Men may greet other men with a strong right handshake and a left hand stroking the greeter's shoulder.

Nonverbal communication plays a vital role in acquiring informed consent for health-care and research procedures and when providing health education and discharge planning. Nonverbal communications among Puerto Ricans may include an affirmative nod with an "aha" response, but this does not necessarily mean agreement or understanding related to the conversation. Using a respectful and friendly approach, health-care providers should seek clarification of the information provided, ask for language preference in verbal and written information, and allow time for the exchange of information with questions and answers when critical decisions need to be made. Puerto Rican patients may prefer to read or share sensitive information, options, and decisions with close family members. Some obtain verbal approval from extended family or community members who are knowledgeable in health matters. When consent is needed from

a woman, the health-care provider should ask if verbal approval or consent from the partner should be obtained first.

Traditional cultural norms discourage an overt sexual-being image for women, but with family assimilation to the mainland, many of these traditional values disappear, in particular for younger Puerto Ricans. When topics such as sex, sexual orientation, sexually transmitted infections (STIs), or other infectious diseases are discussed, an environment built on *confianza* and *personalismo* must be established if these sensitive issues are to be effectively addressed. Voice volume and tone, the degree of eye contact, spatial distancing, and time are variables that can have an impact on discussions of sensitive topics with Puerto Ricans.

The meaning and cultural value placed on direct eye contact has changed over time. Among younger Puerto Ricans and those born on the mainland, eye contact is maintained and is often encouraged among those who believe in a nonsubmissive and assertive portrayal. However, among more traditional Puerto Ricans born and raised in rural areas of Puerto Rico, limited eye contact is preferred as a sign of respect, especially with older people, who are seen as figures of respect and great wisdom.

Temporal Relationships

Most Puerto Ricans are present oriented, having a relativistic and serene view and way of life. This relaxed attitude often frustrates business people and health-care providers. Those unaware of this cultural nuance

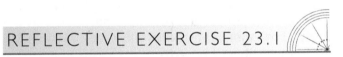

REFLECTIVE EXERCISE 23.1

Paco and Estrellita Lopez bring their 3-year-old son to the clinic. They both speak some English and the nurse speaks no Spanish. The nurse looks at Estrellita holding Pacquito, who is crying, and asks how she can help them. Estrellita looks at her husband and speaks to him in Spanish. Paco tells the nurse that Pacquito ate well until 2 days ago, but now cries while eating. The nurse continues to look at Estrellita and asks if the child has any other health problems.

Estrellita looks at her husband while speaking to him in Spanish, after which the husband tells the nurse that the boy was born with a heart problem. Again, the nurse asks Estrellita if she knows what type of heart problem it is.

Paco looks at his wife and speaks in Spanish to her, then turns to the nurse and says that they can go to La Mirada Clinic to get help for their son.

1. How is the concept of *machismo* displayed in this scenario?
2. How is the concept of *marianismo* displayed in this scenario?
3. Why did the parents leave?

may misinterpret this view as fatalistic. Health-care providers should respect this view and assist in identifying options, choices, and opportunities to empower individuals to change health-risk behaviors.

Most Puerto Ricans have a relativistic view of time, which may interfere with being on time for appointments. This flexible time orientation and relaxed attitude may extend to health-care appointments and interfere with the ability to provide health services in a time-limited, cost-containment environment. At the beginning of an interview, health-care providers should carefully explain the expectation of being on time for appointments and the time limits.

Format for Names

Respect for adults, parents, and older people is highly valued among Puerto Ricans. Respect is reflected in the way children talk, look, and refer to adults and older people. Rather than *Señora* (Mrs.) and *Señor* (Mr.), children and adults are expected to use the terms *Doña* (Mrs.) and *Don* (Mr.) for most adults. Aunts and uncles have their name preceded by *tití* or *tío* (auntie/uncle) and *madrina* or *padrino* (godmother or godfather). These prefixes are symbols of respect and position in the family. In health-care settings, individuals expect to be addressed as Sr., Sra., Don, and Doña. Health-care providers should maintain their respect by using this format for names and by avoiding calling Puerto Rican patients by their first names or using terms such as "honey" or "sweetheart."

Similar to other people of Hispanic heritage, Puerto Ricans have a complex system for addressing individuals, specifically women. Single women prefer to use their father's and mother's surnames, in that order. For example, a single woman may use her name as follows: Sonia López Mendoza, with López being her father's surname and Mendoza her mother's. When she is married, the husband's last name, Pérez, is added with the word *de* to reflect that she is married. This woman's married name would be Sonia López de Pérez; the mother's surname is eliminated. In business and health-care organizations, Señora López de Pérez is the correct formal title to use when promoting conversation or building a relationship. Younger or more acculturated women may change their last names to that of their husbands. The importance and respect given to these prescriptive name formalities are perpetuated when friendly verbal and nonverbal gestures accompany the greeting.

Family Roles and Organization
Head of Household and Gender Roles

Despite many socioeconomic changes and changes in the position and role of Puerto Rican women, many traditional patriarchal values still define women in terms of their reproductive roles. Gender-role expectations are strikingly different among more acculturated families. Traditional and newly migrated families may have expectations and view women as lenient, submissive, and always wanting to please men. Men demand respect and obedience from women and the family. Nevertheless, women play a central role in the family and the community, and the Puerto Rican family is moving toward more egalitarian relationships. Moreover, in Puerto Rico, women make significant contributions to society by participating in politics and traditional male-oriented roles. Many of these changes in family and gender roles have resulted from the acculturation process and the increased participation of Puerto Rican women in the workforce.

Through historical, social, and personal conditions, a new identity is emerging, and Puerto Rican feminist voices are calling for changes in family structure, values, power, and authority. More Puerto Rican families are sharing the economic and social responsibilities of the household. However, *machismo,* a sense of masculinity that stresses virility, courage, and domination of women, including the need to display physical strength, bravery, and virility, continues to be the source of confrontations. Many Puerto Rican women are negotiating for power to equalize the dynamics of sexual relationships with Puerto Rican men, who believe women must be submissive and obedient to men in all matters. When assessing health risks and relationships, health-care providers must consider these issues and assess families for their unique patterns of relating to identify appropriate interventions.

Prescriptive, Restrictive, and Taboo Behaviors for Children and Adolescents

Children are the center of Puerto Rican family life. From childhood through adolescence, children are socialized to have respect for adults, especially the elderly. Great significance is given to the concept of **familism**, and any behavior that shifts from this ideal is discouraged and may be perceived as a disgrace to the family. Families who expect children not to contradict, argue, or disagree with their parents may have difficulties when adolescents raised in the Americanized Puerto Rican culture seek independence and struggle between traditional and contemporary family values. Many of these cultural expectations may become a serious threat to the health and educational future of young Puerto Rican adolescents. Among others, teen pregnancy, substance abuse, delinquent behaviors, and depression have been associated with these issues (National Coalition of Hispanic Health and Human Services Organizations [COSSMHO], 1999). Mental health-care providers addressing family conflict must work within the context of the family to resolve adolescents' mental health issues rather than using individual approaches.

Several prescriptive cultural values surround health and weight. Many families believe that a healthy child is one who is *gordita* or *llenito* (diminutive for fat or overweight) and has red cheeks. Massara's (1989) early work on weight, body image perceptions, and health argued that an oversized body image may be perceived as a mirror of physical and financial wealth, even among adult women. Young mothers are often encouraged to add cereal, eggs, and *viandas* (see Nutrition) to their infant's milk bottles. Nurses are in an excellent position to educate mothers about these practices and the health risks for children who are overweight.

Many families socialize male children to be macho, powerful, and strong with healthy sexual appetites. This *macho* behavior encourages dominance over women; values obtaining social privileges; and emphasizes the pursuit of high-paying careers for their financial advantage. Although many families wish for the education of their children, a few still want educated housewives, not necessarily educated professional working women. Female children are socialized with a focus on home economics, family dynamics, and motherhood, which places women in a powerful social status. Consequently, the value placed on motherhood may be a precursor to teenage pregnancy among Puerto Rican adolescents who are seeking power, support, and cultural recognition (Orshan, 1996).

Some families abide by cultural prescriptions that encourage the initiation of sexual behaviors before marriage, extramarital sexual activity, and control by men over sexual relationships. Girls are socialized to be modest, sexually ingenuous, respectful, and subservient to men, a cultural script related to *marianismo* (Orshan, 1996). Discussions about sexuality are considered taboo for many families, who use the term *tener relaciones* (to have relations) rather than the word *sex*. Modesty is highly valued, and issues such as menstruation, birth control, impotence, STIs, and infertility are rarely discussed.

Less-educated families and those from rural areas may have great difficulty educating young women about sexuality and reproductive issues. Thus, many Puerto Rican adolescents depend on educational organizations to learn about menstruation and the reproductive system. However, this is often not the case for preadolescents or adolescents, who are exposed to information through the media, schools, and peers. Cultural respect for the role of health-care providers as educators places them in an excellent position to educate the family about sexuality issues. This respect gains them entrance into a familiar and trusted family environment that must be valued for its cultural traditions and practices.

Most families expect their children to stay home until they get married or pursue a college education. Families want to care for their young and provide them with emotional and financial support to the extent that it is feasible. Children are expected to follow family traditions and rules. The mother is expected to assume an active role disciplining, guiding, and advising children.

Most fathers expect to be consulted, but they see themselves mainly as financial providers. Puerto Rican families are often very rigorous with their children's discipline. Traditional punishments include making the child who has told a lie kneel on rice until the truth is told, washing the mouth vigorously with soap for using profanity, and spanking the buttocks or lower extremities with a belt. Puerto Rican mothers tend to be very protective of their children and may use physical punishment. Many Puerto Rican mothers use threats of punishment, guilt, and discipline, which can create stress and difficulties for adolescents as they struggle with the more permissive cultural patterns of the United States, such as dating. Health-care providers should assess families for these patterns and provide counseling that promotes stability. The cultural definition of physical abuse is challenging, and health-care providers must assess each situation before determining child abuse.

Family Goals and Priorities

Family roles and priorities among Puerto Ricans are based on the concept of *familism*. Puerto Ricans value the unity of the family. *La familia* is the nucleus of the community and the society. The family structure may be nuclear or extended. Family members include grandparents, great-grandparents, married children, aunts, uncles, cousins, and even divorced children with their children. Two families may live in the same household.

After marriage, children live away from their parents but are expected to maintain very close ties with their families, especially the women. Most Puerto Rican families want a daughter because daughters traditionally are caretakers when parents reach advanced ages. In addition, women continue family traditions. Male children, who are usually more independent, are valued because they continue the family name.

Because children are the center of the family, close and extended family members are expected to participate in the care of children, give support, and encourage the maintenance of cultural and religious traditions. Grandparents assume an active role in rearing grandchildren, supporting the family, babysitting, teaching traditions, disciplining, and enforcing educational activities. If the woman works outside the home, family goals and priorities may change, which often results in social and emotional burdens for women. Health-care providers can use and encourage older Puerto Ricans to introduce health-promotion and disease-prevention education within their families.

As women become older, they gain status for their wisdom. Often, older women have a covert power over spouses, children, and the family. Dependent older people are expected to live with their children and be cared for emotionally and financially. Informal and formal support systems are considered critical factors in promoting the health of older Puerto

Ricans, particularly older women. All members of the family provide support for financial and manpower efforts needed to keep older people at home. Those who have higher financial liquidity may take financial responsibility in exchange for the manpower and physical efforts of those who cannot provide financially. Placements in nursing homes and extended-care facilities may be seen as inconsiderate to older people, and family members who must use these organizations may feel guilty and experience depression and distress. Thus, health-care providers must be sensitive to these issues by exploring alternatives for care and providing information to all family members involved in this decision-making process. Discharge planning, hospice care, and other situations can be addressed in a "conference-style" approach to develop strategies for providing emotional support and assistance to family members.

Friends, neighbors, and close and distant family members are expected to visit a person during times of illness, support the family, and take an active role in family decisions and activities. A family member is expected to be at the bedside of the sick person. Health-care providers should ask the name of the family spokesperson and document it in the patient's chart. Nurses may need to set boundaries with patients' families about visitation, personal space, and privacy matters.

Alternative Lifestyles

Since the early 1980s, Puerto Rican families have experienced an increased incidence of pregnancy among teenagers and unmarried women. This trend is believed to be the result of the increased number of women in the labor force, high divorce rates, poverty, and the increased number of households headed by women. For health-care services to be effective in identifying appropriate interventions, health-care providers must assess social-support factors and the socioeconomic status of individuals.

Homosexuality continues to be a taboo topic that carries a great stigma among Puerto Ricans. Same-sex behavior is often undisclosed to avoid family rejection and preserve family links and support. Unfortunately, the literature does not include information about these families and their lifestyles. When caring for gays and lesbians, health-care providers must inquire about their "disclosed or undisclosed status" and act according to patient preferences and support resources.

Workforce Issues

Culture in the Workplace

In general, Puerto Rican men and women readily assimilate into the U.S. work environment, which is similar to their native work environment in Puerto Rico. Nurses are among the latest group of Puerto Rican

professionals who have come to the United States seeking better employment and educational opportunities. They often seek employment opportunities at federal health facilities such as the Army, Navy, Air Force, and Veterans Administration.

Despite stereotypical views of Puerto Ricans as people who do not work and depend solely on the U.S. welfare system, most Puerto Ricans are hardworking, like to be competitive, and often make extended efforts to please their employers. Many Puerto Ricans in the labor force place a high value on their occupations, positions, and businesses. They strive for high performance even in the face of oppression; they offer little resistance and maintain the ability to be happy even when confronting oppressive situations.

Several cultural differences among Puerto Ricans— such as education; the value placed on honesty, integrity, personal relationships; and relativistic views of time—may have an influence in the workplace. The educational system in Puerto Rico emphasizes theoretical and practical content as well as neatness. Consequently, whereas most migrant Puerto Ricans are task oriented and meticulous about the presentation of their work, some have a relativistic view of time and may not value regular attendance and punctuality in the workforce. Most Puerto Ricans are cheerful, have a positive attitude, and value personal relationships at work. Work is perceived as a place for social and cultural interactions, which may include listening to background music while performing job activities. This practice can lead to loud, cheerful, and noisy conversations that may require the employer's attention.

For many women, family responsibilities, pregnancy, and the health of their children and other family members take priority over work. For others, access to the welfare system becomes more convenient than the pride of having a secure job. In Puerto Rico, women are given a lengthy maternity leave because of the emphasis and value placed on the well-being of working women and their infants. In the U.S. labor force, many working Puerto Rican women resent the limited maternity leave supported by the American culture.

Employers may need to negotiate more lexible work responsibilities among Puerto Ricans during religious holiday celebrations such as Easter and Christmas. In Puerto Rico, schools are closed, and the community celebrates a spiritual and religious recess from day-to-day activities and work responsibilities. The great solemnity and religious commitment among all religious groups bring Puerto Rican families to a societal halt for almost 6 weeks. Schools recess from early December to the middle of January, waiting for the Epiphany, *Los Tres Reyes Magos*, on January 6, and the *Octavitas*, a post-Epiphany traditional musical and cultural celebration that extends the Christmas celebration 8 more days. Many Puerto Ricans on the mainland wish to use vacation and unpaid leave to spend time with their families in Puerto Rico. Traditional music, food, and folk activities during these celebrations are used to uphold ethnic pride. Holiday seasons may challenge employers, who need to manage absenteeism, increased consumption of alcohol, requests for vacation, leave without pay, and decreased productivity.

Issues Related to Autonomy

Puerto Rican families have traditionally socialized men into aggressive, domineering, and outspoken roles. Thus, many men display confidence at work and assume leadership positions with autonomy. However, more recent male immigrants who are less educated and have language difficulties may be reluctant to assume leadership roles, may be shy and not as outspoken, and may hesitate to challenge authority and workplace norms. Changing the conduct of these recent male immigrants in the workforce is related to the passivity and docile behaviors learned in the U.S. and Puerto Rican educational systems. These immigrants are more likely to conform to the behavioral norms of the workplace and avoid personal conflict or confrontations in an effort to maintain positive relationships.

Women from rural areas and traditional families are more likely to come from a submissive and noncompetitive environment. Thus, they may be perceived as less determined, less confident, and less outspoken than other American women in managerial and supervisory capacities. Some women find themselves in conflict with traditional values when in a competitive, assertive work environment. Their ability to succeed in the workforce may depend on their employers' support of assertiveness and on-the-job training. In addition, women who wish to climb the career ladder may benefit from an environment that provides information, promotes confidence, fosters positive interpersonal relationships, and teaches strategies for resolving conflict.

Although most Puerto Ricans are bilingual, some may speak broken English, street English, or Puerto Rican **Spanglish** such as "I must pay billes [bills] and find dinero [money]." Younger and urban Puerto Ricans are usually more fluent in English, a skill that facilitates integration into the labor market. Older adults and people who come from a rural background may have less education, lower literacy levels, decreased English proficiency, and increased difficulty assimilating into the labor force.

Biocultural Ecology

Skin Color and Biological Variations

The heritage of Puerto Ricans is a mixture of Native Indian, African, and Spanish heritage. Some may have dark skin; thick, kinky hair; and a wide, flat nose. Others are white-skinned with straight, auburn hair and hazel or black eyes. Certain traits such as skin coloring require health-care providers to vary their techniques when assessing individual Puerto Ricans for anemia and jaundice.

Limited information is available about the biocultural variations among Puerto Ricans. Although no scientific evidence exists, some posit that diseases such as hypertension and diabetes mellitus, major illnesses among Puerto Ricans in Puerto Rico and on the mainland, are the result of indigenous Indian and African heritage. Consequently, health-care providers should assess each person as a unique individual with awareness that standards developed for the dominant American population do not necessarily apply to the Puerto Rican population.

Disease and Health Conditions

The health conditions of Puerto Ricans on the mainland and in Puerto Rico are similar, with the leading causes of death being heart disease, malignant neoplasms, diabetes mellitus, unintentional injuries, and AIDS (National Alliance for Hispanic Health, 2011). Life expectancy for Puerto Ricans females is 82.71 years, and for men it is 75.31 years (*CIA World Factbook*, 2011b). Puerto Ricans have decreased mortality rates for lung, breast, and ovarian cancers and an increased incidence of stomach, prostate, esophageal, pancreatic, and cervical cancers. In Puerto Rico, prostate, colon, and breast cancer, in that order, are the leading causes of cancer-related deaths, followed by tracheal and lung cancers (Puerto Rico Department of Health, 2009). Although the overall cancer mortality rate among Puerto Ricans is lower than that for other groups, health-care providers should continue to educate Puerto Rican families about cancer prevention. Smoked, pickled, and spiced foods should be discouraged, whereas traditional meals, fruits, and vegetables should be encouraged.

Puerto Ricans on the mainland face a high incidence of chronic conditions such as mental illness among younger adults and cardiopulmonary and osteomuscular diseases among the elderly. Acute conditions among Puerto Ricans include a disproportionate number of acute respiratory illnesses, injuries, infectious and parasitic diseases, and diseases of the digestive system.

Puerto Rican women in the United States have a high incidence of being overweight; in particular, this prevalence increases with age and among women from lower socioeconomic levels. Obesity and centralized body fat among these women increase the incidence of, and mortality from, diabetes, the third leading cause of death for Puerto Rican women on the mainland. Men have a lower incidence of obesity than women, and men from rural areas have lower rates of diabetes than men from urban areas. Health-care providers need to develop interventions that are appropriate to gender, age, and socioeconomic status, while giving consideration to their rural or urban living arrangements.

Dengue fever, a mosquito-transmitted disease caused by any of the four viral serotypes of the *Aedes aegypti* mosquito, is an endemic disease that migrants may bring to the mainland. Health-care providers need to advise Puerto Rican patients and families traveling to Puerto Rico to avoid exposure to endemic areas and to use mosquito repellent and protective clothing at all times. Health-care providers should become familiar with the signs, symptoms, and current treatment recommendations for dengue fever.

Puerto Rico has a higher HIV (human immunodeficiency virus) infection rate than any state in the United States. Compared with other ethnic groups in the United States, Puerto Ricans have the highest incidence of HIV. Among Puerto Ricans with HIV, 20 percent are male-to-male homosexual (compared with 43 percent overall in the United States), 39 percent are intravenous drug users (compared with 25 percent overall in the United States), 37 percent are heterosexual (compared with 25 percent overall in the United States), and 5 percent are other (compared with 6 percent overall in the United States) (Centers for Disease Control and Prevention, 2006).

Variations in Drug Metabolism

Literature searches reveal no information regarding differences in drug metabolism among Puerto Ricans. Health-care providers must be aware that pharmaceutical studies conducted with European Americans may not yield the same results with Puerto Ricans; thus, individual assessments with accurate documentation of observations are imperative. Because of the African heritage of many Puerto Ricans, drug absorption, metabolism, and excretion differences experienced by African Americans and American Indians may hold true for black Puerto Ricans. Given that some Puerto Ricans are short in stature and have higher subscapular and triceps skin folds, long trunks, and short legs, therapeutic dosages calculated for the European American population may not be appropriate for Puerto Ricans.

High-Risk Behaviors

Puerto Ricans are at high risk for illnesses, with increased mortality and morbidity rates related to alcoholism, smoking, illicit drug use, physical inactivity, poor dietary practices, sex-related behaviors, and underutilization of preventive health-care services. Alcoholism is the precursor of increased unintentional injuries, family disruption, spousal abuse, and mental illness among Puerto Rican families. According to Centers for Disease Control (2008), 80 percent of Puerto Rican men and 29 percent of Puerto Rican women have high rates of alcohol consumption. Alcohol consumption among Puerto Ricans is attributed, in part, to acculturation into the mainstream U.S. culture and to psychosocial factors (Torres & Villaruel, 1996).

The prevalence of smoking among Puerto Ricans is lower than that of European Americans but higher than that for other Hispanic subgroups. Puerto Rican women have a higher prevalence of smoking than Cuban and Mexican American women, and when age is adjusted, Puerto Rican women younger than age 40 have the highest prevalence of smoking among all women in the United States. Health-care providers should consider gender and acculturation issues and build on previous successful intervention programs to develop specific programs for decreasing smoking among Puerto Rican populations. Providers must be aware that Puerto Rican adolescents—in particular females—are at higher risk of starting and continuing to smoke than other Hispanic and ethnic subgroups including African Americans and Asians (Epstein, Botvin, & Diaz, 1998).

Drug use is a significant public-health problem for many Puerto Ricans, whose rate of marijuana and cocaine use is often higher than that of the European American population. The last research decade clearly indicates that issues related to acculturation, peer factors, individual, family, parental, and gender-role issues are the most important risk factors in need of early health provider interventions to decrease susceptibility to drug addiction and delinquency. Acculturation, as measured by language use, is significantly associated with marijuana and cocaine use. Many studies have shown that the longer one lives in the United States and the more acculturated one becomes, the higher the rate of use of marijuana, smoking, and cocaine. Among Puerto Rican men, social barriers, family demoralization, and other life problems are significant precursors for illicit drug use. However, acculturation, family factors, peer domains, language, and place of birth do not explain these patterns of illicit drug use in adolescents or men as well as they do for Puerto Rican women (Torres & Villaruel, 1996). Issues such as acculturation, self-esteem, self-concept, depression, hopelessness, and maladaptive coping behaviors are significant factors influencing the pattern and prevalence of Puerto Rican women's drug use. Health-care providers should develop programs that promote early interventions for the use of illicit drugs. Interventions should focus on individual psychological differences, gender issues, and other contributing factors.

Because many Puerto Ricans support *machismo* and submission of women, these roles foster high-risk behaviors that impede the prevention and increase the transmission of HIV. In traditional Puerto Rican culture, most men are given free will over sexual practices, including the approval and initiation of sex before marriage and extramarital affairs with other women. Some men may perceive that sexual intercourse with men is a sign of virility and sexual power rather than a homosexual behavior. Puerto Rican women are often found in a paradoxical position, because they have to deal with cultural beliefs and health-protective practices. Knowledge about HIV, beliefs about health and illness, and beliefs and practices related to condom use are common concerns encountered by health-care providers in the prevention and transmission of HIV.

Lack of condom use is perhaps one of the most significant risk behaviors that need immediate attention and intervention from health-care providers. Issues such as embarrassment, cost, gender or power struggles, and abuse are among the barriers encountered by Puerto Rican women. Some men fear that if they use condoms, they portray a less *macho* image, have decreased sexual satisfaction, or indicate that they have an STI or HIV. In addition, the Catholic Church's opposition to the use of condoms, lower educational levels, lower socioeconomic status, and acculturation are significant variables related to the high rates of AIDS and HIV among Puerto Ricans and other Hispanics. Health-care providers must be aware of these barriers, assess individual perceptions of high-risk behaviors, and intervene with programs designed to meet the particular needs of clients who are at high risk for HIV infection or other STIs.

Nutrition

Meaning of Food

Puerto Ricans celebrate, mourn, and socialize around food. Food is used to honor and recognize visitors, friends, family members, and health-care providers; as an escape from everyday pressures, problems, and challenges; and to prevent and treat illnesses. Puerto Rican patients may bring homemade goods to health-care providers as an expression of appreciation, respect, and gratitude for services rendered. Refusing these offerings may be interpreted as a personal rejection.

Some Puerto Ricans believe that being overweight is a sign of health and wealth. Some eat to excess, believing that if they eat more, their health will be better, whereas others pay no attention to weight control or dietary practices. Many Puerto Ricans perceive that European Americans are more preoccupied with how they look than how healthy they are. Efforts by American health-care providers directed at weight control may be seen as the Americans' excessive preoccupation with a thin body image.

Common Foods and Food Rituals

Traditional Puerto Rican families emphasize having a complete breakfast that begins with a cup of strong coffee or *café con leche* (coffee with milk). Some drink strong coffees such as espresso with lots of sugar; others boil fresh milk (or use condensed milk) and then add the coffee. Many families introduce children to coffee as early as 5 or 6 years of age. A traditional Puerto Rican breakfast includes hot cereal such as oatmeal; cornmeal; or rice and wheat cereal cooked with vanilla, cinnamon, sugar, salt, and milk. Although less common, traditional Puerto Ricans may eat corn pancakes or fritters for breakfast.

Lunch is served by noon, followed by dinner at around 5 or 6 p.m. A cup of espresso-like coffee is also enjoyed at 10:00 a.m. and 3:00 p.m. Rice and stew *habichuelas* (beans) are the main dishes among Puerto Rican families. Rice may be served plain or cooked and served with as many as 12 side dishes. Rice cooked with vegetables or meat is considered a complete meal. *Arroz guisado* (rice stew) is seasoned with *sofrito*, a blend of spices such as cilantro, *recao* (a type of cilantro), onions, green peppers, and other nonspicy ingredients. Rice is cooked with chicken, pork, sausages, codfish, calamari, or shrimp, as well as corn, several types of beans, and *gandules* (green pigeon peas), a Puerto Rican bean rich in iron and protein. Rice with *gandules* is a traditional Christmas holiday dish that is accompanied by *pernil asado* (roasted pork) and *pasteles*, made with root vegetables, green plantain, bananas, or condiments and then filled with meat and wrapped with plantain leaves. Fritters are also common foods.

Puerto Ricans eat a great variety of pastas, breads, crackers, vegetables, and fruits. *Tostones*, fried green or ripe plantains, are a favorite side dish served with almost every meal. Puerto Rican families eat a variety of roots called *viandas*, vegetables rich in vitamins and starch. The most common *viandas* are celery roots, sweet potatoes, dasheens, yams, breadfruit, breadnut, green and ripe plantains, green bananas, tanniers, cassava, and chayote squash or christophines. A list of common Puerto Rican meals is presented in Table 23-1. Because

▌▌▶ Table 23-1 Common Puerto Rican Meals

Puerto Rican Meal	English Translation
Alcapurrias	Green plantain fritters filled with meat or crab
Arepas de maíz y queso	Cornmeal and cheese fritters
Arroz con pollo	Rice with chicken
Arroz con gandules	Rice with pigeon peas
Arroz blanco (con aceite)	Plain rice (with oil)
Arroz guisado básico	Plain stewed rice
Asopao de pollo	Soupy rice with chicken
Bacalaitos	Codfish fritters
Bocadillo	Grilled sandwich
Mondongo	Tripe stew
Paella de mariscos	Seafood paella
Pastelillos de carne, queso, o pasta de guayaba	Turnovers filled with meat, cheese, or guava paste
Pollo en fricase con papas	Stewed chicken with potatoes
Relleno de papa	Potato ball filled with meat
Sancocho	*Viandas* and meat stew
Sofrito	Condiment
Surullo de queso	Cornmeal fritters filled with cheese

Puerto Rican meals are flavorful, patients in the health-care setting may find more traditional American meals to be flavorless and unattractive. However, more acculturated Puerto Ricans are changing their traditional food practices and often follow mainland U.S. dietary practices. Health-care providers who work with traditional Puerto Rican patients should become familiar with these foods and their nutritional content to assist families with dietary practices that integrate their traditional or preferred food selections.

Dietary Practices for Health Promotion

Many Puerto Ricans ascribe to the hot-cold classifications of foods for nutritional balance and dietary practices during menstruation, pregnancy, the postpartum period, infant feeding, lactation, and aging. Some of the hot-cold classifications are presented in Table 23-2. Health-care providers should become familiar with these food practices when planning culturally congruent dietary alternatives.

Understanding that iron is considered a "hot" food that is not usually taken during pregnancy can assist health-care providers to negotiate approval and educate Puerto Rican women about the importance of maintaining adherence to daily iron recommendations, even during pregnancy and lactation. An additional summary of Puerto Rican cultural food habits, reasons for practices, and recommendations for health-care providers during such developmental stages is presented in Table 23-3.

With the advent of alternatives to hormone replacement therapy (HRT) (Taylor, 1999), many Puerto Rican women are using a variety of herbal and botanical remedies. Many are using relaxation, massage, acupuncture, guided imagery, chelation, biofeedback, and therapeutic touch in addition to or as an alternative to HRT. Black cohosh, evening primrose, St. John's wort, gingko, ginseng, valerian root, sarsaparilla, chamomile, red clover, and passion flower are the most common herbs and botanical alternatives used by Puerto Rican women.

▌▶ Table 23-2 **Puerto Rican Hot-Cold Classification of Selected Foods, Medications, Herbs, and Health-Illness Status**

Hot-Cold Classification	Health-Illnesses Status	Western Medications	Traditional Herbs	Foods
Hot	Gastrointestinal illnesses (constipation, diarrhea, Crohn's colitis, ulcer, bleeding)	Syrups	Teas	Cocoa products
	Gynecological issues (pregnancy, menopause)	Dark-colored pills	Cinnamon	Alcoholic beverages
	Skin disorders (rashes, acne)	Aspirin	Dark-leaf teas	Caffeine products
	Neurological disorders (headache)	Anti-inflammatory agents	Teas	Hot cereals (wheat, corn)
	Heart disease	Prednisone		Salt
	Urological illnesses	Antihypertensives		Spices and condiments
		Castor oil		Beans
		Cinnamon		Nuts and seeds
		Vitamins (iron)		
		Antibiotics		
Cold	Osteomuscular illnesses (arthritis, rheumatoid arthritis, multiple sclerosis)	Diuretics	Orange-lemon chamomile	Rice
	Menstruation	Bicarbonate of soda	Linden	Rice and barley water
	Respiratory illnesses	Antacids	Mint	Milk
		Milk of magnesia	Anise	Sugar and sugar products
				Root vegetables
				Avocado
				Fruits
				Vegetables
				White meat
				Honey
				Onions

▐▌ Table 23-3   Puerto Rican Cultural Nutrition and Health Beliefs and Practices During Particular Stages

Behavioral Period	Dietary and Health Practices	Cultural Justification	Recommendation for Health-Care Professionals
Menstruation	*Food taboos:* Avoid spices, cold beverages, acid-citric fruits and substances, chocolate, and coffee.	May induce cramps, hemorrhage, clots, and physical imbalance. May produce acne during menstruation.	Assess individual beliefs and acknowledge them.
	Foods encouraged: Plenty of hot fluids, such as cinnamon tea, milk with cinnamon and sugar. Teas such as chamomile, anise seed, linden tea, mint leaves.	Fluids encourage body cleaning of impurities. Hot beverages encourage circulation and reduce abdominal colic, cramps, and pain. Teas are soothing to all body systems.	Incorporate traditional beliefs in treatments as required in nonsteroidal anti-inflammatories for dysmenorrhea.
	Health practices: Avoid exercise and practice good hygiene. Do not walk barefoot. Avoid wind and rain. Stay as warm as possible.	Exercise may increase pain and bleeding. Good hygiene is important for health. Walking barefoot during menstruation may cause rheumatoid arthritis and other inflammatory diseases. Warm temperatures promote circulation and the health of the reproductive system as well as prevent cramps.	Encourage passive exercise. Provide information about the role of exercise in the reduction of menstrual discomfort. Support other practices.
Pregnancy	*Food taboos:* Hot food, sauces, condiments, chocolate products, coffee, beans, pork, fritters, oily foods, and citrus products.	May cause excess flatus, acid indigestion, bulging, and constipation. Chocolate and coffee may cause darker skin in fetus. Some believe citrus products may be abortive.	Encourage healthy food habits. Provide information about chocolate and coffee myths. Encourage fruits.
	Foods encouraged: Milk, beef, chicken, vegetables, fruits, *ponches.*	Considered healthy and nutritious. Increases hemoglobin, strengthens and promotes good labor.	Discourage the use of raw eggs in beverages because of possibility of *Salmonella* poisoning.
	Health practices: Rest and get plenty of sleep. Eat plenty of food. Follow diet cautiously. Many avoid sexual intercourse early in pregnancy. Practice good hygiene and take warm showers.	Enhances health and prevents problems during birth. Sex may cause problems with baby or preterm labor.	Encourage use of food recommended for pregnancy. Provide information about sexual activity. Encourage a balanced plan of exercise with emphasis on weight control and health of the baby.
Lactation	*Food taboos:* Avoid beans, cabbages, lettuce, seeds, nuts, pork, chocolate, coffee, and hot food items at all times.	These foods cause stomach illnesses for infant and mother, including baby colic, diarrhea, and flatus.	Include a dietary plan that is balanced with substitute food items. Clarify any myths about infant diarrhea, colic, and flatus.
	Foods encouraged: Milk, water, *ponches,* chicken soup, chicken, beef, pastas, hot cereals.	Improve health and increase hemoglobin and essential vitamins. Protect mother and infant from illnesses. Fluids and *ponches* increase milk supply. Red meats reduce cravings.	As above with raw eggs.
	Health practices: Avoid cold temperatures and wind. A few may avoid showering for several days during the *cuarentena* after birth. Great attention is paid to health of the mother.	Cold temperatures and winds are believed to cause stroke and facial paralysis in a new mother. Showering may cause respiratory diseases. Mother is believed to be at risk and fragile.	Provide information about reasons for stroke and facial paralysis. Provide time to ask questions and reduce anxiety during winter season deliveries.
Infant feeding	*Food taboos:* Beans, too much rice, and uncooked vegetables.	Believed to cause stomach colic, flatus, and distended abdomen. Too much rice causes constipation.	Provide information about appropriate dietary patterns for infant.

Continues on page 418

▶ Table 23-3	**Puerto Rican Cultural Nutrition and Health Beliefs and Practices During Particular Stages** *Continued from page 417*		
Behavioral Period	Dietary and Health Practices	Cultural Justification	Recommendation for Health-Care Professionals
	Foods encouraged: Hot cereals, *ponches*, chicken broth or *caldos*. Fresh fruits, cooked vegetables, *viandas*. Raw eggs, cereals, baby foods in milk bottle. Fresh fruit juices. Mint, chamomile, and anise tea. Sugar and honey used for hiccups.	Believed to be nutritious and healthy and to decrease hunger. *Caldos* are fortifying and prevent illness. Cooked vegetables are healthy and prevent constipation. Bottle food fills the baby. Fresh juices and fruits refresh the stomach. Teas help baby sleep and cure flatus. Sugar and honey have curing properties.	Instruct about infant diet and timely introduction of food items to diet. Explain consequences of excessive weight in infants. Discourage food in bottle to prevent choking.
	Health practices: Keep baby warm while feeding.	Warm babies eat, chew, and digest food better, and choking is decreased.	Discourage raw eggs because of the risk of *Salmonella* and egg allergies and the use of honey because of the risk of botulism. Teas are harmless and provide additional fluid when used in moderation without sugar.
			Provide information about babies and choking.

Health-care providers should understand and be able to discuss the safety and efficacy of the most frequently used alternatives. The use of HRT alternatives should be included in routine health assessment among women in this stage.

An infant is believed to be healthy if it is *gordito* (a little fat) and has red cheeks. Consequently, many mothers add ground root vegetables, eggs, hot cereals, rice, canned baby foods, and fruits and vegetables to the infant's bottle at an early age. Traditionally, when children are introduced to soft foods and vegetables, parents boil and grind root vegetables for the infant. For some, these dietary practices have changed with the availability of canned baby food. Many mothers tend to feed whole cow's milk or canned milk (Carnation) earlier than recommended in Western practice, believing that canned milk produces healthier babies. Health-care providers must educate families regarding the nutritional content of canned milk versus fresh milk, breastfeeding, and formula.

For older Puerto Ricans, a good diet includes meats, traditional meals, and vitamin supplements. Beverages such as fresh-squeezed orange juice, grape juice, and *ponches* (punches) are used as additional nutritional support, particularly for those who are immunosuppressed or chronically or terminally ill. If the older individual is believed to have low blood pressure and is weak or tired, a small daily portion of brandy may be added to black coffee to enhance the work of "an old heart." If the health-care provider criticizes these practices, it may deter the client from seeking follow-up care and decrease trust and confidence in health-care providers. Health-care providers must

inquire about these practices and should incorporate harmless or nonconflicting practices into the diet.

During illness, Puerto Ricans pay close attention to dietary practices. Chicken soups and *caldos* (broth) are used as a hot meal to provide essential nutrients. A mixture of equal amounts of honey, lemon, and rum is used as an expectorant and antitussive. A malt drink, *malta* (grape juice), or milk is often added to an egg yolk mixed with plenty of sugar to increase the hemoglobin level and provide strength. Ulcers, acid indigestion, and stomach illnesses are treated with warm milk, with or without sugar. Herbal teas are used to treat illnesses and to promote health. Most herbal teas do not interfere with medical prescriptions. Incorporating their use with traditional Western medicine may enhance adherence to treatment.

Nutritional Deficiencies and Food Limitations

Most Puerto Ricans moving to the mainland locate in areas with Puerto Rican or Hispanic communities and where preferred foods are readily available. Traditional cooking and food practices do not necessarily change. Instead, European American foods are quickly integrated into the dietary practices, thereby increasing food diversity. Fresh fruits and juices are consumed in large quantities.

Few studies have shown significant data about nutritional deficiencies among Puerto Ricans. Studies that include small samples of Puerto Ricans show that Puerto Rican children have nutritional statuses similar to those of Mexican American and African American children in terms of malnutrition, obesity, and short stature. Low-income Puerto Rican children and adolescents have been found to have anemia and tooth decay related to consumption of less than the recommended daily allowances of iron, folacin, thiamin, niacin, and vitamin C. Menstruation is viewed as a time when women must care for themselves and adhere to certain dietary practices to promote health. From the onset of menstruation, young girls are encouraged to avoid foods believed to produce flatus, abdominal cramps, and colic. Hot drinks are encouraged to increase circulation and promote the elimination of metabolic waste.

Pregnancy and Childbearing Practices

Fertility Practices and Views Toward Pregnancy

Marital status, knowledge, attitudes, beliefs about the reproductive system, the role of motherhood, sexuality, and contraceptive use are factors that need to be considered when assessing and implementing culturally congruent maternal–infant interventions and educational programs. Compared with 1990 data, Puerto Rican women are improving their access to prenatal care (National Center for Health Statistics, 2011). Health-care providers should be aware that social support has been found to be one of the most significant factors related to perinatal outcomes among Puerto Rican women. Among others, social support has been found to have significant implications for stress, health behaviors, and infant health (Landale & Oropesa, 2001). Among adolescents, culturally imposed male behaviors and lack of parental guidance or supervision have been listed as predictors of teenage pregnancy (COSSMHO, 1999). The infant mortality rate for Puerto Rican women is 8.07 percent (*CIA World Factbook,* 2011a). Teen pregnancy remains high at 6.9 percent compared with an overall U.S. rate (all races) at 3.4 percent. Ten percent of Puerto Rican births are low weight (National Center for Health Statistics, 2011).

Puerto Rican women do not commonly use birth control methods such as foams, creams, and diaphragms because the Catholic Church, which condones only the rhythm method and sexual abstinence, sees them as immoral. According to the HHANES study, in the United States, fertility control methods used by Puerto Rican women were tubal ligation, called *La Operación* (the surgery) with 23 percent, followed by oral contraceptives with 8.7 percent, hysterectomies with 3.5 percent, and oophorectomies with 3.2 percent (Stroup-Benham & Treviño, 1991).

Prescriptive, Restrictive, and Taboo Practices in the Childbearing Family

Hygiene is highly valued during pregnancy, labor, and the postpartum period. Pregnancy is a time of indulgence for Puerto Rican women. Favors and wishes are

REFLECTIVE EXERCISE 23.2

Rosa Medina, age 33, is 3 days postpartum. She has brought 3-day-old Juanita to the maternal-child clinic because the baby has been crying continuously.

The nurse greets Mrs. Medina and asks how she and her family are getting along with Juanita. Mrs. Medina says that things are "mostly okay" and that her mother and sister help take care of the other children, while her husband was able to keep his job after a lot of people at the market were fired.

The nurse asks if the problem is with Mrs. Medina or her daughter Juanita, and Mrs. Medina says that Juanita has been crying all day, but nothing seems to help. They don't have any chamomile tea to offer the child either.

Nurse: When did she first start crying?
Mrs. Medina: Yesterday morning, right after I gave her the bottle.
Nurse: Was she taking her bottle okay up to that time?
Mrs. Medina: I am not sure. I have been kind of tired since the birth, and my mother has been feeding her most of the time. My mother says that she does not eat as much as she should. My mother never thinks babies eat enough.
Nurse: Can you help me examine her belly?
Mrs. Medina: Yes, but she cries every time I touch her belly. I think she has *empacho*.
Nurse: I notice you have this cloth wrapped around her belly. Can I take it off?
Mrs. Medina: Oh, of course.
Nurse: You have a coin over Juanita's belly. What purpose does it serve?
Mrs. Medina: To keep the bad spirits away and help the cord heal.
Nurse: And the cloth holds the coin in place?
Mrs. Medina: The cloth keeps her belly button from sticking out when she cries.
Nurse: Did you do this with your other children?
Mrs. Medina: Yes. Everyone in our family does this, and we all have flat belly buttons.
Nurse: You know it really is not necessary to put the cloth on her.

1. How is *familism* displayed in this scenario?
2. What is the culture-bound syndrome *empacho*? What is the equivalent Western concept of *empacho*?
3. Should the nurse actively discourage Mrs. Medina from placing the coin on the infant's umbilicus? Why? Why not?
4. Should the nurse actively discourage Mrs. Medina from using the abdominal cloth? Why? Why not?

granted to women for their well-being and the health of their babies. Men are socialized to be tolerant, understanding, and patient regarding pregnant women and their preferences. Pregnant Puerto Rican women are encouraged to rest, consume large quantities of food, and carefully watch what they eat. Many young Puerto Rican families prefer to attend birthing classes.

Some expect women to "get fat" and place little emphasis on weight control. Strenuous physical activity and exercise are discouraged, and lifting heavy objects is prohibited. Women are strongly discouraged from consuming aspirin, Alka-Seltzer, and malt beverages because these substances are believed to cause abortion.

Many women refrain from *tener relaciones* (sexual intercourse) after the first trimester to avoid hurting the fetus or causing preterm labor. Some men view this time as an opportunity for extramarital sexual affairs. Health-care providers should inquire in a nonconfrontational manner about this possibility and educate men regarding the dangers of STIs and HIV.

Women prefer the bed position for labor, wish to have their bodies covered, and prefer a limited number of internal examinations. They welcome their husbands, mothers, or sisters to assist during labor. Men are expected to be supportive. During labor, women may be loud and verbally expressive, a culturally accepted and an encouraged method for coping with pain and discomfort. Pain medications are welcomed. Health-care providers should respect these wishes and explain the necessity of invasive interventions during labor. Most women oppose having a cesarean section because it indicates a "weak woman." The health-care provider should discuss the possibility of a cesarean section early in the pregnancy.

Postpartum women receive care from their family and friends. Their first postpartum meal should be homemade chicken soup to provide energy and strength. Women are encouraged to avoid exposure to wind and cold temperatures, not to lift heavy objects, and not to do housework for 40 days after delivery (the *cuarentena*). Some traditional women do not wash their hair during this time. Because the mother is believed to be susceptible to emotional and physical distress during the postpartum period, family members try not to contribute to stress or to give bad news to the new mother. Fathers may be reluctant to tell the new mother about a problem with the newborn. However, most Puerto Rican women want to be told immediately about any problems. This is a critical issue during the postpartum period, especially with premature babies, given the belief that a healthy baby is a "symbol of father's virility and a time for the woman to demonstrate her fertility, strength, and success during and after birth" (Crouch-Ruiz, 1996).

Some mothers might ask to talk to the pediatrician, rather than to a nurse, about infant problems. Because of the value placed on family and children, women who need to return to work early may experience great distress when they do not follow some of these cultural values or norms. Health-care providers should assess for individual perceptions and dissatisfaction with the working role and birth recuperation. Mothers who breastfeed are encouraged to drink lots of fluids such as milk and chicken soup, and if they are feeling weak or tired, to drink *ponches*, beverages consisting of milk or fresh juices mixed with a raw egg yolk and sugar. Hot foods such as chocolate, beans, lentils, and coffee are discouraged because they are believed to cause stomach irritability and flatus for the mother and colic for the infant.

Early studies on breastfeeding and Puerto Rican women show that only 10 to 11 percent of Puerto Rican women breastfeed (Stroup-Benham & Treviño, 1991). However, traditional Puerto Rican mothers and those from rural areas may prefer to breastfeed their babies for the first year. Mothers who work outside the home may select breastfeeding or formula or both. However, with the introduction of formula through U.S. food stamp programs, two generations of Puerto Rican mothers have been inclined to relinquish breastfeeding and adopt formula as the primary source of infant nutrition. Because some Puerto Rican women believe that breastfeeding increases their weight, disfigures the breast, and makes them less sexually attractive, they undervalue the benefits of breastfeeding. Health-care providers need to provide information about these beliefs and educate women about breastfeeding myths and misconceptions. Because maternal grandmothers have a great influence on practices related to breastfeeding, they should be included along with significant others in educational programs that encourage this practice.

Death Rituals

Death Rituals and Expectations

Death is perceived as a time of crisis in Puerto Rican families. The body is considered sacred and guarded with great respect. Death rituals are shaped by religious beliefs and practices, and family members are careful to complete the death rituals. News about the deceased should be given first to the head of the family, usually the oldest daughter or son. Because of cultural, physical, and emotional responses to grief, health-care providers should use a private room to communicate such news and have a clergy or minister present when the news is disclosed. Family privacy at this time is highly valued.

Providers should allow time for family to view, touch, and stay with the body before it is removed. Traditionally, some Puerto Rican families keep the body in their home before burial. Cultural traditions and financial limitations influence this decision. Consequently, some older adults may wish to follow these death rituals. For some, funeral homes are viewed as impersonal, financially unnecessary, and detrimental to the mourning process because they detract from family intimacy.

Although the family may prefer to have all death rituals finished within a reasonable timeframe, it is important to extend burial rituals until all close family members can be present. The head of the family is expected to coordinate the arrival of family members, which usually creates a delay in death rituals and burial time and an emotional burden and stress on family members. Health-care providers should ensure that members of the family are provided with support, resources, and information regarding differences in U.S. legal requirements. These requirements are often confusing and are considered insensitive, particularly with a stillbirth or when an autopsy is necessary. Authorization from several family members might be essential. Because of the spiritual and religious importance of burial traditions and rituals during these events, cremation is rarely practiced among Puerto Ricans. Among Catholics, the head of the family or other close family member is expected to organize the religious ceremonies, such as the praying of the rosary, the wake (*velorio*), and the novenas, the 9 days of rosary following the death of the family member. Family may meet at the deceased's home for several days, sometimes weeks, to support the family and talk about the deceased. Food is served throughout the day as a symbol of gratitude for those who come to pay their respects.

Responses to Death and Grief

It is culturally acceptable for the family of the deceased to freely express themselves through loud crying and verbal expressions of grief. Some may talk in a thunderous way to God. Others may express their grief through a sensitive but continuous crying or sobbing. Some believe that not expressing their feelings could mean a lack of love and respect for the deceased. Similar to the reaction to other crisis events, some may develop psychosomatic symptoms, and others may experience nausea, vomiting, or fainting spells as a result of a nervousness attack—*ataque de nervios*. Health-care providers should be nonjudgmental with mourners' psychosomatic or other expressions of grief by providing a private environment and helping to minimize interruptions during that period.

Spirituality

Dominant Religion and Use of Prayer

Religious beliefs among Puerto Ricans influence their approach to health and illness. Most Puerto Ricans are Catholic (85 percent), and the remainder are Protestant Evangelical religious affiliations. A few practice *espiritismo*, a blend of Native Indian, African, and Catholic beliefs that deal with rituals related to spiritual communications with spirits and evil forces. *Espiritistas*, individuals capable of communicating with spirits, may be consulted to promote spiritual wellness and treat mental illnesses.

Upon immigration, many Puerto Ricans may feel out of place and need support resources. Many join Evangelical churches because these offer a more personal spiritual approach. These religious groups provide social support and promote harmony and spiritual–physical well-being. Health-care providers should reinforce these spiritual practices, while incorporating prescribed medications, health activities, and the prevention of risk behaviors. *Espiritistas* treat patients with mental health conditions and are often consulted to determine folk remedies compatible with Western medical treatments. Health-care providers should be aware that the elderly, those who have limited access to health care, and those who are dissatisfied with or distrust the Western medical system commonly use spiritual healers.

Among Catholics, candles, rosary beads, or a special patron or figurine might accompany the patient to the health-care facility and be used during prayer rituals. To provide timely and appropriate interventions to Catholic families, health-care providers should inquire about the family's wishes regarding the Sacrament of the Sick. Special prayers and readings are believed to be necessary at the moment of death, and families expect to be present to recite these prayers.

Meaning of Life and Individual Sources of Strength

Puerto Ricans consider life sacred, something that individuals should preserve. Many see the quality of life as a harmonious balance among the mind, the body, and the spirit. Spirituality helps Puerto Ricans gain strength to deal with illness, death, and grief and ultimately promotes well-being. Most Puerto Ricans are very religious, and when confronted with situations related to health, illness, work, death, or the prognosis of a terminal illness, they maintain their trust in spiritual forces. Spiritual forces assist in controlling and managing social and economic constraints. Their own personal actions are perceived as inconsequential or trivial without the trust and confidence in God's will, *Si Dios quiere* (if God wants). Rather than a fatalistic approach to life during illness, death, or health promotion, Puerto Ricans use coping mechanisms such as religious practices that are instrumental in providing control in their lives. For example, the role of religion in the lives of Puerto Ricans with chronic illnesses or with disabled children has been described as a critical source of support and a mechanism that allows for appropriate interpretation of health and illness (Skinner, Correa, Bailey, & Skinner, 2001). God, who is their highest source of strength, guides life. For some, scripture readings, praise, and prayer bring inner spiritual power to the soul, *el alma*.

Spiritual Beliefs and Health-Care Practices

Spiritual practices influenced by religious groups have a great impact on the health status of Puerto Ricans because churches have had a great influence on the health of individuals by discouraging high-risk behaviors and promoting health. Through prayer, church attendance, and worship, many Puerto Ricans discover spiritual courage and inner strength to avoid high-risk behaviors such as smoking and substance abuse. Clergy and ministers are a resource for spiritual wisdom and help with a host of spiritual needs.

Although amulets have lost their popularity, some Puerto Ricans still use them. An *azabache* (small black fist) or a rabbit's foot might be used for good luck, to drive away bad spirits, and to protect a child's health. Rosary beads and patron saint figures may be placed at the head or side of the bed or on the patient to protect him or her from outside evil sources. Health-care providers should ask permission before removing, cleaning, or moving these objects. A benediction may be requested before removing amulets or religious objects, giving the Sacrament of the Sick, or providing spiritual support. These objects are often used as a means of dealing with a crisis or as an expression of hope. The health-care provider should assess individual and family religious preferences and support spiritual resources according to the patient's or family's request.

Health-Care Practices

Health-Seeking Beliefs and Behaviors

Most Puerto Ricans have a curative view of health. They tend to underuse health-promotion and preventive services such as regular dental or physical examinations and Pap smears (Marks, Garcia, & Solis, 1990). Many use emergency health-care services rather than preventive health-care services for acute problems. Acculturation, age, access to health care, education, and income influence health-seeking beliefs and behaviors. Health-care providers must develop mechanisms to integrate individual, family, and community resources to encourage a focus on health promotion and enhance early health screening and disease prevention. In particular, a great deal of attention must be provided to improve interpersonal processes of care among providers and Puerto Rican patients. In a study with Puerto Rican women, Davis and Flannery (2001) reported that women experienced negative interactions with providers who were perceived as the "least helpful resource." Health-care providers that offer weekend, evening, and late-night health-care services in community-based settings may increase the use of preventive services.

Good hygiene is a basic concept for health promotion among Puerto Ricans. Daily showers are essential for good health and personal appearance. Exceptions are made during illnesses such as colds, flu, or viral infections. After surgery, some prefer to bathe using a basin of water instead of taking a shower or tub bath. Most prefer to shower and wash their hair daily; however, some women may avoid doing these activities during menstruation. During hospitalization, some refrain from having a bowel movement if they have to use a bedside commode or bedpan. Nurses are in a unique position to respectfully explore those beliefs and practices and to provide a private, nonintrusive environment for the patient.

Responsibility for Health Care

Most Puerto Ricans believe in family care rather than self-care. Women are seen as the main caregivers and promoters of family health and are the source of spiritual and physical strength. Health-care providers should incorporate the participation of the family in the care of the ill.

Natural herbs, teas, and over-the-counter medications are often used as initial interventions for symptoms of illness. Many consult family and friends before consulting a health-care provider. Moreover, pharmacists play a vital role in symptom management. Although Puerto Rico is subject to U.S. Food and Drug Administration regulations and practices, many Puerto Ricans are able to obtain controlled prescriptions from their local pharmacist in Puerto Rico. When they are on the mainland, they try to obtain the same kind of services from local pharmacists, creating distress and frustration for both the patient and the pharmacist.

Over-the-counter medications and folk remedies are often used by Puerto Ricans to treat mental health symptoms, acute illnesses, and chronic diseases. Health-care providers should inquire about those practices and encourage patients to bring their medications to every visit. Engaging in a friendly conversation encourages patients to reveal their use of folk treatments, over-the-counter medications, and concurrent use of folk healers. Since the early 1980s, Puerto Ricans have become accustomed to the use of extended-care facilities and nursing homes. However, they prefer to keep chronically or terminally ill family members at home.

Folk and Traditional Practices

Espiritismo and **Santería** are magico-religious and folk-healing practices used by some Puerto Ricans. *Espiritistas* solve problems by communicating with spirits. The *Santería* focuses on health promotion and personal growth and development. Clients who use these folk practices visit **bótanicas** (folk religious stores) and use natural herbs, aromatic incenses, special bathing herbs, prayer books, prayers, and figurines for treating illness and promoting good health. Providers must examine their own views about traditional practices and healers and refrain from making prejudicial comments that may inhibit collaboration with folk healers.

Puerto Ricans may use folk practices for shortness of breath, nausea, and vomiting. Asphyxia or shortness of breath is believed to be caused by lack of air in the body. Fanning the face or blowing into the patient's face is believed to provide oxygen and relieve dyspnea. Some may use tea from an alligator's tail, snails, or *savila* (plant leaves) for illnesses such as asthma and congestive heart failure.

Nausea and vomiting may be embarrassing and cause alarm to many Puerto Rican patients. Many believe that smelling or rubbing isopropyl alcohol (*alcolado*) may help alleviate these symptoms. Some place a damp cloth on the forehead to refresh the "hot" inside the body and relieve nausea. Some put the head between the legs to stop vomiting. Mint, orange, or lemon tree leaves are boiled and used as tea to relieve nausea and vomiting. Rectal suppositories are believed to induce diarrhea. Health-care providers should provide clear information about suppositories and the etiologic cause of symptoms.

Barriers to Health Care

The medically indigent in Puerto Rico receive free health-care services through the Department of Health. On the mainland, accessing health-care services is a complex issue for many Puerto Ricans. A recent analysis of insurance coverage and use of health services showed that 26 percent of Puerto Ricans are uninsured, and those who are insured are likely to receive services through public health insurance coverage (Puerto Rican Health News, 2007). Lack of access to health care limits the use of preventive health-care services such as routine dental and physical examinations, prenatal care, postpartum care, and the prevention and treatment of chronic illnesses such as hypertension, diabetes, and cancer. Additional barriers to using health-care services include poor English-language skills, low acculturation, poor socioeconomic status, and lack of transportation and child care.

Cultural Responses to Health and Illness

When a family member is ill, other family members and friends become a source of support and care. Puerto Ricans may be loud and outspoken in expressing pain. Health-care providers should not censure this expression of pain or judge it as an exaggeration. This expressive behavior is a socially learned mechanism to cope with pain. *Ay!* is a common verbal moaning expression for pain (*dolor*). Because rural older individuals might have difficulty interpreting and quantifying pain, the use of numerical pain-identifying scales may be inappropriate. Most people prefer oral or intravenous medications for pain relief rather than intramuscular injections or rectal medications. In addition, herbal teas, heat, and prayer are used to manage pain.

Because mental illness carries a stigma, obtaining information or talking about mental illness with Puerto Rican families may be difficult. Some might not disclose the presence or history of mental illnesses, even in a trusting environment. In addition, Puerto Ricans may have a different cultural perception about the etiology, meaning, and treatment of mental illnesses. A mental illness may result from a terrible experience, a crisis, or the action of evil forces or spirits. Some perceive that symptoms of mental illness result from *nervios* (nerves), having done something wrong, or breaking God's commandments. When someone is anxious or overcome with emotions or problems, she or he is just *nervioso*. Similarly, someone who is experiencing despair, anorexia, bulimia, melancholy, anxiety, or lack of sleep may be *nervioso(a)*, or suffering from *ataque de nervios* rather than being clinically depressed, manic-depressive, or mentally ill. These conditions may be used to camouflage mental illness. Given the high incidence of depression (Munet-Vilaro, Folkman, & Gregorich, 1999; Oquendo, Ellis, Greenwald, Malone, Weissman, & Mann, 2001), this is a critical mental health issue for Puerto Ricans. Providers must acknowledge the confidentiality of information when obtaining a history. If trust is developed, health-care providers may get a more accurate response to their questions.

Health-care providers must become familiar with the vocabulary used to describe signs and symptoms of mental illnesses among this group. Families must be provided with clear and relevant information about the diagnosis, treatment, and etiology of mental illnesses to enhance adherence to treatment and follow-up care. In addition, health-care providers should be aware of traditional healing practices and be sensitive to mental health services for Puerto Rican families. Community-based settings such as churches, schools, and child care centers are excellent environments for promoting physical and mental health among Puerto Ricans.

Genetic or physical defects among Puerto Ricans may be seen as a result of heredity, suffering, or lack of care during pregnancy. Less-educated individuals may place guilt and blame on the mother or father. Caregivers must provide information about the causes of genetic defects and reduce stress and guilt for parents. For decades, some Puerto Rican families cared for impaired family members in a covert environment, away from the eyes of the community. At present, families are more open about these family members and care for the physically and mentally challenged at home, which is preferred over acute- or long-term-care facilities. The role of familism is of particular importance for Puerto Ricans because they provide caregiving in an interdependent network of extended family members who provide social support, solidarity, *cariño*, and resources for the family. Sociocultural differences exist in parental beliefs and attitudes when caring for children with disabilities. Puerto Rican parents develop a sense of interdependence and overprotection that is expressed through extreme nurturing behaviors and positive caring behaviors. As a result, conventional test scores for family functioning may not be

REFLECTIVE EXERCISE 23.3

Mrs. Martínez, a 37-year-old beauty salon worker from Puerto Rico, has been visiting her brother, who is a student at Central University. The following is the conversation that she has with a nurse at a clinic in her brother's town:

Nurse: Good afternoon. Why have you come to the clinic?

Mrs. Martínez: Shouldn't I be here?

Nurse: What is wrong with you that you came here?

Mrs. Martínez: I think that I am having a miscarriage.

Nurse: What is your name?

Mrs. Martínez: Lucero Martínez de Estrada y Rodríguez.

Nurse: That is a very long name.

Mrs. Martínez: Yes, I am from Puerto Rico, and we have longer names than you do on the mainland.

Nurse: What makes you think you are having a miscarriage?

Mrs. Martínez: I am 3 months pregnant, and I started bleeding this afternoon.

Nurse: How much bleeding are you having?

Mrs. Martínez: Oh, a lot.

Nurse: Well, do you have insurance?

Mrs. Martínez: Yes, I have insurance through my work.

Nurse: I do not know if we take insurance from Puerto Rico.

Mrs. Martínez: I can pay if I need to.

Nurse: Are you married?

Mrs. Martínez: Oh, yes, I am married.

Nurse: Where is your husband?

Mrs. Martínez: Back in Puerto Rico taking care of our daughter. I am here visiting my brother.

Nurse: Are you taking any medicine?

Mrs. Martínez: (Takes a bottle out of her purse.) Just these that I got from the pharmacist.

Nurse: I do not recognize these pills. They are in Spanish. You know you should not be taking any medicine unless it is prescribed by a doctor.

Mrs. Martínez: He is a pharmacist. And he prescribed these pills.

Nurse: Since this is not a big emergency, it might be a long wait to see the doctor.

Mrs. Martínez: I'll call my brother and tell him where I am.

1. Did the nurse approach Mrs. Martinez with *simpatia*?
2. In what ways did the nurse display *respeto*?
3. What evidence in this scenario can be construed as the nurse not displaying *respeto*?
4. What might the nurse have done to determine the English equivalent of the medicine prescribed by the pharmacist?
5. How common is it for pharmacists to prescribe medications in Puerto Rico?
6. How common is it for pharmacists to prescribe medications in the United States?
7. Does the mainland United States accept insurance from Puerto Rico?

appropriate to interpret child development and family adaptation. Health-care providers should be aware of these differences and act with caution when interpreting these results (Gannotti, Handwerker, Groce, & Cruz, 2001). Caregivers' stress should be a key component of the health assessment of these families. Health-care providers should supply information about community resources, support groups, and culturally appropriate mental health services.

Blood Transfusions and Organ Donation

For many Puerto Ricans, organ donation is seen as an act of good will and a gift of life. However, autopsy may be seen as a violation of the body. When discussions regarding autopsies and organ donations are necessary, the health-care provider must proceed with patience and provide precise and simple information. A clergy or minister may be helpful and may be expected to be present at the time of death. Although no proscriptions exist against blood donation and blood transfusion, many Puerto Ricans may be reluctant to engage in these procedures for fear of contracting HIV. Health-care providers need to carefully explore these beliefs and dispel myths.

Health-Care Providers

Traditional Versus Biomedical Health-Care Providers

Many Puerto Ricans use traditional and folk healers such as *espiritistas* and *Santeros* along with Western health-care providers. Some *espiritismo* practices are used to deal with the power of good and evil spirits in the physical and emotional development of the individual. *Santeros*, individuals prepared to practice *santería*, are consulted in matters related to the belief of object intrusion, diseases caused by evil spirits, the loss of the soul, the insertion of a spirit, or the anger of God.

Modesty is a highly valued quality. An intimate and unobtrusive environment is preferred for disclosing health-related concerns. Individuals expect a respectful environment; a soft tone of voice; and time to be heard, explain concerns, and ask questions when discussing health matters. Rooms without doors are considered disrespectful and conspicuous, particularly if the visit requires the removal of clothing. Some Puerto Ricans may have a gender or age bias against health-care providers. Men prefer male physicians for care and may feel embarrassed and uncomfortable with a female physician. A few individuals discount the academic and intellectual competencies of female physicians and may distrust their judgment and treatment. Some Puerto Rican women feel uncomfortable with a male physician, whereas a few prefer a male doctor. Elderly Puerto Ricans may prefer older health-care providers because they are seen as wise and mature in matters related to health, life experiences, and the use of folk practices and remedies. To build the patient's confidence, younger and female health-care providers must demonstrate an overall concern for the patient and develop respect and understanding by acknowledging and incorporating traditional healing practices into treatment regimens.

Status of Health-Care Providers

Puerto Ricans hold health-care providers in high regard because they are seen as wise authority figures. Distrust may develop if the health-care provider lacks respect for issues related to traditional health practices, ignores personalism in the relationship, does not use advanced technological assessment tools, and has a physical or personal image that differs from the traditional "well-groomed, white-attire" image. Overall, however, Puerto Ricans are well-educated health consumers and expect high-quality care blended with traditional practices and reliable technological approaches.

REFERENCES

Caraballo, R.S., Yee, S.L., Gfroerer, J., & Mirza, S.A. (2008). Adult tobacco use among racial and ethnic groups living in the United States, 2002–2005. *Preventing Chronic Disease 5*(3). Retrieved from http://www.cdc.gov/pcd/issues/2008/jul/07_0116.htm

Centers for Disease Control and Prevention. (2006). *HIV among Hispanics.* Retrieved from http://www.cdc.gov/hiv/latinos/index.htm

Centers for Disease Control and Prevention. (2008). *State-specific alcohol consumption rates.* Retrieved from http://www.cdc.gov/ncbddd/fasd/monitor_table2008.html

CIA World Factbook. (2011). *United States.* Retrieved from https://www.cia.gov/library/publications/the-world-factbook/geos/rq.html

CIA World Factbook. (2011). *Puerto Rico.* Retrieved from https://www.cia.gov/library/publications/the-world-factbook/geos/rq.html

Crouch-Ruiz, E. (1996). The birth of a premature infant in a Puerto Rican family. In S. Torres (Ed.), *Hispanic voices: Hispanic health educators speak out* (pp. 26–28). New York, NY: National League for Nursing.

Davis, R.E., & Flannery, D.D. (2001). Designing health information delivery systems for Puerto Rican women. *Health Education and Behavior, 28*(6), 680–695.

Epstein, J.A., Botvin, G.J., & Diaz, T. (1998). Ethnic and gender differences in smoking prevalence among a longitudinal sample of inner-city adolescents. *Journal of Adolescent Health, 23,* 160–166.

Gannotti, M.E., Handwerker, W.P., Groce, N.E., & Cruz, C. (2001). Sociocultural influences on disability status in Puerto Rican children. *Physical Therapy, 81*(9), 1512–1523.

Landale, N.S., & Oropesa, R.S. (2001). Migration, social support and perinatal health: An origin-destination analysis of Puerto Rican women. *Journal of Health and Social Behaviors, 42*(2), 166–183.

Marks, G., Garcia, M., & Solis, J. (1990). Health risk behaviors of Hispanics in the United States: Results from the HHANES 1982–1984. *American Journal of Public Health, 80*(Suppl.), 20–26.

Massara, E.B. (1989). *!Que gordita!: A study of overweight among Puerto Rican women.* New York: AMS Press.

Munet-Vilaro, F., Folkman, S., & Gregorich, S. (1999). Depressive symptomatology in three Latino groups. *Journal of Nursing Research, 21*(2), 209–224.

National Alliance for Hispanic Health. (2011). Retrieved from http://www.hispanichealth.org/

National Center for Education Statistics. (2007). *Elementary/secondary education.* Retrieved from http://nces.ed.gov/fastfacts/

National Center for Health Statistics. (2011). *Puerto Rico facts.* Retrieved from http://www.cdc.gov/nchs/fastats/popup_pr.htm

National Coalition of Hispanic Health and Human Services Organizations (COSSMHO). (1999). *The state of Hispanic girls.* Washington, DC: COSSMHO Press.

Oquendo, M.A., Ellis, S., Greenwald, S. Malone, K., Weissman, M.M., & Mann, J. (2001). Ethnic and sex differences in suicide rates relative to major depression in the United States. *American Journal of Psychiatry, 158*(10), 1652–1658.

Orshan, S.A. (1996). Acculturation, perceived social support, and self-esteem in primigravida Puerto Rican teenagers. *Western Journal of Nursing Research, 18,* 460–473.

Puerto Rico Department of Health. (2009). Retrieved from http://minorityhealth.hhs.gov/templates/content.aspx?ID=8064&lvl=2&lvlID=6

Puerto Rican Health News. (2007). *Health insurance coverage.* Retrieved from http://health.einnews.com/puertorico/

Skinner, D.G., Correa, V., Bailey, D., & Skinner, M. (2001). Role of religion in the lives of Latino families with young children with developmental delays. *American Journal of Mental Retardation, 106*(4), 297–213.

Stroup-Benham, C.A., & Treviño, F.M. (1991). Reproductive characteristics of Mexican-American, Puerto Rican and Cuban-American women. *Journal of the American Medical Association, 265,* 222–226.

Taylor, M. (1999). Alternatives to conventional hormonal replacement therapy. *Contemporary OB/GYN, 12*(3), 23–54.

Torres, S., & Villaruel, A. (1996). Health risk behaviors for Hispanic women. *Annual Review of Nursing Research, 5,* 293–319.

U.S. Census Bureau. (2009). *Educational attainment by race and Hispanic origin.* Retrieved from http://www.census.gov/compendia/statab/2011/tables/11s0225.pdf

DavisPlus For reflective exercises, review questions, and additional information, go to

http://davisplus.fadavis.com

Chapter 24

People of Russian Heritage

Karen J. Aroian, Galina Khatutsky, and Alexandra Dashevskaya

Overview, Inhabited Localities, and Topography

Overview

Russia, also known as the *Russian Federation*, was the largest part of the former Soviet Union before the Soviet Union collapsed in 1991. Presently, Russia is the largest country in the world, nearly twice the size of the United States. It covers 11 time zones. The climate ranges from temperate and humid to arctic. Ethnically, 80 percent of those living in Russia are Russian, 3.8 percent are Tartars, 2 percent are Ukrainian, and 14.4 percent are other smaller groups. Between 15 and 20 percent of Russians are Russian Orthodox, 10 to 15 percent are Muslim, and 2 percent belong to other Christian groups. Only about 500,000 Russians are Jews. In 2005, Russian Orthodoxy became the official religion and enjoys a privileged position with the current government (Library of Congress, 2010). However, a large number of Russians are either nonreligious or nonpracticing, which is the result of over 7 decades of religious suppression under communist rule. The population of Russia is about 139 million and is declining, with 1.6 deaths for each birth (*CIA World Factbook,* 2010). This high death rate is related to high-risk behaviors such as smoking, alcoholism, heart disease, traffic accidents, and low education about sexually transmitted infections. The average life expectancy is 59 and 73 years for Russian men and women, respectively. A low fertility rate (1.4 per women of reproductive age) adds to this population decline (*CIA World Factbook,* 2010; Library of Congress, 2010; Marquez, 2005). The two largest cities—Moscow, which is Russia's capital, and St. Petersburg—have 10 million and 4.5 million people, respectively. Although major cities are heavily populated, 27 percent of Russians live in very rural areas (*CIA World Factbook,* 2010; Library of Congress, 2010).

In 1917, the imperial Czar was overthrown and Vladimir Lenin took power, replacing imperial rule with communism. The overthrow, referred to as the Bolshevik revolution, was due to the discontent that ensued after the horrific defeat of the Russian armies during World War I. Josef Stalin took power after Lenin, further strengthening and unifying communist rule and infusing it with brutality. During this time, the Soviet Union was comprised of 15 ethnically and culturally diverse republics, the largest of which was the Republic of Russia.

On August 24, 1991, the Soviet Union collapsed and Russia became an independent country. Each of the other republics of the former Soviet Union also developed into independent nations. This collapse led to Russia adopting a new constitution in 1993 and three branches of government: the executive, the legislative, and the judiciary. The 1990s were a period of intense democratic reform and the development of a market economy. However, many important democratic reforms made in the 1990s have been overturned. Political bribery and corruption are rampant today.

Russia's poverty rate is 13.1 percent, with a 6.7 percent inflation rate (*CIA World Factbook,* 2010). The number of adults who are unemployed (7.6 percent) or underemployed is high (*CIA World Factbook,* 2010). Crime rates are also high. Police have low pay, low status, and are highly corrupt.

Economically, Russia has some of the most abundant natural resources, including rich deposits of oil, natural gas, coal, timber, and minerals such as diamonds, nickel, aluminum, and platinum. Over 20 percent of the world's forests are in Russia (Library of Congress, 2010). However, water, land, and air pollution is high (Energy Information Administration [EIA], 2010; Library of Congress, 2010).

Heritage and Residence

According to the Russian 2002 census, the largest ethnic group was Russian, accounting for 80 percent of the total population. Ethnic minority groups with significant numbers (about 1 million in each group) include Tartar, Ukrainian, Bashkir, Chuvash, Chechen, and Armenian. These minority groups are the result of their homelands being former republics of the Soviet Union. During the period of Soviet rule (1917 to 1991), Soviet citizens moved, leaving their own culture and birthplace to work and live in another republic. Since the fall of the Soviet empire, non-Russians in Russia have been migrating back to their homelands, in part because of growing intolerance in Russia against its ethnic minorities (Library of Congress, 2010).

International migration includes the United States, Israel, Canada, and Australia as major destinations (Vishnevsky & Zayonchkovskaya, 1994). In fact, in the 1990s, immigrants from the former Soviet Union were one of the fastest-growing ethnic groups in the United States, with a 254 percent increase in the Russian-speaking population (U.S. Department of Homeland Security, 2005a). Another source of population growth came from adopting Russian children (U.S. Department of Homeland Security, 2005b). According to the U.S. Census Bureau, (2000), over 2.6 million Russians live in the United States. However, in the last decade, the immigration from Russia to the United States is slowing. From 2001 to 2009, about 14,277 Russian immigrants came to the United States (U.S. Department of Homeland Security, 2010).

Almost 90 percent of Russian immigrants in the United States live in urban areas such as New York City and the Tri-State area (24 percent), Boston, Philadelphia, Baltimore, Miami, Atlanta, Cleveland, Chicago, Detroit, Denver, Houston, Los Angeles, San Diego, San Francisco, Seattle, and Portland, Oregon (Allied Media Corp., n.d.). Florida has also become an increasingly popular destination for Russian immigrants who are close to retirement age (U.S. Department of Homeland Security, 2005c). In Canada, Russian-speaking immigrants primarily live in Toronto, Vancouver, and Montreal (Aroian, 2003).

Classifying Russian immigration is complicated by several facts. First, until the Soviet Union collapsed, people from Russia and other former republics of the Soviet Union were often referred to and classified as one group regardless of where they were from. Second, the definitions vary widely; some are based on the country of origin, some on primary language, and some on the ethnic or religious affiliation. Third, the immigrants from the former Soviet Union are presently classified as from independent republics, such as Armenia, Russia, and Azerbaijan. Thus, when the term *Russian immigrant* is used in the literature, it may refer broadly to Russian-speaking immigrants of multiple nationalities from the former Soviet Union (one group under Soviet rule with Russian as the official language uniting them) or to people specifically from Russia.

Given the complicated history of Russian immigration to the United States, this chapter should be read with an important qualifier in mind. Most of what is written pertains to immigrants who emigrated in the latter part of the 20th century. These immigrants were reared under communism. Later arrivals, those who came after the Soviet Union collapsed, left a very different homeland. These immigrants were more apt to be familiar with the English language and a market economy. In addition, as is the case for most immigrant groups, immigrants become more acculturated over time. This is particularly true for immigrants who are younger and go to school and/or work in the new country. Although most of this chapter pertains to a given wave of migration, generational and cohort differences as well as acculturation trends will be noted when applicable.

Reasons for Migration and Associated Economic Factors

Migration to the United States from Russia or the former Soviet Union occurred in four waves (Hobbs, 2002). The first wave of Christian Orthodox Russians fleeing religious and political persecution was between 1900 and 1914 (Hobbs, 2002). The second wave began in 1914 and primarily included middle- or upper-class Russians fleeing the Bolshevik revolution and the onset of communism. After the Bolshevik revolution of 1917, thousands of expropriated wealthy Russians and middle-class professionals and army officers fled their homeland. About 20,000 Russian refugees, enslaved workers, or war prisoners from Germany entered the United States from 1947 to 1952 (Hobbs, 2002). As the first and second waves of Russian immigration to the United States, Jews from Ukraine and other bordering countries were also migrating to escape the pogroms (Abramson, 1991). The third wave began in the 1970s, when the United States granted refugee status to religious and ethnic minorities because of their persecution by the Soviet government (Aroian, 2003). This wave was comprised primarily of Soviet Jews, but it also included Soviet Armenians, Pentecostals, and Evangelicals (Aroian, 2003). The fourth wave of immigration started in 1991 with the dissolution of the Soviet Union, which resulted in much more freedom to immigrate. One motivation for this fourth wave of immigration included harsh economic conditions. When communism transitioned to a free-market system, economic conditions were particularly difficult for researchers, scientists, and physicians. Salaries were fixed and well below poverty levels, causing a desperate migration in hopes of improved quality of life. Motivation for the fourth wave also included family reunification, political turmoil, and greater overtly expressed Russian nationalism and anti-Semitism (Bistrevsky, 2005). Presently, emigration from Russia has slowed considerably. Only about 3 percent of the Russian population emigrated in 2010 (*CIA World Factbook,* 2010).

Educational Status and Occupations

The average age for U.S. Russian immigrants is 42 years, and nearly one-fourth of the total U.S. Russian immigrant population is 65 years of age or older. Almost two-thirds (64 percent) of these immigrants are married, with 1.6 children per couple. Of adults over age 25, 1 million have at least a bachelor's degree, and over 18 percent have graduate degrees. The average adult Russian in the United States works in a professional area, is well educated, and has a better-than-average income (Media Corp, n.d.). However, it is important to note that more recently arrived Russian-speaking immigrants tend to be less well educated and more likely to pursue technical and service occupations (Minnesota Department of Employment and Economic Development [MDEED], 2006).

Of note is that Russia has a 99.4 percent literacy rate, which is one of the highest literacy rates in the world. Men and women are equally literate. Russian-speaking immigrants highly value education. In the former Soviet system, education was strongly promoted for both genders, and prestige was tied to occupational status, which in turn was determined by education (Aroian, 2003). Given these values, it is not uncommon in the United States for extended Russian immigrant families to work additional hours and pool their financial resources to provide a good education for their children.

However, the value on education is in transition. By the mid-1990s, making money by being an entrepreneur became another venue for self-respect and prestige in Russia (Library of Congress, 2010). The current focus on commercialization will likely influence the cultural values of immigrants from future waves of immigration.

Teaching/learning systems in Russia are rigid compared with U.S. standards. Until recently, learning English was not a priority. As a result, Russian immigrants, especially older people and those who came to the United States before English became part of the standard curriculum, are likely to have difficulty with the English language. Recently, English has grown more popular in Russia owing to the Internet and other forms of media, including Western films, music, and advertising. Thus, younger, more recent immigrants are likely to have some English ability.

Some Russian immigrants in the United States receive public assistance such as Medicaid, Supplemental Security Income, subsidized housing, or food stamps. This assistance offsets low income because of disability, age, and inability to find work commensurate with pre-migration work experience. Most Russians immigrants receiving public assistance, including older immigrants, have a college education (Hobbs, 2002).

Many Russian immigrants, particularly those who came in the latter third of the 20th century, were highly trained professionals, employed in fields such as engineering, math, medicine, biotechnology, computer science, and education. Unfortunately, full-time and well-paying positions in these fields were unavailable to many of these professionals due to language, licensing, and credentialing barriers in the United States. Language barriers and unfamiliar legal regulations were also salient for Russian-speaking immigrants who attempted to start their own small businesses (Hobbs, 2002). Thus, occupational status demotion was a common component of the initial immigrant experience for Russian immigrants (Aroian & Norris, 2003). Most Russian immigrants were able to overcome this initial occupational status demotion, but this was not the case for Russians who emigrated at an older age.

Communication

Dominant Language and Dialects

Russian is a living language that is rich and expressive. It is one of the world's major languages, the most pervasive of all Slavic languages, and the primary language for over 150 million people. It is also one of the six official languages of the United Nations. As the official language of the former Soviet Union, it unified the 15 Soviet republics and Soviet-controlled satellite nations. Although each republic and Soviet-controlled satellite nation had its own language and culture, schoolchildren under Soviet rule were required to take many years of Russian-language courses.

According to the U.S. Census Bureau (2007), 850,000 persons over age 5 spoke Russian at home. Of these, only 43 percent could speak English very well, 29 percent could speak English well, 21 percent could not speak English well, and 6 percent could not speak English at all. Even with limited English proficiency, many Russian-speaking immigrants can read and write English better than speak it.

Most Russian immigrants, with the exception of older ones, eventually become proficient in English. However, large urban centers with a concentrated number of Russian speakers have their own newspapers and television and radio programming. These are self-maintained communities with numerous Russian-language services, including health care. Immigrants in these communities usually get by despite having very limited English proficiency, speaking both Russian and their own native languages (e.g., Ukrainian, Georgian). This is especially true for older Russians immigrants who intentionally live in Russian-language communities even when their adult children move to outlying areas. Living in a Russian-speaking enclave allows older Russian immigrants to purchase food and supplies from Russian retailers and socialize with their Russian-speaking peers. Such communities provide little incentive to learn English.

Written Russian uses the Cyrillic alphabet, which is derived from but not the same as the Greek alphabet. Russian is considered phonetic and includes five vowels and numerous consonants that are considered hard or soft. Interestingly, Russian does not include articles (e.g., "the") and is often called a *house green* language ("the" and "is" are omitted).

Cultural Communication Patterns

Russians enjoy intellectual conversations that focus on political, economic, cultural, and social issues. Word of mouth and advice among Russian speakers are strong influencing factors for making decisions regarding health care and major purchases (Aroian, Khatutsky, Tran, & Balsam, 2001). Russians seek emotional support from spouses, relatives, and friends, and report not trusting religious advisors, teachers, social service workers, or community leaders. However, they report a willingness to talk with physicians and other health-care providers, especially when these workers are able to speak Russian (Hobbs, 2002).

Russians tend to speak loudly (MDEED, 2006). They have great insight into their own and others' feelings and often communicate on an emotional level. Russians make eye contact, nod their head in a gesture of affirmation or approval, and are respectful in their verbal and nonverbal behaviors toward older people and persons of perceived rank or authority ("Culture Tips," 2000; MDEED, 2006).

Russian men shake hands firmly, and this symbol of agreement is considered more binding than paper documents. The doorway of a Russian home is considered the spirit center of the house, and it is a bad omen to shake hands over the threshold. Shoes are often removed prior to entering the home (MDEED, 2006).

Behavior in public is formal and respectful. Russians do not appreciate casual gestures such as standing with hands inserted into pockets, arms crossed over the chest or behind the head, slouching posture, and putting feet up on a desk. These behaviors are particularly insulting if they occur when they are being interviewed for a job. Shaking a fist shows anger or disagreement, and pointing with the index finger is considered rude (Hobbs, 2002; MDEED, 2006).

Russians often require less personal space than European Americans. Russians freely touch friends and family members. Greeting close friends by kissing each cheek is common. Russians are social diplomats and will "bend" the truth for the sake of politeness or to soften bad news (Birch, 2006).

Russians have a sense of duty, self-sacrifice, and genuine caring toward others ("Culture Tips," 2000). They perceive themselves as spontaneous and emotional, able to be extremely empathetic toward the suffering of others. They are emotionally strong and have a long and distinguished history of enduring great hardship and adversity. Thus, Russians may present a pervasive attitude of endurance with comments such as "We have overcome many troubles and we can overcome these troubles because we are strong; we are Russians." They look to others for the same level of respect and recognition of social order as they give.

Temporal Relationships

Russians who have immigrated to the United States tend to be both present and future oriented. This is not the case, however, among nonimmigrants. Russians living in Russia live in the present, as demonstrated by a comment the chapter authors and book editor heard frequently: "Because we have no future." Russian immigrants are punctual and value this attribute. For appointments, Russians will arrive either early or right on time. However, being punctual is less important for social occasions. Social occasions typically last late into the night, so late arrivals are not disruptive.

Format for Names

Russians use titles such as Mr., Mrs., Dr., professor, aunt, and grandfather to show the appropriate respect ("Culture Tips," 2000; Hobbs, 2002). Even when friendships are established, they often ask to be addressed by their first name plus their patronymic. The patronymic is the first name of their father with either a feminine or a masculine ending, depending on the person's gender. An example of a preferred name format might be Oleg Vasilievich (Oleg, son of Vasily).

Family Roles and Organization

Head of Household and Gender Roles

In Russia, younger adults and youth depend on the wisdom of their parents and grandparents whenever important decisions need to be made. In the United States, these roles are often reversed because of an English-language barrier whereby older Russian-speaking immigrants often have to depend on their children and grandchildren to guide decision making (Aroian, Khatutsky, & Dashevskaya, 2006). Role reversal may be particularly difficult for older Russians if they are not living in the United States by choice.

Unlike many other immigrant groups, Russian immigrants arrived in the United States in multigenerational family units. This emigration pattern occurred, in part, because the Soviet regime did not allow families to emigrate unless they took older family members with them (Aroian et al., 2006).

Although women are an important part of the workforce in Russia, the roles of mother and homemaker are also valued. Russian women pursue education and careers, but they often juggle multiple roles, fulfilling cultural expectations for home and child-care responsibilities (Aroian, 2003; Aroian, Norris, & Chiang, 2003; Remennick, 1999).

It is important to note that Russians will be reluctant to sign consent forms and other documents without first consulting their family members (Keefe, 2006). Family members will often attend health-care appointments in order to provide cognitive as well as affective support (Aroian, 2003).

Prescriptive, Restrictive, and Taboo Behaviors for Children and Adolescents

Russian children are taught to obey their parents and older people, as well as to achieve high grades in school and complete a university education. Children are expected to care for family members who are ill and in need of care ("Culture Tips," 2000). Older people are expected to raise their grandchildren, especially if both parents are employed.

Sexual topics such as contraception and sex education are not considered appropriate topics for public discussion. Sexual activity outside of marriage is not sanctioned even though the age of sexual consent in Russia is 16. If teen girls get pregnant, abortion is the primary intervention (Aroian, 2003). Older Russian immigrants tend to be more modest, disliking public displays of affection (Aroian, 2003).

Family Goals and Priorities

Collectivism has been part of Russian society for centuries. Russians view family, group, and communal needs as more important than individual needs. Extended family and friends are highly important. Relationships are very close. Russians depend on and trust family, neighbors, friends, and colleagues. Love and support from family and friends are expected and forthcoming during crises. Spouses consult each other ("Culture Tips," 2000). Russians contrast their personal relationships with Americans' tendency to reserve close, intimate ties for immediate family members and are struck by Americans' individualism and independence.

Russian young people are expected to do household chores. Household chores are gender-specific, with girls doing tasks such as cooking and cleaning and boys doing more physical labor. Grocery shopping is an exception; it is a task for both boys and girls. Although education and a good job are considered important for Russian women, finding a good husband is even more important. Being an "old maid" is socially frowned upon (Aroian, 2003).

Domestic violence is a rising concern in Russia. Because of long-standing distrust of authority figures, Russian immigrants may not report domestic violence. Russian women will only rarely admit to and report being raped. This cultural tendency may also be operative after immigration. Domestic violence is often tied to alcohol abuse.

Alternative Lifestyles

Divorce rates in Russia are high, and small families are typical because of economic hardships. Russian immigrants also have high divorce rates, perhaps because of the stress of immigration. For example, Russian immigrant women grow more independent as they acculturate, and differential rates of acculturation can cause family problems (Aroian, Spitzer, & Bell, 1996). On the other hand, Russian women may wait to reach their new country before ending an unhappy marriage.

Religion seldom plays a role in the lives of most Russian immigrants, most likely because of the antireligion dogma of communism. (Exceptions include Russian Pentecostals and other religious fundamentalist groups in Russia.) Therefore, divorce does not negatively affect social status. Divorced men in Russia are rarely awarded child custody, and although they pay child support, they do not often remain active in their children's lives (Aroian, 2003). This tendency may also be noted with Russian immigrants.

Russian women with fertility problems are not considered desirable spouses (Aroian, 2003). Although Russian women are expected to marry by age 25 and have children, they are also expected to continue to pursue education and career paths. This is possible because grandmothers become primary caregivers for young children. Men are seldom expected to fulfill child-care responsibilities.

The Russian penal code was revised in 1997, and homosexuality is no longer a crime. In July 1997, the first gay and lesbian pride festival occurred in Moscow. Even so, alternative lifestyle choices are still stigmatized by a large part of the population. Overtly expressed antigay graffiti is still commonly seen in Russia ("News About Gay Russia," n.d.). Given the lack of acceptance about same-sex relationships, gay and lesbian Russians in the United States are likely to remain closeted, even with health-care providers, unless significant trust is developed. Similarly, same-sex behavior is not typically disclosed to family members or friends.

Workforce Issues
Culture in the Workplace

When communicating in the workplace, Russians embrace the value of positive social communication. Politeness is a key component of positive social communication, as well as saying nice things to connote acceptance, offer support and empathy, and just to avoid negative discourse. When negotiating compromise in the workplace, Russians invest time and effort to provide information that supports their decisions and requests. Russians expect to be specifically asked for this kind of information (Bergelson, 2003). This communication style is in contrast with the more direct communication Russians employ with friends. Direct communication with friends is considered to be a sign of sincerity.

Russian-speaking health professionals in the United States serve a large group of older Russian immigrants who do not speak English or do not speak it well. If the health-care professionals were trained in the former Soviet Union, they are used to an authoritarian work environment. The training for nurses in the former Soviet Union has been likened to that of American licensed practical nurses (LPNs) (Alaniz, 2001). These nurses are not used to critical thinking and are used to hierarchical relationships with physicians, which conflicts with expectations in the United States for nurses to be part of a health-care team (Alaniz, 2001). A positive characteristic of health professionals trained in the former Soviet Union is that they reflect the Russian emphasis on holism and holistic health care.

Issues Related to Autonomy

In the United States, nurses and physicians work as a team. Yet each member maintains independence. In Russia, the physician makes the decisions and does the problem solving. Thus, the nursing profession gets limited status and respect from Russians (Alaniz, 2001). One Russian immigrant explained, "What do we expect from a nurse? We don't expect anything; we only expect something from a doctor. A nurse is just someone who obeys" (Smith, 1996). Russian immigrants in other professions may also be used to hierarchical work relationships based on authority.

Biocultural Ecology

Skin Color and Other Biological Variations

Ethnic Russians are Caucasian. Stature and skin color for ethnic Russians are similar to other North American groups, with the exception of high rates of obesity among Russians and Russian immigrants.

Diseases and Health Conditions

Common health disorders seen in Russian immigrants include hypertension, coronary disease, gastrointestinal disorders, and diabetes. Common disabilities include the results of diabetes (e.g., sensory impairment) and other chronic health disorders, such as hypertension, psychosocial disorders, arthritis, lung disease, and cancer (Keefe, 2006; MDEED, 2006; Shpilko, 2006). There is also some evidence of a higher than average rate of colorectal polyps (Vadlamani et al., 2001).

A number of studies suggest that health status is poorer among Russian immigrants than it is for other immigrant and nonimmigrant groups. For example, Russian Jews who immigrated to Israel between 1989 and 1992 reported an average of 3.5 chronic diseases—a much higher rate than that reported among immigrants from other countries (Rennert, Luz, Tamir, & Peterburg, 2002). These findings are similar to findings from a comparative study of low-income Russian immigrant and nonimmigrant older persons in the United States (Aroian & Vander Wal, 2007). In this study, Russian immigrants had more

health problems than their nonimmigrant counterparts even though the nonimmigrant group was significantly older than the Russian immigrant group.

Older Russian immigrants are also prone to depression, particularly when they live alone and do not speak English well (Aroian et al., 2001; Shpilko, 2006; Tran, Khatutsky, Aroian, Balsam, & Conway, 2000). In Russia, older people often live with their adult children and have family responsibilities, such as caring for grandchildren. In the United States, because of language barriers, older people are more apt to live in elder housing with other Russian-speaking older immigrants rather than with their children and grandchildren.

Other groups of Russian immigrants at risk for psychological distress include those with less education and greater immigration demands, such as difficulty with English (Aroian, Norris, Patsdaughter, & Tran, 1998; Miller & Chandler, 2002; Miller, Sorokin, Wang, Feetham, Choi, & Wilbur 2006). Russian immigrants who feel alienated in the United States or do not possess resilient personalities also experience more psychological distress (Miller et al., 2006). In a longitudinal study of depression trajectories over time, Russian immigrants who remained depressed past the initial resettlement period were less likely to have family in the area or to have the highest immigration demands at both time points (Aroian & Norris, 2003).

There is also some indication that Russian immigrant children are at risk. Goodman, Slobodskaya, and Knyazev (2005) found that emotional and behavioral disorders were nearly 70 percent higher in Russian immigrant children compared to other children in Great Britain. The most predictive factors in this study were the child's school performance, the mother's mental health, having a close relative with alcohol addiction, and witnessing domestic violence.

A number of anecdotal reports and empirical studies suggest that Russians somaticize psychological disorders (Belozersky, 1990; Brod & Heurtin Roberts, 1992; Levav, Kohn, Flaherty, Lerner, & Aisenberg, 1990). For example, Russians may present with vague complaints of skeletal or gastrointestinal problems when they are suffering from depression. This tendency to somaticize has been attributed to the stigma of mental illness in Russia, Soviet ideology that recast psychiatric disorders as neurological, and prior psychiatric abuses by the Soviet regime. However, it is important to note that Aroian and Norris (1999) found that somatization was more common among Russian immigrants who were not highly educated and those who were older.

Variations in Drug Metabolism

According to Gaikovitch (2003), who investigated variability in genetic polymorphism and drug metabolism, the allele distribution of important metabolizing enzymes in Russians is not significantly different from that of other Caucasians. In other words, there are no genetic differences to suggest that medications are rendered more water-soluble and more readily excreted in urine in Russians. Thus, drug side effects and efficacy in Russians are likely similar to other European populations.

The metabolism of alcohol may be the exception. According to Gabriel (2005), Russians may have inherited a genetic characteristic from Mongolian invaders that prevents processing ethanol derived from fruit or potatoes. Gabriel believes that this genetic trait makes Russians more susceptible to alcoholism, especially when the alcoholic beverage is cognac or vodka.

High-Risk Behaviors

Nutritional issues are a major contributing factor toward the number of chronic diseases experienced by Russians. According to some studies, over half of Russian adults have high blood cholesterol, obesity, or hypertension (Marquez, 2005; Mehler, Scott, Pines, Gifford, Bigerstaff, & Hiatt; 2001). Nearly half of the sample in one study (Mehler et al., 2001) had two or more cardiovascular risk factors. All of these chronic illnesses are related to Russians' nutritional habits, specifically high-salt, carbohydrate, and fat intake (Keefe, 2006).

Hard liquor, mostly vodka and cognac, are served routinely at family gatherings and celebrations, and heavy alcohol consumption is a part of daily life in Russia. Russian statisticians estimate that over 30 percent of deaths in Russia are directly related to alcohol (Nemtsov, 2005; Nicholson, Bobak, Murphy, Rose, & Marmot, 2005). Russian authorities appear indifferent to these statistics, as they have no official plan to address the problem of alcoholism.

Alcoholism is far less prevalent among Russian religious groups and women (Aroian, 2003). This fact most likely accounts for lower rates of alcoholism among Russian immigrants relative to the population in Russia. A disproportionate number of those who emigrated from Russia are Jews or Christian fundamentalists, and these groups are known to have lower rates of alcoholism.

Smoking is prevalent in Russia. Russia is one of the few countries that currently do little or nothing to curb tobacco use. Nearly 63 percent of Russian men and 15 percent of Russian women smoke, and this number increases by about 2 percent per year. Although 60 percent of current smokers want to quit, no state-supported programs exist to help them do so (Parfitt, 2006). This may explain, in part, why the male life expectancy in Russia is just above 59.8 years (*CIA World Factbook,* 2011). Like alcoholism, smoking is less prevalent in Russia's ethnic minorities. Russian immigrants, who are comprised of a disproportionate number of Russian ethnic minorities, do not demonstrate the same level of smoking behaviors as their native-born counterparts. However, more recent Russian immigrants are likely to engage in these behaviors at higher rates than earlier Russian immigrants because current migration from Russia includes fewer ethnic and religious minorities (Hasin et al., 2002).

Based on high rates of injection drug use in Russia, there is some evidence that Russian immigrants are at risk. A preliminary study conducted in New York City on this topic found that Russian immigrants have unique drug abuse patterns and behaviors, including rapid transition to injection drug use (Isralowitz, Straussner, & Rosenblum, 2006). This study also found that Russian immigrants are suspicious of traditional drug treatment approaches.

Russians are reluctant to immunize, and this reluctance may also be considered a high-risk behavior. In Russia, immunizations are available but are of poor quality. Reports of hepatitis- and HIV-positive–contaminated immunization needles have created fear and distrust. Thus, Russian immigrant parents may not immunize their children unless they receive sufficient assurances that immunizations are safe.

Another high-risk behavior is the medication behavior of many Russian immigrants. These behaviors include sharing leftover prescriptions with family and friends, not informing health-care providers that they are using herbal remedies, and polypharmacy from augmenting prescriptions with Russian pharmaceuticals (Aroian, 2003). Russian grocery stores in Russian immigrant communities or people traveling to and from Russia are both ample sources of Russian pharmaceuticals and herbs. Adverse health consequences from polypharmacy are a well-known problem, and some common herbal remedies interact dangerously with prescribed medications.

According to one study, high-risk sexual behavior is increasing among Russia immigrant adolescent girls, with greater risk among girls who are more acculturated to American culture (Jeltova, Fish, & Revenson, 2005). The association between risky behavior in adolescents and acculturation is not unique to Russian immigrants or girls. Mostly likely the association between acculturation and greater risky behavior results from the erosion of traditional family practices as youths acculturate to the United States.

Nutrition
Meaning of Food

Many Russians grew up with serious food shortages. Thus, food carries a lot of meaning. When entertaining, Russians can use food as a demonstration of their love and respect for their visitors, spending days purchasing and preparing food for their guests. Presently, this practice appears to be limited by time constraints and increased acculturation to the United States.

Common Foods and Food Rituals

Older Russian immigrants have little interest in American food. As previously stated, traditional Russian diets contain high levels of saturated and hydrogenated vegetable fats, salt, and carbohydrates (Keefe, 2006). Typically, Russian immigrants eat three meals a day, with their largest meal in the middle of the day. Russians enjoy snacks and tea, water, and fruit juices without ice. Russian grocery stores and restaurants were quite popular in Russian immigrant communities, but these venues are losing business as Russian immigrants, particularly younger ones, are acculturating to American diets.

Dietary Practices for Health Promotion

When Russians are ill, they prefer soup and broths, bland foods, chicken, potatoes, fruit and vegetables, and yogurt. Tea with honey and milk is considered medicinal (Hobbs, 2002).

Nutritional Deficiencies and Food Limitations

Russian Jews, if observing kosher dietary restrictions, do not eat pork or shellfish or combine milk and meat products (Hobbs, 2002).

REFLECTIVE EXERCISE 24.1

Inna Scheider is an 87-year-old woman residing in a long-term-care facility. She has multiple chronic diseases, including advanced congestive heart failure (CHF) and is very frail. Inna had balance problems and had multiple falls in the past year, which resulted in numerous hospitalizations. In addition, she has moderate dementia. Currently, Inna exhibits some behavioral problems and does not follow directions. Inna does not speak English and can communicate with her health-care providers only through an interpreter or when her sons are present. One of the certified nursing assistants (CNAs) in the facility is Russian-speaking and often stops by to help calm her down when her family is not present. Inna has two sons who live in the area and visit often. Both are very devoted to their mother and are very involved in her care.

In the past, when Inna lived at home with her children, she was a great cook and spent a significant amount of time preparing family meals. Making multicourse meals was a very important daily family ritual. In the United States, Inna developed a great fondness for local Russian grocery stores that sell foods that were not available during severe food shortages in the Soviet Union.

After several months in the long-term-care facility, Inna developed weakness and dizziness. Her physician suspects that she had internal gastrointestinal bleeding. Her physician was also concerned about risk of aspiration. As a result, Inna was put on a soft food diet and receives some of her food with added thickeners. However, the facility staff noticed that her sons repeatedly brought Inna ready-prepared Russian food from a local Russian grocery store. One son was observed trying to feed her pieces of hard salami, herring with black bread, and a diced beet salad. Inna was choking from her difficulty swallowing some of the items. When confronted by the staff, the son responded that this was the food that Inna loved and it would make her feel better.

1. What cultural trait in food attitudes is exhibited by Inna's sons?
2. What educational efforts are needed by the health-care team to educate the family about Inna's condition and the need for a special diet?
3. How can Inna's care plan be integrated to balance her health-care needs with the need to validate her tastes and preferences?

Pregnancy and Childbearing Practices

Fertility Practices and Views Toward Pregnancy

Marriage and childbearing are acceptable starting at age 20. Childbearing and child rearing are highly valued. Infertility is perceived by Russians as a health problem, disappointment, and even punishment for some feminine wrongdoing (Aroian, 2003).

Russian women are responsible for contraception and often make contraception decisions without consulting their male partners. These decisions often relate to access, cost, safety, and partner issues. Contraception for Russian women is allowed without sanctions or taboos. Even so, many Russian immigrants are afraid of birth control pills and refuse to take them. Possible reasons for this reluctance are the poor quality and high dosage of oral contraceptives in Russia. To compound this problem, condoms in Russia were poorly made, and many jokes have evolved about the routine breakage of Russian-made condoms. Furthermore, Russian men believe that condoms hinder sexual pleasure and many refuse to wear them. Most Russian men also refuse vasectomies (Aroian, 2003).

Abortion was and is one of the most common forms of birth control in Russia. Russia has one of the world's highest abortion rate, with the average woman having three or more abortions in her lifetime. In 1990, there were 1972 abortions per 1000 live births. In 2002, this number dropped to 1276 abortions per 1000 live births (World Health Organization [WHO], 2005). Self-induced abortions are not uncommon. Frequent abortions contribute to the high rate of infertility in Russian women. Infertility issues may lead to marital discord and divorce.

Beliefs about menstruation are based on biomedical principles. Nonetheless, young Russian women are discouraged from strenuous exercise, including swimming, while menstruating (Aroian, 2003). This practice may have evolved from the former unavailability of tampons in Russia.

Prescriptive, Restrictive, and Taboo Practices in the Childbearing Family

Pregnant Russian women do not engage in heavy lifting and often commit to bed rest if it is prescribed. Russian women who are pregnant receive more respect. When born, boys are dressed in blue and girls in pink. Breastfeeding is encouraged, and nursing women are told to drink tea with milk and eat nuts to improve their milk supply (Aroian, 2003).

Owing to religious beliefs, Russian Jews circumcise their male infants. Ethnic Russians do not circumcise their newborn boys.

Death Rituals

Death Rituals and Expectations

Flowers are used to beautify caskets and funeral services. Caskets are typically closed, and stones are put on graves instead of flowers. Food and beverages are usually served during wakes and funerals. Friends and family come to pay their respects for 7 days postmortem, but the expected total period of official mourning is 1 full year. A full year is considered the minimal appropriate time for a surviving spouse to wait before remarrying. Close relatives of the deceased dress in black. Russians do not hesitate to cry and sob at funerals, but overt wailing is often confined to the home of the deceased (Aroian, 2003).

A family will hold vigil day and night if their loved one is dying. All relatives and friends are expected to visit a dying patient and often sit with the person for hours. Depending on religious affiliation, the placing of hands on the ill person's forehead may occur as a ritual gesture of blessing. Religious symbols may also be placed at the ill person's bedside, and a spiritual advisor may be present when death is impending. Russian Orthodox families pay vigil to terminally ill and deceased persons, praying for mercy on their souls and their entry into heaven (Yehieli, Lutz, & Grey 2005). Spiritual leaders from the Russian Orthodox religion institute a special prayer vigil, called *panikhida*, over the deceased, a vigil that includes chants, prayers, singing of hymns, and gospel readings (Yehieli et al., 2005). Regardless of religious affiliation, once a person dies, his or her mouth and eyes are closed, and mirrors are covered with black fabric (University of Washington Medical Center, 2005).

If the patient and family are Russian Orthodox, cremation is unlikely (University of Washington Medical Center, 2005). Cremation is forbidden in the Jewish tradition. However, some Russian immigrants may choose cremation so the deceased's ashes can be shipped back to "Mother" Russia (Yehieli et al., 2005). Russian Jews bury the dead within 24 hours except during holidays, on Saturdays, or if awaiting the arrival of additional friends and family (University of Washington Medical Center, 2005).

Responses to Death and Grief

Russians are reluctant to disclose terminal illness or poor prognosis to patients and believe that talking about death is a bad omen (Aroian et al., 2006; Birch, 2006; MDEED, 2006; Norman, 1996). Family members feel responsible for protecting their loved one from the psychological turmoil that could result from disclosing a poor prognosis. They tend to feign cheeriness in the presence of a dying person rather than openly grieve in front of a sick or dying loved one. This behavior stems from the belief that the stress of bad news increases morbidity and perhaps even causes death (Norman, 1996). Two additional explanations for not disclosing a poor prognosis are that the dying person would lose hope and succumb to the illness and the prognosis could be wrong. Therefore, it is important to carefully and diplomatically talk with the family first, prior to disclosure of bad news to the patient (MDEED, 2006).

Consistent with the value on collectivism, Russians believe that a problem for one family member is a problem for the entire family. However, discussions about end of life are better addressed by identifying a spokesperson from the family. When discussing end-of-life decisions, it is also important to note that morphine or other potent analgesics may be perceived as hopelessness or abandoning the patient (University of Washington Medical Center, 2005).

Compared with Americans, being in control of decisions at the end of life is less important for Russian immigrants. Therefore, requests for living wills or durable powers of attorney, as well as consents for withholding or withdrawing treatment, are usually declined by Russian patients and family members (University of Washington Medical Center, 2005). One reason for this is that Russians have great faith in U.S. medical care and therefore expect that everything possible will be done to restore health, even when their expectations are at odds with a grave prognosis (Aroian et al., 2006). However, evidence suggests that culturally sensitive educational efforts can be productive in increasing family decisions for palliative care of Russian older adults (Dashevskaya, 2004).

Spirituality

Religious Practices and Use of Prayer

Preferred religious practices for Russian immigrants vary. Many Russians have no religious affiliation, which is likely the consequence of antireligious dogma of the former Soviet Union. Prior to the overthrow of Czarist Russia, ethnic Russians were predominantly Russian Orthodox. However, during the Soviet era,

REFLECTIVE EXERCISE 24.2

During the admission to the long-term-care facility, the health-care team approached Inna and her sons to complete health-care proxy forms and make some end-of-life decisions. During the admission interview, it became clear that Inna's sons do not fully understand the extent of their mother's physical and cognitive impairment and would like the health-care team to pursue a very aggressive approach in treating her. Inna did not participate in the discussion fully and deferred all decision making to her sons. As a result, Inna's treatment plan included "full code" instructions to health-care providers. One day while visiting, one of the sons observed a team treating Inna during an acute CHF episode. He was distraught by how much his mother suffered from the brutality of the medical intervention. Afterward, he asked the health-care team to change "full code" instructions to Do Not Resuscitate (DNR) but declined Do Not Hospitalize (DNH) instructions, stating that he did not have the heart to institute this instruction.

1. What attitudes and cultural trends were demonstrated by Inna's sons during her admission to the long-term facility?
2. How should the facility admission team have approached the discussion regarding Inna's end-of-life wishes?
3. How should the discussion about DNR and DNH have been framed to demonstrate respect for Inna's sons' values and traditions?
4. What type of educational materials would be helpful for Inna's sons to help them consider how to address quality of life and end-of- life goals in her treatment plan?

religious practices of all types were condemned, and people caught practicing their religion risked being punished severely. With the resurgence of Russian nationalism, the Russian Orthodox Church has resumed a major role in the life and politics of the Russian people. As evidence of this renewed emphasis, Russian Orthodox Churches are being restored.

Religious practices among ethnic/religious minorities in present-day Russia also vary. Russian Jews may or may not be religious, but Pentecostals tend to be devout.

Meaning of Life and Individual Sources of Strength

Although self-professed atheism has had a dramatic decline since 1991, religion is still not prominent in many Russians' lives. Russians, including Russian immigrants, often lead secular lives and tend to gain spiritual strength, stability, and meaning through their associations with family and friends.

Spiritual Beliefs and Health-Care Practices

Seriously ill patients and family members who are religious consider prayer an essential and powerful tool toward health and healing (University of Washington Medical Center, 2005). Members of the Russian Orthodox faith believe in the heavenly position of saints as well as religious miracles.

Health-Care Beliefs and Practices

Russians define health as the absence of disease. Although they embrace biomedical explanations for disease, their approach to health is holistic. They endorse the notion that stress, including family and economic stress, is a causative factor in disease. Additional causative factors include getting chilled and not having fresh air, sunlight, and nutritious food. Given their holistic perspective, they expect their health-care providers to holistically diagnose the etiology of health problems. A common complaint is that Western medicine places too much emphasis on medications and laboratory results and not enough on clinical diagnosis and holistic care.

Russians consider health an important resource and are active in maintaining their health (Aroian et al., 2001). Russian immigrants generally keep health-care appointments and adhere to prescribed treatments (Aroian, 2003). On the other hand, the general belief is that more professional input is superior to relying on a single health provider. Thus, Russians often combine prescribed treatments from many providers, and providers are often unaware of multiple treatment plans. In addition, Russians often supplement prescribed treatments with homeopathic and herbal remedies.

Mental illnesses are highly stigmatized in Russia. As a result, Russian immigrants may not provide truthful answers to questions regarding a family or personal history of mental illness (University of Michigan Health System, 2007).

Russians often self-diagnose, seeking out and reading Russian-language health articles related to their disorders. One important method of receiving health-care information is through mass media and the Internet. *Rulist.com* is a search engine that provides a kind of Russian yellow pages with information on health and wellness. Russian immigrants may also subscribe to the *Russian Health Magazine,* a magazine geared toward increasing the medical awareness of Russian-speaking people in the United States. It is also noteworthy that a significant portion of Russian immigrant men and women who emigrated in the latter part of the 20th century were physicians. Although some of the older people from this group never practiced medicine in the United States, they provide informal health information to Russian immigrants.

Russian immigrants have a very different view of obesity than the dominant U.S. culture. Generally, they are more accepting of excess weight and obesity, perhaps because excess weight and obesity are common due to a high caloric diet and low levels of exercise. For example, Stevens and colleagues (1997) compared attitudes and behaviors related to body size and other parameters among black, white, and Russian adolescents. Russian adolescent girls were less likely than black and white adolescent girls to identify obese and overweight status as a concern.

Health-Seeking Beliefs and Behaviors

Clinical and anecdotal reports describe Russians as demanding patients who overuse health care. It is true that Russians are not passive in voicing their health-care needs (Aroian, 2003). However, empirical data about their health care use illustrate that their use is not always disproportionate to their health needs (Aroian & Vander Wall 2007). It is also important to consider that the Russian immigrant community in the United States is diverse, with much variation in many of the characteristics that affect health-care use, such as education, language ability, age, and insurance coverage. For example, Ivanov and Buck (2002) found that younger Russian immigrant women only used health care for emergencies, reportedly because of lack of time and third party insurance. In contrast, the older Russian immigrant women in their sample had much heavier use, presumably because they were retired and covered by Medicaid. There is also geographic variation in the number of Russian-speaking health-care providers and transportation barriers for accessing health care. Geographical differences may account for why Wei and Spigner (1994) found that Russian immigrants had lower rates of clinic use than Southeast Asian refugees in Portland, Oregon, whereas Aroian and colleagues (2001) found very high health-care use among Russians in Boston, Massachusetts. Portland had comparatively fewer language barriers for Southeast Asians than for Russians, whereas Boston had almost no language barrier for Russians. Russian-speaking physicians in Boston also purposefully set up practices close to dense Russian-speaking communities so as to minimize transportation barriers.

There are mixed findings about how satisfied Russian immigrants are with their health-care providers. In one study, Russian immigrants expressed dissatisfaction with family physicians, perceiving them as lacking professionalism (Ivanov & Buck, 2002). They were dissatisfied with the general appearance of health-care providers and how difficult it is to distinguish between the nurse and the janitor. In contrast, another study that compared Russian immigrants with nonimmigrants found no differences in satisfaction with providers, but did find that Russians were less satisfied with appointment availability and physical access (Aroian & Vander Wall, 2007). Dissatisfaction with appointment availability and physical access may be related to the fact that Russians were used to having health care readily available in Russia through walk-in clinics located in convenient settings where people

live and work. Russians were also used to physicians making home visits in Russia when people are too ill or frail to travel for health care (Aroian et al., 2001).

Russians perceive male physicians as more skilled and competent and as having more status than female physicians (Ivanov & Buck, 2002). Nonetheless, they are used to having female physicians. Women in Russia have been practicing medicine in large numbers for decades.

Responsibility for Health Care

Russians believe that individuals are responsible for their health and that disabilities and negative health events result when individuals do not take care of themselves (Aroian et al., 2001; Aroian & Vander Wal, 2007). Most Russians take an active role in their health and health care. They use alternative and homeopathic remedies and commit to self-care.

Even though Russians acknowledge personal responsibility for their health, they are used to authoritarian health encounters. They expect health-care providers to be directive, telling them exactly what to do to get or stay well (Aroian et al., 2006; Ivanov & Buck, 2002). They are unlikely to schedule preventive screening unless a health-care provider directs them to do so (Ivanov & Buck, 2002).

Folk and Traditional Practices

Homeopathic and traditional medicines have been used for centuries in Russia and continue to be used widely, often simultaneously with those of Western medical science. Russians, especially older individuals, use herbal teas, tinctures, mud baths, massage, saunas, and other alternative medicines and healing practices (Yehieli et al., 2005). Additional home remedies include rubbing oils and ointments, enemas, saunas and whirlpools, mineral water (for soaking as well as drinking), herbal teas, hot and cold soups, liquors, and mud plasters (Bistrevsky, 2005). "Cupping," a technique whereby the inside of a glass cup is heated and placed on a person's back, shoulder, or chest, is used for respiratory problems such as bronchitis and asthma. In Russia, physicians and nurses go to patients' homes to perform cupping.

Barriers to Health Care
Awareness and Attitudes

Russians expect their health-care providers to look and act professional. Russian immigrants also expect health-care providers to be nonjudgmental about herbal and homeopathic treatments. Russians are very involved with the care of their family members, which can conflict with providers who approach care by only involving the patient, either as a means of promoting autonomy or protecting the patient's privacy. Owing to social and political sanctions against psychiatric illness in Russia, Russian immigrants may also be reluctant to disclose mental health issues and a family history of mental disorders. Therefore, providers need to approach the subject carefully and with full assurances of confidentiality.

Russians are unaccustomed to the concept of managed care. They want direct access to multiple, sophisticated tests and procedures and to health-care specialists of their choice. They believe the additional step of needing a referral by a primary care provider is not only expensive and wasteful but also detrimental to their health because it reduces timeliness to care. Recent Russian immigrants may also be unfamiliar with concepts such as defensive health care and medical malpractice.

Affordability

Russians are egalitarian and believe in an equal distribution of health-care benefits (Culture Tips, 2000). In the former Soviet Union, health care was free. Therefore, concepts like private pay, co-pay, and insurance premiums are difficult for many Russian immigrants to understand. They may need help to understand U.S. health-care systems, including Medicaid and Medicare programs. However, the Russian health system underwent significant transformation after the fall of communism. Therefore, recent immigrants are more familiar with the notion of paid health care and the need to have health insurance coverage.

In the United States, about 85 percent of Russian immigrants carry some kind of health insurance

REFLECTIVE EXERCISE 24.3

When Inna was admitted to the long-term-care facility, the admission staff obtained a list of her prescribed medications from her primary care provider. During one of the visits by Inna's other son, the staff observed that he was giving Inna pills to take with her meal. In the facility, Inna receives several medications, and they are administered in a crushed form due to her soft food diet and difficulty swallowing. The staff was worried and informed Inna's physician that her son was giving her additional medications. When the physician called Inna's son, the son explained that the pills were "natural," were recommended by his alternative health-care provider, and were likely to help his mother. He takes the same pills to boost his energy level. However, he does not know what the pills contain.

1. What cultural responses to health and illness are demonstrated by Inna's son?
2. What was the missing element in the admission process in terms of Inna's medication history?
3. What discussion should have taken place when Inna's care team discussed her medication regimen and her treatment plan with her family?

coverage, including employer-based private insurance or government plans such as Medicaid, Medicare, or both (Ethnic Population, 2003). Due to low income, a lot of older immigrants are dual eligible: enrolled in Medicare as their primary insurance and also enrolled in Medicaid to help pay for co-payments and deductibles. In cases of chronic illness and frailty, dual enrollment provides coverage for home and community-based services and nursing home care. Even with coverage, cost can be a major barrier to health care. Copayments can compete with money needed for food and other household essentials (Ivanov & Buck, 2002).

Language Proficiency

There are generational differences in language proficiency. Older immigrants have a lesser command of English than younger immigrants who went to school in the United States and/or are working for American employers. Therefore, younger family members often act as interpreters for the elderly. However, Russian immigrants who are not proficient in English strongly prefer Russian-speaking health-care providers and will actively look for them.

Depending on geographical area, there are a large number of Russian-speaking health providers and health services in the United States. For example, some nursing homes have "Russian units" staffed by Russian-speaking nurses. It is also noteworthy that Russian medical and dental associations have been established in the United States and are a testimony to the language- and culture-specific health-care resources that are available to Russian immigrants who speak only Russian. The Russian American Medical Association (RAMA) was founded in 2002 and has a peer-reviewed journal and a Web site with information relevant to all Russian-speaking health-care providers (RAMA, 2007). As previously mentioned, there is also a good amount of Russian-language health literature available for Russian lay audiences (e.g., the *Russian Health Magazine* and Web sites like Rulist.com). There is also a Web site called RussianDoctor.com, which allows Russian immigrants to locate Russian-speaking dentists and physicians by specialty and location (city/state).

Accessibility

For every 1000 people in Russia, there are 4.25 physicians compared with 2.56 physicians in the United States (WHO, 2006). Although the United States has more nurses and more nurses in expanded practice roles than Russia, Russian immigrants perceive that health care is far less accessible than what they were used to (Aroian & Vander Wall, 2007; Benisovich & King, 2003). Russian immigrants complain about needing to wait many weeks or months before getting a health-care appointment. As mentioned above, Russians were used to much greater accessibility in the former Soviet Union, including conveniently located walk-in clinics and home visits by physicians. Transportation is another barrier, even in geographical settings where Russian-speaking health-care providers have intentionally set up practices in Russian-speaking neighborhoods. In addition, in the Soviet Union, people were hospitalized for minor illnesses. Therefore, Russian immigrants may be less used to traveling back and forth for outpatient visits and multiple appointments in different locations.

Cultural Responses to Health and Illness

Russian immigrants often have unrealistic expectations of U.S. health-care providers (Aroian et al., 2001). They expect that a rich country like the United States should be able to cure disease easily, regardless of disease state. When one physician is unable to meet expectations, the patient will likely seek the services of others. Treatments prescribed by one health-care provider may not be disclosed to another, which raises concerns about negative health effects from polypharmacy (Aroian, 2003). In addition, Russians are accustomed to health-care providers placing a greater emphasis on treatment than prevention. Long in-patient hospitalizations were the norm in Russia. Thus, Russian immigrants are dismayed by short hospital stays in the United States (Aroian et al., 2001).

Blood Transfusion and Organ Donation

Owing to contaminated blood supplies in Russia and the former Soviet Union, health-care providers may have difficulty convincing Russian immigrants to consent to giving or receiving human blood products.

Health-Care Providers

Traditional Versus Biomedical Care

In Russia, health care was more holistic, with biomedical providers prescribing homeopathic treatments as supplements to biomedical approaches. As previously mentioned, Russian immigrants are disappointed by the lack of holism in American health care.

Status of Health-Care Providers

Physicians are considered to be the most knowledgeable of all health-care providers and "in charge" of health care.

REFERENCES

Abramson, H. (1991). Jewish representation in the independent Ukraian governments of 1917–1920. *Slavic Review, 50*(3), 542–550.

Alaniz, J. (2001, September 11). Crossing cultures: Russian nurses navigate the unfamiliar U.S. health care system, finding career advantages and obstacles. *NurseWeek*. Retrieved from www.nurseweek.com/news/features/01-09/cultures_print.html

Allied Media Corp. (n.d.). Television for Russian Americans RTVI. (Author). *Multicultural communication*. Retrieved from www.allied-media.com/RussianMarket/rtvi.htm

Aroian, K.J. (2003). Russians (former Soviets). In P. St. Hill, J. Lipson, & A.I. Meleis, (Eds.), *Caring for women cross-culturally* (pp. 249–263). Philadelphia: F. A. Davis.

Aroian, K.J., Khatutsky, G., & Dashevskaya, A. (2006). Cross-cultural health care for older Russian-speaking Americans. In R.N. Adler & H.K. Kamel (Eds.), *Doorway thoughts: Cross-cultural health care for older Russian-speaking Americans* (Vol. 2, pp. 152–166). Boston, MA: Jones and Bartlett.

Aroian, K.J., Khatutsky, G., Tran, T.V., & Balsam, A.L. (2001). Health and social service utilization among elderly immigrants from the former Soviet Union. *Journal of Nursing Scholarship, 33*(3), 265–271.

Aroian, K.J., & Norris, A.E. (1999). Somatization and depression among former Soviet immigrants. *Journal of Cultural Diversity, 6*(3), 93–101.

Aroian, K.J., & Norris, A.E. (2003). Depression trajectories in relatively recent immigrants. *Comprehensive Psychiatry, 44*(5), 420–427.

Aroian, K.J., Norris, A.E., & Chiang, L. (2003). Gender differences in psychological distress among immigrants from the former Soviet Union. *Sex Roles, 48*(1/2), 39–51.

Aroian, K.J., Norris, A., Patsdaughter, C.A., & Tran, T.V. (1998). Predicting psychological distress among former Soviet immigrants. *International Journal of Social Psychiatry, 44*(2), 284–294.

Aroian, K.J., Spitzer, A., & Bell, M. (1996). Family support and conflict among former Soviet immigrants. *Western Journal of Nursing Research, 18*(6), 655–674.

Aroian, K.J., & Vander Wal, J.S. (2007). Health service use in Russian immigrant and nonimmigrant older persons. *Family and Community Health, 30*(3), 213–223.

Belozersky, I. (1990). New beginnings, old problems: Psychocultural frame of reference and family dynamics during the adjustment period. *Journal of Communal Services, 67,* 124–130.

Benisovich, S.V., & King, A.C. (2003). Meaning and knowledge of health among older adult immigrants from Russia: A phenomenological study. *Health Education Research, 18*(2), 135–144.

Bergelson, M.B. (2003). *Russian cultural values and workplace communication. III International RCA Conference–2006 "communication and (re) making social worlds."* Retrieved from http://www.russcomm.ru/eng/rca_biblio/b/bergelson03_eng.shtml

Birch, D. (2006, August 27). In Russia, the truth is optional [Electronic version]. *The Baltimore Sun*, opinion section.

Bistrevsky, T. (2005, Summer). Insight into Spokane's Russian families. *ABCD and ABCDE Newsletter*. Spokane Regional Health District. Retrieved from www.SRHD.org

Brod, M., & Heurtin Roberts, S. (1992). Older Russian emigres and medical care. *The Western Journal of Medicine, 157,* 333–336.

CIA World Factbook. (2011). *Russia.* Retrieved from www.cia.gov/library/publications/the-world-factbook/index.html

Culture tips: Understanding the Russian culture and individual. (2000). *Cross Cultural Connection, 5*(4), 3–4.

Dashevskaya, A. (2004). Aging well together across cultures. Presented at a workshop for health providers, Lynn, Massachusetts, April 14, 2004.

Energy Information Administration [EIA]. (2010). *Russia Energy Profile.* Retrieved from http://www.eia.doe.gov/cfapps/country/country_energy_data.cfm?fips=RS

Ethnic Population. (2003, July 30). *Russian market in USA.* Retrieved from www.inforeklama.com/market.htm

Gabriel, R. (2005, March). A commentary on pharmacogenomics: What can it do? *Medical Laboratory Observer*. Nelson Publishing/Gale Group.

Gaikovitch, E.A. (2003, July 14). *Genotyping of the polymorphic drug metabolizing enzymes cytochrome P450 2D6 and 1A1, and N-acetyltransferase 2 in a Russian sample.* Dissertation, Humbolt University, Berlin, Germany.

Goodman, R., Slobodskaya, H., & Knyazev, G. (2005). Russian child mental health: A cross-sectional study of prevalence and risk factors. *European Child and Adolescent Psychiatry, 14,* 28–33.

Hasin, D., Aharonovich, E., Liu, X., Mamman, Z., Matseoane, K., Carr, L., & Li, T-K. (2002). Alcohol and ADH2 in Israel: Ashkenazis, Sephardics, and recent Russian immigrants. *American Journal of Psychiatry, 159*(8), 1432–1434.

Hobbs, R. (2002, July 16). *Knowledge of immigrant nationalities: Russia.* Retrieved from www.immigrantinfo.org/kin/russia.htm

Isralowitz, R.E., Straussner, S.L., & Rosenblum, A. (2006). Drug abuse, risks of infectious diseases and service utilization among former Soviet Union immigrants: A view from New York City. *Journal of Ethnicity and Substance Abuse, 5*(1) 91–96.

Ivanov, L.L., & Buck, K. (2002). Health care utilization patterns of Russian-speaking immigrant women across age groups. *Journal of Immigrant Health, 4*(1), 17–27.

Jeltova, I., Fish, M.C., & Revenson, T.A. (2005). Risky sexual behaviors in immigrant adolescent girls from the former Soviet Union: Role of natal and host culture. *Journal of School Psychology, 43*(1), 3–22.

Keefe, S. (2006, August 21). Russian-speaking home care nurses help bridge language and cultural barriers among Brooklyn's Russian immigrants. *ADVANCE* Newsmagazines: Merion Publications. Retrieved from http://nursing.advanceweb.com/common/editorial [Requires registration]

Levav, I., Kohn, R., Flaherty, J.A., Lerner, Y., & Aisenberg, E. (1990). Mental health attitudes and practices of Soviet immigrants. *Israeli Journal of Psychiatry and Related Sciences, 27,* 131–144.

Library of Congress. (2010, July). *Country profile: Russia.* Library of Congress—Federal Research Division, Library of Congress call number: DK510.23. R883 1998. Retrieved from http://memory.loc.gov/frd/cs/rutoc.html

Marquez, P.V. (2005). *Dying too young: Addressing premature mortality and ill health due to non-communicable diseases and injuries in the Russian Federation.* Washington, DC: World Bank.

Mehler, P.S., Scott, J.Y., Pines, I., Gifford, N., Biggerstaff, S., & Hiatt, W.R. (2001). Russian immigrant cardiovascular risk assessment. *Journal of Health Care for the Poor and Underserved, 12*(2), 224–235.

Miller, A.M., & Chandler, P.J. (2002). Acculturation, resilience, and depression in midlife women from the former Soviet Union. *Nursing Research, 51,* 26–32.

Miller, A.M., Sorokin, O., Wang, E., Feetham, S. Choi, M., & Wilbur, J. (2006). Acculturation, social alienation, and depressed mood in midlife women from the former Soviet Union. *Research in Nursing and Health, 29,* 134–146.

Minnesota Department of Employment and Economic Development [MDEED]. (2006). *Russian immigrants in Minnesota.* Minnesota State Services for the Blind. Retrieved from www.mnssb.org/rcb/moc/russian.htm

Nemtsov, A. (2005). Russia: Alcohol yesterday and today. *Addiction, 100,* 146–149.

News about gay Russia. (n.d.). Retrieved from http://russia.bi.org/news.html

Nicholson, A., Bobak, M., Murphy, M., Rose, R., & Marmot, M. (2005). Alcohol consumption and increased mortality in Russian men and women: A cohort study based on the mortality of relatives. *Bulletin of the World Health Organization, 83*(11), 812–819.

Norman, C. (1996). Breaking bad news: Consultations with ethnic communities. *Australian Family Physician, 25*(10), 1583–1587.

Parfitt, T. (2006). Campaigners fight to bring down Russia's tobacco toll. *The Lancet, 368,* 633–634.

Remennick, L.I. (1999). Women of the "sandwich" generation and multiple roles: The case of Russian immigrants of the 1990's in Israel. *Sex Roles, 40,* 347–378.

Rennert, G., Luz, N., Tamir, A., & Peterburg, Y. (2002). Chronic disease prevalence in immigrants to Israel from the former USSR. *Journal of Immigrant Health, 4*(1), 29–33.

Russian American Medical Association (RAMA). (2007). Retrieved from www.russiandoctors.org/

Shpilko, I. (2006). Russian-American health care: Bridging the communication gap between physicians and patients. *Patient Education and Counseling, 64,* 331–341.

Smith, L.S. (1996). New Russian immigrants: Health problems, practices, and values. *Journal of Cultural Diversity, 3*(3), 68–73.

Stevens, J., Alexandrov, A.A., Smirnova, S.G., Deev, A.D., Gershunskaya, Y.B., Davis, C.E., & Thomas, R. (1997). Comparison of attitudes and behaviors related to nutrition, body size, dieting, and hunger in Russian, black-American, and white-American adolescents. *Obesity Research, 5,* 227–236.

Tran, T.V., Khatutsky, G., Aroian, K., Balsam, A., & Conway, K. (2000). Living arrangements, depression, and health status among elderly Russian-speaking immigrants. *Journal of Gerontological Social Work, 33*(2), 63–77.

U.S. Census Bureau. (2000). *Fact sheet: United States. Census 2000 demographic profile highlights: Selected population group: Russian* (pp. 148–151). Summary file 4(SF4).

U.S. Census Bureau. (2007). *Language use in the United States.* Retrieved from http://www.census.gov/hhes/socdemo/language/data/acs/ACS-12.pdf

U.S. Department of Homeland Security. (2005a). *Table 3: Legal permanent resident flow by region and country of birth: Fiscal years 1995 to 2005.* Retrieved from www.uscis.gov/graphics/shared/statistics/yearbook/LPRO5.htm

U.S. Department of Homeland Security. (2005b). *Table 12: Immigrant orphans adopted by US citizens by gender, age, and region and country of birth: Fiscal year 2005.* Retrieved from www.uscis.gov/graphics/shared/statistics/yearbook/LPRO5.htm

U.S. Department of Homeland Security. (2005c). *Supplemental Table 2: Legal permanent resident flow by leading core-based statistical areas (CBSAs) of residence and region and country of birth: Fiscal year 2005.* Retrieved from www.uscis.gov/graphics/shared/statistics/yearbook/LPRO5.htm

U.S. Department of Homeland Security. (2010). *Yearbook of Immigration Statistics: 2009.* Retrieved from http://www.uscis.gov/graphics/shared/statistics/yearbook/LPRO5.htm

University of Michigan Health System. (2007). *Cultural competency.* Patient Education. Ann Arbor. Retrieved from http://www.uofmhealth.org/health-library

University of Washington Medical Center. (2005, April). *Communicating with your Russian patient.* Culture clues: Staff Development Workgroup, Patient and Family Education Committee. Seattle.

Vadlamani, A., Maher, J.F., Shaete, M., Smirnoff, A., Cameron, D.G., Winkelmann, J.C., & Goldberg, S.J. (2001). Colorectal cancer in Russian-speaking Jewish émigrés: Community-based screening. *American Journal of Gastroenterology, 96*(9), 2755–2760.

Vishnevsky, A., & Zayonchkovskaya, Z. (1994). Emigration from the former Soviet Union: The fourth wave. In H. Fassman & R. Munz (Eds.), *European migration in the late twentieth century: Historical patterns, actual trends, & social implications* (pp. 239–285). Aldershot, UK: Edward Elgar Publishing Limited.

Wei C., & Spigner, C. (1994). Health status and clinic utilization among refugees from Southeast Asia and the Former Soviet Union. *Journal of Health Education, 25*(3), 266–273.

World Health Organization (WHO). (2005, January 14). *Country profile*. WHO Regional Office for Europe. Retrieved from http://www.who.int/countries/rus/en/

World Health Organization (WHO). (2006). *Health workers: A global profile. The world health report 2006: Working together for health*. Annex table 4, pp. 197–199. Retrieved from http://www.who.int/whr/2006/en/

Yehieli, M., Lutz, G., & Grey, M. (Eds.). (2005, November). Russians and other immigrants from the former Soviet Union. *Health disparity factsheets*. Cedar Falls, IA: Center for Health Disparities, University of Northern Iowa.

DavisPlus *For case studies, review questions, and additional information, go to*
http://davisplus.fadavis.com

Appendix

Cultural, Ethnic, and Racial Diseases and Illnesses

Causes are grouped into three categories—genetic, lifestyle, and environment.

Lifestyle causes include cultural practices and behaviors that can generally be controlled—for example, smoking, diet, and stress.

Environmental causes refer to the external environment (e.g., air and water pollution) and situations over which the individual has little or no control (e.g., presence of malarial mosquitos, exposure to chemicals and pesticides, access to care, and associated diseases).

Cultural/Racial Group	Diseases/Disorders	Causes
Black Populations	**AFRICAN AMERICANS**	
	Sickle cell disease	Genetic, environment
	Hypertension	Genetic, lifestyle
	Systemic lupus erythematosus	Genetic with an environmental trigger
	Diabetes mellitus	Genetic, lifestyle
	Glaucoma	Genetic
	Cardiovascular disease	Genetic, environment, lifestyle
	Lung, colon, and rectal cancer	Environment and lifestyle
	Prostate cancer	Genetic, environment
	Lead poisoning	Environment
	Asthma	Environment and lifestyle
	HIV/AIDS	Lifestyle
	Hemoglobin C disease	Genetic
	Hereditary persistence of hemoglobin F	Genetic
	Glucose-6-phosphate dehydrogenase deficiency	Genetic
	β-Thalassemia	Genetic
	HAITIANS	
	Malaria	Environment
	Tuberculosis	Lifestyle, environment
	Diabetes mellitus	Genetic, environment, lifestyle
	Hypertension	Genetic, lifestyle
	SOMALI	
	Depression, post-traumatic stress disorder	Environment, lifestyle
	Tuberculosis	Environment, lifestyle
	Hepatitis B	Environment, lifestyle
	Helicobacter pylori, intestinal parasites	Environment, lifestyle
	Malaria	Lifestyle

Continues on page 442

Cultural/Racial Group	Diseases/Disorders	Causes
	Trichuris trichuria, Enterobius vermicularis, Entamoeba histolytica, Dientamoeba fragilis, Ascaris lumbricoides, and Schistosoma mansoni	Environment, lifestyle
	Lactase deficiency	Genetics
	KENYANS	
	Nasopharyngeal cancer	Lifestyle
	Esophageal cancer	Lifestyle, environment?
	ZAIRIANS & UGANDANS	
	Stomach cancer	Lifestyle
	Duodenal ulcers	Unknown
	ZIMBABWEANS	
	Stomach cancer	Lifestyle
	SUB-SAHARAN AFRICANS	
	Liver cancer	Environment
	100 DEGREES NORTH AND SOUTH OF THE EQUATOR	
	Burkitt lymphoma	Environment
Hispanics/Latinos	**BRAZILIANS**	
	Tuberculosis	Lifestyle, environment
	Dengue fever	Lifestyle, environment
	Malaria	Lifestyle, environment
	Trypanosomiasis	Lifestyle, environment
	Schistosomiasis	Lifestyle, environment
	Chagas disease	Lifestyle, environment
	Yellow fever	Lifestyle, environment
	Intestinal parasites	Lifestyle, environment
	Cancers	Lifestyle, genetics
	CUBANS	
	Hypertension	Genetic, lifestyle
	Coronary artery disease	Genetic, lifestyle
	Obesity	Environment, lifestyle
	Diabetes mellitus	Genetic, lifestyle
	Lung cancer	Lifestyle, environment
	GUATEMALANS	
	Lactase deficiency	Genetic
	Gastritis	Environment, lifestyle
	Malaria	Environment, lifestyle
	Tuberculosis	Environment, lifestyle
	Eye disorders	Lifestyle
	MEXICANS	
	Lactase deficiency	Genetic
	Diabetes mellitus	Genetic, lifestyle
	Cleft lip/palate	Lifestyle
	Dental caries	Lifestyle, environment
	Cardiovascular disease	Genetic, environment, lifestyle
	Tuberculosis	Environment, lifestyle
	Hypertension	Genetic, environment, lifestyle
	COSTA RICANS	
	Malignant osteoporosis	Environment? Genetic?
	PUERTO RICANS	
	Cardiovascular disease	Genetic, environment, lifestyle
	Hypertension	Genetic, environment, lifestyle
	Dengue fever	Environment
	Breast cancer	Genetic, lifestyle
	Prostate cancer	Genetic, environment, lifestyle

Cultural/Racial Group	Diseases/Disorders	Causes
Arabs/Middle Easterners	Familial Mediterranean fever	Genetic
	Familial paroxysmal polyserositis	Genetic
	Tuberculosis	Environment, lifestyle
	Malaria	Genetic, environment
	Trachoma	Environment, lifestyle
	Typhoid fever	Environment
	Glucose-6-phosphate dehydrogenase deficiency	Genetic
	Sickle cell disease	Genetic, environment
	Thalassemia	Genetic
	Hepatitis A and B	Environment, lifestyle
	Schistosomiasis (bilharzia)	Environment, lifestyle
	Familial hypercholesterolemia	Genetic, lifestyle
	IRANIANS	
	Dubin-Johnson syndrome	Genetic
	Epilepsy	Genetic
	IRAQIS	
	Ichthyosis vulgaris	Genetic
	YEMENIS	
	Phenylketonuria	Genetic
	Glucose-6-phosphate dehydrogenase deficiency	Genetic
	LEBANESE	
	Dyggve-Melchior-Clausen syndrome	Genetic
	Familial hypercholesterolemia	Genetic
	EGYPTIANS	
	Schistosomiasis	Lifestyle, environment
	Trachoma	Environment, lifestyle
	Typhoid fever	Environment
	Tuberculosis	Lifestyle, environment
	β-Thalassemia	Genetic
	SAUDI ARABIANS	
	Metachromatic leukodystrophy	Genetic
Asian/Pacific Islanders	**CHINESE**	
	α-Thalassemia	Genetic
	Glucose-6-phosphate dehydrogenase deficiency	Genetic
	Lactase deficiency	Genetic
	Nasopharyngeal cancer	Environment, lifestyle
	Liver cancer	Environment, lifestyle
	Stomach cancer	Unknown, lifestyle and/or environment
	Cardiovascular disease	Genetic, lifestyle, environment
	Hepatitis B	Genetic, lifestyle, environment
	Tuberculosis	Environment, lifestyle
	Diabetes mellitus	Genetic, lifestyle, environment
	JAPANESE	
	Vogt-Koyanagi-Harada syndrome	Genetic
	Cardiovascular disease	Genetic, lifestyle, environment
	Asthma	Lifestyle, environment
	Takayasu disease	Genetic
	Acatalasemia	Genetic
	Cleft lip/palate	Lifestyle, genetic
	Oguchi disease	Genetic
	Lactase deficiency	Environment, lifestyle
	Stomach cancer	Genetic, lifestyle, environment
	Hypertension	Genetic, lifestyle, environment

Continues on page 444

Cultural/Racial Group	Diseases/Disorders	Causes
	ASIAN INDIANS	
	Cancer of the cheek	Lifestyle
	Ichthyosis vulgaris	Genetic
	Tuberculosis	Lifestyle, environment
	Malaria	Environment
	Rheumatic heart disease	Environment
	Cardiovascular disease	Genetic, lifestyle, environment
	Sickle cell disease	Genetic
	FILIPINOS	
	Diabetes mellitus	Genetic, environment, lifestyle
	Hyperuricemia	Lifestyle
	Cardiovascular disease	Genetic, lifestyle, environment
	Hypertension	Genetic, lifestyle, environment
	Thalassemia	Genetic
	Glucose-6-phosphate dehydrogenase deficiency	Genetic
	THAILANDERS	
	Glucose-6-phosphate dehydrogenase deficiency	Genetic
	Thalassemia	Genetic
	Lactase deficiency	Genetic
	VIETNAMESE	
	Nasopharyngeal cancer	Lifestyle, environment
	Lactase deficiency	Genetic
	Post-traumatic stress disorder	Environment
	Tuberculosis	Lifestyle, environment
	Malaria	Environment
	Hepatitis B	Environment, lifestyle
	Melioidosis	Environment, lifestyle
	Paragonimiasis	Environment, lifestyle
	Leprosy	Genetic
	HMONGS AND LAOTIANS	
	Nasopharyngeal cancer	Lifestyle, environment
	Lactase deficiency	Genetic
	Tuberculosis	Environment, lifestyle
	Hepatitis B	Genetic, environment, lifestyle
	KOREANS	
	Stomach cancer	Lifestyle
	Liver cancer	Genetic, environment
	Hypertension	Genetic, lifestyle, environment
	Schistosomiasis	Environment, lifestyle
	Hepatitis A and B	Environment, lifestyle
	Lactase deficiency	Genetic
	Osteoporosis	Genetic, lifestyle
	Peptic ulcer disease	Lifestyle, environment
	Lactose intolerance	Genetic
	Tuberculosis	Environment and lifestyle
	Astestosis	Environment
	Insulin autoimmune deficiency disease	Genetic
	Renal failure	Lifestyle
European American Ethnic White Populations	Skin cancer	Environment, lifestyle
	Appendicitis	Unknown
	Diverticular disease	Lifestyle, genetic?
	Colon cancer	Lifestyle, genetic?
	Hemorrhoids	Lifestyle, unknown

Cultural/Racial Group	Diseases/Disorders	Causes
	Cardiovascular disease	Genetic, lifestyle, environment
	Varicose veins	Genetic
	Diabetes mellitus	Genetic, lifestyle
	Multiple sclerosis	Environment
	Obesity	Lifestyle
ENGLISH		
	Cystic fibrosis	Genetic
	Hereditary amyloidosis, type III	Genetic
	Rosacea	Genetic
ESTONIANS, LATVIANS, LITHUANIANS		
	Tuberculosis	Environment, lifestyle
	Alcohol misuse	Environment, lifestyle
FRENCH CANADIANS		
	Sickle cell disease	Genetic, environment
	Osteoporosis	Lifestyle, genetic
	Osteoarthritis	Genetic
	Cardiovascular disease	Genetic, lifestyle, environment
	Lung cancer	Environment, lifestyle
	Breast cancer	Genetic, lifestyle
	Cystic fibrosis	Genetic
	Phenylketonuria	Genetic
	Tyrosinemia	Genetic
	Morquio syndrome	Genetic
	Familial hypercholesterolemia	Genetic, lifestyle
	Breast and ovarian cancer	Genetic, environment
	Spastic ataxia Charlevoix-Saguenay type	Genetic
	Cytochrome lipase deficiency	Genetic
	Phenylketonuria	Genetic
GERMANS		
	Myotonic muscular dystrophy	Genetic
	Hereditary hemochromatosis	Genetic
	Sarcoidosis	Genetic, environment
	Dupuytren's disease	Genetic
	Peyronie's disease	Genetic
	Cholelithiasis	Genetic, lifestyle
	Stomach cancer	Genetic, lifestyle, environment
	Cystic fibrosis	Genetic
	Hemophilia	Genetic
POLISH		
	Cardiovascular diseases	Environment, lifestyle
	Diabetes mellitus	Genetic, lifestyle
	Alcohol misuse	Environment, lifestyle
	Cancer	Environment, lifestyle
	Pulmondary disorders	Environment, lifestyle
GREEKS		
	Tay-Sachs disease	Genetic
	Cardiovascular disease	Genetic, environment, lifestyle
	Malaria	Environment
	Tuberculosis	Environment, lifestyle
	Glucose-6-phosphate dehydrogenase deficiency	Genetic
	Hepatitis A and B	Environment, lifestyle

Continues on page 446

Cultural/Racial Group	Diseases/Disorders	Causes
	FINLANDERS	
	Stomach cancer	Lifestyle, environment
	Congenital nephrosis	Genetic
	Generalized amyloidosis, type V	Genetic
	Polycystic liver disease	Genetic
	Retinoschisis	Genetic
	Aspartylglycosaminuria	Genetic
	Diastrophic dwarfism	Genetic
	Choroideremia	Genetic
	ITALIANS	
	Vogt-Koyanagi-Harada syndrome	Genetic
	β-Thalassemia	Genetic
	Recurrent polyserositis	Genetic
	Hypertension	Lifestyle, genetic
	Nasopharyngeal cancer	Lifestyle
	Stomach cancer	Lifestyle
	Liver cancer	Lifestyle
	Familial Mediterranean fever	Genetic
	Glucose-6-phosphate dehydrogenase deficiency	Genetic
	JEWS	
	Lactase deficiency	Genetic
	Werdnig-Hoffmann disease	Genetic
	Mucolipidosis IV	Genetic
	Phenylketonuria	Genetic
	Kaposi sarcoma	Genetic
	Gaucher disease	Genetic
	Niemann-Pick disease	Genetic
	Tay-Sachs disease	Genetic
	Riley-Day syndrome	Genetic
	Torsion dystonia	Genetic
	Factor XI plasma thromboplastin antecedent (PTA) deficiency	Genetic
	Cystinuria	Genetic
	Ataxia-telangiectasia	Genetic
	Familial Mediterranean fever	Genetic
	Metachromatic leukodystrophy	Genetic, unknown
	Bloom syndrome	Genetic, lifestyle
	Myopia	Genetic, lifestyle
	Polycythemia vera	Genetic
	Hypercholesterolemia	Genetic
	Breast cancer	Environment, lifestyle
	Diabetes mellitus	Genetic, lifestyle, environment
	POLES	
	Phenylketonuria	Environment
	Respiratory diseases	Environment, lifestyle
	Cardiovascular diseases	Lifestyle
	APPALACHIANS	
	Black lung	Environment, lifestyle
	Emphysema	Unknown, environment, lifestyle
	Tuberculosis	Genetic, lifestyle, environment
	Hypochromic anemia	Environment, lifestyle
	Cardiovascular disease	Genetic, lifestyle
	Sudden infant death syndrome	Genetic
	Diabetes mellitus	Genetic
	Otitis media	Lifestyle

Cultural/Racial Group	Diseases/Disorders	Causes
	SCANDINAVIANS	
	Cholelithiasis	Genetic, lifestyle
	Sjögren-Larsson syndrome	Genetic
	Krabbe disease	Genetic, environment, lifestyle
	Phenylketonuria	Genetic
	IRISH	
	Phenylketonuria	Genetic
	Neural tube defects	Genetic
	Cardiovascular disease	Genetic
	Alcoholism	Genetic, environment, lifestyle
	Skin cancer	Genetic
	AMISH	
	Limb-girdle muscular dystrophy	Genetic
	Ellis–van Creveld syndrome	Genetic
	Dwarfism	Genetic, unknown
	Polydactylism	Genetic
	Cartilage hair hypoplasia	Genetic
	Phenylketonuria	Genetic
	Glutaric aciduria	Genetic
	Manic-depressive disorder	Genetic
	Pyruvate kinase deficiency	Genetic
	Hemophilia B	Genetic
	RUSSIANS	
	Alcoholism	Lifestyle, genetic, environment
	Hypertension	Lifestyle, environment
	Pulmonary disorders	Lifestyle, environment
	Hyperlipidemia	Lifestyle, genetic
	Diabetes mellitus	Lifestyle, genetic
	Depression	Lifestyle, environment
	Gastrointestinal disorders	Lifestyle
Native Americans/	Diabetes mellitus	Genetic, lifestyle, environment
Alaskan Natives	Cholelithiasis	Lifestyle
	Lactase deficiency	Genetic
	Liver disease	Environment, lifestyle
	Hepatitis B	Environment, lifestyle
	Nasopharyngeal cancer	Environment, lifestyle
	Tuberculosis	Environment, lifestyle
	Alcoholism	Lifestyle, genetic
	NAVAJOS	
	Ear anomalies	Genetic
	Arthritis	Genetic
	Severe combined immunodeficiency syndrome	Genetic
	Navajo neuropathy	Genetic
	Albinism	Genetic
	Tuberculosis	Environment, lifestyle
	HOPIS	
	Tyrosinase-positive albinism	Genetic
	Trachoma	Environment, lifestyle
	PUEBLOS	
	Albinism	Genetic
	ZUNIS	
	Tyrosinase-positive albinism	Genetic

Continues on page 448

Cultural/Racial Group	Diseases/Disorders	Causes
	ESKIMOS	
	Hereditary amyloidosis	Genetic
	Congenital adrenal hyperplasia	Genetic
	Methemoglobinemia	Genetic
	Lactase deficiency	Genetic
	Pseudocholinesterase deficiency	Genetic
	Haemophilus influenza type B	Genetic?
	TURKS	
	Sickle cell	Genetic, environment
	Goiter	Genetic, environment
	Helminthiasis	Environment, lifestyle
	Behçet's disease	Genetic
	Thalassemias	Genetic
	Lactase deficiency	Genetic
	Tuberculosis	Environment, lifestyle
	Cardiovascular disease	Genetic, lifestyle
	Diabetes mellitus	Genetic, lifestyle

Abstracts

American Indians and Alaska Natives

Olivia Hodgins and David Hodgins

The Bureau of Indian Affairs (BIA) recognizes 556 different tribes of American Indians and Alaska Natives (AI/ANs) that extend throughout the United States. Most live on reservations created on undesirable lands that European Americans did not view as valuable. Because of severe economic conditions and high unemployment rates, significant migration occurs into and out of the reservations. Many who leave the reservation experience culture shock, and some return due to lack of social support systems and loss of identity and self-esteem. In contrast to other cultures, competitiveness is generally discouraged among AI/AN populations. Group achievements are more important than individual achievement.

Health-care providers must be extremely careful when attempting to speak an AI/AN language because minor variations in pronunciation may change the entire meaning of a word or phrase. The willingness of AI/ANs to share their thoughts and feelings varies from group to group and from individual to individual. In addition, no set pattern exists regarding their willingness to share tribal ceremonies. However, suspicion always exists because earlier government and church groups banned tribal ceremonies and events.

AI/ANs are collectivist cultures with a focus on the group that promotes reliance and a close bond with family members, community, and tribe. Older adults are looked on with clear deference and play an important role in maintaining rituals and in instructing children and grandchildren. Elders transmit the ancestral knowledge to the youth of their tribe, the community at large, and, specifically, their family. Time is not viewed as a constant or something that one can control, but rather as something that is always with the individual. Planning for the future may be viewed as foolish.

A primary social premise is that no person has the right to speak for another. Parents tend to be more silent, noninterfering, and permissive in their child-rearing practices. Children are allowed to make decisions that other cultures may consider irresponsible. For example, children may be allowed to decide whether they want to take their medicine and if they would like to live with extended family members.

Many AI/ANs remain traditional in their practice of religious activities, often taking time from work or school. The needs of the individual must be weighed against organizational requirements in the development of a reasonable solution. IHS is the only organization allowed to discriminate in hiring practices; it is required to hire an AI/AN when possible. This law is referred to as the *Indian Preference Law*.

Skin color among AI/ANs varies from light to very dark brown, depending on the tribe. Newborns and infants commonly have Mongolian spots on the sacral area.

Historically, most diseases affecting AI/ANs were infectious such as tuberculosis, smallpox, and influenza. In the past, contact with settlers who had communicable diseases eliminated entire tribes because they had no acquired immunity. Common diseases related to living in close contact with others include upper respiratory illnesses and pneumonia. Diseases of the heart, malignant neoplasm, unintentional injuries, diabetes mellitus, and cerebrovascular disease are the leading causes of AI/AN deaths.

Other conditions include a high incidence of **severe combined immunodeficiency syndrome (SCIDS)**, which results in a failure of the antibody response and cell-mediated immunity. Thus far, studies indicate that SCIDS is unique to the Navajo population. **Navajo neuropathy** has been researched since 1974, and in 2006 it was discovered to be the result of a mutation of the MPV17 gene. Characteristics of this disease include poor weight gain, short stature, sexual infantilism, serious systemic infections, and liver derangement. Manifestations include weakness, hypotonia, areflexia, loss of sensation in the extremities, corneal ulcerations, acral mutilation, and painless fractures. Individuals who survive have many complications and are ventilator dependent; none have survived past 24 years old.

Most AI/AN tribes exhibit high-risk behaviors related to alcohol misuse, with its subsequent morbidity and mortality. Many accidents are attributed to driving while under the influence of alcohol. Although alcohol is illegal on most reservations, many purchase it off the reservation, and bootleggers make money selling it on reservations at grossly inflated prices. Spousal abuse is frequently related to alcohol use. The wife is the usual recipient of the abuse, but occasionally, the husband is abused.

Food has major significance beyond nourishment in AI/AN populations. Food is offered to family and friends or may be burned to feed higher powers and those who have died. Life events, dances, healing, and religious ceremonies evolve around food. Corn is an important staple in the diet of American Indians and is used in many rituals.

AI/AN diets may be deficient in vitamin D because many members suffer from lactose intolerance or do not drink milk. Isolated tribes lack electricity for refrigeration. Therefore, they have difficulty storing fresh vegetables or milk. Distances from settlements or villages to larger off-reservation towns limit the availability of fresh food items because of shipping and storage issues.

The definitive goal for a woman in AI/AN societies is being a mother and rearing a healthy family. Traditional AI/ANs do not practice birth control and often do not limit family size.

Death rituals vary among tribes, maintaining and adapting them to their regional environments. Most AI/AN tribes believe that the souls of the dead pass into a spirit world and become part of the spiritual forces that influence every aspect of their lives. Some tribes maintain their traditional practices but use a mortuary or the IHS morgue to prepare their dead. The Pueblo tribes prepare their own dead, and only certain family members are allowed to prepare the body. Hopis bury their dead before the next setting of the sun and bury them in upright sitting positions. After the Zuni burial ceremony, the members must take off 3 days from work for a cleansing ceremony.

The individual's source of strength comes from the inner self and depends on being in harmony with one's surroundings. Spirituality cannot be separated from the healing process in ceremonies. Illnesses, especially mental illnesses, result from not being in harmony with nature, from the spirits of evil persons such as a witch, or through violation of taboos. Healing ceremonies restore an individual's balance mentally, physically, and spiritually. The following are core concepts to traditional Indian medicine:

- AI/ANs believe in a Supreme Creator.
- Each person is a threefold being composed of mind, body, and spirit.
- All physical things, living and nonliving, are a part of the spiritual world.
- The spirit existed before it came into the body and it will exist after it leaves the body.
- Illness affects the mind and the spirit as well as the body.
- Wellness is harmony with nature and spirits
- Natural unwellness is caused by violation of a taboo.
- Unnatural wellness is caused by witchcraft.
- Each of us is responsible for our own health.

Through existing treaties, the federal government assumed responsibility for the health-care needs of AI/ANs. However, with the Indian Self-Determination Act, many tribes have contracted for this money to operate their own health-care systems. Few tribal members have traditional health insurance.

Since the early 1980s, an increase has occurred in wellness-promotion activities and a return to past traditions such as running for health, avoiding alcohol, and using purification ceremonies. Mental-health programs are not well funded and are understaffed in IHS. Physicians are oriented to traditional healing practices, but if patients perceive reluctance to accept these practices, they do not reveal their use. This is especially true among older people who seek hospital or clinic treatments only when their conditions become life-threatening. Younger generations seek treatment sooner and use the health-care system more readily than do older people. However, if their parents are traditional, they may combine native traditional medicine with Western medicine.

Medicine men, diagnosticians, crystal gazers, and shamans tell them how to restore harmony. The medicine man is expected to diagnose the problem and prescribe necessary treatments for regaining health. AI/ANs receiving care within the context of Western medicine are concerned about obtaining adequate pain control. Frequently, pain control is ineffective because the intensity of their pain is not obvious to the health-care provider because patients do not request pain medication. Older adult AI/AN's view pain as something that is to be endured and may not ask for analgesics or may not understand that pain medication is available. At other times, herbal medicines are preferred and used without the knowledge of the health-care provider.

AI/AN healers are divided primarily into three categories: those working with the power of good, those working with the power of evil, or both. Generally, medicine people are from specific clans and promote activities that encourage self-discipline and self-control and involve acute body awareness. Within these three categories are several types of practitioners. Some are endowed with supernatural powers, whereas others have knowledge of herbs and specific manipulations to "suck" out the evil spirits.

Treatment regimens prescribed by a medicine man not only cure the body but also restore the mind. Acceptance of Western medicine is variable, with a blending of traditional health-care beliefs. Experienced IHS providers understand the concepts of holistic health for AI/ANs, and behavioral health specialists are beginning to make referrals to the medicine man.

People of Baltic Heritage: Estonians, Latvians, and Lithuanians

Rauda Gelazis

The Baltic countries today are democratic, growing economically, and successful when compared with many other former Soviet Union countries where poverty and dictatorships have been predominant. All three Baltic countries have established strong ties to Western democratic countries and have been accepted into the North Atlantic Treaty Organization (NATO) and the European Union. Since the mid-1990s, the Baltic countries have experienced a "brain drain" to some extent, because many of their highly educated people have emigrated to the United States and Europe.

People of Baltic descent share thoughts and feelings readily. The stereotype of quiet, stoic individuals is not borne out by observation or research. Older individuals from these cultural groups are generally first-generation Americans or immigrants who came to the United States after World War II. Many individuals are not as acculturated as younger people and often prefer to speak their own languages. Health-care providers need to be sure that any instructions given to these patients are well understood. The father or father figure is the head of the household in the typical family of Baltic heritage, although both men and women in the family may have jobs and discuss major decisions. Health-care and other major decisions are often made jointly by both spouses. Because both spouses tend to work, child care may be shared by grandparents and should be included in health teaching.

People of Baltic descent adapt readily to American values of timeliness in the workplace. Most have no difficulty maintaining their sense of autonomy and readily assume work roles and responsibility for decision making. They usually do not like to directly confront those in authority and find ways to deal with difficult situations or people through the use of humor or deference. Recent immigrants who have lived under the Soviet regime may not be accustomed to making decisions for themselves or acting autonomously, and this must be considered when they are hired.

Recent immigrants from Estonia, Latvia, and Lithuania may be at risk for cancer because of the current industrial pollution, including radiation exposure resulting from the Chernobyl nuclear disaster in 1988. Some immigrants are survivors of political torture, having spent years in prison labor camps in Siberia. When performing health assessments, health-care providers need to be alert to ill health resulting from the conditions that immigrants endured because of the political situations in their countries of origin.

Americans of Baltic descent are health conscious and believe that a well-balanced lifestyle maintains health and well-being. For example, well-being among Lithuanian Americans is typically described as a holistic concept—that is, a state of being in which the person's physical, spiritual, psychological, and social health are in balance. Moderation is perceived as desirable for living a healthy life. Natural foods are preferred, and whenever possible, vegetables and fruits are homegrown.

Americans of Baltic descent use modern Western medicine practices, are likely to obtain early prenatal medical care, and are likely to be receptive to health teaching for prenatal and postnatal care. Because they prefer natural processes, some women and families prefer natural childbirth and breastfeeding.

Grief is expressed by sadness, crying, and talking about the deceased with fondness and respect. Emotions are readily expressed but not in highly dramatic ways. Decorum is maintained in public and with strangers. Estonian Americans and Latvian Americans are predominantly Lutherans but include some Catholics. Lithuanian Americans are predominantly Roman Catholic. Most Americans of Baltic descent consider prayer an individual expression of their faith. The nurse or health-care provider should allow the patient and family to take the lead with regard to prayer. Because prayer is individualized, some patients welcome time for individual or shared prayer, whereas others do not wish to pray. Many have been sustained through hardships by their strong religious faith and continue to have strong religious needs. Patients find considerable comfort in speaking with the clergy in times of crises and serious illness.

Some stigma is attached to mental illness, but medical care is sought. The family encourages adherence to prescription medications and treatments. Most people of Baltic descent accept physical handicaps, mental illness, and mental retardation. The family usually cares for the individual at home. The community is also supportive. Americans of Baltic descent do not enjoy the sick role and avoid it when possible. People of Baltic descent are used to both men and women giving direct physical care. Physicians in the Baltic countries may be female. Health-care providers need to provide for privacy and consider the modesty needs of female and male patients of these cultures as they would for any patient.

People of Brazilian Heritage

Marga Simon Coler and Maria Adriana Felix Coler

Brazilians are a mixture of Portuguese, French, Dutch, German, Italian, Japanese, Chinese, African, Arab, and native Brazilian Indians. Information about Brazilian culture is unidentifiable in the professional health-care literature, which tends to incorporate Brazilians into aggregate data on Hispanics. Most Brazilians in the United States are concentrated in communities around Boston; New York; Newark, New Jersey; and Miami.

Portuguese is the official language of Brazil and continues to dominate the Brazilian communities in the United States. Brazilians, in general, are not punctual, arriving late—from minutes to hours—especially for social occasions. However, those in professional circles are punctual. Health-care providers may need to carefully explain the necessity of showing up on time for health appointments.

Gender roles vary according to socioeconomic class and education. Brazilian society is one of machismo, with the middle and upper classes being patriarchal in structure. As women assert their equality, more egalitarian relationships are becoming evident. However, lower-socioeconomic households tend to be more matriarchal in nature. Godparents are a very important family extension to Brazilians. Poor families frequently ask their *patron* or *patrona* (employer and his wife) to be godparents to their child. Godparent responsibilities include clothing, schooling, and caring for the child if the parents die. Health-care providers need to be nonjudgmental regarding Brazilian family decision-making patterns.

Brazilians value diplomacy over honesty, as shown in their tendency to promise to attend to something the next day, knowing that it will be impossible. This is due in part to their fatalistic beliefs and in part to the need to save face. Most Brazilians in the workforce show up for work on time and generally respect authority. They are more comfortable in employment situations in which rules and job specifications are well defined. Brazilians often have a lesser sense of responsibility than is seen in the dominant American culture. When educated people believe that they can do something

more efficiently, they are apt not to ask permission from their supervisor to do what they believe is required to complete the job.

Specific diseases related to the regional topography and climate of Brazil include dengue fever, meningitis, rabies, and yellow fever. In addition, Chagas disease, schistosomiasis, typhoid fever, Hansen's disease, hepatitis, and tuberculosis are present in various parts of Brazil. Because intestinal worms are common in Brazilian immigrants, parasitic diseases should be considered during health assessments.

The undocumented status of Brazilian immigrants places them at a high risk for nonassimilation into the culture of the community in which they live. Brazilians in America have become vitamin and health food conscious. The preference, especially among young Brazilian women, is to rely on vitamins instead of a heavy diet to help them remain thin. Undocumented Brazilians who are here to earn fast money may experience malnutrition.

Brazilian immigrants generally practice birth control so that pregnancy will not interfere with their reason for leaving Brazil. At times, single women become pregnant to facilitate their chance of remaining permanently in their new country. This opportunity is greatly enhanced if the child is born in the United States and has been able to attend school. Many restrictions are related to pregnancy. Women are encouraged not to do heavy work or swim. Taboos also warn against having sexual relations during pregnancy. During pregnancy, some foods are to be avoided and other specific foods are recommended.

The meaning of life is found in religion, economy, fatalism, and reality. The greatest source of strength for Brazilians is their immediate and extended families. Tradition and folk religion are other sources of strength.

Most Brazilians do not talk about their illnesses unless these are very serious. Generally, illness is discussed only within the family. Many Brazilians feel that talking about an illness such as cancer negatively influences their condition. Because many Brazilians tend to shun hospitals, when they are hospitalized, their families accompany them and stay around the clock. Brazilian families are eager to participate in patient care and, thus, can be taught various procedures and care activities.

Responses to death and grief depend on the family. To a poor family, a continuously suffering person is rescued. The fatalistic expression "It was God's will" helps the grieving among the rich and the poor. Older people wear black for various lengths of time, depending on the relationship of the family member. Frequently, the final portrait is hung in the family chapel or near the family altar, and prayers are recited. An eternal light burns.

The Brazilian culture is rich in folk practices that depend on geographic region, ethnic background, socioeconomic factors, and generation. Traditional and homeopathic pharmacies are supplemented by *remedios populares* (folk medicines) and *remedios caseiros* (home medicines). Health-care providers need to specifically ask about their use. Brazilians generally do not like to talk about pain. However, once the emotional barrier is removed, they feel relieved to be able to discuss their discomfort. Many pain-relieving medicines are available without a prescription in Brazil. Frequently, a person requiring these on a regular basis will request that friends or friends of friends bring a supply from Brazil.

The folk health field has many types of health-care practitioners for Brazilians. *Curandeiros* are divinely gifted; *rezadeiras* (praying women) help exorcise an illness; card readers can predict fortunes; espiritualistas are able to summon souls and spirits; conselheiros are counselors or advisors; and *catimbozeiros* are sorcerers. All have the power to heal their believers. Health-care providers need to specifically ask Brazilian patients about their use of folk healers and the treatments prescribed.

People of Egyptian Heritage
Afaf Ibrahim Meleis and Mahmoud Hanafi Meleis

Egypt is considered part of 22 Arabic-speaking countries in North Africa and as a Middle Eastern country. Scholarly literature about Egyptians in the United States is limited. Most Egyptians Americans are Sunni Muslims but are diverse in many ways. However, only the most common patterns of responses and experiences of Egyptian Americans with regard to health and illness are presented in this chapter. An influential part of modern Egyptian history is the Arab-Israeli conflict. The conflict between Egypt and Israel ended in 1979 when the two countries signed the Camp David Accords. Another important turning point for Egyptians, as well as Egyptian Americans, in their identity and connection to their cultural heritage is the February 2011 revolution that ousted President Hosni Mubarak. Egyptians have immigrated to the United States to escape economic stagnation, for educational opportunities, for career options, and for economic incentives that reward hard-working individuals.

The terrorist attacks in New York, Pennsylvania, and Washington, DC, and the tragic consequences of September 11, 2001, have rendered many newly immigrated Egyptian Americans vulnerable to profiling and stereotyping in the United States of America. Therefore, a newly acquired sense of stigma tends to influence their patterns of responses in ways that were not manifested previously.

The dominant language of Egyptians is **Arabic**. The written Arabic language is the same in all Arab countries, but spoken Arabic is dialectal and does not necessarily follow proper Arabic grammar. A number of Arabic dialects are spoken in Egypt. Despite these different dialects and their distinct vocabularies, neither Egyptians nor Egyptian Americans have any noticeable communication barriers among themselves.

Several values govern interaction patterns among Egyptians. The first is respect, ***ihteram***, which is expected when speaking with those who are older and those in higher social positions. A second important value, politeness, ***adab***, is related to what is appropriate, expected, and socially sanctioned. Truth and reality may be sacrificed for what is appropriate and polite. Politeness results in a preference for more indirect modes of communication. Sharing negative news directly or asking for things directly is not polite. Therefore, a poor prognosis of an illness is not immediately shared; calamities should be slowly and deliberately introduced and shared in stages.

Egyptian Americans tend to be in touch with their inner feelings and are highly expressive of them; however, this expression is governed by external orientation, spontaneity, and the differences between private and public spheres. Because their personal space boundaries tend to be small, they stand and sit very close to one another. Most speak with expressive words and facial expressions, gesticulating with hands and using body movements. Devout Muslim men and women do not touch each other; even a handshake is not practiced.

Respect for individuals is demonstrated in the use of certain titles: *inta* (you) for those in equal or lower positions, and *hadretak* (you) for those in higher-ranking positions or for older people. Older people should never be called by their first names without an adjective or title attached to the name. The man is formally considered the head of the household; however, the demands of life on immigrants and nuclear families force couples to share responsibilities and decision making. Egyptian American family roles change considerably after immigration.

Children are treasured and viewed as security for their parents' future. During their early years, they are expected to be studious and goal oriented, respectful, and loyal to the family. When they become adults, they are expected to take care of their parents. However, second-generation Egyptians tend to blend with other Americans. The greatest calamity that may happen in a Christian or Muslim Egyptian American household is to have a daughter lose her virginity prematurely. This fear stems from a potential lack of marriageability of the daughter, loss of face for the father, and gossip within the Egyptian American community.

Although Egyptians in their own country have extended families, Egyptian American families tend to be more nuclear. They also prefer family gatherings to adult gatherings where they often include extended family and their new networks of friends.

Egyptian immigrants tend to be team players and effective contributors to the society at large. They are usually punctual and follow work rules and procedures. Being well assimilated, they create a close network of colleagues.

Pap smears for unmarried women are discouraged and considered totally unacceptable because of the expectations for preserving virginity until marriage. Gynecological examinations are given only to married women, usually during the checkup for a first pregnancy.

Egyptians entertain lavishly and enjoy good food, which represents nurturing. The more food one provides, the more love is portrayed. Egyptians develop trust in one another by having a meal together. The more food a person eats, the greater the potential for being healthy. Thus, children tend to be overfed. Food is associated with generosity and giving. To offer food and to accept food are indications of friendship. Mealtime is for eating and for socializing but not for conducting business or discussing issues.

Most devout Muslims do not consume pork or drink alcohol. Egyptian Copts may consume both in moderation. Ramadan calls for a month of fasting to experience the plight of the poor and the underprivileged. Fasting precludes taking anything by mouth or intravenously and abstaining from sexual activities. Even Egyptian Americans who do not follow and abide by the teachings of Islam during the year consider this month holy, and they become more devout during Ramadan.

Women are advised to curtail physical activities during pregnancy for fear of miscarriage. Women are also advised to eat more because they are feeding two. Some Egyptian American women have strong cravings for certain foods. They believe if these foods are not consumed, babies may be marked with the shape of the foods that were craved.

Egyptians react vigorously and dramatically to the loss of a family member, expressing their grief outwardly. Wailing and public crying occur when first learning of death. This public reaction is an expected demonstration of their grief; otherwise, the community may regard them as lacking affection for the deceased. Among Muslims, the burial ritual includes cleaning the body and wrapping it in a white cotton cloth.

Prayers, even for the nondevout Muslim or Christian, are significant during times of illness. Egyptian Americans may bring the *Qur'an* or the Bible to their hospital beds and usually put it under the pillow or on the bedside table. Prayers may be recited by the individual or in groups.

Whereas Egyptian Americans are usually well educated, their views are colored by beliefs about the influence of imbalances, the evil eye, and Islamic beliefs about the role God plays in their illness. However, they are firm believers in Western medicine's miraculous ability to treat and cure illnesses.

Cleanliness and hygiene are integral to practicing Muslims. A number of elaborate prayer rituals are also related to health care and prevention of illness. For example, before praying, Muslims must engage in a purification ritual, which consists of washing every exposed body part. Prayer, required five times daily, consists of elaborate bending and kneeling movements in systematic ways, increasing a person's range of movements, limbering stretches, and meditative poses.

Typically, Egyptian Americans experiencing a health problem consult family members and friends before visiting a trusted health-care provider. Once in the health-care system, they prefer immediate, personalized attention. They value tests and prescriptions for their illnesses and follow medical regimens and prescriptions carefully, particularly if they consist of oral medications, injections, or both. Egyptian Americans tend to share medications freely and use Western medications and home remedies such as herbs, hot compresses, and hot fluids and foods. They also believe that vitamins given intramuscularly and intravenously are more effective than vitamins taken in pills.

Egyptians believe the evil eye is responsible for personal calamities. The evil eye is cast by those who have blue eyes, by those who tend to speak of an admired person or object in a boastful manner, or by the mere description of beauty, wealth, or health without saying some verses from the *Qur'an* or Bible. These verses protect the person from losing whatever good they possess. Some use blue beads or religious verses inscribed on charms to protect them or their children from the evil eye. Children are particularly at risk for the evil eye and need more protection than adults.

Egyptians avoid pain at all costs by seeking prompt interventions. They tend to be verbally and nonverbally expressive about pain; moaning, groaning, sighing, and holding the painful body part tightly are common expressions of pain. Although they tend to be more constrained in front of health-care providers or other "strangers," they are quite expressive in front of family members. Egyptian descriptions of pain may not be as specific as the Western health-care system prefers. Egyptians present a more generalized description of pain, regardless of whether it is localized. They usually describe general weakness, dizziness, or overall tension and stress associated with pain. They also use metaphors reflecting humoral medicine such as earth, rocks, fire, heat, and cold to describe their pain.

Mental and emotional issues tend to be expressed somatically; psychosomatic interventions are more effective than psychologically based interventions. They also do not like to call treatments "psychotherapy" or "analysis" but prefer to call it "counseling." Disabilities are usually hidden from public view. Whereas there are public sympathy and acceptance of people with disabilities, families still tend to be protective and shield them from public display.

Egyptian Americans have no taboos against blood transfusions or organ transplants. All measures needed to heal, cure, or prolong life are welcomed.

Accustomed to Egyptian physicians whose clinical judgments and skills have been developed within a system that lacks adequate resources for meticulous diagnoses, some may misperceive an American physician's thoroughness as a lack of experience or appropriate knowledge. Therefore, they may shop for physicians whose clinical judgments are congruent with their cultural expectations of a prompt and firm diagnosis.

Sharing the intimate details of their health history is enhanced if the health-care provider is the same gender. Egyptian Americans may also view older female physicians as more experienced and, therefore, more trustworthy than younger female physicians. The physician's age, years of experience, and position in the organization may indicate better qualifications.

People of French Canadian Heritage

Myriam Gauthier and Ginette Lazure

Canada, with a population of 34 million and an area of more than 3,800,000 square miles, is larger than the entire United States but has only one-ninth the population. One-quarter of the population uses French as their mother tongue, and the rest speak French as a second language. The **Métis**, descendants of Native Americans and Europeans, are mainly, though not entirely, French-speaking. Some regard the Métis as a historically and culturally distinct people in their own right. Another major portion of Canada's French-speaking population is the **Acadians**, descendants of the early French colonists. Canadians whose first language is French are called **Francophones**.

Canada has two official languages, French and English. Regional differences exist in accent, vocabulary, and degree of Anglicization. Oral communication, in particular, has undergone assimilation. Indian words have been added, and English words are incorporated into a syntax and grammar that is essentially French, resulting in a dialect, **Joual** in Québec and **Chiac** in New Brunswick.

Among French Canadians, a conversation may be conducted with high voice crescendos that do not necessarily mean anger or violence. Volume can increase with the importance and the emotional charge invested in the content of the message. Nonverbal communication patterns for French Canadians encourage sharing thoughts and feelings. Acadians are more reserved, quieter, shy, even self-effacing, and are less likely to share their thoughts and feelings than people from Québec. The use of hand gestures for emphasis when speaking is common.

When in the intimacy zone, people may touch frequently and converse in close physical space; however, they tend to avoid physical contact in public. When greeting another person, men usually shake hands, an approach recommended for health-care providers. Eye contact is an important way for the health practitioner to acknowledge whether the person has understood or is following what is being said.

Under Québec law, a woman keeps her maiden name throughout her lifetime, although in other parts of Canada, the husband and wife decide what name the wife will use. A Québécois family of two spouses and two children may well include four different surname combinations: One child may have the father's surname or the mother's surname alone or a hyphenated or nonhyphenated surname composed of those of the father and mother. For a second child, the surnames are the same, but in reverse order. The decision for using surnames rests entirely with the parents and must appear on the birth certificate.

Traditionally, the Catholic Church dictated the parameters of sexual behavior, with a high priority placed on marriage and the begetting and raising of children. In the years before 1960, abstinence from premarital sex was encouraged, and a sexual double-standard existed, whereas the 1970s and 1980s witnessed a liberalization of sexual norms and the establishment of more egalitarian relationships between young men and women. In 1996, the Canadian government extended health, relocation, and other job benefits to same-sex partners of federal employees. During the same year, the Ontario Court of Appeals ruled that same-sex couples must be treated as common-law couples under the Family Leave Act. Canada is one of the few countries in the world where same-sex marriage is legalized.

The primary causes of death among the Québec population are cancer, with an increase in lung cancer in women, and cardiovascular diseases. Prostate cancer is high among the Francophone population of Québec. Genetic susceptibility to breast and ovarian cancer is high among French Canadians. The suicide rate in Québec is higher than in any other province and occurs more often in rural areas than in urban areas. Few countries surpass the Québec mortality rate by suicide. Eighty percent of all suicides reported in 1991 involved men. The population's osteoarthritic disorders and the prevalence of multiple sclerosis are among the highest in the world.

A number of hereditary and genetic diseases are more common among Québécois, including spastic ataxia Charlevoix-Saguenay type, cystic fibrosis, tyrosinaemia, and cytochrome lipase deficiency (COX), to name a few. Familial chylomicronemia resulting from the lipoprotein lipase (LPL) deficiency, hyperlipoproteinemia type I, is the highest frequency worldwide. A rare genetic disease among French Canadian newborns is phenylketonuria (PKU). In addition, increased incidences of cystic fibrosis and muscular dystrophy occur among French-speaking Canadians.

The French population has a long-standing appreciation of alcohol, with wine being their beverage of choice. Alcohol consumption has increased since the early 1990s, particularly among men; drinking and driving among young men has reached a summit despite the legal implications. Impaired driving is still the leading cause of fatalities on Québec roads.

Good health practices are more prevalent among Canadian men under the age of 25 years and over the age of 65 than among men in their middle adult years. In contrast to men, the prevalence of good health practices among Canadian women increases until the age of 65 and then decreases. These practices were positively correlated with levels of education in both sexes, adequate income for women, and managerial or professional occupations for men.

Food is associated with hospitality and warmth and is part of all meetings and celebrations. Common vegetables enjoyed by French Canadians include potatoes, turnips, carrots, asparagus, cabbage, lettuce, cucumbers, and tomatoes. Apart from citrus fruits, all other edible fruits, particularly apples and berries grown in gardens or in the wild, are prepared and preserved by French Canadians for the winter. Meat choices are mainly beef, pork, and poultry. Lately, however, lamb has gained popularity. In Acadia, owing to the proximity of the coastal areas, fresh fish and seafood are part of the diet.

Until the middle of the 20th century, French Canadians maintained high fertility rates, which is uncommon for a population living in an industrialized country. The "overfertility" of French Canadians appears to be a response to socialization that is distinguished by the prevalence of extended family ties. However, as education increases, the fertility rate within the Francophone group decreases, whereas the contrary is observed within the English group, meaning that as education level increases, so does the fertility rate. For many years, French Canadian fertility practices have been closely tied to the Catholic religion. The number of children per family started to decline from 3.1 in 1965 to 1.5 in 1990, with a current record of 1.1 children per family.

Midwives have officially been accepted by the government, but the use of midwives and maternity centers is far from being customary, mostly because of a fear of problematical labor. More women are talking about the desire to deliver at home, but the actual use of a midwife throughout labor and delivery at home is quite low. Fathers are encouraged to be present in the delivery room. They are invited to assume an active role by assisting the mother and the physician, receiving the baby, cutting the cord, and "kangaroo's father care"—placing the infant in direct skin-to-skin contact. With the advent of birthing rooms, more women are delivering their babies in half-sitting or side-lying positions.

Rooming-in of the mother and child is a relatively new practice. Breastfeeding has regained importance after years of bottle-feeding. The mother's general hesitation to breastfeed relates to not having sufficient milk, experiencing sore nipples, losing breast firmness, and muscle wasting after the breastfeeding period. In practice, once the mother has made a decision regarding breastfeeding, the father's support and encouragement are key for a successful outcome.

French Canadians' issues related to death and death rituals are closely related to Christian religious practices. If death is expected, part of the preparation is the vigil, where a family member will stay with the dying person. During this time, in devout families, people will usually recite prayers, and a priest is often called in to deliver the Sacrament of the Sick. During the viewing, if the person was religious, a relative might be designated to say the rosary. Religious services are either full funeral masses held in the deceased's parish church or a more intimate service at the funeral home. Graveside rites are generally brief and include a few prayers and a blessing.

Traditionally, French Canadians buried their dead according to Roman Catholic rites. Over the last few decades, however, cremation has become a common alternative to burial. Ashes are usually buried in the cemetery or placed in a mausoleum. Grief is usually expressed with "restrained sincerity." Genuine grief is viewed with compassion, but displays of keening and wailing are usually seen as unsincere and overly dramatic.

Whereas most French Canadians identify themselves as Roman Catholic and are baptized at birth, they may or may not remain active church members. A growing number of births are registered through civil channels rather than through the traditional Catholic registry and baptism. Despite the sharp decline in actively practicing Catholics, most people from all socioeconomic levels turn to their church for important life events such as marriage and funerals.

Older adults are more inclined to use prayers for finding strength and for adapting to difficult physical, psychological, and social health problems. In times of illness and tragedy, many French-speaking Canadians use prayer to help recovery. The younger generation is not strongly influenced by religious values, beliefs, and faith practices. They tend to turn to spirituality rather than religion. Renewed interest in spirituality across Canada is being recognized as a source of physical and psychological health.

The health beliefs, values, and practices of the French Canadian population are very similar to those of other Canadians. Being healthy is described as having reached balance in one's life, taking into consideration the relationship among the physical, mental, social, and spiritual aspects of the person. Health-seeking behaviors span the gamut of diet, exercise, sleep, home remedies, a belief in a spiritual being, and consulting health-care providers. Canada's government-administered health system ensures free, universal health coverage at any point of entry into the system. However, many people in the upper socioeconomic classes call on their family physicians instead of the local community service centers. Among the lower-socioeconomic classes of Québec and the Maritimes, many do not seek health care until their health becomes a crisis situation. French Canadians have no official proscription against receiving blood or blood products. Those who are members of a religious group that prohibits the acceptance of a blood transfusion are rare in Canada. The decision to donate or receive an organ or a tissue is an individual decision.

Health-care providers hold a favorable status in the eyes of French Canadians, especially among older people. Today, folk and traditional practitioners are almost nonexistent.

People of Greek Ancestry

Irena Papadopoulos and Larry D. Purnell

The Greek and Greek Cypriot diaspora is of considerable size and is spread to all continents and numerous countries. The largest Greek community outside Greece is in America, whereas the largest Greek Cypriot community outside Greece is in Britain. The characteristics of Greek and Greek Cypriot communities vary considerably according to the time of immigration; rural, island, or urban residence; and other variant cultural characteristics.

Despite considerable temporal and geographic variation, several core themes are common to people who retain affiliation with a Greek community: emphasis on family, honor, religion, education, and Greek heritage. The core values of honor, respect, and shame are key when considering the experience of Greeks and Greek Cypriots. Because Greeks and Greek Cypriots value warmth, expressiveness, and spontaneity, northern Europeans are often viewed as "cold" and lacking compassion. Eye contact is generally direct, and speaking and sitting distances are closer than those of other European Americans. Whereas innermost feelings such as anxiety or depression are often shielded from outsiders, anger is expressed freely, sometimes to the discomfort of those from less-expressive groups. Thus, health-care providers must not take personal offense with verbal and nonverbal communication practices that are different from theirs.

Greek children are included in most family social activities and tend not to be left with babysitters. The child may be disciplined through teasing, which is thought to "toughen" children and make them highly conscious of public opinion. Providers must interpret these child-rearing practices within their cultural context.

Treatment of older people reflects the themes of closeness and respect within the family. Grandparents tend to participate fully in family activities. Families feel responsible to care for their parents in old age, and children are expected to take in widowed parents. Failure to do so results in a sense of dishonor for the son and guilt for the daughter. Health-care providers need to thoroughly assess the family beliefs when considering long-term care.

In regard to the workforce, probably no single characteristic applies so completely to members of the Greek and Greek Cypriot communities as the emphasis on self-reliance within a family context. Greeks and Greek Cypriots in North America, Britain, Australia, and Sweden stress this trait, seen as reluctance to be told what to do and given as a major reason for their pattern of establishing their own businesses as soon as possible.

Two important genetic conditions, thalassemia and glucose-6-phosphate dehydrogenase (G-6-PD), are seen in relatively high proportions among Greek populations. Drugs such as aspirin, primaquine, quinidine, thiazolsulfone, dapsone, furzolidone, nitrofural, naphthalene, toluidine blue, phenylhydrazine, and chloramphenicol can induce a hemolytic crisis. This threat is sufficiently severe that the World Health Organization recommends that all hospital populations in areas with high proportions of Greeks and Greek Cypriots be screened for G-6-PD deficiency before drug therapy is offered.

Fasting is an integral part of the Greek Orthodox religion. General fast days are Wednesdays and Fridays; nowadays, these are observed only by some older people. Greek Orthodox wishing to take Holy Communion observe at least 3 days of fasting. However, people with health conditions and small children are exempt from fasting. The prevalence of lactose maldigestion among Greek adults is about 75 percent; however, milk intolerance is rarely seen in children. Health-care providers should use this knowledge when counseling clients with these conditions.

If a pregnant woman remarks that a food smells good, or if she has a craving for a particular food, it should be offered to her; otherwise, the child may be "marked." This is the usual explanation for birthmarks.

After a death in the Greek community, pictures and mirrors may be turned over. During a wake, women may sing dirges or chant. In some regions, people practice "screaming the dead," in which they cry a lament, the *miroloyi*. This ritual may involve screaming, lamenting, and sobbing by female kin. After death, family and close relatives, who stay at home, mourn for 40 days. Close male relatives do not shave, as a mark of respect.

The Greek Orthodox religion emphasizes faith rather than specific tenets. Easter is considered the most important of holy days, and nearly all Greeks and Greek Cypriots in America and Britain attempt to honor the day. Women often consider faith an important factor in regaining health. Family members may make "bargains" with saints, such as promises to fast, be faithful, or make church donations if the saint acts on behalf of an ill family member.

Three traditional folk healing practices are particularly notable: those related to *matiasma* (bad eye or the evil eye), *practika* (herbal remedies), and *vendouses* (cupping). Matiasma results from the envy or admiration of others. Whereas the evil eye can harm a wide variety of things, including inanimate objects, children are particularly susceptible to attack. Common symptoms of matiasma include headache, chills, irritability, restlessness, and lethargy; in extreme cases, matiasma has resulted in death.

Ponos (pain) is the cardinal symptom of ill health and an evil that needs eradication. The person in pain is not expected to suffer quietly or stoically in the presence of family. The family is relied on to find resources to relieve the pain or, failing that, to share in the experience of suffering. However, in the presence of outsiders, the lack of restraint in pain expression suggests lack of self-control. Although the experience of physical pain is acknowledged publicly, emotional pain is hidden within the privacy of the family.

Many Greeks and Greek Cypriots display a general distrust of all professionals and may "shop around" for physicians and other health-care providers to obtain additional opinions. The use of several physicians simultaneously may result in untoward drug interactions from conflicting multiple drug use.

People of Guatemalan Heritage

Tina A. Ellis and Larry D. Purnell

People of Guatemalan heritage compose a growing number of Hispanic/Latino populations in the United States. Whereas some Guatemalans may share a common Spanish language with other Hispanic ethnic groups, they are, nonetheless, a unique cultural group. Guatemala continues to be plagued by "abject" poverty, resulting in more than 600,000 legal and undocumented Guatemalan immigrants in the United States. Most Guatemalans are a mixture of Spanish and Mayan Indian heritage. A small group of black Guatemalans have an ancestry from the Caribbean and Africa. This accounts for variations in skin color, facial features, hair, body structure, and other biological variations.

Although many Guatemalans speak Spanish, many speak one of 23 Amerindian languages, including Quiche, Cakchiquel, Kekchi, Mam, Garifuna, and Xinca. Each Mayan ethnic group speaks one dialect as their primary language. Most Guatemalan people tend to value the past and live in the present, being more concerned with today than the future because the future is uncertain for many.

Because work is such a priority in the life of many Guatemalans, they seek health care only when their illness has progressed to the point of preventing them from working or carrying out their duties or roles within the family. Taking time to go to the doctor means time lost from work and loss of pay.

Guatemalans who have a Hispanic heritage use the Spanish format for names. At birth, a child is given a first name (Ovidio), followed by the surname of his father (Garcia), and then the surname of his mother (Salvador), resulting in Ovidio Garcia Salvador. When referring to him as Mr. (*señor*), it would be appropriate to use Señor Garcia. Men's names remain the same through their lifetime. However, when a woman named Jovita Garcia Salvador marries Francisco Vasquez Gutierrez, she then becomes Jovita Garcia de Vasquez or simply Jovita Garcia Vasquez. She should be addressed as Mrs. (*señora*) Vasquez.

To convey respect, health-care providers should address Guatemalans in a formal manner unless otherwise requested by the patient. Male children and adults are referred to as Mr. (*señor*). Females are referred to as Ms. or Miss (*señorita*) or Mrs. (*señora*). Highly respected persons in the community are often referred to as *Don* (male) or *Doña* (female), followed by the person's first name. For example, one respected gentleman is referred to as *Don* Martin and a respected nurse is referred to as *Doña* Alma. Guatemalans are customarily greeted with a handshake.

In rural areas, people shake hands softly. A firm handshake indicates aggressive behavior. Guatemalans avoid direct eye contact with others, including health-care providers, which is a way of demonstrating respect and should not be misinterpreted as avoidance, low self-esteem, or disinterest. They speak softly in public. Speaking loud is considered rude. Many Guatemalan families follow traditional roles for husbands, wives, and children, although this is changing for some, especially in the United States.

Guatemalans place a high value on the family and the extended family. Most families are nuclear—comprising a father, mother, and children. Extended family is important to Guatemalans and may include grandparents, aunts, uncles, and cousins. Children are taught to be obedient and demonstrate respect for older people.

Most Guatemalans in the United States work in agriculture, housekeeping, or the restaurant business. Guatemalans may miss work owing to an illness of a loved one, a need for transportation to an appointment, or a lack of child care. Because punctuality is not valued in Guatemala, the Guatemalan employee in the United States may arrive for work late. Some may not wear a watch, be able to tell time, or understand the importance of punctuality in the United States.

Guatemalans tend to respect persons in positions of authority. Those of lower socioeconomic status and/or with formal education and English-language skills usually acquire positions with responsibility but little authority.

Men who immigrate to the United States from Guatemala for work may find themselves drinking alcohol excessively, even if they did not prior to migration. This may be due to such factors as the stress of living in another country illegally; being away from family, friends, and support systems; fears of inadequate work and deportation; and illness and being victims of violence and injury. They may live with other men they hardly know.

Food to Guatemalans signifies physical, spiritual, and cultural wellness. Foods vary among Guatemalans based on cultural traditions and accessibility. Guatemalans value corn because it brings good health. Corn is eaten at every meal, most often in the form of tortillas. The Mayan diet primarily consists of maize, black beans, rice, chicken, squash, tomatoes, carrots, chilies, beets, cauliflower, lettuce, cabbage, chard, leeks, onions, and garlic.

Guatemalans value life beginning from conception; a baby is a gift from God. For religious reasons, most do not believe in contraception or abortion. Mayan women do not believe in lying down to give birth or delivering in a hospital. Following delivery, the placenta has to be burned, not buried, because it is disrespectful to the earth to do so. Guatemalan women may continue breastfeeding until the child reaches the age of 5 years. Moreover, they may be breastfeeding a new baby while continuing to breastfeed a toddler.

Some Guatemalans relate their illness to "punishment" or impending death to "God's will" and refuse an intervention or heroic measures to reverse the outcome. Guatemalans believe in burial; they do not practice cremation. Yellow is the color of mourning. When a Guatemalan dies in the United States, the family may request repatriation, because it is important for the final resting place to be the home country. Often, immediate and extended family will pool their resources to send the body home.

Most Guatemalans are Roman Catholic. Many integrate aspects of Catholicism into their lives, while continuing to believe in the spirituality of their ancestors in private. Family provides Guatemalans with meaning in their lives. Life revolves around the nuclear and extended family. Whether Catholic, Protestant, or traditional Maya, many believe that life's events happen for a reason. The reason may be attributed to favor from God or the gods when positive experiences occur and to punishment or disfavor from God or the gods when negative events occur. Some feel nothing can be done to change the outcome of these experiences. This belief is referred to as *fatalism*.

The preferred mode of treatment among Guatemalans is medication administered by hypodermic injection. For example, if an infant has a cold, Guatemalans believe an injection is necessary to treat it effectively. If someone has the flu, an IV infusion is preferred. Intramuscular medications are preferred to those taken orally.

Health-care seeking among Guatemalans generally occurs by first seeking advice from a mother, grandmother, or other respected elder. If this approach is unsuccessful, then the family usually seeks health care from folk healers. Many are fearful of hospitals. In Guatemala, when hospital care is necessary, patients are often seriously ill, resulting in death, which perpetuates the belief that "hospitals are places where patients go to die."

Guatemalans tend to view health and illness in relation to their ability to perform duties associated with their roles. As long as women are functioning in their role of caring for the home and family, and men are functioning in their job, then they feel "healthy." When an illness prevents normal functioning required for their roles, then Guatemalans view it seriously.

The cause of debilitating illness or disease may be viewed as punishment from God rather than lack of prevention or early detection. Sometimes early warning signs of illness or disease are ignored in hopes they will go away on their own. When symptoms persist, fear may keep the Guatemalan patient from seeking medical attention. Some Guatemalans fear venipuncture because taking blood leaves the body without enough blood to keep them strong and healthy.

Guatemalans have great respect and admiration for health-care providers, who are viewed as authority figures with clinical expertise. Guatemalans expect their health-care provider to have the appearance and manners of a professional. When this is not the case, Guatemalans may lose confidence in the provider. Guatemalans are very private and are not accustomed to discussing issues and concerns openly. It may take a while to develop the necessary trust in and rapport with the provider for them to share. They fear disclosure may result in deportation or rejection. Patients also fear confidentiality will not be maintained in the health-care setting.

Guatemalan women are usually very modest. They may refuse to discuss personal issues or receive an examination by a male health-care provider. Likewise, a male Guatemalan patient may refuse a female health-care provider. Because Guatemalans dislike conflict, they may not actually refuse care, but they may withhold personal information owing to discomfort with the health-care provider. Incorporating these preferences into the encounter with Guatemalan patients enhances the development of relationships that result in effective and meaningful care.

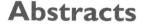

People of Iranian Heritage

Homeyra Hafizi and Hydeh Hafizi

Iran is a geographically and ethnically diverse, non–Arabic-speaking Muslim country. Iran's 1979 Revolution generated a steady wave of immigration to North America, Europe, and Australia. Since the 1979 Revolution, Iran's socioeconomic and political instability and the most recent power shifts in the Middle East have spurred emigration. Many Iranian immigrants face considerable ethnic bias in the United States, with an intensity directly linked to the ongoing events in the Middle East. Over 400,000 Iranians live in the United States, although unofficially the estimate may be over 1 million. The political climate discourages some Iranian immigrants from disclosing their native origin; hence, they self-identify as "other" or "white." **Farsi** is the national language of Iran; however, nearly half the country's population speaks different languages and dialects, such as Turkish, Kurdish, Armenian, or Baluchi.

Even though the focus of this chapter is on cultural commonalities and aggregate data, health-care providers must recognize that Iranians are a highly diverse population. Overemphasis on culture, religion, and ethnicity as the defining factors in the expression of health and illness, treatment-seeking behaviors, and health-maintenance practices can lead to stereotyping.

A central tenet of the Iranian social life and personal development is the boundary between inside/private (**baten**) and outside/public (**zaher**). The most private and true self is always kept for intimate spaces and trusted relations. "Inside" and "outside" define both individuals and families, in which honor and social shame play powerful roles. Challenges particular to the older population of Iranian immigrants have been learning the language, adapting to the new culture and lifestyle, and redefining the relationship between parent and child.

Iranians greatly value education and expect their children to do well. Iranian immigrants strive to maintain a social façade of affluence and upper-class status because family judgment and social shame weigh heavy on their decision making. Many immigrants who held white-collar positions in Iran are unable to find comparable work in the United States.

Not verbalizing one's thoughts is viewed as a customary and useful defensive behavior. This form of communication, also known as **ta'arof**, can effectively hinder open exchange of feelings with the health-care provider.

More traditional married couples do not publicly display outward affections to each other; however, most are vocal in expression of love for their children. Greeting is often accompanied by a kiss on each cheek (maybe three kisses) and/or a handshake. A slight bow or nod while shaking hands shows respect. Crossing one's legs when sitting is acceptable, but slouching in a chair or stretching one's legs toward another person is considered offensive. Nonverbal beckoning is done by waving the fingers with the palm mostly up. Tilting the head up quickly means no and down means yes. Extending the thumb (like thumbs-up) is considered a vulgar sign.

As in other Mediterranean cultures, personal distance is generally closer than that of Americans or Northern Europeans. The strength of the relationship affects how freely participants touch one another. Iranians maintain intense eye contact between intimates and equals of the same gender. This behavior may be observed less in traditional Iranians.

Time orientation is a combination of emphasis on the present and on the future. The ideal is to maintain a balance between enjoying life to the fullest and ensuring a comfortable future.

Iranians refrain from calling older people and those in higher status by their first names. Traditional, and many nontraditional, women do not take the surname of their husbands. Iranians give their name with the given name (first name) first followed by their surname (last name).

Consistent with traditional collectivistic cultures, Iranian families value harmony within an established patriarchal hierarchy. Also valued are avoidance of open conflict, unconditional respect for parents, and indirect and figurative communication to maintain social hierarchy and group harmony. In the father's absence, the oldest son has authority.

Young women are expected to remain sexually inactive until they marry, but sexual activity by men outside marriage is tolerated. Dating is not allowed in the most traditional Iranian families but is tolerated in more acculturated families. Many Iranian adolescents in the United States resemble their American counterparts in dress and outward behavior; they often behave more respectfully toward family members, particularly older people and other highly respected individuals and members of the family.

Religious women living outside Iran may avoid bright colors, cover their arms and legs, and conceal their heads with head covers or scarves (**hijab**). In Iran, wearing the *hijab* is mandatory because of the ruling Islamic Republic.

Although homosexuality undoubtedly occurs in Iranians as frequently as in any other group, it is highly stigmatized. Iranian gays and lesbians do not easily disclose their sexual orientation because they would be against both a religious and a cultural norm. The punishment is death if the participants are consenting adults of sound mind. In contrast to the older generation, younger Iranians in the United States are increasingly tolerant of alternative lifestyles.

Iranians may perceive and actually experience a degree of bias at work. There is a general lack of understanding that the countries of the Middle East and their people are very different in ethnic identity and culture. More acculturated immigrant professionals respond flexibly in the workplace. Efficiency and efficacy supersede personal communication and human connection.

In the United States, many Iranians experience stress-related health problems from cultural conflict and loss, homesickness, and the previous conditions of war. Iranians' high-risk health behaviors are similar to those in the general population. Among both men and women, smoking is more prevalent in Iran than in the immigrant population residing in the United States. Alcohol is prohibited by the **Qur'an**, the Holy Book of the Islamic faith. However, Iranians who are not devoutly religious drink socially, only in private places, and sometimes to excess.

Iranian food is flavorful, with a lengthy preparation time. Presentation is important. At any given table, a pleasing mixture of foods of different colors and ingredients, composed of a balance of **garm** (hot) and **sard** (cold). Islam has a strict set of dietary prescriptions, **halal**, and proscriptions, **haram**. Slaughter of poultry, beef, and lamb must be done in a ritual manner to make the meat *halal*. Strict Muslims avoid pork and alcoholic beverages; a few avoid shellfish. Historically, pork was prohibited for hygienic reasons. Compliance with proscriptive food and beverage items is seen less frequently among the younger generations.

Based on humoral theory, Iranians classify foods into one of two categories: *garm* (hot) and *sard* (cold). The categories sometimes correspond to high- and low-calorie foods. The key to humoral theory is balance and moderation. The belief is that too much of any one category can cause symptoms of being "overheated" or "chilled."

Food cravings during pregnancy are believed to result from the needs of the fetus; thus, cravings must be satisfied. Special attention is given to the balance of hot and cold food items. Heavy work is believed to cause miscarriage.

During the birthing process, in the more traditional families, the father is usually not present. The postpartum period can be as long as 30 to 40 days. Some families believe in keeping an infant home for the first 10 to 15 days, after which time the infant is strong enough to handle environmental pathogens.

Family members and friends gather to support the dying person and one another. Among devote Muslims, the deathbed, or at least the patient's face, is turned to face Mecca. Withdrawal of life support may be considered as "playing God." This is not to say that Iranians absolutely defy withdrawal of life support. There may be no objection to beginning life support, viewing it as a gift of medical technology. Cremation is not practiced in Iran. It is unlikely for Iranians in other countries to practice cremation, but cases of personal choice have been documented.

Grieving may be expressed outwardly and loud. Black is the customary color for clothing. On the anniversary of the death, the family gathers again.

During the month of **Ramadan**, devout Muslims fast from sunrise to sunset, although certain individuals are exempt from fasting, such as those whose health is in jeopardy. Prayer is observed five times per day by those who have a strong faith.

The sacred traditions include beliefs in the evil eye and *jinns* as evil spirits. Healing is reached through eliminating impurities from the body or by prayers. Galenic medicine is a way of life, a daily practice in health promotion and wellness, illness, disease, and injury prevention; and health promotion and wellness. Modern medicine is viewed more curative in nature. Biomedicine and humoral medicine complement each other.

Among Iranians, *narahati* is a general term used to express a wide range of undifferentiated, unpleasant emotional or physical feelings such as feeling depressed, uneasy, nervous, disappointed, or, generally speaking, not well. Iranians may use somatization to communicate emotional distress in a way that is culturally sanctioned and socially understood. In some instances, a sudden ailment may be attributed to the evil eye, **cheshm-i-bad**, the belief that negative thoughts and jealousy can cause illness. *Cheshm-i-bad* can be the result of an intentional or unintentional projection of a thought. Acculturated immigrants use the terminology in everyday speech and encounters; however, most do not fully believe in the concept.

Self-medication is common, with prescription medications, over-the-counter remedies, and homemade herbal preparations used simultaneously. When ill, Iranians rely heavily on family members for support and assistance. The patient may behave passively while the family appears persuasive in medical encounters. If a patient is hospitalized, visiting is frequent, sometimes excessive according to U.S. standards.

Most Iranians are expressive about their pain. Some justify suffering in the light of rewards in the afterlife. Blood transfusions, organ donations, and organ transplants are widely accepted among Iranians. In Iran, donation of organs has become a business transaction: if a kidney is needed, it can be purchased.

Iranians appreciate state-of-the-art facilities, high-technological equipment, and skilled professionals. Many Iranian clients expect to receive a definitive diagnosis and a clear road map for treatment, including prescriptions and therapies. They may not ask too many questions or inquire about different modalities, believing that the provider knows best. The most respected health-care provider is an educated and experienced physician.

Abstracts

People of Irish Heritage

Sarah A. Wilson

The history of the Irish in America has not been harmonious. Early immigrants were subjected to religious persecution and economic discrimination. Irish Americans are a diverse group, and health-care providers must be careful to avoid generalizations or assumptions, such as the Irish being superstitious, heavy drinkers, and practical jokers, because these do not apply to all Irish. Religious persecution and deplorable economic conditions were primary reasons for early immigration to America. Ireland had a population of 8.5 million until the Great Potato Famine of 1846 to 1848, when the population decreased to 3.4 million. During the famine, thousands of Irish died from malnutrition, typhus epidemics, dysentery, and scurvy, and millions immigrated to America.

The Irish use low-context English, in which many words are used to express a thought. This low-contextual use of the language has its roots in the Celtic folk tradition of storytelling. Humility and emotional reserve are considered virtues. Displays of emotion and affection in public are avoided and often difficult in private. They often rely on humor and teasing as expressions of affection and may use this form of humor with health-care providers.

Kinship and sibling loyalty are important to the Irish. Irish families emphasize independence and self-reliance in children. Boys are allowed and expected to be more aggressive than girls. Girls are raised to be respectable, responsible, and resilient. Children are expected to have self-restraint, self-discipline, and respect and obedience for their parents and older people. Over time, the Irish have made a place for themselves in the workforce in the United States or wherever they have migrated and are represented in all occupations and professional roles.

Most Irish are either dark-haired and fair-skinned or have red hair, rosy cheeks, and fair skin. However, as with other ethnic groups, variations in hair and skin color exist. The fair complexion of the Irish places them at risk for skin cancer. The major cause of infant mortality in Ireland is congenital abnormalities. Other conditions with a high incidence among the Irish are phenylketonuria (PKU), neural tube defects, and alcoholism. Most states require screening all newborns for PKU; health-care providers may need to encourage women who give birth at home to seek PKU screening for their infants.

Alcohol problems in Ireland are among the highest internationally. In their multinational review of the literature on alcohol use, Purnell and Foster reported that the percentage of people in the United States, Ireland, and England who drink is the same; however, behavior problems are greater among the Irish. Because drinking may be a way of coping with problems, the health professional needs to assist Irish American clients to explore more effective coping strategies and caution them against the dangers of mixing alcohol with medications.

The Irish believe that not eating a well-balanced diet or not eating the right kinds of food may cause the newborn to be deformed. In addition, the Irish share the belief common to many other ethnic groups that the mother should not reach over her head during pregnancy because the baby's cord may wrap around its neck. A taboo behavior in the past, which some women still respect, is that if the pregnant woman sees or experiences a tragedy during pregnancy, a congenital anomaly may occur.

The Irish reaction to death is a combination of their pagan past and current Christian beliefs. The Celts denied death and ridiculed it with humor. The Irish are fatalists and acknowledge the inevitability of death. The American emphasis on technology and dying in the hospital may be incongruent with the Irish American belief that family members should stay with the dying person. The Irish wake continues as an important phenomenon in contemporary Irish families and is a time of melancholy, rejoicing, pain, and hopefulness.

The predominant religion of most Irish is Catholicism, and the church is a source of strength and solace for many Irish Americans. In times of illness, Irish Catholics receive the Sacrament of the Sick, which includes Anointing, Communion, and a blessing by the priest. Prayer is an individual and private matter. In

469

the health-care setting, patients should be given privacy for prayer, whether or not a clergy member is present. Some Irish Americans wear religious medals to maintain health. These emblems provide them with solace and should not be removed by the health-care provider.

The Irish's fatalistic outlook and external locus of control influence health-seeking behaviors. Irish Americans use denial as a way of coping with physical and psychological problems. Many Irish limit and understate symptoms when ill. For some Irish Americans, illness behavior does little to relieve suffering and perpetuates a self-fulfilling prophecy. Illness or injury may be linked to guilt and the result of having done something morally wrong. The behavioral response of the Irish to pain is stoic, usually ignoring or minimizing it.

In most Irish families, nuclear family members are consulted first about health problems. Mothers and older women are usually the family members who possess the knowledge of folk practices to alleviate common problems such as colds. When home remedies are not effective, the Irish seek the care of biomedical health-care providers.

People of Italian Heritage

Sandra M. Hillman

This chapter describes the beliefs and practices of Italian Americans from the mainland of Italy, although some of these characteristics may be shared by Italian Americans with a heritage from Sicily and Sardinia.

The willingness to share thoughts and feelings among family members is a major distinguishing characteristic of the Italian American family. Many times, a fluctuating emotional climate exists within the family, with expressions of affection erupting briefly into what appears to an outsider as anger or hostility. Italians are sentimental and not afraid to express their feelings, and this extends into the health-care environment. Even though traditional roles remain strong in Italian American families, a trend toward more egalitarian relationships is evolving. Families maintain close relationships: daughters have close ties with both parents, particularly as they approach old age.

Most Italians believe strongly in the work ethic, are punctual, and rarely miss work commitments owing to a cold, headache, or minor illnesses. If completing their work requires staying later, they do so. Although the family is of utmost importance to Italians, work takes priority over family unless serious family situations arise. This cultural predisposition parallels the North American work ethic.

People of Italian ancestry have some notable genetic diseases, such as familial Mediterranean fever, Mediterranean-type glucose-6-phosphate dehydrogenase (G-6-PD) deficiency, and β-thalassemia. Thus, administration of sulfonamides, antimalarial agents, salicylates, and naphthaquinolones should be avoided. A recommendation is to screen all people of Italian heritage for these conditions before administering medications.

A close association between food and mothering results in some predictable problems. Many Italians believe that bigger babies are healthier. The size of the baby is perceived as an index of the successful maintenance of maternal and wifely responsibilities. The belief that a mother does not conceive while nursing continues to be held by many Italian women. Among traditional Italians, a postpartum woman is not allowed to wash her hair, take a shower, or resume her domestic chores for at least 2 or 3 weeks after birth so she can rest. New mothers are expected to breastfeed, restoring the health of the reproductive organs and keeping the mother and baby free of infections.

In the Italian American family, death is a great social loss and brings an immediate response from the community. Sending food and flowers (chrysanthemums), giving money, and congregating at the home of the deceased are expected. The funeral procession to the cemetery is a symbol of family status. There is great pride in the size of the event, which is determined by the number of cars in the procession. Although there is a tendency today to decrease the elaborateness of the funeral, it remains very much a family and community event.

Emotional outpourings can be profuse. Women may mourn dramatically, even histrionically, for the whole family. They do not merely weep; they may rage against death for the harm it has done to the family. Family members may moan and scream for the deceased throughout the church. Screaming is an effort to ensure that Jesus, Mary, and the saints hear what the bereaved are thinking and feeling.

Their predominant religion, Roman Catholicism, includes folk religious practices. Most Italians pray to the Virgin Mary and the saints in addition to God. Many traditional first-generation and newer Italian American families display shrines to the Blessed Virgin in their backyards. God is an all-understanding, compassionate, and forgiving being. Prayer and having faith in God and the saints help Italian Americans through illnesses. The health-care provider may need to help the client obtain the basic rites of the Sacrament of the Sick, which includes Anointing, Communion, and if possible, a blessing by the priest.

The concept of family, the most dominant influence on the individual, is the most credible source of health-care practices. Italians believe that the most significant moments of life should take place under their own roofs. The extended family is the front-line resource for intensive advice on emotional problems.

Mental health providers are frequently perceived as inappropriate agents for meeting problems that are beyond the expertise of the family and local community.

Individuals can protect themselves from the evil eye by using magical symbols and by learning the rituals of the *maghi*, which means "witch." Amulets are worn on necklaces or bracelets, held in a pocket, or sewn into clothing. *Cornicelli*, "little red horns," can still be purchased as good luck charms. These should not be removed from patients' bedsides or from their clothing because they provide significant solace for some.

Both age and gender mediate ethnic differences in the expression of pain for Italian Americans. Older Italian Americans, especially women, are more likely to report pain experiences, express symptoms to the fullest extent, and expect immediate treatment. Italians tend to be more verbally expressive with chronic pain. The sick role for many Italian Americans is one not entered into without personal feelings of guilt; thus, they may keep sickness a secret from family and friends and are not inclined to describe the details because they blame themselves for the health problem.

People of Somali Heritage

Richard Adair and Yurub Jama

Somali people are united by a common language, Somali; religion, Sunni Muslim; and culture that are influenced by their Arabic neighbors. Although minority languages exist in Somalia, the majority of the inhabitants speak Somali.

After the collapse of the Somali government in 1991, at least 1 million Somali people fled to neighboring counties. Many of these refugees have now resettled in the United States, Canada, Europe, Australia, and New Zealand. Others are still living in refugee camps, especially in one large camp on the outskirts of Nairobi, under difficult and somewhat unsafe conditions. Some children and adolescents have spent most of their lives in these camps.

Children are encouraged to speak Somali at home, but it is recognized that learning English is important. Somalis are polite and appreciate full introductions of everyone in the room, including interpreters and family members. Somalis follow Muslim traditions regarding social touching. Somali women typically greet one another with a hug and a kiss on the cheek.

Voice volumes are not noticeably different from American cultural norms. Many use their hands to make gestures when speaking. Women and men are not shy about the process of obtaining medical care, and often they will ask detailed/direct questions until they are satisfied. Although the use of family members is not recommended, most Somali prefer close family member to interpret. They may want to use an interpreter who is of the same gender, especially in issues such as sex or genital exam visits.

A man or woman may not touch a person of the opposite gender except for spouses or close relatives. This includes handshaking with the opposite gender. However, in the exam room, it is understood that touching is permitted because there is a specific medical reason. Maintaining eye contact in considered polite when speaking with someone. Punctuality is not expected in a social context, but Somali people are generally quick to adapt to new cultures and learn that they are expected to be on time for appointments.

Somalis do not have surnames in the Western sense. To identify a Somali, three names must be used: a given name, followed by the father's given name, and then the grandfather's name. Women, therefore, do not change their names at marriage.

A Somali nuclear family is considered to include father, mother, children, and grandchildren. The father is the head of the family and the final decision maker in family affairs. Family relations are based on hierarchical respect, as the Qur'an expects children to be unconditionally obedient to their parents. Children are also expected to care for their parents when they are in need, especially in times of sickness, aging, or financial hardship.

For all Somalis, the family is the ultimate source of personal security and identity. When Somalis meet one another, they don't ask "Where are you from?" but *"Whom* are you from?" Most Somalis in the United States help support their family members in Somalia or in refugee camps in neighboring countries. Same-sex relationships are hidden and not discussed. Marrying and producing children are expected.

Somali people tend to have thinner frames, lighter skin, and more Arabic-looking faces than West Africans, the ancestors of the majority of today's African Americans. Men are quite lean, and women less so.

Many Somali immigrants have significant depression or post-traumatic stress disorder related to war, family disruption, and long years in refugee camps. Many patients are uncomfortable with the word "depression" and respond better to simpler explanations like too much stress, not enough sleep, *or* a reaction to the past.

Tuberculosis is by far the most important infectious disease in Somali immigrants; extrapulmonary tuberculosis, especially in lymph nodes, is more common than pulmonary tuberculosis and often presents with fever alone or with vague other symptoms. Other common infectious diseases are hepatitis B, *Helicobacter pylori*, intestinal parasites, and malaria. Remember that most arrivals are coming from refugee camps in countries other than Somalia, especially Kenya and Ethiopia.

Lactase deficiency occurs in adulthood but is not a common cause of symptoms. Rates of obesity and diabetes among Somalis have increased dramatically, especially among women adjusting to the availability of food in Western countries and decreased physical activity due to being in cold climates or fear of going outdoors in high-crime neighborhoods.

Common foods are rice, pasta, bread, potatoes, corn, beans, and sugar. Meat products include goat, lamb, beef, camel, and fish. Fruits include banana, mango, papaya, grapefruit, oranges, lemons, grapes, and dates. Beverages include milk from goats, cows, and camels; tea and coffee; and soda.

A typical breakfast includes *angelo*, a flour product resembling crepes, to which oil with sugar can be added, and tea. At midday, curry rice or pasta with sauce is consumed and often includes vegetables such as onions and potatoes. For dinner, meat is usually not consumed, but a mixture of beans and corn called *ambulo* is consumed with added sugar and oil. Pork of any kind is forbidden.

Somali families tend to be large by American and European standards. Children and pregnancy are invariably considered a precious gift. Abortion is prohibited. Expectant and newly delivered mothers benefit from a strong network of women within Somali culture. During pregnancy, women are expected to eat well and avoid heavy exertion or lifting.

After childbirth, a period of 40 days is observed where the woman stays home, eats well, is assisted by her family and neighbors, and abstains from sexual intercourse. During this time, the mother wears earrings made from string placed through a clove of garlic, and the baby wears a bracelet made from string and the herb *malmal* in order to ward away the evil eye. Incense (myrrh) is burned twice a day in order to protect the baby from the ordinary smells of the world, which are felt to have the potential to make him or her sick.

Breastfeeding for as long as possible, usually up to 2 years, is a religious obligation. Newborn care includes warm water baths, sesame oil massages, and passive stretching of the baby's limbs. *Malmal* is applied to the umbilicus for the first 7 days of life. *Malmal* is available in the United States in some Asian markets.

When a person is dying, a religious person such as the imam from the local mosque may visit the person in the hospital, offer prayers, and help mobilize community support. As faithful Muslims, Somalis believe that Allah will determine how long a person will live. For this reason, discussing end-of-life care or advance directives is taboo and may be misunderstood.

In Somalia there are no confidentiality laws, and the family is informed instead of the patient. The family may feel distrustful of health-care providers if they are not informed of their family member's prognosis. Somalis feel it is important to tell the immediate family first if there is a poor prognosis so they can be prepared

to work together and comfort the patient. After death, the funeral home cooperates with the mosque in preparing the body, washing it, wrapping it in white cloth, and delivering it to the mosque for a prayer service.

Essentially all Somalis are devout Sunni Muslims. Prayers (*Salat*) are performed five times daily, in any location, facing Mecca. These specified prayers take about 3 minutes apiece and involve kneeling and touching the forehead to the ground.

Strict fasting occurs during the lunar month of Ramadan. During this time, all people age 15 years and older refrain from taking food or drink from sunrise to sunset. Sometimes this is interpreted to include medication, including insulin. Exceptions can be made in the event of illness, travel, menstruation, pregnancy, and so forth. Many Somalis will give January 1 of the year they were born when asked by immigration authorities or Western medical records systems.

Traditional Somali healing practices include ritual reading or reciting of verses from the Qur'an; creating superficial skin burns on the abdomen, chest, or head; superficial cutting of the skin (especially used for jaundice in children from hepatitis A); *Mingis* (or *Saar*), which consists of ceremonial drumming, singing, and dancing around the sick person; and herbs that may be consumed or used as a poultice. Such practices are guided by a traditional healer. Some traditional healers specialize in setting fractures or trephine procedures for subdural bleeding.

In Somalia, prepubertal girls are circumcised by removing the clitoris, labia minora, and labia majora. The vaginal orifice is then narrowed by sutures, leaving room for menstruation. At the time of marriage, these sutures are removed. In another variation of this practice, only the clitoris is removed. While these practices seem extreme to Western medical providers, they are accepted as normal by many Somali women who value chastity and tradition. In the United States, this practice is illegal. In response, some families arrange for their children to travel to Africa for circumcision.

There are no restrictions on accepting blood products when needed. Organ donation at the time of death is traditionally not practiced in Somalia. Traditionally, Somalis believe the body should be buried intact. Donating an organ while still alive or receiving a transplanted organ may be considered more acceptable. Since there are no specific codes on transplant and organ donation in Islamic law, there are different approaches to treatment.

Somali people sometimes seek healing from traditional and religious healers first. But they do not hesitate to go to the physician when symptoms persist or are alarming.

A Somali traditional healer, usually an older man, is called an *alaqad*. Traditional healing may include participation by a large group of people. Respect for medical education and expertise is the rule; physicians and nurses are valued as professionals.

Abstracts

People of Thai Heritage

Ratchneewan Ross and Jeffrey Ross

Siam, the land of the musical *The King and I*, is the former name of Thailand and is the only Southeast Asian country that has never been colonized by Westerners. Thailand began a tradition of emulating Western political, economic, and cultural ideas in the late 19th century. Over 150,000 Thais live in the United States, with most living in Los Angeles, California. The first two Thai immigrants in the United States were Eng and Chang Bunker, the famous Siamese twins who captured the world's attention because of their conjoined chests and whose career was a public exhibition.

The standard Thai dialect, which is a fixed tonal language with five tones, is the official language in Thailand. Thus, the same phonetic sound can have different meanings depending on the tone. The written alphabet is a complicated system of 44 letters with over 33 vowels or vowel combinations. The north, northeast, and southern regions of Thailand have their own unique dialects.

A Thai female uses the word "*Kah*," and a Thai male uses "*Kraab*" at the end of a sentence to add politeness in a conversation. Looking in a person's eyes and conversing quietly reflect respect and politeness. A distance of 1½ to 2 feet between two speakers is preferable. Thais usually greet each other with the "*Wai*" motion—putting the palms of both hands together in a prayer-like gesture and bowing the head slightly. This gesture is used by both men and women of all age groups. Respect for older people, an important aspect of Thai culture, is always signaled by a younger person gesturing with the "*Wai*" to the older person first.

Traditional Thai families are nuclear in nature. When older people in a Thai family are unable to care for themselves, younger members are morally required to care for them. Most Thais have long first and long last names. A Thai is usually referred to by his or her first name, even in an official setting like school or work. In general, when a woman marries, she usually takes her husband's last name. A couple's children also take their father's last name. When Thai names are transcribed in English, the spelling is merely a kind of phonetic translation from its spelling in the Thai alphabet. Because Thai is a tonal language, however, the correct pronunciation of names cannot be ascertained from their spelling in English. Importantly, almost all Thais have a short nickname used by their family and close friends and often by colleagues at work. Nicknames normally have no relationship with first names. They are often humorous to Thais themselves. Nicknames are usually either Thai or English words. They might be derived from names of colors, body types, fruits, or any number of other things.

A man is the head of the household in a traditional Thai family, usually being the breadwinner and managing important tasks. In most Thai families, responsibilities involving household chores and taking care of children belong to a woman. However, more Thai families today have begun to divide household chores between men and women. Thai female adolescents have traditionally been expected to protect their virginity until marriage. Dating with a chaperone present is preferable to parents. However, more and more Thai adolescents date on their own today.

Children are the center of the family for Thais. Many Thai children sleep with their parents from birth until some point in time before they reach adolescence. Often, children are spoon-fed by adults until they are 6 to 7 years old.

Most Thais try to avoid personal conflicts at work and are hard workers. Although the family is deemed very important for Thais, in many circumstances, especially for economic reasons, work comes before family. Thai Americans respect their supervisors because seniority is strongly valued in their culture. Thus, they might not be assertive at work. Therefore, supervisors may be wise to provide open discussions and expression of opportunities for their Thai American colleagues. English proficiency among some Thais is low. Therefore, with Thai Americans who are learning English as their second language, the language used in the workplace should be clear. Slang expressions should be avoided. If used, slang expressions need to be clarified.

Glucose-6-phosphate dehydrogenase deficiency (G6PD) and thalassemia are common genetic disorders among Thais. Some recent literature reports some variations in drug metabolism between Thais and non-Thais associated with antiretroviral medications.

In general, an individual portion of a Thai dish is about one-third to one-fifth of a typical U.S. dish in terms of volume. As a result, most Thais are slim owing to these smaller portions and also the types of food they eat. Thais believe that foods containing adequate essential nutrients help to maintain life and growth and delay illness later in life. A Thai balanced diet usually includes low-fat/low-meat dishes with a large percentage of vegetable and legumes. Rice and fish are main staples. Overall, pork or chicken is eaten more than beef. All meats are consumed more sparingly in proportion to vegetables when compared with a Western diet.

Communal eating is an essential part of the Thai culture. Friends and families eat seated together either on the floor or at a table. Either way, when rice is part of the meal, Thais will begin with a large amount of rice on their plates and reach to central communal plates of combined meat and vegetable recipes to add to their rice. Hot or warm foods or drinks are considered healthier than cold ones. This idea is based in part on a belief in "cold and hot" or "Yin and Yang." Some herbs are considered a panacea. Therefore, Thai dishes usually contain some kind of herbs, particularly garlic and hot chilies.

Thai women view pregnancy as a special time in their lives when they need extra care physically and emotionally. Ideally, the age of 20 years is the optimal time for pregnancy owing to the women's physical and emotional maturity. Owing to modesty, especially during a vaginal examination, Thai women prefer female healthcare providers over their male counterparts. In general, Thai pregnant women are discouraged from visiting a hospitalized person (regardless of the kind of sickness), attending a funeral ceremony, or visiting a house where there has been a death. Some new mothers might be advised to not eat eggs, chicken, or buffalo meat, believing that the new mother's perineum may not heal. Eggs are avoided by some mothers, believing that they could cause a big scar on the perineum.

Thai Buddhists believe that after a person dies, the person will be reborn somewhere else based on that person's *Karma*. "*Karma* means 'action' and . . . refers to the process by which a person's moral behavior or actions have consequences for the person's future, either in the present or later life." Most Thai Buddhists follow the custom of cremation. Many people believe that if the deceased is not given a proper burial or if a sanctified tombstone is not placed on the grave, then the soul of the deceased will wander to the four corners of the world and weep and wail and sometimes even return to disturb the relatives.

During the funeral ceremony, the family gets together. The sons of the deceased are expected to be ordained for a short period of time, ranging from 1 week to 3 months. The ordination is believed to help the dead go to heaven. Female relatives normally wail quietly. The family members pray quietly to the dead before the cremation to ask for forgiveness and wish the dead to be reborn in a happy and peaceful home.

Most Thais are Buddhist, and the rest are Muslim, Christian, Hindu, or other. Buddhism is an exceptionally tolerant religion with its roots in Hinduism. Family support along with Buddhism is a crucial source of strength. The ultimate goal for a Buddhist Thai is to reach *Nirvana*. This is the end of reincarnation or the cycle of rebirths. When there is no rebirth, there is no suffering. They are either happy or suffering. "Peace" is the ultimate goal.

Many Thais believe that unwholesome *Karma* from their past life has caused them to become ill in the present life. They believe that the illness can be improved by following the Five Precepts, similar to the Christian Ten Commandments, which stress abstinence from killing, stealing, lying, sexual misconduct, and illicit drugs and alcohol consumption. Meditation and prayer are ways for many Thais to cope with an illness.

Health promotion and disease prevention among the Thais are very limited. Many Thais believe that bad *Karma* and/or negative supernatural power causes mental illness. Therefore, folk therapies from traditional healers are the first resource for many. Folk therapies may include healing ceremonies, using shamans (as a mediator) to converse with supernatural beings (such as black magic, evil beings, and/or ancient/natural spirits) and negotiating with them to release the sick person from his or her illness. Stigmatization attached to mental illness and beliefs in animism and *Karma* tend to prevent some Thais from seeking professional help when mental health problems arise. Some may not seek assistance from healthcare providers until they realize that traditional healers, shamans, cannot help them.

Many Thais may appear stoic in trying to withhold expressions of pain or suffering from their illness. No religious beliefs against blood transfusion exist for Thais. Although donating and receiving organs are acceptable among many Thais, belief in their rebirth might prevent some from donating their organs, for fear they might not have the organ in the next life.

Abstracts

People of Turkish Heritage

Marshelle Thobaben and Sema Kuguoglu

The 202,000 people of Turkish descent in the United States live in 42 states, with over half living in New York, California, New Jersey, and Florida. Just over half of the individuals in this group were born outside the United States, and most arrived since 1980. Most Turks practice Islam and come from a collectivist culture in which an individual's behavior is expected to conform to the norms or traditions of the group, which has important implications for health-care providers advocating health promotion and wellness; illness, disease, and injury prevention; and health-maintenance restoration.

Modern Turkish women tend to be more Westernized than some of their Middle Eastern or Muslim counterparts, resulting in more egalitarian decision making. Older people in Turkish culture are attributed authority and respect until they become weak or retired, at which time their authoritative roles diminish. However, respect always remains a factor. Individuals are socialized to take care of older parents, regarding it as normal rather than an added burden. Grandparents play a significant role in raising their grandchildren, especially if they live in the same home.

Turkey is known for its high-power distance (the psychological and emotional distance between superiors and subordinates), respect for authority, centralized administration, and authoritarian leadership style. In Turkish culture, a manager's authoritative control is often more important than the achievement of organizational goals; thus, the U.S. workforce culture must be explained to ensure satisfactory work relationships.

Helminthiasis (intestinal worms), hepatitis, tuberculosis, and malaria have not been fully eradicated in Turkey. Endemic goiter associated with iodine deficiency is a major health problem among Turks. Turkey also has some of the highest rates of occupational diseases and work accidents in Europe. Thus, health-care providers may need to provide education regarding safety issues in occupational health and assess newer Turkish immigrants for intestinal parasites, tuberculosis, malaria, and other health conditions found in Turkey.

Turkish cuisine is influenced by the many civilizations encountered by nomadic Turks over the centuries, as well as by a mixture of delicacies from different regions of the vast Ottoman Empire. Therefore, food choices are varied and tend to provide a healthy, balanced diet. Food is a highly valued symbol of hospitality and communicates love and respect to those for whom it is prepared. The Islamic tradition of Ramazan is a month of fasting observed by practicing Muslims throughout the world. During Ramazan, one is not allowed to eat or drink anything from sunrise to sunset, necessitating adjustments in medication administration. Generally, pregnant and postpartum women, travelers, and those who are ill are excused from fasting.

Motherhood, and therefore pregnancy, is accorded great respect, and pregnant women are usually made comfortable in any way possible, including satisfying their cravings. Pregnant women may continue their daily activities or work as long as they are comfortable. In traditional Turkish culture, one of the most important desires of a married woman is to have a child. A woman who has not had a child is faced with social pressure and accusations and, thus, may try to use some traditional practices to increase fertility. Newborns are treated as cherished gifts. A small blue bead, *nazar boncuk,* protects the child from the "evil eye" and is usually placed on the child's left shoulder. This practice protects the child from the evil angel whispering in the left ear, often portrayed in Christian religious art.

Traditional rituals after death are closing the eyes of the deceased, tying the chin, turning the head toward Mecca, putting the feet next to each other, putting the hands together on the abdomen, and removing clothing. After the burial, the deceased is honored with a meal that signifies moving the deceased into the afterlife, emphasizing the need to eat and drink, and filling the void that will occur in the community. If these rituals are not completed, the spirit of the deceased will be left behind.

Turks who emigrate to the West tend to be very moderate Muslims. Traditional prayer is practiced five times each day and can take place anywhere as long as one is facing the holy city of Mecca. A special small rug is used for praying. Health-care providers may need to assist patients to prepare for prayers.

Most Turks rely on Western medicine and highly trained professionals for health and curative care. However, remnants of traditional beliefs have an impact on health-care practices. A common explanation for the cause of illness is an imbalance of hot and cold. For example, diarrhea is thought to come from too much cold or heat; pneumonia results from extreme cold.

Terminally ill patients are generally not told the severity of their conditions. Informing a patient of a terminal illness may take away the hope, motivation, and energy that should be directed toward healing, or it may cause the patient additional anxiety related to the fear of dying and concern about those being left behind. Thus, the health-care provider should discuss a terminal illness with the family spokesperson before informing the patient.

Depression is a major public health problem in Turkey; high-risk groups include women, individuals in middle adulthood, and those in nuclear rather than extended families. Such groups may well describe a large portion of Turkish immigrants in the United States, requiring careful assessments. Physicians, and to a lesser extent nurses and midwives, have historically been held in very high esteem. Moreover, health-care providers should ask about a same-gender health-care provider for those who practice Islam.

People of Vietnamese Heritage

Susan Mattson

Well over 1 million Vietnamese live in the United States. Vietnamese immigrants confront a unique set of problems, including dissimilarity of culture, lack of family or relatives to offer initial support, and a negative identification with the unpopular Vietnam War. Many Vietnamese are involuntary immigrants. Their expatriation was unexpected and unplanned, and their departures were often precipitous and tragic. Escape attempts were long, harrowing, and, for many, fatal. Survivors were often placed in squalid refugee camps for years.

Whenever confronted with a direct but delicate question, many Vietnamese cannot easily give a blunt "no" as an answer, because such an answer may create disharmony. Self-control, another traditional value, encourages keeping to oneself, whereas expressions of disagreement that may irritate or offend another person are avoided. Expressing emotions is considered a weakness and interferes with self-control. At times of distress or loss, they often complain of physical discomforts, such as headaches, backaches, or insomnia.

A person's age is calculated roughly from the time of conception; most children are considered to already be a year old at birth and gain a year each Tet, the Asian Lunar New Year. A child born just before Tet could be regarded as 2 years old when only a few days old by American standards. Because the practice of determining age is so different in Vietnam, many immigrants may have difficulty determining their exact birth date and are often given January 1 as a date of birth for official records.

The traditional Vietnamese family is strictly patriarchal and is almost always an extended family structure, with the man having the duty of carrying on the family name through his progeny. Young people are expected to respect their elders and to avoid behavior that might dishonor the family. As a result of the effects of their exposure to Western cultures, a disproportionate share of young people have difficulty adapting to this expectation. A conflict often develops between the traditional notion of filial piety, with its requisite subordination of self and unquestioning obedience to parental authority, and the pressures and needs associated with adaptation to American life.

Most Vietnamese respect authority figures with impressive titles, achievement, education, and a harmonious work environment. They may be less concerned about such factors as punctuality, adherence to deadlines, and competition. Other traditions include a willingness to work hard, sacrificing current comforts, and saving for the future to ensure that they assimilate well into the workforce. Because many fear losing their jobs if they speak out about inequities, they are likely to be taken advantage of by some more unscrupulous employers.

The Vietnamese family may try various home remedies, allowing the condition to become serious before seeking professional assistance. Once a physician or nurse has been consulted, the Vietnamese are usually quite cooperative and respect the wisdom and experience of health-care providers. Hospitalization is viewed as a last resort and is acceptable only in case of emergency, when everything else has failed. With respect to mental health, Vietnamese do not easily trust authority figures, including treatment staff, because of their refugee experiences.

A predominant aspect of the traditional Asian system of health maintenance is the principle of balance between two opposing natural forces, known as *am* and *duong* in Vietnamese. These forces are represented by foods that are considered hot (duong) or cold (am). Illness or trauma may require therapeutic adjustment of hot-and-cold balance to restore equilibrium. The am-and-duong balance of forces continues during pregnancy and postpartum. Because body heat is lost during delivery, Vietnamese women avoid cold foods and beverages and increase consumption of hot foods to replace and strengthen their blood. Ice water and other cold drinks are usually not welcome, and most raw vegetables, fruits, and sour items are taken in lesser amounts.

Most Vietnamese have an aversion to hospitals and prefer to die at home. Some believe that a person who dies outside the home becomes a wandering soul with no place to rest. Family members think that they can provide more comfort to the dying person at home. Vietnamese families may wish to gather around the body of a recently deceased relative and express great emotion. Traditional mourning practices include the wearing of white clothes for 14 days, the subsequent wearing of black armbands by men and white headbands by women, and the yearly celebration of the anniversary of a person's death.

Vietnamese religious practices are influenced by the Eastern philosophies of Buddhism, Confucianism, and Taoism. Confucianism stresses harmony through maintenance of the proper order of social hierarchies, ethics, worship of ancestors, and the virtues of chastity and faithfulness. Taoism teaches harmony, allowing events to follow a natural course that one should not attempt to change. These beliefs have contributed to an attitude characterized by maintenance of self-control, acceptance of one's destiny, and fatalism toward illness and death that may be perceived as passive by Westerners.

Good health is achieved by having harmony and balance with the two basic opposing forces, am (cold, dark, female) and duong (hot, light, male). An excess of either force may lead to discomfort or illness. The belief that life is predetermined is a deterrent to seeking health care. For many Vietnamese, diagnostic tests are baffling, inconvenient, and often unnecessary. Common treatments practiced in Vietnam and continued, to some degree, in the United States are *cao gio*, *giac*, *be bao*, *xong*, moxibustion, and acupuncture. Fatalistic attitudes and the belief that problems are punishment may reduce the degree of complaining and expression of pain among the Vietnamese, who view endurance as an indicator of strong character. One accepts pain as part of life and attempts to maintain self-control as a means of relief.

Traditional Asian male practitioners do not usually touch the bodies of females and sometimes use a doll to point out the nature of a problem. Young and unmarried women are more comfortable with female health-care providers.

Glossary

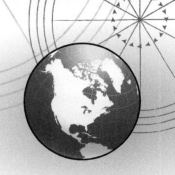

A

aagwachse Amish folk illness, referred to in English as livergrown, with symptoms of abdominal distress believed to be caused by too much jostling, especially occurring in infants during buggy rides.

abnemme Amish folk illness characterized by "wasting away"; usually affects infants or young children who seem to be too lean and not active.

abwaarde Amish term for ministering to someone by being present and serving when someone is sick in bed.

Acadia Part of the Canadian Maritime Provinces.

Acadian Early French settler of Acadia; a French dialect spoken by people in Acadia.

acculturate To modify or give up traits from the culture of origin as a result of contact with another culture.

achegewe Amish term for warm hands.

adab Egyptian term for politeness.

afatanbah Somali term for after childbirth.

alaqad Somali traditional healer.

Allah Greatest and most inclusive of the names of God. Arabic word used to describe the God worshipped by Muslims, Christians, and Jews.

am Pervasive force in Vietnamese traditional medicine, associated with cold conditions and things that are dark, negative, feminine, and empty.

Anabaptist Adherent of the radical wing of the Protestant Reformation who espouses baptism of adult believers.

Anatolia Geographic and historical term denoting the westernmost protrusion of Asia, comprising the majority of the Republic of Turkey.

antyesti Hindu equivalent of last rites.

apocopation Dropping the first vowel when one word ends with a vowel and the next word begins with a vowel.

Arabic Semitic language of the Arabs.

arwah Egyptian term for spirits.

Ashkenazi Descended from Eastern Europe and Russia.

assimilate To gradually adopt and incorporate the characteristics of the prevailing culture.

attitude State of mind or feeling with regard to some matter of a culture.

!Ay bendito! Frequently used Puerto Rican phrase expressing astonishment, surprise, lament, or pain.

Ayurveda Traditional Asian Indian medicine.

B

barrenillos Spanish term for obsessions.

baten Iranian term for inner self.

be bao or bat gio Vietnamese folk practice in which the skin is pinched in order to produce ecchymosis and petechiae; practiced to relieve sore throats and headaches.

boat people Haitian or Cuban immigrants who arrive in small boats; usually of undocumented status.

Boricua Puerto Rican term used with great pride; name given to Puerto Rico by the Taino Indians.

botanica Traditional Cuban or other Spanish store selling a variety of herbs, ointments, oils, powders, incenses, and religious figurines used in Santería.

brauche Folk healing art common among Pennsylvania Germans.

braucher Amish practitioner of brauche, a folk healer.

bris or brit milah Ritual circumcision of a male Jewish child.

Bureau of Indian Affairs (BIA) Federal agency responsible for ensuring services to Native Americans, Alaskan Indians, and Eskimo tribes.

C

caida de la mollera Condition of fallen fontanelle, believed to occur because the infant was withdrawn too harshly from the nipple; common among some Spanish-speaking populations.

Cami Turkish word for mosque.

cao gio Vietnamese practice of placing ointments or hot balm oil across the chest, back, or shoulders and rubbing with a coin; used to treat colds, sore throats, flu, and sinusitis.

cariñoso(a) Hispanic term for caring, in both verbal and nonverbal communications.

catimbozeiros Portuguese word for sorcerer; can be a folk practitioner.

Celtic Belonging to a group of Indo-European languages: Irish, Welsh, or Breton.

Chasidic (or Hasidic) Ultra-Orthodox Jewish sect.

cheshm-i-bad Iranian term for evil eye.

Chiac or ciac French dialect used in New Brunswick.

cho Haitian word for cold.

Chondo-Kyo Korean naturalistic religion that combines Confucianism, Buddhism, and Daoism.

choteo Cuban term for a lighthearted attitude, involving teasing, bantering, and exaggeration.

collectivism Moral, political, or social outlook that stresses human interdependence.

comadre Portuguese term for godmother.

community Group of people having a common interest or identity; goes beyond the physical environment to include the physical, social, and symbolic characteristics that cause people to connect.

compadrazgo Spanish term for a system of personal relationships in which friends or relatives are considered part of the family whether or not there is a blood relationship.

compadre Portuguese term for godfather.

confianza Hispanic term for trust developed between individuals; essential for effective communication and interpersonal interactions in health-care settings.

Conservative Jewish term for the religious group between Reform and Orthodox in terms of religious practice.

contadini Italian term for peasants.

cornicelli Italian charm with little red horns worn for good luck.

Creole Rich and expressive language derived from two other languages, such as French and Fon, an African tongue.

cultural awareness Appreciation of the external signs of diversity such as the arts, music, dress, and physical characteristics.

cultural competence Having the knowledge, abilities, and skills to deliver care congruent with the patient's cultural beliefs and practices. (See Chapter 1 for a more extensive definition.)

cultural humility Focuses on the process of intercultural exchange, paying explicit attention to clarifying the professional's values and beliefs through self-reflexion.

cultural imperialism Practice of extending the policies and practices of one organization (usually the dominant one) to disenfranchised and minority groups.

cultural imposition Intrusive application of the majority cultural view onto individuals and families.

cultural leverage A process whereby the principles of cultural competence are deliberately invoked to develop interventions.

cultural relativism Belief that the behaviors and practices of people should be judged only from the context of their cultural system.

cultural safety Expresses the diversity that exists within cultural groups and include the social determinants of health, religion, and gender in addition to ethnicity.

cultural sensitivity Having to do with personal attitudes and not saying things that may be offensive to someone from a cultural or ethnic background different from the health-care provider's background.

culture Totality of socially transmitted behavior patterns, arts, beliefs, values, customs, lifeways, and all other products of human work and thought characteristics of a population of people that guides their worldview and decision making. Patterns may be explicit or implicit, are primarily learned and transmitted within the family, and are shared by the majority of the culture.

curandeiro Portuguese folk practitioner whose healing powers are divinely given.

curandero Traditional folk practitioner common in Spanish-speaking communities; treats traditional illness not caused by witchcraft.

D

daadihaus Amish grandparents' cottage adjacent to farmhouse.

dan wei Functional unit of Chinese society; work unit or neighborhood unit responsible to and for the Chinese people's way of life.

dao Balance between yin and yang.

dayah Arab midwife.

decensos Spanish term for fainting spells.

demut German term for humility, a priority value for the Amish, the effects of which may be seen in details such as the height of the crown of an Amish man's hat, as well as in very general features such as the modest and unassuming bearing and demeanor usually shown by Amish in public. This behavior is reinforced by frequent verbal warnings against its opposite, hochmut, pride or arrogance, which is to be avoided.

Deitsch/Duetsch Pennsylvania German (sometimes incorrectly anglicized as Pennsylvania Dutch); American dialect derived from several uplands and Alemanic German dialects, with an admixture of American English vocabulary.

docte fey Haitian word for leaf doctor.

docte zo Haitian word for bonesetter.

doule Haitian word for pain.

dulse Iodine-rich edible seaweed used in clarifying beer and wine and as a suspension medium in some medicines; also known as Irish moss.

duong Vietnamese force used in traditional health practice, associated with things positive, masculine, light, and full.

E

Eid Arabic, Iranian, and Somali term for celebration of a feast—for example, Eid Gorgan (day/feast ending pilgrimage to Mecca); 'Eid Fetr (last day of the month of Ramadan).

Eire Gaelic name for Ireland.

el ataque/ataque de nervios Hyperkinetic spasmodic activity common in Spanish-speaking groups. The purpose is to release strong feelings or emotions. The person requires no treatment, and the condition subsides spontaneously. It is an expression of deep anger or depression.

empacho Condition common among some Spanish-speaking populations; believed to be caused by a bolus of food stuck in the gastrointestinal tract. Massage of the abdomen is believed to relieve the condition.

enculturation A natural conscious and unconscious conditioning process of learning accepted cultural norms, values, and roles in society.

endropi Greek term for shame.

espiritista (espiritualista) Spanish or Portuguese folk practitioners who receive their talent from "God"; treat conditions believed to be caused by witchcraft.

estampitas Spanish for little statues of saints.

ethic of neutrality Avoiding aggression and assertiveness, not interfering with others' lives unless asked to do so, avoiding dominance over others, and avoiding arguments and seeking agreement.

ethnic group Group of people who have had experiences different from those of the dominant culture in status, background, residence, religion, education, or other factors that functionally unify the group and act collectively on one another. Pertains to a religious, racial, national, or cultural group.

ethnocentrism Universal tendency for human beings to think that our own ways of thinking, acting, and believing are the only right, proper, and natural ones and to believe that those who differ greatly are strange, bizarre, or unenlightened.

F

familism Social pattern in which family solidarity and tradition assume a superior position over individual rights and interests.

Falasha Black Jews originating from Africa.

fam saj Haitian Creole word for lay midwife.

Farsi The national language of Iran.

fatalism Acceptance that occurrences in life are predetermined by fate and cannot be changed by human beings.

Francophone People living in Canada using French as their first language.

freindschaft Amish three-generational extended family network of relationships.

fret Haitian word for cold.

G

Gaelic The language spoken in Ireland.

garm Iranian term for hot.

garmie Iranian digestive problem caused from eating too much hot food.

gelassenheit Amish term for submission, yielding, surrender of self and ego to the higher will of the group or deity.

Gemeinschaft German word for community.

generalization Reducing numerous characteristics of an individual or group of people to a general form that renders them indistinguishable. Generalizations have to be validated by the individual.

giac Vietnamese dermabrasive procedure performed with cup suctioning.

giagia Greek term for grandma.

Global society Seeing the world as one large community as people travel and interact.

Great Eid Islamic feast of 4 days.

guanxi Chinese term defining how relatives are expected to help one another through connections, used by Chinese society in a manner similar to the use of money in other cultures.

Gullah Creole language spoken by African Americans who reside on or near the islands off the coasts of Georgia and the Carolinas.

H

Hasidic (or Chasidic) Ultra-Orthodox Jewish sect.

hadith Oral tradition of the Prophet Muhammad; collection of words and deeds that form the basis of Muslim law.

Hajji (Hajj an haji) Annual pilgrimage to Mecca.

halal The lawful—that which is permitted by Allah; also, the term used to describe ritual slaughter of meat.

hanbang Traditional Korean medical-care system.

hanui Korean word for oriental medicine doctor.

hanyak Korean traditional herbal medicine used to create harmony between oneself and the larger cosmology; a healing method for body and soul.

haram The unlawful—that which is prohibited by Allah; anyone who engages in what is prohibited is liable to incur punishment in the hereafter (as well as legal punishment in countries that incorporate Islamic law into legal codes).

Hasidic Jewish ultra-Orthodox sect.

Hebrew Language of Israel and of Jewish prayer.

hejab Iranian term for any behavior that expresses modesty in public—for example, in women, modest attire (loose dress or head scarf) or shy, self-limiting behavior in relating to the other gender.

hijab Modest covering of a Muslim woman; conceals the head and the body, except for the hands and face, with loosely fitting, nontransparent clothing.

hilot Filipino folk healer and massage therapist.

Hindi Primary language of India.

Hispanic American of Spanish or Latin American origin.

Hochmut Amish term for pride and arrogance.

hogan Earth-covered Navajo dwelling.

honor Spanish term for goodness or virtue; can be diminished or lost by an immoral or unworthy act.

hot-and-cold theory Hispanic concept that illness is caused when the body is exposed to an imbalance of hot and cold; foods are also classified as hot or cold.

hwa-byung Korean traditional illness that occurs from repressing anger or other strong emotions.

hwangap Significant celebration in Korean society—at the age of 60, a person starts the calendar cycle over again.

I

ideology Thoughts and beliefs that reflect the social needs and aspirations of an individual or an ethnocultural group.

Ihteram Egyptian Arabic word for respect.

il mal occhio Italian term for the evil eye.

imam Muslim leader of the prayer; usually the most learned member of the local Islamic community.

Indian Health Service Federal agency that has the responsibility for providing health services to Native Americans.

Indids Asian Indians who have a light brown skin color.

individualism Term used to describe a moral, political, or social outlook that stresses human independence and the importance of individual self-reliance, and freedom.

individuality The sense that each person has a separate and equal place in the community and where individuals who are considered "eccentrics or local characters" are tolerated.

Indochinese Individuals originating from Vietnam, Cambodia, or Laos.

Insallah or Insh'Allah Arabic and Turkish word for "if God wills."

Islam Monotheistic religion in which the supreme deity is Allah; according to Muslim belief, God imparted his final revelations—the Holy Qur'an—through his last prophet, Mohammed, thereby completing Judaism and Christianity.

issei First-generation Japanese immigrant.

itami Japanese term for pain.

itheram Egyptian term for respect.

J

jenn Egyptian term for the devil.

jerbero Spanish folk practitioner who specializes in treating health conditions through the use of herbal therapy.

Jinn Arabic term for demons.

Joual French dialect incorporating English words into a syntax and grammar that is essentially French.

Judaism Refers to a religion, people, and a culture.

K

kaddish Jewish prayer said for the dead.

kampo Japanese term for East Asian or Chinese medical practices and botanical therapies.

karma Hindu term for actions performed in the present life and the accumulated effects from past lives.

kashrut or kashrus Jewish laws that dictate which foods are permissible under religious law.

ki Korean term for the energy that flows through living creatures.

Koran See Qur'an.

kosher Kashrut laws in the Jewish religion.

koumbari Greek term for coparents.

kut Korean shamanistic ceremony to eliminate the evil spirits causing an illness.

L

la gente de la raza Phrase denoting a genetic determination to which all Spanish-speaking people belong, regardless of class differences or place of birth.

lace curtain Irish Name given to Irish in America who left inner-city enclaves and moved to the suburbs.

Latino(a) Person from Latin America.

laub Hmong dish made with raw pork and vegetables and spices.

laying on of hands Spiritual practice of placing one's hands on an individual for the purpose of healing.

lien Vietnamese concept that represents control over and responsibility for moral character.

M

maalesh Arabic term meaning never mind, it doesn't matter; substantial efforts are directed at maintaining pleasant relationships and preserving dignity and honor; hostility in response to perceived wrongdoing is warded off by an attitude of maalesh.

machismo Sense of masculinity that stresses virility, courage, and domination of women; includes the need to display physical strength, bravery, and virility.

madichon Haitian term used when children are disrespectful; it means that their future will be marred by misfortune.

maghi Italian word for witch.

magissa Greek folk healer.

mal ojo Spanish term for the evil eye, a hex condition with unspecific signs and symptoms believed to be caused by an older person admiring a younger person; condition can be reversed if the person doing the admiring touches the person being admired.

Marielitos Cuban immigrants who arrived in 1980 on a massive boatlift from Muriel Harbor, Cuba, to Key West, Florida.

masallah Turkish term for God bless and protect.

matiasma Greek term for the evil eye.

Métis People of mixed Native American and European, especially French Canadian, heritage.

mestizo(a) Person of mixed Spanish and Native American heritage.

mezuzah Container with biblical writings; placed on the doorpost of homes or hung around the neck on a necklace.

mien Vietnamese concept based on wealth and power.

Mohammed Prophet of God and founder of Islam.

mohel Ritual circumciser in the Jewish faith.

moreno Portuguese Brazilian individual who has black or brown hair and dark eyes.

morita therapy Indigenous Japanese school of psychotherapy.

Moslem See Muslim.

mosque Muslim place of worship.

moxibustion Vietnamese health-care practice in which pulverized wormwood is heated and placed directly on the skin at specified meridians to counter conditions associated with excess cold.

mukrah Arabic term for undesirable but not forbidden.

Mulatto Person of mixed European and African heritage.

mundang Korean folk healer who has special abilities for communicating with the spirits and in treating illnesses after all other means of treatment are exhausted.

Muslim Person who follows the Islamic faith, the world's second-largest religion.

N

naharati Iranian term for generalized distress.

Naikan therapy Japanese indigenous psychotherapy of reflection on how much goodness and love are received from others.

Navajo neuropathy Neurological condition confined to Navajo Indians; characterized by a complete absence of myelinated fibers resulting in short stature, sexual infantilism, systemic infection, hypotonia, areflexia, loss of sensation in the extremities, corneal ulcerations, acral mutilation, and painless fractures.

nazar Turkish term for envy.

nazar boncuk Small blue bead used among Turkish people to protect a child from the evil eye.

nervioso(a) Hispanic term used to describe signs and symptoms of nervousness, anxiety, sadness, and grief.

nevra Greek folk illness.

Niuyoricans Puerto Ricans born in New York.

Nihon/Nippon Japanese name for Japan.

Nihonjin Japanese term that denotes a strong sense of nationalism and pride in ethnic purity.

nisei Japanese term for the second generation of an immigrant family.

O

Old Order Amish Most conservative and traditionalist group among the followers of Jacob Ammann; today simply called Amish, but technically known as Old Order Amish Mennonite to distinguish them from other related Amish and Mennonite groups.

oppression Haitian ailment related to asthma; describes a state of anxiety and hyperventilation.

ordnung Codified rules and regulations that govern the behavior of a local Amish church district, or congregation; local consensus of faith and practice; also the German term for order.

orishas Gods or spirits in Santería.

Orthodox Traditional Judaism.

P

Padrone or capo di famiglia Italian word for master, head of the family.

Paj ntaub (pan dow) Form of embroidery that Hmong women do to decorate their clothing and make historical story cloths.

pappous Greek word for grandfather.

parve Jewish term used for foods that are neutral and can be eaten with meat or milk products.

Pasah Dai Dialect in southern Thailand.

Pasah Isaan Dialect in northeastern Thailand.

Pasah Nua Dialect in northern Thailand.

personalismo Spanish word for emphasis on intimate, personal relationships as more important than impersonal, bureaucratic relationships.

philptimo Greek term for respect.

phylacto Greek amulet worn to ward off envy.

pidgin Simplified language used for communicating between speakers of different languages.

pikirist Haitian word for injectionist.

pogrom Organized persecution or massacre of a minority group.

Polonia Communities heavily occupied by Polish immigrants and descendants of Polish nationals. Also the medieval name for Poland.

Ponos Greek word for pain.

practika Greek herbal remedies.

pseudofamilies Vietnamese households made up of close and distant relatives and friends that share accommodations, finances, and fellowship.

pu tong hua Recognized language of China.

Q

qi One of five substances or elements of traditional Chinese medicine; encompasses the foundation of the energy of the body, environment, and universe; includes all sources and expenditures of energy.

quinceñera A Hispanic/Latino girl's 15th birthday that celebrates her passage into womanhood.

Qur'an or Koran Muslim holy book; believed by Muslims to contain God's final revelations to humankind.

R

rabbi Jewish religious leader.

Ramadan or Ramazan The 9th month of the Islamic year during which Muslims are required to fast during daylight hours for 30 days.

Reconstructionism Mosaic of the three main branches of Judaism; is an evolving religion of the Jewish people; seeks to adapt Jewish beliefs and practices to the needs of the contemporary world.

Reform Liberal or Progressive Judaism.

remedios caserios Portuguese (Brazilian) home medicine or remedy.

remedios populares Portuguese (Brazilian) folk medicine practices.

respeto Hispanic term denoting respect; refers to the qualities developed toward others such as parents, the elderly, and educated people who are expected to be honored, admired, and respected.

restavec Haitian term to denote children who are sent to live with a nonparent family for the purposes of improving their lives economically.

Rezadeiras Brazilian spiritual leaders.

S

Sabra Jew who was born in Israel.

sansei Japanese term for the third generation of an immigrant family.

Santería 300-year-old Afro-Cuban religion that syncretizes Roman Catholic elements with ancient Yoruba tribal beliefs and practices.

santero Practitioner of Santería.

sard Iranian term for cold.

sardie Iranian digestive problem; occurs from eating too much cold food.

sensei Japanese term for master; used to address teachers, physicians, or those in seniority in a corporate setting.

Sephardic Jewish term for being descended from Spain, Portugal, the Mediterranean, Africa, or Central or South America.

severe combined immune deficiency syndrome Immune deficiency syndrome (unrelated to AIDS), characterized by a failure of antibody response and cell-mediated immunity.

shanty Irish Term for Irish who lived in urban Irish ethnic enclaves.

sheikhs The most learned individuals in an Islamic community.

Shinryo Naika Japanese indigenous therapy focusing on bodily illnesses that are emotionally induced.

Shinto Indigenous religion of Japan.

simpatia Spanish term for smooth interpersonal relationships; characterized by courtesy, respect, and the absence of harsh criticism or confrontation.

Small Eid Islamic holy feast of 3 days.

sobador Spanish folk practitioner, similar to a chiropractor, who treats illnesses and conditions affecting the joints and musculoskeletal system.

Solidarnosc "Solidarity" Union of interests, purposes, and sympathies promoting fellowship with Polish nationals.

Spanglish Sentence structure that includes both English and Spanish words.

stereotyping Oversimplified conception, opinion, or belief about some aspect of an individual or group of people.

sto lat Polish phrase meaning that the celebrant should live a hundred years.

subculture Group of people who have had experiences different from those of the dominant culture in status, ethnic background, residence, religion, education, or other factors that functionally unify the group and act collectively on one another.

susto "Magical fright," a condition believed to be caused by witchcraft; symptoms can be quite varied and include both mental and physical concerns.

Synagogue, temple, or shul Jewish house of worship.

T

T'ai chi Chinese system of exercise for mind and body control.

ta'arof Iranian ritual expressing courtesy.

tae-kyo Korean term, literally fetus education, with the objective being health and well-being of the fetus and the mother through art, beautiful objects, and a serene environment.

tae-mong Korean term signifying the beginning of pregnancy; the pregnant woman dreams of conception of the fetus.

Tagalog Filipino national language.

Tesbih Turkish small beads traditionally used for praying, now take a more secular meaning and are often referred to as worry beads.

Tet Asian Lunar New Year; celebrated in January or February.

Torah Five books of Moses; referred to in the Jewish faith.

treyf Jewish term for forbidden or unclean.

tribe Native American social organization comprising several local villages, bands, districts, lineages, or other groups who share a common ancestry, language, and culture.

Tridosha Theory that the body is made up of five elements: fire, air, space, water, and earth.

tu txiv neeb Hmong shaman who is a religious leader and health healer.

tudo bom Portuguese word for great, often said in a stoical sense.

two spirit Term to used among AI/AN populations to connote diverse gender and sexual identities.

V

variant cultural characteristics Determine a person's adherence to beliefs and values of his or her dominant culture. Includes nationality, race, color, gender, age, religious affiliation, educational status, socioeconomic status, occupation, military experience, political beliefs, urban or rural residence, enclave identity, marital status, parental status, physical characteristics, sexual orientation, gender issues, and reason for migration (sojourner, immigrant, or undocumented status).

velorio Spanish term for a wake; a festive occasion following the burial of a person.

vendouses Greek practice of cupping.

verguenza Spanish term for a consciousness of public opinion and the judgment of the entire community.

via nuova Italian for new way.

via vecchia Italian for old way.

Viddui Jewish personal confession recited when death is imminent.

visiting High-frequency custom of family-to-family home visits that help to maintain kinship and church ties and the flow of information within the Amish community.

voudou or voodoo Vibrant religion born from slavery and revolt; the term means sacred in the African language of Fon.

W

wake Watch over a deceased person before burial; usually accompanied by a celebration, which may include feasting.

warm hands Healing art related to therapeutic touch; regarded by Amish as a gift to be applied for the good of others in need of healing; a form of brauche.

worldview Way an individual or group of people look upon their universe to form values about their life and the world around them.

Y

yang In Chinese belief system, one of two opposing principles of the balance of life; can be either a single phenomenon or a state of being of a phenomenon. See yin.

yarmulke Jewish head covering worn by men.

yerbero See jerbero.

Yiddish Language often spoken by elderly Jews.

yin In Chinese belief system, one of two opposing principles of the balance of life; can be either a single phenomenon or a state of being of a phenomenon. See yang.

Z

zaher Iranian term for public persona.

zar Egyptian transmeditative ceremony.

Zhong guo The Chinese name for China and means "middle kingdom."

zong Vietnamese herbal preparation; relieves motion sickness or cold-related problems.

Index

NOTE: Page numbers followed by *f* refer to figures; *t* refer to tables